Huntington's Disease: Causes, Diagnosis and Treatment

Huntington's Disease: Causes, Diagnosis and Treatment

Editor: David Mercury

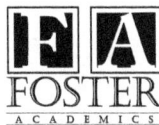

FA
FOSTER
ACADEMICS

www.fosteracademics.com

www.fosteracademics.com

FA FOSTER
ACADEMICS

Cataloging-in-Publication Data

Huntington's disease : causes, diagnosis and treatment / edited by David Mercury.
    p. cm.
Includes bibliographical references and index.
ISBN 978-1-63242-893-6
1. Huntington's disease. 2. Huntington's disease--Etiology. 3. Huntington's disease--Diagnosis.
4. Huntington's disease--Treatment. 5. Chorea. 6. Genetic disorders. I. Mercury, David.
RC394.H85 H86 2020
616.851--dc23

Foster Academics,
118-35 Queens Blvd., Suite 400,
Forest Hills, NY 11375, USA

ISBN 978-1-63242-893-6 (Hardback)

Contents

Preface

Every book is initially just a concept; it takes months of research and hard work to give it the final shape in which the readers receive it. In its early stages, this book also went through rigorous reviewing. The notable contributions made by experts from across the globe were first molded into patterned chapters and then arranged in a sensibly sequential manner to bring out the best results.

Huntington's disease (HD) is an inherited disorder that causes death of brain cells. The progression of the disease presents itself with increasingly debilitating signs such as lack of coordination, unsteady gait, jerky body movements, inability to talk and dementia. HD is considered to be an inherited disease, but 10% of all cases of HD may be due to acquired mutations of genes. It is caused due to an autosomal dominant mutation in either of the two copies of the Huntingtin gene of an individual. There exists no cure for HD. Towards the later stages of the disease, the patient requires full-time care. Nutrition management becomes increasingly important as dysphagia and muscle discoordination lead to eating difficulties and weight loss. Therapy seeks to relieve symptoms and improve quality of life. Tetrabenazine, neuroleptics and benzodiazepines are certain medications with proven results for treatment of chorea in HD. This book presents the causes, diagnosis and therapeutic advances in Huntington's disease in the most comprehensible language. Different approaches, evaluations, methodologies and advanced studies on HD have been included in this book. As the field of neurology is emerging at a fast pace, this book will help the readers to better understand the latest research and therapeutic advances.

It has been my immense pleasure to be a part of this project and to contribute my years of learning in such a meaningful form. I would like to take this opportunity to thank all the people who have been associated with the completion of this book at any step.

Editor

Allele-Specific Silencing of Mutant Huntingtin in Rodent Brain and Human Stem Cells

Valérie Drouet[1,2][9], Marta Ruiz[1,2][9], Diana Zala[3,4,5], Maxime Feyeux[6,7], Gwennaëlle Auregan[1,2], Karine Cambon[1,2], Laetitia Troquier[9], Johann Carpentier[1,2], Sophie Aubert[8], Nicolas Merienne[9], Fany Bourgois-Rocha[6,7], Raymonde Hassig[1,2], Maria Rey[9], Noëlle Dufour[1,2], Frédéric Saudou[3,4,5], Anselme L. Perrier[6,7], Philippe Hantraye[1,2], Nicole Déglon[1,2,9]*

1 Institute of Biomedical Imaging (I2BM) and Molecular Imaging Research Center (MIRCen), Atomic Energy Commission (CEA), Fontenay-aux-Roses, France, 2 URA2210, Centre National de Recherché Scientifique (CNRS), Fontenay-aux-Roses, France, 3 Institut Curie, Orsay, France, 4 UMR3306, Centre National de Recherché Scientifique (CNRS), Orsay, France, 5 U1005, Institut National de la Santé et de la Recherche Médicale (INSERM), Orsay France, 6 U861, Institut National de la Santé et de la Recherche Médicale (INSERM), AFM, Evry, France, 7 UEVE U861, I-STEM, AFM, Evry, France, 8 CECS, I-STEM, AFM, Evry, France, 9 Department of Clinical Neurosciences (DNC), Lausanne University Hospital (CHUV), Lausanne, Switzerland

Abstract

Huntington's disease (HD) is an autosomal dominant neurodegenerative disorder resulting from polyglutamine expansion in the huntingtin (HTT) protein and for which there is no cure. Although suppression of both wild type and mutant *HTT* expression by RNA interference is a promising therapeutic strategy, a selective silencing of mutant *HTT* represents the safest approach preserving WT *HTT* expression and functions. We developed small hairpin RNAs (shRNAs) targeting single nucleotide polymorphisms (SNP) present in the *HTT* gene to selectively target the disease *HTT* isoform. Most of these shRNAs silenced, efficiently and selectively, mutant *HTT in vitro*. Lentiviral-mediated infection with the shRNAs led to selective degradation of mutant *HTT* mRNA and prevented the apparition of neuropathology in HD rat's striatum expressing mutant HTT containing the various SNPs. In transgenic BACHD mice, the mutant *HTT* allele was also silenced by this approach, further demonstrating the potential for allele-specific silencing. Finally, the allele-specific silencing of mutant *HTT* in human embryonic stem cells was accompanied by functional recovery of the vesicular transport of BDNF along microtubules. These findings provide evidence of the therapeutic potential of allele-specific RNA interference for HD.

Editor: David Blum, Inserm U837, France

Funding: This work was supported by the Agence Nationale de la Recherche [ANR-2006-MRAR-043-01], FP6-NeuroNe [LSHM-CT-2004-512039], FP6-Clinigene [LSH-2004-1.2.4-3], the Atomic Energy Commission, FP6 STEM-HD, DIM-STEM POLE Region Ile-de-France fellowship to [F.B-R] and the Swiss National Science Foundation. The funders had no role in study design, data collection and analysis, decision to publish, or preparation of the manuscript.

Competing Interests: The authors have declared that no competing interests exist.

* E-mail: nicole.deglon@chuv.ch

9 These authors contributed equally to this work.

Introduction

HD is an autosomal dominant neurodegenerative disease that affects 1 in 10,000 adults [1]. The symptoms, which include progressive motor, psychiatric and cognitive dysfunctions, are associated with the degeneration of the major population of striatal neurons, the GABAergic spiny projection neurons. The mutation underlying HD is an expansion of a trinucleotide CAG repeat which encodes a polyglutamine (polyQ) tract in the N-terminal region of the HTT protein [2]. This mutation confers a new toxic function on the protein, in part through the production of short N-terminal fragments carrying the polyglutamine and the accumulation of misfolded HTT [3].

Gene silencing techniques, aiming to reduce intracellular levels of polyglutamine-encoding mRNA, have the potential to halt, or at least delay, the process of neuronal death at its source and are therefore promising for the treatment of polyglutamine (polyQ) diseases [4]. However, most *in vivo* studies have been performed with small interfering RNAs (siRNAs) that do not discriminate

between the WT and mutant alleles. Several groups including ours demonstrated that non allele-specific silencing of *HTT* with shRNA is well tolerated up to 9 months in a lentiviral-based HD model [5] and in transgenic N171-82Q mice [6] but leads to transcriptomic changes; the functional consequences of these changes are currently unknown. Thus, an allele-specific silencing of mutant *HTT* is potentially the optimal solution for blocking polyQ pathogenesis.

Recently, strategies based on chemically modified single-stranded RNAs targeting the CAG expansion were developed to selectively target mutant *HTT* [7–9]. As an alternative strategy, single nucleotide polymorphisms (SNP) have been used to discriminate between WT and mutant transcripts associated with polyglutamine disorders [10–12]. Studies with HD patients indicate that the level of heterozygosity of a limited number of SNP is sufficient to select most HD patients, confirming the feasibility of the approach [13–15]. Two studies showed that targeting three SNP would be sufficient to treat 75% of their respective HD cohort [13]. Note that a large proportion of patients of European origin clusters in a single haplotype with a specific set of SNPs [16–18].

One challenge is that available HD animal models are not entirely appropriate for assessing the therapeutic efficacy and selectivity of shRNAs targeting SNPs. Knock-in mice do not express the human *HTT* gene [19] and transgenic models expressing short N-terminal fragments of human HTT (R6/2, N171-82Q) or viral-based HD models do not contain the corresponding SNPs [20,21]. Transgenic mice expressing full-length *HTT* possess only one human allele [22,23], allowing analysis of efficacy but not selectivity, which is an important aspect of this strategy. Only lately, one fully humanized transgenic mouse model of HD was created, containing two human *HTT* alleles, but it was not available at the time we started the study [24]. Therefore, we developed new HD models based on lentiviral expression of a chimeric mutant *HTT* reporter system. Using these new tools and neural derivatives of HD human embryonic stem cells (hESCs), we tested the efficacy and selectivity of shRNAs targeting SNPs in exons 39, 50, 60 and 67 of the human *HTT* gene and functional recovery associated with this silencing.

Materials and Methods

Plasmids and lentiviral vector production

We selected four SNPs within the *HTT* gene: rs363125 (exon 39, A or C), rs362331 (exon 50, C or T), rs2276881 (exon 60, A or G) and rs362307 (exon 67 C or T). We designed eight small-hairpin RNA (shRNA) targeting these *HTT* isoforms and cloned them in lentiviral vectors (Materials and Methods S1, Table S1). To assess the efficacy and the selectivity of these shRNAs, we produced constructs encoding chimeric mutant *HTT*, consisting of the sequence of the first 171 amino acids of the human *HTT* with 82 CAG repeats and fused to a part of *HTT* exons containing the SNP (SIN-W-PGK-htt171-82Q-exon; Materials and Methods S1, Table S2). Each chimeric mutant *HTT* construct contains one SNP of interest.

Lentiviral vectors encoding the various shRNAs and the eight chimeric HTT were produced in 293T cells using a 4-plasmid system as previously described [25]. The particle content of viral batches was determined by p24 antigen ELISA (RETROtek, Gentaur, France). The stocks were stored at −80°C until use.

In vivo experimental design and animals

Two sets of *in vivo* experiments were carried out. First, we validated the chimeric targets and tested shRNAs in 200 g adult male Wistar rats (Iffa Credo/Charles River, Les Oncins, France). Second, BACHD mice expressing full-length mutant HTT with 97Q [23] were used to validate the shRNA therapeutic strategy. BACHD mice were genotyped to identify *HTT* isoform present at SNPs studied. Stereotaxic injections of the lentiviral vectors are described in the Materials and Methods S1.

The animals were housed in a temperature-controlled room and maintained on a 12 h day/night cycle. Food and water were available *ad libitum*. All experiments were carried out in accordance with the European Community directive (86/609/EEC) for the care and use of laboratory animals as well as the Swiss animal welfare laws under the authorization n° VD 2486 and 2487 from the Service de la consommation et des affaires vétérinaires du Canton de Vaud, Switzerland.

Laser Capture Microdissection and punches

Four weeks after co-infection of chimeric *HTT* construct with fully matched or mismatched shRNA, or shCtrl, the animals were sacrificed by administration of an overdose of sodium pentobarbital. Processing of the brains for laser capture microdissection and RT-qPCR were conducted as previously described with human specific primers [5] (platform profileXpert: www.profilexpert.fr). BACHD mice injected with matched shRNA and shCtrl were sacrificed. One millimeter-thick fresh brain slices were obtained using a mouse brain matrix and punches were sampled from the GFP-positive area under a fluorescent microscope and were quickly lyzed in Trizol and stored at −80°C until RNA extraction.

Quantitative real-time PCR from 293T cells or BACHD striata

Total RNA was extracted with Trizol reagent 48 hrs post-transfection of 293T cells or 4 weeks post-injection of BACHD mice. RT-qPCR was performed in triplicate with random-primed (Invitrogen, Cergy Pontoise, France) cDNAs generated from 0.3-1 µg total RNA. Quantitative PCR was carried out in a 20 µl reaction volume containing Platinum SYBR Green qPCR super Mix-UDG (Invitrogen Cergy Pontoise, France), and 10 µM of both forward and reverse primers recognizing a sequence of human *HTT* present in the first part of all chimeric constructs and in the BACHD human allele (sequences in Table S3) using a Realplex thermal cycler (Eppendorf). Three to 5 samples from cells and 4–10 samples from the striatum punches were subjected to RT-qPCR analyses. Values for *HTT* mRNA were normalized to a reference: β-actin (*ACTB*) or peptidyl propyl isomerase A (*PPIA*) and are expressed as mean percentages ± SEM relative to the control condition.

Histological processing

Four to 8 weeks post-lentiviral injection, the animals were given an overdose of sodium pentobarbital and were transcardially perfused with a phosphate solution followed by 4% paraformaldehyde (PFA, Sigma-Aldrich, St. Louis, Missouri, United States) and 10% picric acid for fixation. The brains were processed as previously described [5] for immunohistochemistry for dopamine and cAMP-regulated phosphoprotein of a molecular mass of 32 kDa (DARPP-32), ubiquitin (Ubi) and mutant HTT (EM-48). Pictures were taken using 4x, 20x or 63x objectives on an Olympus AX70 microscope.

Quantification of DARPP-32 lesions and formation of inclusions

The loss of DARPP-32 expression was analyzed by collecting digitized images of twelve sections per animal (separated by 300 µm) with an optic bench and by quantifying the lesion areas in mm^2 with image analysis software (MCID Core 7.0, InterFocus Imaging, GE Healthcare Niagara Inc.). Lesion areas in each section were determined as regions poor in DARPP-32 staining relative to the surrounding tissue. The lesion volume for each animal is expressed in mm^3, calculated as the sum of the total lesion area in mm^2 of all sections multiplied by the inter-section distance (300 µm). For estimation of the number of ubiquitin-positive HTT inclusions, 12 serial coronal sections of the striatum (separated by 300 µm) were scanned with a 10x objective using a Zeiss Axioplan2 imaging microscope equipped with an automated motorized stage and acquisition system (Mercator Pro V6.50, ExploraNova). All ubiquitin-positive objects with an apparent cross-sectional area comprised between 1 and 50 $µm^2$ were measured as previously reported [5]. The same parameters were applied for EM-48 aggregates quantification. Bravais-Pearson correlation was performed to validate the use of Ubiquitin staining as a measure of HTT aggregation (Statistica, Statsoft, Maisons-Alfort, France).

Neural Stem Cells culture and nucleofection

Neural stem cells (NSCs) were obtained and maintained as described previously [26]. NSC lines were differentiated from the following human ES lines: SA-01 (WT XY, passages 30-83, Cellartis AB, Sweden), H9 (WT XX, passages 40-60, WiCell Research Institute), VUB05 (HD XY, 44 CAG, passages 35-130, AZ-VUB, Belgium [27]), SIVF017 (HD, XY, 40 CAG, passages18-35, Sydney IVF Stem Cells, Australia [28]), SIVF018 (HD XX, 46 CAG, passage 18-30, Sydney IVF Stem Cells, Australia [28]) and Huez2.3 (HD XX, 44 CAG, passages 25-47, IGBMC, Strasbourg [29]).

Genotypes for SNP rs362331 of Huez2.3, VUB05 and SIVF018 NSC lines were analyzed by sequencing the PCR product encompassing this SNP generated using the following primers: 5′-CCCAAACGAAGGTACACGA and 5′-CCTGTTGGCC-ATCTCTCACC.

For videomicroscopy analysis, NSCs were electroporated with 1 µg BDNF-mCherry, a gift from G. Banker (Oregon Health and Science University) and 4 µg SIN-CWP-GFP-TRE-H1-shCtrl (controls: shLUC or shUNIV), -sh50T or -sh50C (see Table S2). NSCs were plated on glass coverslips previously coated with Poly-L-ornithine and Laminin (Sigma, St. Louis, Missouri, United States). Live videomicroscopy was carried out seven to ten days after transfection using an imaging system as previously described [30] with little modifications (Materials and Methods S1). After videomicroscopy experiments, the neuronal cultures were processed for immunofluorescence for anti-HTT-2166 (Materials and Methods S1).

Results

Development of SNP-specific shRNA for the treatment of HD

To distinguish the normal and disease HTT alleles in HD patients, we developed shRNAs targeting the disease isoform of heterozygous single-nucleotide polymorphisms (SNP). We produced eight shRNAs corresponding to four SNP present within the HTT gene: in exons 39, 50, 60 and 67 (**Fig. 1A**). The selection was based on their presence in HTT exons and a high frequency of heterozygosity in the human population (http://www.ncbi.nlm.nih.gov/snp and [13,14,16]). DNAs encoding the shRNAs targeting each SNP (shSNPs: sh39A, sh39C, sh50C, sh50T, sh60A, sh60G and sh67C, sh67T) were inserted into a lentiviral vector [5] (**Fig. 1B**). The SNP was localized at 10 (p10, exons 39, 60 and 67) or 11 (p11, exon 50) bases from the 5′ end of the guide strand of the shRNA to ensure selective cleavage of the target sequence [31]. All the exons selected correspond to the 3′ part of the HTT mRNA. As the transcript (>10 kb) is too long for the entire sequence to be inserted into lentiviral vectors, we created a chimeric HTT gene to test the efficacy and selectivity of our shSNPs. The chimeric HTT contains a N-terminal fragment of mutant HTT corresponding to the first 171 amino acids with 82 glutamines (Htt171-82Q) fused in frame to the part of the protein encoded by the exons carrying the SNP of interest (**Fig. 1A** and Materials and Methods S1). A sequence encoding the HA tag was added to 3′ the end to facilitate detection of the resulting fusion proteins.

We tested the ability of the lentiviral vectors encoding the shSNPs to silence their corresponding chimeric constructs. 293T cells were co-transfected with the plasmids expressing the chimeric HTT and the shRNA, and mutant HTT levels were analyzed by quantitative RT-PCR (**Fig. 2a**) and western blotting (**Fig. 2B**). The presence of fully matched shSNP was associated with robust degradation of the chimeric HTT mRNA (**Fig. 2A**), with the shSNP targeting exons 39 and 67 being the most potent (around 80% of degradation of the targeted mRNA). In contrast, HTT mRNA levels were only modestly reduced (10% of silencing in most cases) following co-transfection with mismatched shSNP (**Fig. 2A**). This demonstrates the capacity of this approach to discriminate between the two HTT alleles. Selectivity was however poorer for sh50T and sh67C/T, with 40-50% degradation of HTT mRNA with the mismatched shRNAs. Additional experiments (n = 3) were performed to demonstrate the correlation between the HTT mRNA and protein levels (Figure S1). HTT protein levels were decreased in all matched and, to a lower extent, in most mismatched conditions. A strong correlation was observed between the HTT mRNA and protein levels, in agreement with published studies [32,33].

Effective allele-specific silencing of mutant HTT in the HD rat model

To evaluate the therapeutic efficacy of this approach in vivo, we needed an appropriate model expressing the SNPs of interest. We injected the various chimeric Htt171-82Q-exon vectors and the pathogenic control Htt171-82Q vector into the striatum of adult rats to induce a local expression of the disease protein, and compared the severity of HD neuropathology. Misfolded HTT labeled with the ubiquitin antibody was detected and the typical lesion with a down-regulation of DARPP-32 expression was observed for all the chimeric constructs (**Fig. 3A**), consistent with previous findings [34]. This ubiquitin staining is faithfully reflecting the accumulation of misfolded HTT protein revealed with the EM48 antibody (Figure S2). After 8 weeks, there was no apparent difference between animals injected with the Htt171-82Q or the other Htt171-82Q-exon vectors (**Fig. 3A**).

To assess the efficacy of allele-specific silencing, we co-injected lentiviral vectors encoding human Htt171-82Q-exon with the corresponding shSNP into the striatum of adult rats. Four weeks post-injection, using the GFP-reporter gene present on the vectors expressing the shSNP to identify the infected cells (mostly neurons as previously reported [35] [36]), the GFP-positive area was laser microdissected and the amount of HTT mRNA was determined by RT-qPCR. All shSNPs efficiently silenced HTT gene expression (**Fig. 3B**). In the same experiment, we then tested the ability of the shRNAs to selectively discriminate SNPs in vivo. The striatum of adult rats was co-injected with Htt171-82Q-exon and the corresponding mismatched shRNAs. The shSNPs targeting exons 50 or 60 efficiently discriminated between the two SNP variants (0 to less than 35% degradation of mismatched HTT mRNA), whereas the shSNPs targeting exon 39 or 67 did not discriminate (around 80% of degradation) (**Fig. 3B**). These experiments demonstrate the efficiency of all shSNPs is accompanied by good specificity for five of the eight shSNPs.

Inhibition of HD neuropathology in matched shSNP-treated lentiviral HD rat model

To further confirm the therapeutic potential of the shSNPs, we investigated the formation of HTT aggregates and striatal neuronal dysfunction. HTT inclusions are a hallmark of the pathology and a reliable marker of the severity of HD pathology. We co-injected the chimeric constructs with either the fully matched or mismatched shSNPs or a shRNA control (shCtrl). Eight weeks later, we quantified the down-regulation of DARPP-32 expression and the number of ubiquitin-positive aggregates.

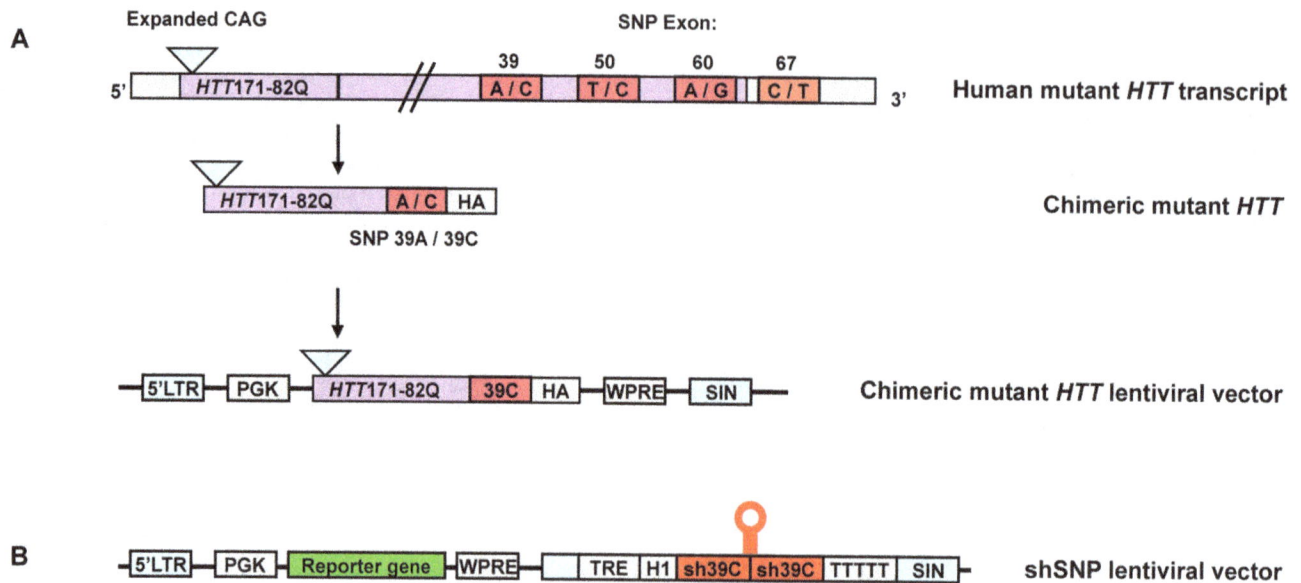

Figure 1. Schematic representation of the chimeric *HTT*- and shSNP-containing lentiviral vectors. (**A**) We chose four SNP within the human *HTT* transcript: exon 39 (rs363125), exon 50 (rs362331), exon 60 (rs2276881) and exon 67 (rs362307). This last SNP is located after the stop codon, in the 3′UTR of the *HTT* gene. The chimeric *HTT* with the exon 39 SNP is illustrated as an example: the sequence surrounding the SNP (A or C) is fused in frame to the 5′ sequence of mutant *HTT* encoding the first 171 amino acids with 82Q. A sequence encoding the HA tag is added at 3′ the end of all fusion proteins to facilitate detection. The fusion construct is then inserted into a SIN transfer vector. (**B**) Representation of a lentiviral vector expressing the shSNP (example of sh39C). The sequence corresponding to the shRNA is inserted downstream from a tetracycline responsive element (TRE) and a H1 promoter in the 3′LTR of the vector. A second expression cassette contains a GFP reporter gene under the control of a PGK promoter. The SNP was located at position 10 or 16 for this particular shSNP, counting from the 5′ end of the guide strand of the shRNA.

DARPP-32 immunostaining (**Fig. 4A**) showed that the lesion size was reduced in the matched conditions, except for the sh39, but not in control and some mismatch injected areas (**Fig. 4C**). This staining indicated that most of the shSNPs in the matched condition inhibited the appearance of an HD neuropathology with very high efficacy. Large numbers of ubiquitin immunostained aggregates were observed in the control and most mismatch injected areas, whereas smaller numbers were found in the matched conditions (**Figs. 4B and 4D**). In the mismatch condition, the SNP discrimination power of sh39 and sh67 was low (not significant; **Figs. 4C and 4D**). Injection of the shSNP only didn't lead to striatal dysfunction based on DARPP32 staining, 8 weeks after injection (data not shown).

Pfister and collaborators have shown that for the SNP in exon 39, placing the mismatch at position 16 rather than 10 improved the discrimination ratio in a luciferase reporter system [13]. We therefore developed new vectors encoding sh39p16 and compared them with the sh39p10 constructs by evaluating *in vitro* mutant *HTT* mRNA levels in 293T cells co-transfected with the chimeric *HTT* and the shRNA (Figure S3A) and *in vivo* lesion volumes and the numbers of ubiquitin-positive aggregates in co-injected rats (Figure S3B and S3C). Sh39p16 efficiently silenced mutant *HTT*, however the selectivity was not improved by placing the mismatched base at position 16 of the shRNA.

Efficient silencing of mutant *HTT* in BACHD mice using matched shSNP

BACHD mice express full-length human mutant *HTT* at physiological levels. Human mutant *HTT* mRNA in these mice is approximately 1.36 fold the level of endogenous WT *HTT* [37]; whereas mutant *HTT* mRNA level in animals injected with lentiviral vectors is about 25 times higher than the endogenous one [5]. We therefore used these animals to measure silencing efficacy

on endogenous full-length *HTT* mRNA in the disease context. Genotyping showed that these mice express exon39C, exon60G and exon67C, and exon50T in agreement with Carroll et al. [15]. The four matched shSNPs and the shCtrl were injected bilaterally into the striatum of these adult and pre-symptomatic transgenic mice (we chose to inject sh39Cp16 because it is more efficacious than sh39Cp10, Figure S3). Four weeks post-injection, the mice were sacrificed and the GFP-positive area of the striatum was grossly punched out from 1 mm-thick striatal slices. *HTT* mRNA was measured by RT-qPCR from these punches to measure the average silencing obtained in the striatum (i.e. infected/treated and non-infected cells) and evaluate treatment efficiency, which can be expected with this gene transfer approach. The data gathered from this *in vivo* experiment and those presented in Figures 3–4 are therefore complementary and provide two distinct types of information on the allele-specific silencing. In striatal punches from BACHD mice, the amounts of mutant *HTT* mRNA (**Fig. 5A**) were lower (around 50%) in mice treated with each of the four shSNPs than shCtrl. There was no significant difference in the mRNA levels of the neuronal marker Neuronal Nuclei (NeuN) between any of the samples (**Fig. 5B**) confirming that they were comparable. To further demonstrate the selectivity of the silencing on full-length human mutant *HTT*, we performed one additional experiment in BACHD mice injected with sh50T, sh50C and shCtrl. As expected, a statistically significant silencing was observed with the sh50T while *HTT* mRNA level in the sh50C group was similar to the control group (**Fig. 5C**). Therefore, the capacity to discriminate the two alleles was confirmed.

Functional recovery after allele-specific silencing of mutant *HTT* in neurons derived from HD-hESCs

To assess the silencing of endogenous *HTT* and the functional recovery, we took advantage of the recent isolation of human

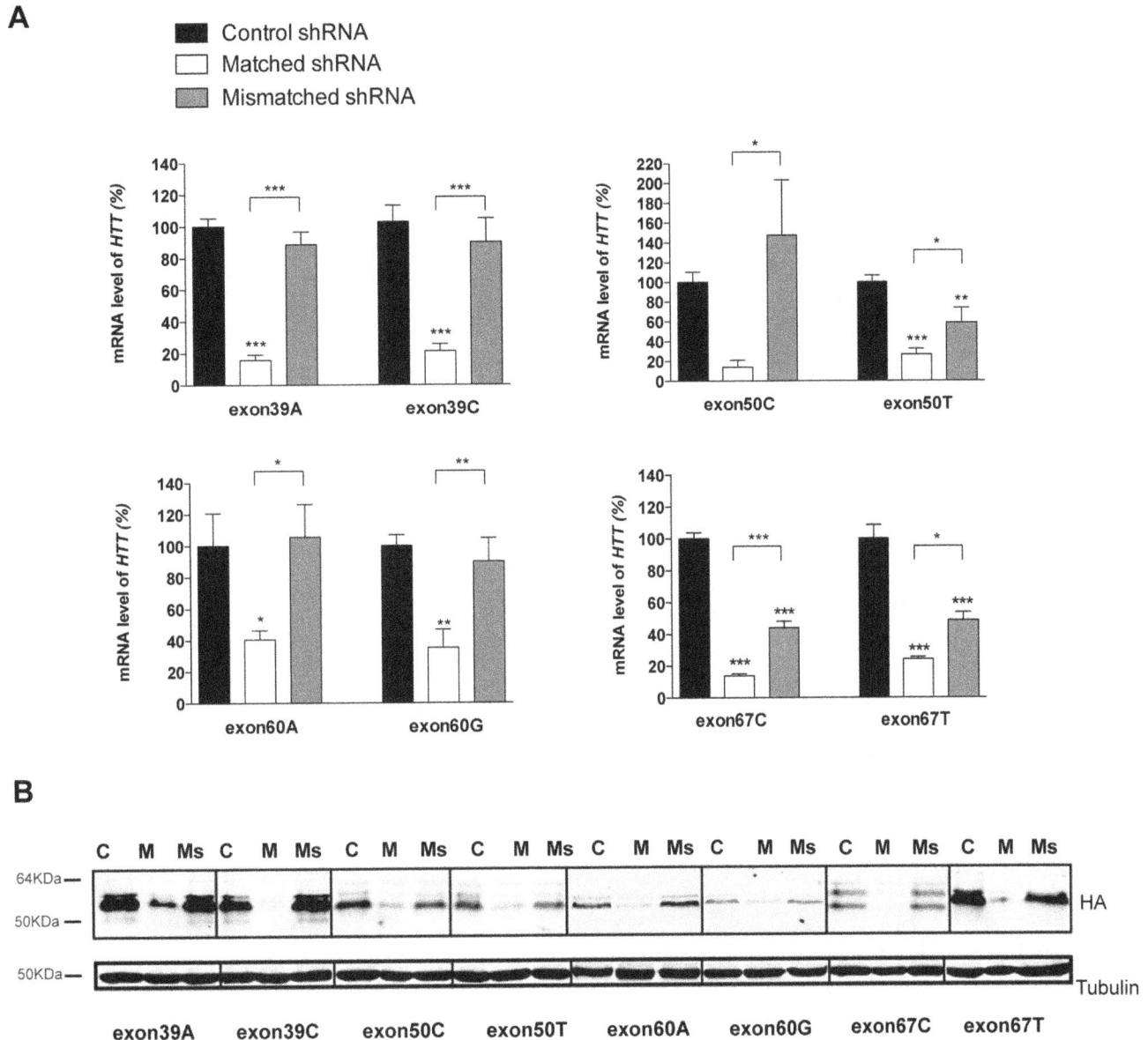

Figure 2. Efficacy and selectivity of the shSNP *in vitro*. (A) Quantitative real-time PCR analyses showing the silencing of *HTT* mRNA in transfected 293T cells co-expressing chimeric *HTT* and shSNP or the control shRNA. Levels of the chimeric *HTT* mRNA were normalized to β-Actin and are reported as mean percentages relative to the control condition (set at 100%) ± SEM (n = 3–5). One-way analyses of variance (ANOVA) were performed for each SNP. Newman-Keuls Post-hoc comparison between the shCtrl groups and shSNP groups indicated significant efficacy for sh39A, sh39C, sh50T, sh67T, sh67C (***$P<0.001$), sh60G (**$P<0.01$) and sh60A (*$P<0.05$) whereas the difference between the control condition and the sh50C condition was not statistically significant. The mismatched shRNA conditions were not significantly different from the control condition except for 50T+sh50C (**$P<0.01$), 67T+sh67C and 67C+sh67T (***$P<0.001$) and they were all significantly different from the matched shRNA conditions showing the selectivity of this approach *in vitro* (sh39A, sh39C, sh67C (***$P<0.001$), sh60G (**$P<0.01$), sh50C, sh50T, sh60A and sh67T (*$P<0.05$). **(B)** Representative western blot (n = 3) with anti-HA antibody illustrating production of the chimeric proteins. The efficacy test lanes (matched shRNA: M) evidence the decrease/absence of the corresponding chimeric proteins, whereas in selectivity lanes (mismatched shRNA: Ms) the mutant HTT is still present as in the control condition (c).

neural stem cells (NSCs) from HD-hESCs [26]. We transfected the HD-NSC line Huez2.3 homozygous for the SNP in exon 50 (T/T) and demonstrated that the silencing obtained with si50T was similar to that with the previously described siHtt6, which targets both alleles [5]. Transfecting the cells with the mismatched siRNA (si50C) had little effect on *HTT* expression, confirming the selectivity of the approach (**Fig. 6A**). Because the CAG expansion is located far from the SNP position, we then developed a new method based on SNP-specific reverse transcription and amplifi-

cation of CAG repeats by PCR, coupled with size detection on a chip, to link the SNP and the mutant allele in the heterozygous HD-hESC. Using this strategy, we found that the mutant CAG expansion (46 or 44 CAG) was associated with the SNP50T in SIVF018 and VUB05 cells. Treatment of these cells with si50T and si50C significantly decreased mutant and WT *HTT* mRNA levels, respectively, and as expected the silencing was more pronounced with siHtt6 (**Fig. 6B**).

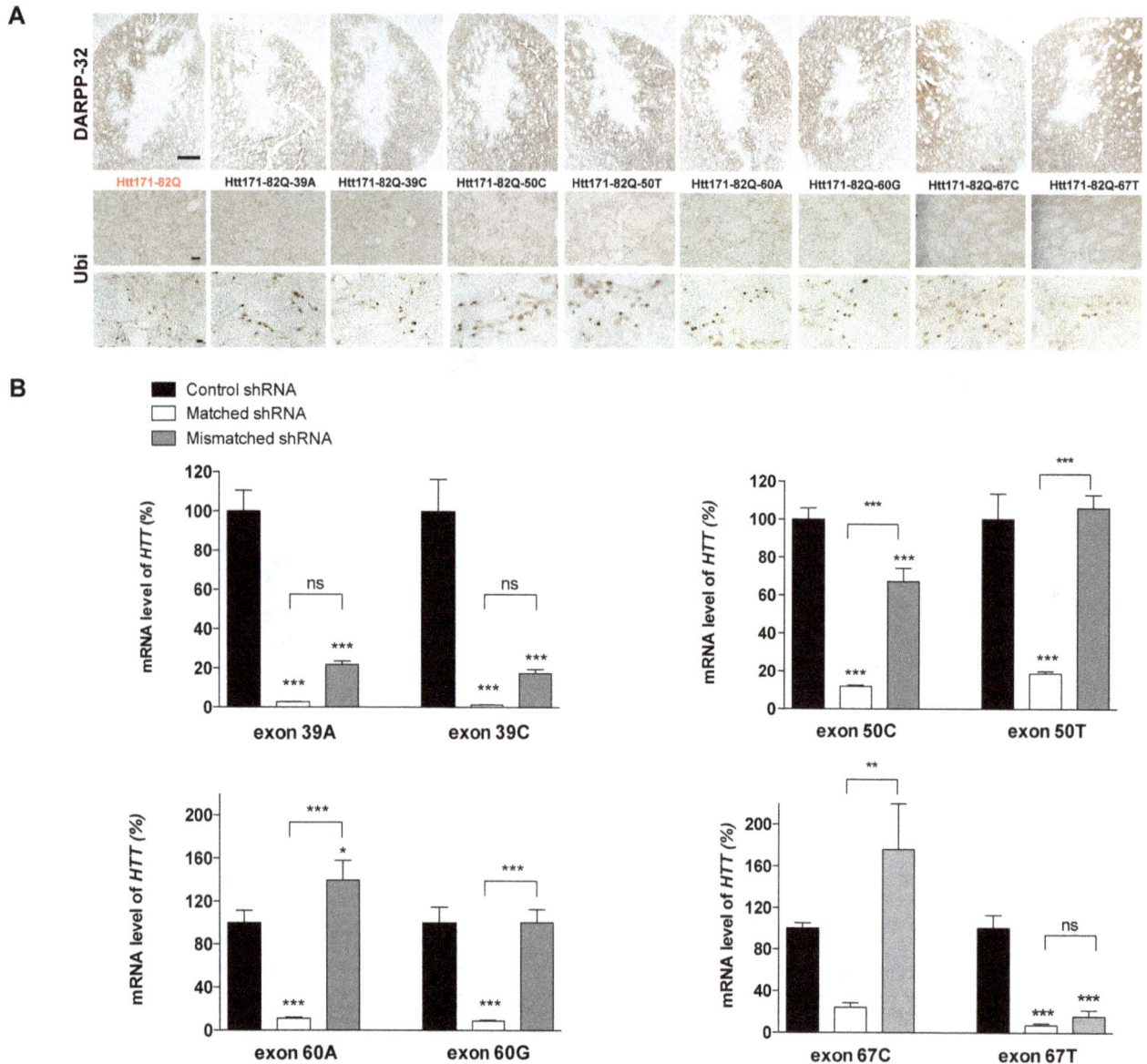

Figure 3. Expression of *HTT* after co-injection of constructs encoding chimeric mutant *HTT* and GFP-shSNPs *in vivo*. (A) Lentiviral vectors expressing the htt171-82Q fragment or the various chimeric mutant *HTT* were injected into the striatum of rats (n = 4 per group). Eight weeks after injection, DARPP-32 and ubiquitin (Ubi) staining (low and high magnification pictures) demonstrated that all the constructs led to HD-like neuropathology (loss of DARPP-32 staining and ubiquitin-positive aggregates), similar to that with the htt171-82Q lentiviral-based model. **(B)** Four weeks after injection, the GFP-positive area was laser-capture microdissected and *HTT* mRNA was assayed by RT-qPCR. Values for *HTT* mRNA were normalized to PPIA and are expressed as mean percentages of the value for the control condition $\pm$ SEM (n = 6). One-way ANOVAs were conducted for each SNP. 39A: ***$P<0.001$; 39C: ***$P<0.001$; 50C: ***$P<0.001$; 50T: ***$P<0.001$; 60A: ***$P<0.001$; 60G: ***$P<0.001$; 67T: ***$P<0.001$; 67C: P> 0.05. Newman-Keuls Post-hoc comparison between the shCtrl groups and matched shRNA groups demonstrates significant silencing of all targeted *HTT* mRNAs, ***$P<0.001$, except for exon 67C. Post-hoc comparison between the shCtrl groups and mismatched shRNA groups revealed no significant differences for sh50T, sh60A or sh60G, a significant difference for sh67C, and highly significant differences for sh39A, sh39C, sh50C and sh67T. This comparison as the matched/mismatched post-hoc provides evidence of the different selectivities of the shSNPs.

We tested whether the allele-specific silencing of mutant *HTT* was associated with a functional recovery. We took advantage of the defect in the vesicular trafficking of the brain-derived neurotrophic factor, BDNF, previously described in primary cultures expressing mutant HTT [30]. We measured BDNF anterograde and retrograde velocity in neurons derived from WT (lines H9 and SA-01) and HD lines (Huez2.3 and SIVF018) (**Fig. 7A**). Direct fluorescence allowed us to select cells co-transfected with BDNF-mCherry and shRNA (GFP) (**Fig. 7B**).

Kymographs showing the spatial positions of BDNF vesicles through time were used to quantify the dynamics in different conditions (**Figs. 7C and 7D**). When differentiated into neurons, both HD-lines (Huez2.3 and SIVF018) displayed vesicular trafficking defects relative to the WT lines (H9 and SA-01) (**Fig. 7A**). This confirms that an expansion as limited as 44 CAG is sufficient to impair transport function [30]. Immunofluorescence staining confirmed that these cells expressed HTT (**Fig. 7B**). We then analyzed mCherry-BDNF transport in the SIVF018 line and

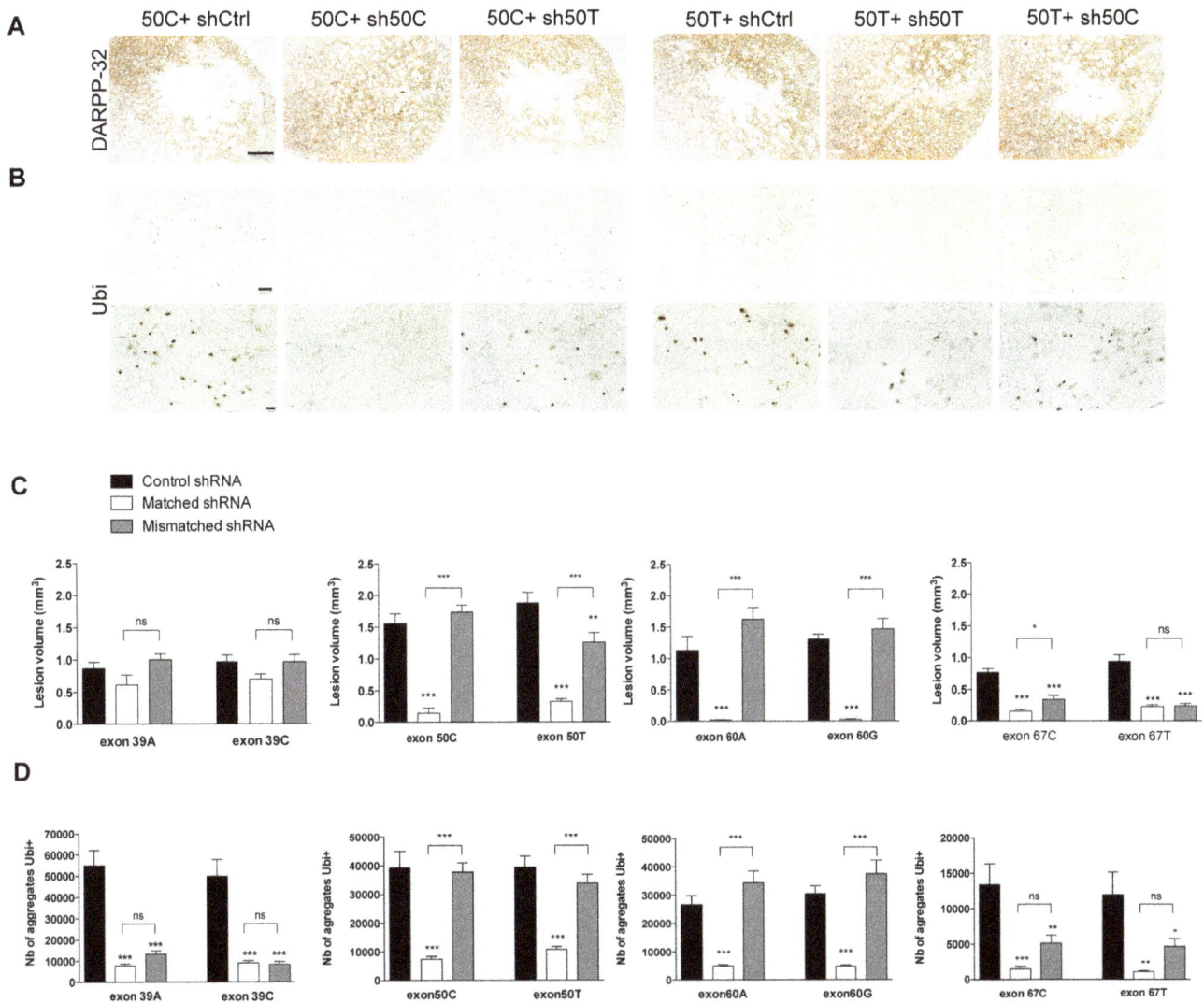

Figure 4. Efficacy and selectivity of the GFP-shSNP *in vivo*. (A) and **(C)** DARPP-32 immunostaining and quantification 8 weeks after injection evidencing loss of this striatal marker in the control and mismatched injected areas but its preservation in the matched conditions, except for sh39 and sh67. The results are expressed as mean volumes in mm³ depleted of DARPP-32 ± SEM (n = 8). One-way ANOVAs were conducted for each SNP: 50C, 50T, 60A, 60G, 67T, and 67C: ***P<0.001. Newman-Keuls Post-hoc comparison between control conditions and test conditions showed a highly effective prevention of DARPP-32 loss for most of the matched shSNPs and also significant, although less so, prevention of loss for the mismatched sh50C and sh67. For the other mismatched conditions, the post-hoc test was not significant, indicating the selectivity of the shSNPs. **(B)** and **(D)** Ubiquitin immunostaining (low and high magnification pictures) and quantification showing large numbers of aggregates in the control and mismatched injected areas and fewer aggregates in the matched conditions. The results are expressed as mean numbers of ubiquitin-positive aggregates ± SEM (n = 8). One-way ANOVAs were conducted for each SNP: 39A, 39C, 50C, 50T, 60A, 60G, and 67T: ***P<0.001; 67C: **P<0.01. Newman-Keuls Post-hoc comparison between control and matched conditions showed highly significant prevention of aggregate formation for all matched shSNPs. For mismatched conditions, the post-hoc test was not significant except for the mismatched sh39 and sh67.

a second HD heterozygous line, VUB05. Both anterograde and retrograde trafficking of BDNF was significantly greater in SIVF018 and VUB05 neurons when the mutant *HTT* was silenced with the sh50T, whereas targeting the WT *HTT* allele with sh50C had no effect (**Figs. 7C and 7D**). Thus, allele-specific silencing of mutant *HTT* in HD cells is associated with a functional recovery of BDNF transport. Also, silencing of the mutant allele is sufficient to alleviate the dominant effect of the mutant *HTT* over the WT *HTT*.

Discussion

Targeting heterozygous SNPs to degrade mutant *HTT* selectively while preserving the WT transcript is an extremely promising approach to HD treatment. However, developing and validating appropriate protocols is challenging. The frequencies and maps of heterozygous SNPs in the population have been established [13–18], and the number of SNP candidates is limited (approximately 40–50) compared to the countless sequences that could be targeted with a non allele-specific strategy. Also, the sequences flanking an SNP are not necessarily optimal for shRNA interaction, and the mismatches in SNPs have different discrimination powers that affect the selectivity of the silencing further

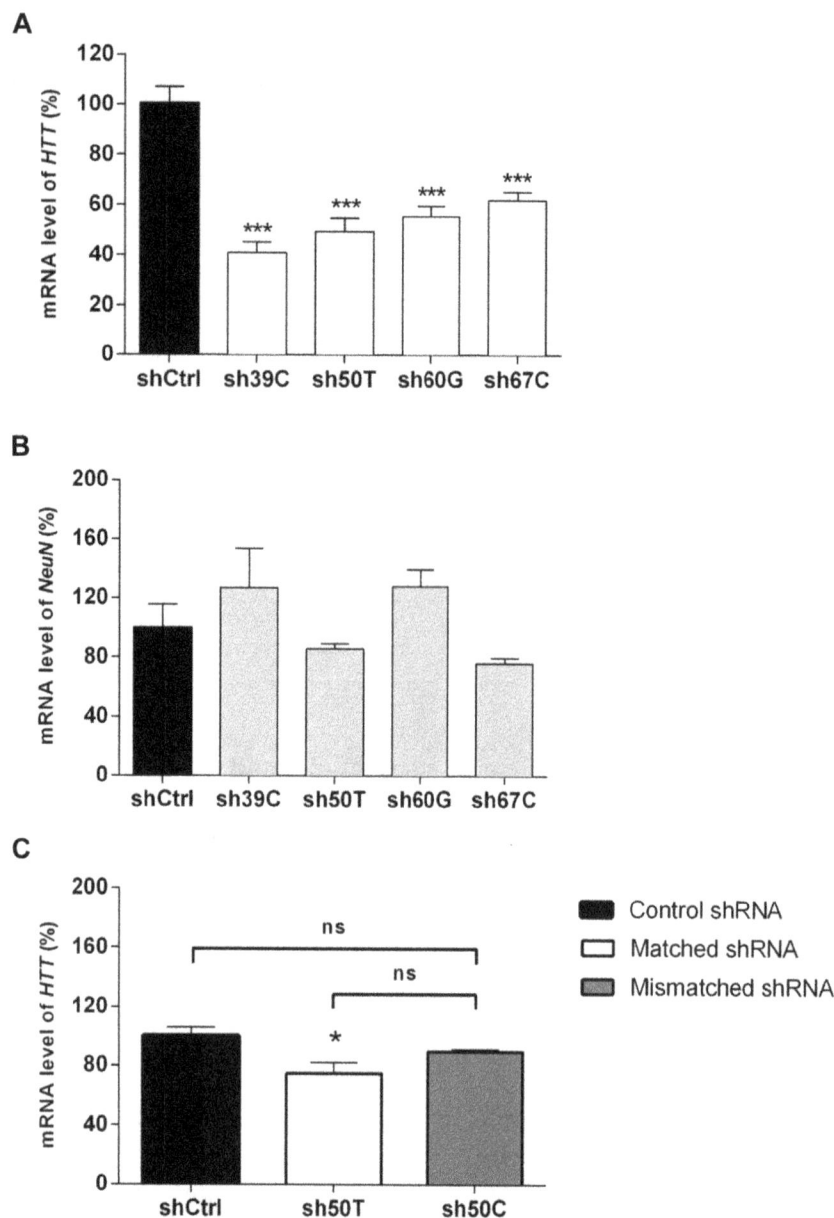

Figure 5. Effective and selective SNP-specific silencing in BACHD mice. (A) Four weeks after injection of constructs encoding fully matched shSNP in BACHD mice striatum, the GFP-positive area was dissected and *HTT* mRNA was assayed by RT-qPCR. Values for *HTT* mRNA were normalized to a reference peptidyl propyl isomerase A (*PPIA*) and are expressed as mean percentages relative to the control condition (set at 100%) ± SEM (n = 10). One-way ANOVAs were conducted for each matched SNP for *HTT* 39C, 50T, 60G, and 67C: ***P<0.001. Newman-Keuls Post-hoc comparison between the shCtrl and matched shRNA groups demonstrate significant silencing of targeted human *HTT* mRNA. (B) Samples all showed similar NeuN gene expression (One-way ANOVAs and Newman-Keuls Post-hoc comparison test). (c) Three weeks after injection of constructs encoding shCtrl, sh50T and sh50C in BACHD mice striatum, 1 mm³ punches of the GFP infected area were dissected and *HTT* mRNA was assayed by RT-qPCR with primers specific for the human *HTT*. Values for *HTT* mRNA were normalized to a reference *PPIA* and are expressed as mean percentages relative to the control condition (set at 100%) ± SEM (n=4–6). One-way ANOVAs were conducted for each groups: *P<0.05. Newman-Keuls Post-hoc comparison between the shCtrl and the sh50T confirm the silencing of human mutant *HTT* mRNA, whereas no statistically significant difference was observed between shCtrl and sh50C groups, demonstrating the selectivity of *HTT* silencing.

reducing the number of possibilities. Furthermore, clinical implementation will undoubtedly require the development and validation of several products to treat the most patients.

Here, we addressed some of these issues by targeting four SNP among the most frequent in the population. We showed that the eight shRNAs covering these SNPs provide efficient and, in most cases, selective silencing of *HTT in vitro* and *in vivo* and hence are good candidates for the treatment of many HD patients.

These findings were obtained with novel models developed specifically for screening shSNPs. The chimeric reporter plasmids expressing the construct encoding human mutant *HTT* fused to the exons containing the various SNP allow large-scale and quick quantitative analysis of the silencing efficacy and selectivity. We reported that the allele-specific silencing demonstrated in 293T cells was reproduced in human NSC derived from HD-hESC lines involving a mutated *HTT* corresponding to that responsible for

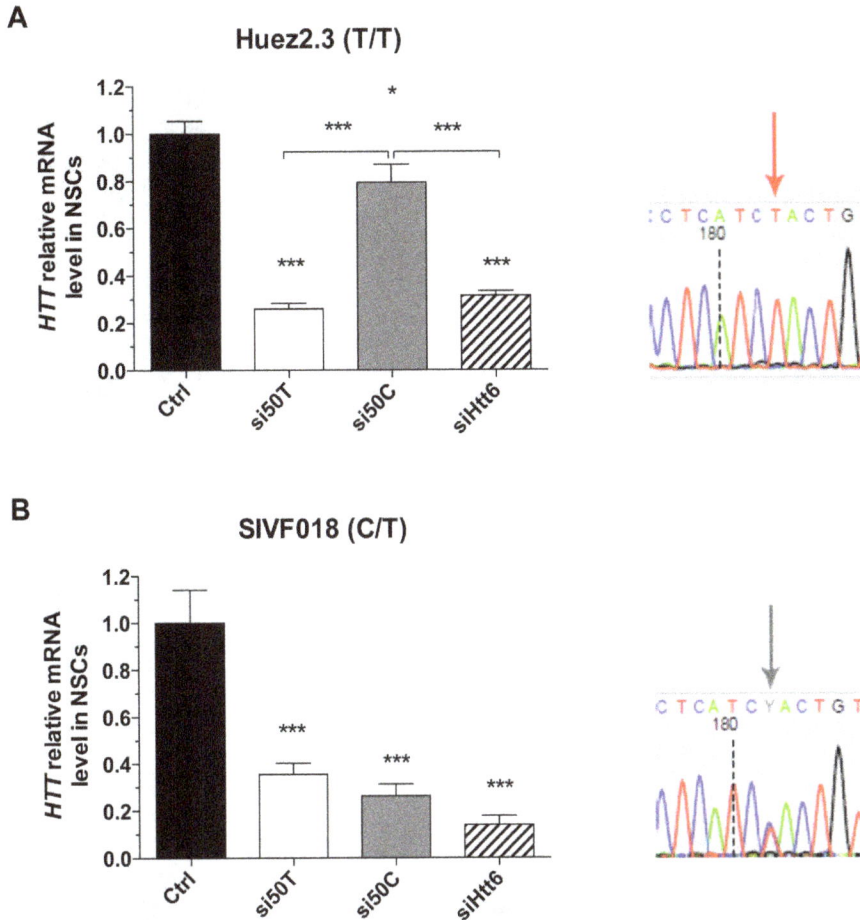

Figure 6. Allele specific knock-down of *HTT* mRNA in human HD NSC. Relative *HTT* mRNA levels normalized to controls (non-targeting siRNA) measured by RT-qPCR in HD-NSCs transfected with pan-allelic (siHtt6) or allele-specific *HTT*-targeting (si50T and si50C) siRNAs. HD-NSCs were derived from two HD-hESC lines, Huez2.3 (**A**) and SIVF018 (**B**), T/T homozygous and C/T heterozygous for SNP rs362331, respectively. n = 4. P-value by one-way ANOVA and Tukey's multiple comparison test; *P<0.05; **P<0.01; ***P<0.001; Error bars depict SEM.

adult onset HD. These experiments showed that the *in vitro* platform based on 293T cells and HD-specific human pluripotent stem cells is suitable for evaluating the effects of allele-specific shRNA. We reported that neurons derived from HD-hESCs reproduce the defect in anterograde and retrograde BDNF vesicular transport associated with HD [30]. Allele-specific silencing of mutant *HTT* restored the mean velocity of BDNF vesicles to control values. Silencing of WT *HTT* in neurons heterozygous for SNP exon 50 did not alter trafficking along microtubules in neurites, as previously reported [38]. The different effects of treatment with sh50T and sh50C suggest that these shSNP are sufficiently potent and selective to modulate axonal vesicular transport in neurons. Importantly, *HTT* mRNA levels in NSC derived from hESC are closer of the values observed in patient brain samples than in HD-derived fibroblasts or lymphoblasts (which are 100x lower), increasing the potential value of this cellular model [26].

Silencing levels were similar to those obtained with shRNA targeting both alleles [5]. Even though the sequences of these shSNP were not selected according to established algorithms and criteria for optimal silencing, all of them efficiently promoted degradation of the target mRNA. In agreement with Lombardi et al. [14], we observed that the sh50C/T led to efficient degradation of the targeted mRNA (74%; fully matched sequence), while a

central mismatch in the shRNA sequence abolished this silencing (21%; mismatched sequence). In contrast, antisense oligonucleotides (ASO) targeting the exon 50 were associated with poor discrimination power in human HD fibroblasts [15]. This discrepancy might be due to differences in the mode of action between shRNA and ASO, the experimental paradigm, method of administration modalities or different concentrations.

HD transgenic mice available when we initiated this study, express only one allele of the human *HTT* gene and only full-length *HTT* genes are suitable for validating the chosen SNP, most of which map in the 3′ part of the gene. We therefore used two approaches for *in vivo* validation. As a first screen to assess the efficacy and selectivity of *HTT* allele-specific silencing, we injected lentiviral vectors encoding the first 171 amino acids of the human mutant *HTT* fused to the exon containing the SNP into the striatum of adult rats [5,34]. Our shSNP recognized only the human *HTT* transcript, because the targeted regions display only limited sequence identity with the rodent *HTT* mRNA. These experiments therefore replicate allele-specific silencing as it would occur in human patients. Four weeks after the injection, the majority of the animals treated with fully matched shRNA showed *HTT* mRNA levels that were 80% lower than control values, and a concomitant reduction of the number of *HTT* aggregates and lesion size at 8 weeks. These experiments confirmed the efficacy

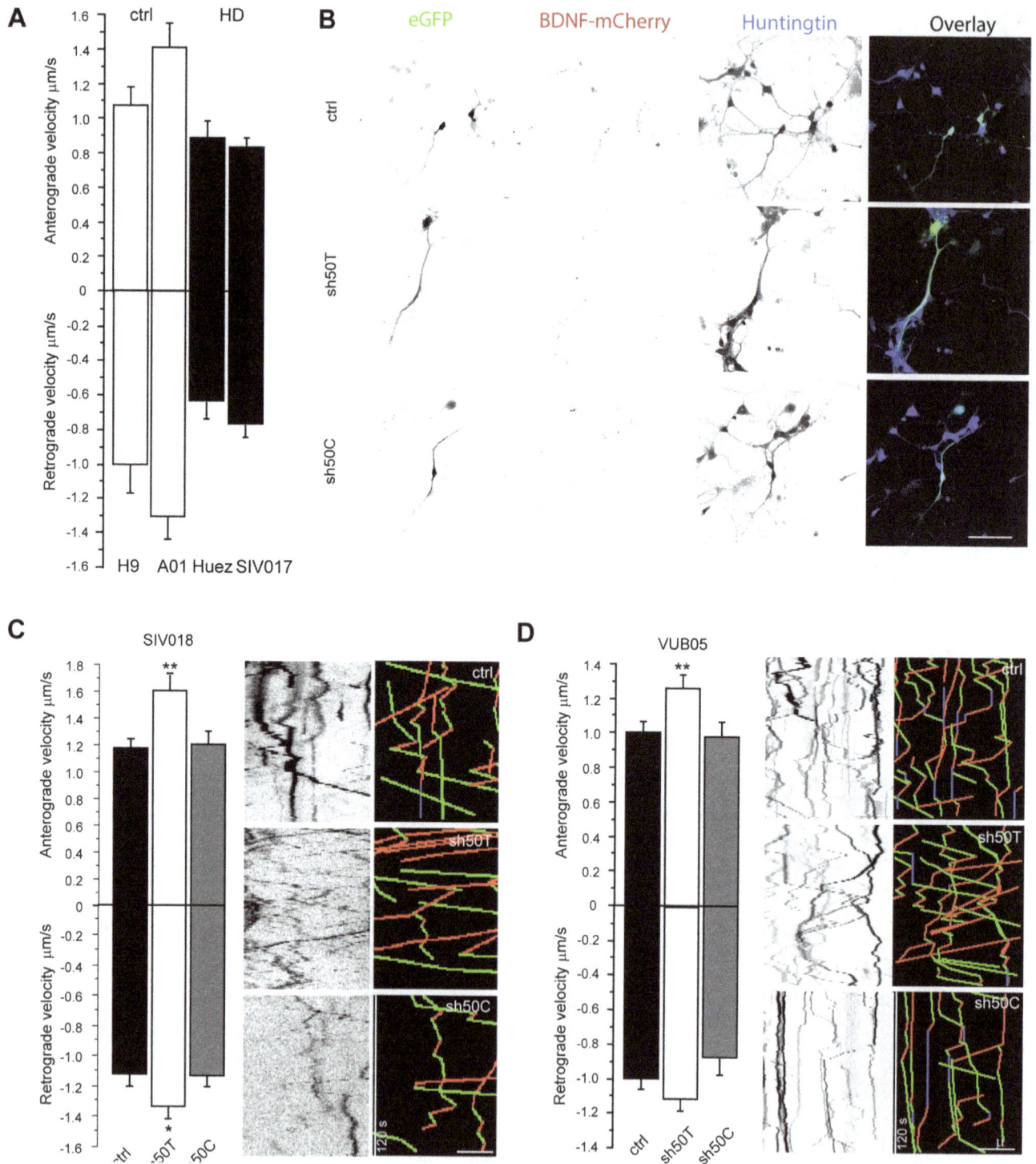

Figure 7. Recovery of BDNF trafficking after allele-specific silencing of mutant *HTT* in neurons derived from HD-hESCs. (**A**) Quantitative analyses of anterograde and retrograde BDNF vesicular velocity in two different WT NSC lines (H9 and SA-01; white bars) and two HD-derived NSC lines (Huez2.3, SIVF017; black bars): anterograde and retrograde velocities are higher in WT neurons than in HD cells. One-way ANOVAs were conducted for anterograde and retrograde velocity separately. Anterograde: ***P<0.001; n = 43 to 170. Retrograde: **P<0.01; n = 43 to 133. (**B**) Direct GFP and mCherry fluorescence and immunofluorescence staining of HTT in transfected neurons derived from one HD-hESC line (VUB05); these cells were used for video-microscopy analyses. (**C, D**) Quantitative analyses of anterograde and retrograde BDNF vesicular velocities in SIVF017 cells (**C**) and VUB05 cells (**D**) with representative kymographs and the analyzed trajectories (green for anterograde, red for retrograde and blue for pausing vesicles). (**C**) One-way ANOVA for anterograde velocity: **P<0.01; n = 50 to 72. Fisher's PLSD Post-hoc test demonstrated significant velocity recovery with respect to the control group in the sh50T group, **P<0.01, but not in the sh50C group. For retrograde: F(2,198) = 3.095, *P<0.05; 55 to 77 events were recorded for each group. Fisher's PLSD Post-hoc test demonstrated significant velocity recovery with respect to the control group in the sh50T group, *P<0.05 but not in the si50C group. (**D**) One-way ANOVAs were conducted for anterograde and retrograde velocity separately. For anterograde: F(2, 329) = 5.494, **P<0.01; 51 to 153 events were recorded for each group. Fisher's PLSD Post-hoc test demonstrated a significant increase in velocity for the sh50T group, **P<0.01 but not the sh50C group, with respect to the control group. For retrograde: F(2,313) = 2.585,

P = 0.077; 44 to 144 events were recorded for each group. There was no significant difference between control group and treated groups for retrograde transport.

and selectivity of the shSNPs targeting Exon50C/T and Exon60G/A. The shSNPs specific for exon 39A/C and exon 67C/T were also extremely effective, although their discriminatory power was not completely preserved. Additionally, besides a strong transgene knockdown by targeting exon 39, as shown by reduction of target RNA and ubiquitin inclusions, there was a limited rescue of the lesion volume. These particular shRNAs could be partially complementary to one or several rat's transcripts and lead to their expression alteration, ultimately causing toxicity. Indeed, Jackson and collaborators [39] reported that 11 consecutive nucleotides could lead to unspecific degradation of off-target mRNA. However, in a human context, the panel of potential targets may be different because of sequence dissimilarities between rodents and human, therefore the shSNP39 could be better tolerated. Unfortunately, we are unable to verify this hypothesis since none of our human neural stem cell lines are heterozygous for SNP39; treating with either shSNP39 would degrade the WT *HTT* allele, which would provoke transcriptomic changes [6]. Work in Aronin's lab suggests that placing the SNP exon 39 at p16 of the shRNA might be more favorable than at p10 to discriminate the two alleles [13]. We tested this *in vivo* and found no improvement in selectivity but, interestingly, the DARPP-32 lesion volume was significantly smaller indicating a better tolerance of this sequence. These experiments demonstrate that most of the shSNP can selectively reduce the expression of the disease-causing *HTT* allele without significantly inhibiting expression of the WT allele *in vitro* or *in vivo*. To assess silencing of the endogenous full-length *HTT* transcript, we injected the lentiviral vectors into the striatum of BACHD mice. BACHD mice have alleles which are present in most HD patients, whereas this is not the case for YAC128 [15]. SNP in exons 39 and 50 are in linkage disequilibrium with each other and with the CAG expansion, and there are no such associations for the SNPs in exon 60 and 67 [14]. RT-qPCR analysis confirmed that all shRNAs targeting the SNPs present in these animals led to efficient degradation of the full-length mutant human *HTT*. It is important to mention that the SNPs 67C/T were in their original context here (i.e. 3′UTR) whereas they were in the coding sequence in the lentiviral HD rat model. Anyhow, it didn't alter its ability to trigger RNA cleavage as showed by decreased levels of *HTT* mRNA in both models. Nevertheless, we can't exclude that part of this effect is mediated by translational repression or mRNA decay mediated by Ago1, 3 and 4 as previously demonstrated [40,41].

The clinical implementation of this type of strategy will require the genotyping of HD patients for the selected SNPs, and, to treat a large proportion of HD patients, the development of eight therapeutic products (shSNP). A growing number of pre-clinical and clinical trials have been launched to assess the use of RNAi for the treatment of autosomal dominant diseases [42]. Both exogenous oligonucleotides and shRNA produced by the target cells are being investigated. Chemically modified siRNAs and ASO have an excellent safety profile and half-life, but the issues of crossing the blood-brain barrier to reach target cells in deep brain areas and long-term administration in general still represent major challenges for these therapeutic agents. Intraventricular infusion allows broad diffusion throughout the brain, but the dose of oligonucleotides needed to achieve efficient silencing are very high and could lead to an oversaturation of the RNAi machinery at the level of the RISC complex [9,43]. An alternative route of entry into the CNS is intraparenchymal administration of appropriate

viral vectors. The design, production, and efficiency of gene transfer vectors, especially for transduction of the central nervous system (CNS), has improved remarkably, and protocols for safe transduction and long-term and robust transgene expression in the brain are now available [21,44-46]. These developments have led to the initiation of several phase I/II clinical trials with adeno-associated vectors (AAV) [47]; more recently trials have started with lentiviral vectors for the treatment of adrenoleukodystrophy [48] and Parkinson's disease [49]. The issue of the safety of shRNA (off target effects) and lentiviral vectors (genotoxicity profile) needs further evaluation. Nevertheless, our study and the rapidly accumulating data evidencing the potential value of this type of approach argue for continued efforts to develop clinical applications of these techniques.

Supporting Information

Figure S1 Correlation between *HTT* mRNA and protein levels in 293T transfected cells. (A) Levels of the chimeric HTT, represented by HA (representative pictures Figure 2B), were normalized to tubulin and are reported as mean percentages relative to the control condition (set at 100%) $\pm$ SEM (n = 3). One-way analyses of variance (ANOVA) were performed for each SNP. Newman-Keuls Post-hoc comparison was conducted between the control shRNA and matched shRNA (***p<0.001: 39A, 50C, 60A, 60G, 67C, 67T; **p<0.01: 50T) and between the matched shRNA and mismatched shRNA (***p<0.001: 39A, 60A, 67C, 67T; **p<0.05: 60G). **(B, C)** Distribution of *HTT* RT-qPCR and western blot data (n = 3) normalized on shUNIV results in 293T cells obtained with all match **(B)** or mismatch **(C)** shRNAs. Results demonstrate a high correlation between the *HTT* mRNA and proteins quantities independently of the exon targeted (for match shRNA: r = 0.63, p<0.01; for mismatch shRNAs: r = 0.66, p<0.001).

Figure S2 Number of Ubiquitin-positive aggregates is highly correlated to the number of HTT aggregates. (A) and **(B)** EM-48 immunostaining and quantification showing large numbers of aggregates in the control and mismatched injected areas and fewer aggregates in the matched conditions for the SNP 50C and 50T (same animals as in **Fig. 4**). The results are expressed as mean numbers of EM-48-positive aggregates $\pm$ SEM (n = 6–7). One-way ANOVAs were conducted for each SNP; 50C and 50T: ***P<0.001. Newman-Keuls Post-hoc comparison between control and matched conditions showed highly significant prevention of aggregates formation for the matched shSNPs. For mismatched conditions, the post-hoc test was not significant compared to control condition. Matched and mismatched conditions were significantly different for the 2 SNP studied (50C: ***p<0.001; 50T: **p<0.01). **(C)** Correlation between the numbers of Ubiquitin- and EM-48-positive aggregates quantified from the same animals. EM-48-positive aggregates are always more numerous but the number is highly correlated to the number of ubiquitin-positive aggregates (Bravais-Pearson correlation coefficient r = 0.93; p<0.001).

Figure S3 Efficacy and selectivity of the sh39A and sh39C with SNP in p10 or p16. (A) Quantitative real-time PCR analyses showing the silencing of *HTT* mRNA in transfected

293T cells co-expressing chimeric *HTT* and shSNP or the control shRNA. Levels of the chimeric *HTT* mRNA were normalized to a reference peptidyl propyl isomerase A (*PPIA*) and are expressed as mean percentages relative to the control condition (set at 100%) ± SEM (n = 3). One-way ANOVAs were performed for each SNP. Newman-Keuls Post-hoc comparison between the shCtrl and shSNP groups indicated significant efficacy for the two SNP in the two positions: sh39Ap10, sh39Ap16 (*P<0.05), sh39Cp10 and sh39Cp16 (**P<0.01). The mismatched sh39p16 conditions were significantly different from the control condition (sh39Ap16 (*P< 0.05) and sh39Cp16 (**P<0.01)). (**B**) and (**C**) Eight weeks post-injection, DARPP32 and ubiquitin immunoreactivity were used to quantify the lesion volume and the number of ubiquitin-positive aggregates after sh39p10 or sh39p16 co-injection with htt171-82-exon39. The results are expressed as means ± SEM (n = 8). One-way ANOVAs were conducted for each SNP (**P<0.01; ***P< 0.001). Newman-Keuls post-hoc comparison between control and matched shRNA groups concerning the size of the lesion showed significant efficacy for the shSNP only in position 16 (**B**). Regarding the number of aggregates (**C**), the four constructs were effective. However, for the mismatched conditions, the post-hoc test also revealed significant differences for both stainings revealing that these shSNP are not selective.

Table S1 Sequences of the primers used to generate fragments of *HTT* gene containing each SNP. The

sequences targeted by the shSNPs are in bold. The position of the SNP is in red.

Table S2 Sequences of the oligonucleotides used to generate the shRNA targeting the SNP and the controls. The sense and anti-sense strands of the shRNA are given in bold. The position of the SNP is in red.

Table S3 Sequences of the primers used for RT-qPCR.

Table S4 List of primer sequences used for SNP sequencing in NSC.

Materials and Methods S1

Acknowledgments

We would like to thank Martine Guillermier, Diane Houitte, Marion Chaigneau and Kévin Gorrichon for expert technical assistance.

Author Contributions

Conceived and designed the experiments: N. Déglon ALP PH FS. Performed the experiments: VD M. Ruiz DZ MF GA KC LT FBR RH JC SA NM M. Rey N. Dufour. Analyzed the data: VD M. Ruiz. Contributed to the writing of the manuscript: VD M. Ruiz N. Déglon.

References

1. Vonsattel JP, Myers RH, Stevens TJ, Ferrante RJ, Bird ED, et al. (1985) Neuropathological classification of Huntington's disease. J Neuropathol Exp Neurol 44: 559–577.
2. The, Huntington's disease collaborative research (1993) A novel gene containing a trinucleotide repeat that is expanded and unstable on Huntington's disease chromosome. Cell 72: 971–983.
3. DiFiglia M, Sapp E, Chase KO, Davies SW, Bates GP, et al. (1997) Aggregation of huntingtin in neuronal intranuclear inclusions and dystrophic neurites in brain. Science 277: 1990–1993.
4. Zhang Y, Friedlander RM (2011) Using non-coding small RNAs to develop therapies for Huntington's disease. Gene Ther 18: 1139–1149.
5. Drouet V, Perrin V, Hassig R, Dufour N, Auregan G, et al. (2009) Sustained effects of nonallele-specific Huntingtin silencing. Ann Neurol 65: 276–285.
6. Boudreau RL, McBride JL, Martins I, Shen S, Xing Y, et al. (2009) Nonallele-specific silencing of mutant and wild-type huntingtin demonstrates therapeutic efficacy in Huntington's disease mice. Mol Ther 17: 1053–1063.
7. Hu J, Liu J, Corey DR (2010) Allele-selective inhibition of huntingtin expression by switching to an miRNA-like RNAi mechanism. Chem Biol 17: 1183–1188.
8. Fiszer A, Mykowska A, Krzyzosiak WJ (2011) Inhibition of mutant huntingtin expression by RNA duplex targeting expanded CAG repeats. Nucleic Acids Res 39: 5578–5585.
9. Yu D, Pendergraff H, Liu J, Kordasiewicz HB, Cleveland DW, et al. (2012) Single-Stranded RNAs Use RNAi to Potently and Allele-Selectively Inhibit Mutant Huntingtin Expression. Cell 150: 895–908.
10. Miller VM, Xia H, Marrs GL, Gouvion CM, Lee G, et al. (2003) Allele-specific silencing of dominant disease genes. Proc Natl Acad Sci U S A 100: 7195–7200.
11. Alves S, Nascimento-Ferreira I, Auregan G, Hassig R, Dufour N, et al. (2008) Allele-specific RNA silencing of mutant ataxin-3 mediates neuroprotection in a rat model of Machado-Joseph disease. PLoS One 3: e3341.
12. Ostergaard ME, Southwell AL, Kordasiewicz H, Watt AT, Skotte NH, et al. (2013) Rational design of antisense oligonucleotides targeting single nucleotide polymorphisms for potent and allele selective suppression of mutant Huntingtin in the CNS. Nucleic Acids Res 41: 9634–9650.
13. Pfister EL, Kennington L, Straubhaar J, Wagh S, Liu W, et al. (2009) Five siRNAs targeting three SNPs may provide therapy for three-quarters of Huntington's disease patients. Curr Biol 19: 774–778.
14. Lombardi MS, Jaspers L, Spronkmans C, Gellera C, Taroni F, et al. (2009) A majority of Huntington's disease patients may be treatable by individualized allele-specific RNA interference. Exp Neurol 217: 312–319.
15. Carroll JB, Warby SC, Southwell AL, Doty CN, Greenlee S, et al. (2011) Potent and selective antisense oligonucleotides targeting single-nucleotide polymorphisms in the Huntington disease gene/allele-specific silencing of mutant huntingtin. Mol Ther 19: 2178–2185.
16. Warby SC, Montpetit A, Hayden AR, Carroll JB, Butland SL, et al. (2009) CAG expansion in the Huntington disease gene is associated with a specific and targetable predisposing haplogroup. Am J Hum Genet 84: 351–366.
17. Warby SC, Visscher H, Collins JA, Doty CN, Carter C, et al. (2011) HTT haplotypes contribute to differences in Huntington disease prevalence between Europe and East Asia. Eur J Hum Genet 19: 561–566.
18. Lee JM, Gillis T, Mysore JS, Ramos EM, Myers RH, et al. (2012) Common SNP-based haplotype analysis of the 4p16.3 Huntington disease gene region. Am J Hum Genet 90: 434–444.
19. Menalled LB (2005) Knock-in mouse models of Huntington's disease. NeuroRx 2: 465–470.
20. Bowles KR, Brooks SP, Dunnett SB, Jones L (2012) Gene expression and behaviour in mouse models of HD. Brain Res Bull 88: 276–284.
21. Lundberg C, Bjorklund T, Carlsson T, Jakobsson J, Hantraye P, et al. (2008) Applications of lentiviral vectors for biology and gene therapy of neurological disorders. Curr Gene Ther 8: 461–473.
22. Slow EJ, van Raamsdonk J, Rogers D, Coleman SH, Graham RK, et al. (2003) Selective striatal neuronal loss in a YAC128 mouse model of Huntington disease. Hum Mol Genet 12: 1555–1567.
23. Gray M, Shirasaki DI, Cepeda C, Andre VM, Wilburn B, et al. (2008) Full-length human mutant huntingtin with a stable polyglutamine repeat can elicit progressive and selective neuropathogenesis in BACHD mice. J Neurosci 28: 6182–6195.
24. Southwell AL, Warby SC, Carroll JB, Doty CN, Skotte NH, et al. (2013) A fully humanized transgenic mouse model of Huntington disease. Hum Mol Genet 22: 18–34.
25. Hottinger AF, Azzouz M, Deglon N, Aebischer P, Zurn AD (2000) Complete and long-term rescue of lesioned adult motoneurons by lentiviral-mediated expression of glial cell line-derived neurotrophic factor in the facial nucleus. J Neurosci 20: 5587–5593.
26. Feyeux M, Bourgois-Rocha F, Redfern A, Giles P, Lefort N, et al. (2012) Early transcriptional changes linked to naturally occurring Huntington's disease mutations in neural derivatives of human embryonic stem cells. Hum Mol Genet 21: 3883–3895.
27. Mateizel I, De Temmerman N, Ullmann U, Cauffman G, Sermon K, et al. (2006) Derivation of human embryonic stem cell lines from embryos obtained after IVF and after PGD for monogenic disorders. Hum Reprod 21: 503–511.
28. Bradley CK, Scott HA, Chami O, Peura TT, Dumevska B, et al. (2011) Derivation of Huntington's disease-affected human embryonic stem cell lines. Stem Cells Dev 20: 495–502.
29. Tropel P, Tournois J, Come J, Varela C, Moutou C, et al. (2010) High-efficiency derivation of human embryonic stem cell lines following pre-implantation genetic diagnosis. In vitro cellular & developmental biology Animal 46: 376–385.

30. Gauthier LR, Charrin BC, Borrell-Pages M, Dompierre JP, Rangone H, et al. (2004) Huntingtin controls neurotrophic support and survival of neurons by enhancing BDNF vesicular transport along microtubules. Cell 118: 127–138.

31. Elbashir SM, Harborth J, Lendeckel W, Yalcin A, Weber K, et al. (2001) Duplexes of 21-nucleotide RNAs mediate RNA interference in cultured mammalian cells. Nature 411: 494–498.

32. Kordasiewicz HB, Stanek LM, Wancewicz EV, Mazur C, McAlonis MM, et al. (2012) Sustained therapeutic reversal of Huntington's disease by transient repression of huntingtin synthesis. Neuron 74: 1031–1044.

33. van Bilsen PH, Jaspers L, Lombardi MS, Odekerken JC, Burright EN, et al. (2008) Identification and allele-specific silencing of the mutant huntingtin allele in Huntington's disease patient-derived fibroblasts. Hum Gene Ther 19: 710–719.

34. de Almeida LP, Ross CA, Zala D, Aebischer P, Deglon N (2002) Lentiviral-mediated delivery of mutant huntingtin in the striatum of rats induces a selective neuropathology modulated by polyglutamine repeat size, huntingtin expression levels, and protein length. J Neurosci 22: 3473–3483.

35. Naldini L, Blomer U, Gallay P, Ory D, Mulligan R, et al. (1996) In vivo gene delivery and stable transduction of nondividing cells by a lentiviral vector. Science 272: 263–267.

36. Deglon N, Tseng JL, Bensadoun JC, Zurn AD, Arsenijevic Y, et al. (2000) Self-inactivating lentiviral vectors with enhanced transgene expression as potential gene transfer system in Parkinson's disease. Hum Gene Ther 11: 179–190.

37. Pouladi MA, Stanek LM, Xie Y, Franciosi S, Southwell AL, et al. (2012) Marked differences in neurochemistry and aggregates despite similar behavioural and neuropathological features of Huntington disease in the full-length BACHD and YAC128 mice. Hum Mol Genet 21: 2219–2232.

38. Zala D, Colin E, Rangone H, Liot G, Humbert S, et al. (2008) Phosphorylation of mutant huntingtin at S421 restores anterograde and retrograde transport in neurons. Hum Mol Genet 17: 3837–3846.

39. Jackson AL, Bartz SR, Schelter J, Kobayashi SV, Burchard J, et al. (2003) Expression profiling reveals off-target gene regulation by RNAi. Nat Biotechnol 21: 635–637.

40. Wei N, Zhang L, Huang H, Chen Y, Zheng J, et al. (2012) siRNA has greatly elevated mismatch tolerance at 3'-UTR sites. PLoS ONE 7: e49309.

41. Wu L, Fan J, Belasco JG (2008) Importance of translation and nonnucleolytic ago proteins for on-target RNA interference. Current biology: CB 18: 1327–1332.

42. Davidson BL, McCray PB Jr. (2011) Current prospects for RNA interference-based therapies. Nat Rev Genet 12: 329–340.

43. Davidson BL, Monteys AM (2012) Singles engage the RNA interference pathway. Cell 150: 873–875.

44. Bowers WJ, Breakefield XO, Sena-Esteves M (2011) Genetic therapy for the nervous system. Hum Mol Genet 20: R28–41.

45. Taymans JM, Vandenberghe LH, Haute CV, Thiry I, Deroose CM, et al. (2007) Comparative analysis of adeno-associated viral vector serotypes 1, 2, 5, 7, and 8 in mouse brain. Hum Gene Ther 18: 195–206.

46. Mandel RJ, Manfredsson FP, Foust KD, Rising A, Reimsnider S, et al. (2006) Recombinant adeno-associated viral vectors as therapeutic agents to treat neurological disorders. Mol Ther 13: 463–483.

47. Mingozzi F, High KA (2011) Therapeutic in vivo gene transfer for genetic disease using AAV: progress and challenges. Nat Rev Genet 12: 341–355.

48. Cartier N, Hacein-Bey-Abina S, Bartholomae CC, Veres G, Schmidt M, et al. (2009) Hematopoietic stem cell gene therapy with a lentivector in X-linked adrenoleukodystrophy. Science 326: 818–823.

49. Palfi S, Gurruchaga JM, Ralph GS, Lepetit H, Lavisse S, et al. (2014) Long-term safety and tolerability of ProSavin, a lentiviral vector-based gene therapy for Parkinson's disease: a dose escalation, open-label, phase 1/2 trial. Lancet 383: 1138–46.

2

Huntingtin is Critical Both Pre- and Postsynaptically for Long-Term Learning-Related Synaptic Plasticity in *Aplysia*

Yun-Beom Choi[1,2], Beena M. Kadakkuzha[5], Xin-An Liu[5], Komolitdin Akhmedov[5], Eric R. Kandel[1,2,3,4]*, Sathyanarayanan V. Puthanveettil[5]*

1 Department of Neuroscience, College of Physicians and Surgeons of Columbia University, New York, New York, United States of America, 2 Department of Psychiatry, College of Physicians and Surgeons of Columbia University, New York, New York, United States of America, 3 Howard Hughes Medical Institute, College of Physicians and Surgeons of Columbia University, New York, New York, United States of America, 4 Kavli Institute for Brain Science, College of Physicians and Surgeons of Columbia University, New York, New York, United States of America, 5 Department of Neuroscience, The Scripps Research Institute, Scripps Florida, Jupiter, Florida, United States of America

Abstract

Patients with Huntington's disease exhibit memory and cognitive deficits many years before manifesting motor disturbances. Similarly, several studies have shown that deficits in long-term synaptic plasticity, a cellular basis of memory formation and storage, occur well before motor disturbances in the hippocampus of the transgenic mouse models of Huntington's disease. The autosomal dominant inheritance pattern of Huntington's disease suggests the importance of the mutant protein, huntingtin, in pathogenesis of Huntington's disease, but wild type huntingtin also has been shown to be important for neuronal functions such as axonal transport. Yet, the role of wild type huntingtin in long-term synaptic plasticity has not been investigated in detail. We identified a huntingtin homolog in the marine snail *Aplysia*, and find that similar to the expression pattern in mammalian brain, huntingtin is widely expressed in neurons and glial cells. Importantly the expression of mRNAs of huntingtin is upregulated by repeated applications of serotonin, a modulatory transmitter released during learning in *Aplysia*. Furthermore, we find that huntingtin expression levels are critical, not only in presynaptic sensory neurons, but also in the postsynaptic motor neurons for serotonin-induced long-term facilitation at the sensory-to-motor neuron synapse of the *Aplysia* gill-withdrawal reflex. These results suggest a key role for huntingtin in long-term memory storage.

Editor: Riccardo Mozzachiodi, Texas A&M University - Corpus Christi, United States of America

Funding: This work is supported by grants from the Howard Hughes Medical Institute (to E.R.K.), National Institutes of Health grant NS053415 (to Y.-B.C.) and Whitehall foundation grant and TSRI start up funds (to S.V.P.). The funders had no role in study design, data collection and analysis, decision to publish, or preparation of the manuscript.

Competing Interests: The authors have declared that no competing interests exist.

* Email: sputhanv@scripps.edu (SVP); erk5@columbia.edu (ERK)

Introduction

Huntington's disease (HD) is caused by a mutation that expands the number of trinucleotides CAG repeats in a gene leading to an expansion of polyglutamine stretch in huntingtin, the encoded protein (The Huntington's Disease Collaborative Research Group, 1993). HD is a neurodegenerative disorder characterized by involuntary movements, emotional disturbance, and cognitive impairment [1]. In HD, early cognitive deficits occur many years prior to overt motor deficits [2], a finding also observed in a transgenic mouse model of HD [3]. At the cellular level, synaptic dysfunction is noted many years before the neuronal cell loss characteristic of neurodegenerative diseases [4,5]. In various transgenic mouse models of HD, there is a deficit in forms of synaptic plasticity thought to contribute to learning and memory. Specifically, transgenic mice containing mutant huntingtin exhibit reduced long-term potentiation (LTP) as well as an abnormal development of NMDA-dependent long-term depression (LTD) in the hippocampus [6–9].

Because of the dominant inheritance pattern of HD, investigation of the pathogenesis of HD has been focused on the mutant huntingtin's gain-of-function. However, huntingtin is highly conserved from *Drosophila* to humans, suggesting that it likely has a central role in cell biological functions of the nervous system and there may be loss-of-function from the reduced wild type protein that also contributes to HD pathogenesis. Indeed, various experimental approaches have been used to investigate wild type huntingtin function and itss possible involvement in the pathogenesis of HD [10–12]. The findings suggesting the role of wild type huntingtin in the pathogenesis of HD include: (1) increased wild type huntingtin expression leads to improved brain cell-survival [13–15] and (2) a removal of the wild type huntingtin generates some of the phenotypes observed in the presence of mutant huntingtin such as neuronal cell death [16].

Huntingtin-knockout mice exhibit embryonic death before day 7.5 suggesting that huntingtin is essential for embryonic development [17–19]. In post-mitotic neurons, it has a scaffolding function and a possible role as a facilitator of signal transduction

[20]. Huntingtin interacts postsynaptically with N-methyl D-aspartate receptors (NMDARs) indirectly by binding to SH3 domain of PSD95, an adaptor protein in the postsynaptic density [21]. Huntingtin is also present presynaptically where it is associated with recycling endosomes, the endoplasmic reticulum, the Golgi complex, and clathrin-coated vesicles and synaptic vesicles [22–24]. Increased expression of wild type huntingtin caused an increased transcription of brain-derived neurotrophic factor (BDNF) in mice [25,26]. *In vitro*, wild type huntingtin stimulates BDNF vesicle trafficking in neuronal cells [27]. Neuronal deletions of *Drosophila* huntingtin using RNAi caused axonal blockage [28], which is characteristic of mutations not only in cytoskeletal motor proteins such as kinesin or dynein that are required for axonal transport, but also proteins that function as binding partners for motor proteins [29,30]. Huntingtin-associated protein-1 also interacts directly with kinesin light chain [31].

The roles of huntingtin in BDNF production and vesicular transport suggest that wild type huntingtin could be important for learning-related synaptic plasticity. However, despite the results showing dysfunction in LTP and LTD in the brains of transgenic mice expressing mutant huntingtin [6–9], the role of wild type huntingtin in long-term learning-related synaptic plasticity has not been studied in detail.

To explore the role of normal huntingtin in long-term learning-related synaptic plasticity, we turned to an elementary neural circuit that underlies a simple form of learned fear in *Aplysia*–sensitization of the gill-withdrawal reflex. Specifically, a critical component of the *Aplysia* gill-withdrawal reflex that contributes importantly to the behavior is a direct monosynaptic connection from the siphon sensory neurons to the gill motor neurons. The sensory-to-motor neuron synapse can be reconstituted in dissociated cell culture and is modulated, as in the intact animal, by serotonin (5-HT), a modulatory transmitter released during the learning of fear [32]. In the sensory-to-motor neuron synapses, one brief application of 5-HT produces short-term facilitation (STF) that lasts minutes, while five spaced applications of 5-HT to these synapses produce long-term facilitation (LTF) that lasts for days and results in growth of new synaptic connections [33,34]. These identified neurons are larger in size and form precise connections with one another facilitating the study of cell biology of huntingtin in specific cells and cellular compartments at high resolution and allowing selective manipulation of either the presynaptic sensory neuron or postsynaptic motor neuron [35]. Previously, *Aplysia* sensory-to-motor neuron synapse as a model system has been used to show that an overexpression of the mutant human huntingtin N-terminal fragment containing 150 glutamine residues tagged with enhanced green fluorescent protein (Nhtt150Q-EGFP) in sensory neurons inhibits 5-HT induced LTF [36].

In this study, we identified a homolog of huntingtin in *Aplysia*. We find that repeated applications of 5-HT upregulate huntingtin transcripts. Furthermore, knocking down huntingtin mRNAs, in either pre- or postsynaptic neurons abolish 5-HT-induced LTF at the sensory-to-motor neuron synapse, but it did not affect STF. Our findings suggest that huntingtin participates in both pre- and postsynaptic regulation of long-term synaptic plasticity that underlies long-term memory.

Results

Aplysia homolog of huntingtin (ApHTT)

Screening the *Aplysia* sequence base (www.aplysiagenetools.org) and the NCBI transcript data base yielded a transcript corresponding to a huntingtin homolog in *Aplysia californica* (accession number: XM_005093588.1). The predicted protein, the *Aplysia* homolog of huntingtin (ApHTT) is 2873 amino acids in length, slightly shorter than human huntingtin (3144 amino acids). Comparison of ApHTT with human huntingtin at the amino acid level reveals that ApHTT is 40% identical to human huntingtin (Figure 1). ApHTT does not have the N-terminal polyglutamine stretch, which is expanded in HD, but much shorter in lower vertebrate and absent in *Drosophila* as in *Aplysia* [37,38]. ApHTT, similar to *Drosophila* and lower vertebrates, also lacks the polyproline region that follows polyglutamine stretch in human or higher vertebrates. However, ApHTT has a high degree of sequence conservation in the first 17 amino acids–12 out of 17 amino acids are identical to human huntingtin – that determine sub-cellular localization and aggregation [39]. In addition, ApHTT has a high degree of sequence conservation in the region of HEAT (Huntingtin, elongation factor 3, regulatory A submit of protein phosphatase 2a and TOR1) repeats, which cluster in three domains in the N-terminal half of human huntingtin, and is thought to be involved in protein-protein interactions [40].

ApHTT is expressed in presynaptic and postsynaptic neurons in *Aplysia*

We first examined the distribution of ApHTT mRNAs in sensory-to-motor neuron co-cultures. Based on the ApHTT transcript sequence information, we sub-cloned a 400 base pair fragment and prepared digoxegenin (DIG) labeled antisense ribo-probes. These probes were used in the mRNA *in situ* hybridization experiment to visualize distribution of ApHTT mRNAs. Consistent with the findings on huntingtin distribution in mammalian brain, we find that ApHTT mRNA is ubiquitously expressed in *Aplysia* sensory neurons, motor neurons and in glial cells (Figure 2). ApHTT mRNA is mostly localized in the cell body cytosol of sensory and motor neurons.

ApHTT mRNAs are induced by repeated applications of 5-HT

Transcriptional changes in expression of specific genes are an important component of long-term memory in addition to changes in translation and axonal transport [41]. As a first step to understand the role of ApHTT in memory storage, we used specific primers in qRTPCR reactions to determine whether the transcript levels of ApHTT would change in response to repeated applications of 5-HT (five pulses of 10 µM). We isolated RNAs from pleural sensory neuron clusters at 0, 30, and 90 minutes after the completion of the 5-HT treatment and quantitated changes in ApHTT mRNA levels. We used expression changes in *Aplysia* CCAAT enhancer-binding protein (ApC/EBP) mRNA as a positive control [42]. As expected we found a robust increase in ApC/EBP transcript levels immediately after the 5-HT treatment, which declines gradually over 90 minutes. In contrast, there were no significant changes in ApHTT expression immediately or at 30 minutes after 5-HT treatment. However, there was a significant increase in ApHTT transcript levels at 90 minutes (Figure 3, fold changes: at 0 minute: ApC/EBP 7.10 ± 0.09, $p=0.0002$, $t=9.0156$, $df=6$; ApHTT 1.41 ± 0.07, $p=0.24$, $t=1.283$, $df=6$; at 30 minutes: ApC/EBP 3.80 ± 0.20, $p=0.0011$, $t=5.8932$, $df=6$; ApHTT 1.44 ± 0.09, $p=0.06$, $t=1.8266$, $df=8$; at 90 minutes: ApC/EBP 3.50 ± 0.26, $p=0.0028$, $t=3.5775$, $df=6$; ApHTT 1.81 ± 0.11, $p=0.01$, $t=3.5775$, $df=6$, Student's t test) suggesting that 5-HT induces a delayed expression of the ApHTT transcripts.

We next carried out RNA *in situ* hybridization experiments using ribo probes in sensory-to-motor neuron co-cultures to confirm qRTPCR findings and to examine whether the upregula-

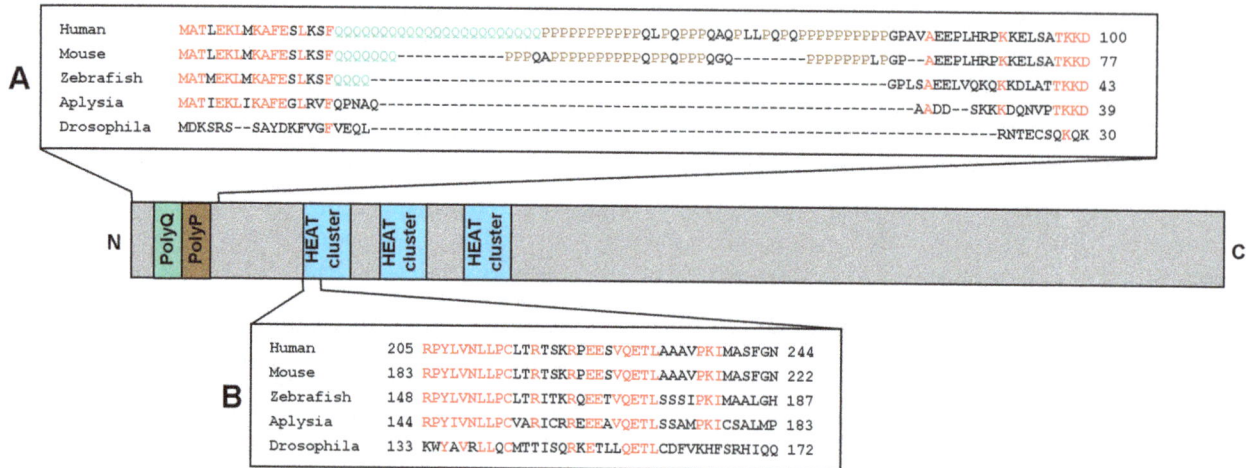

Figure 1. Sequence comparison between an *Aplysia* homolog of huntingtin (ApHTT) and huntingtin from other species. Comparison of the deduced amino acid sequences of ApHTT with huntingtins from other species at (A) the N-terminal end and (B) the first HEAT repeat region. Red letters denote identical amino acid residues. Sequences are from NCBI protein database. Human: NP_002102.4, Mouse: NP_034544.1, Zebrafish: NP_571093.1, *Aplysia*: XP_005093645.1, *Drosophila*: NP_651629.1. The domain structure of human huntingtin is shown as a reference. PolyQ: polyglutamine stretch, PolyP: polyproline region, HEAT cluster: clusters of HEAT repeats.

tion of ApHTT occurs only in sensory neurons or both in sensory neurons and in motor neurons. The possibility that 5×5-HT regulated ApHTT in both pre- and post synaptic neurons will further inform us about function of huntingtin in neural circuits. We find that ApHTT mRNA expression is induced both in the cell body and neurites of sensory neurons and motor neurons at 90 minutes after 5-HT treatment (Figure 4, % change when compared to control: Soma, motor neuron: 482.42±7.13%, t = 8.9364, df = 5, p = 0.0004; neurites, motor neuron: 626.95%±5.41% t = 14.0046, df = 6, p = 0.001; soma, sensory neuron: 365.42%±4.00%, t = 12.3577, df = 6; neurites, sensory neuron: 174.30±12.49%, t = 3.8020, df = 6, p = 0.0001 for both soma and neurites, N = 4 for all except for soma of control motor neuron where N = 3).

Injection of ApHTT anti-sense oligonucleotides into the presynaptic sensory neuron does not affect STF

We next turned to study role of ApHTT in learning-related synaptic plasticity. We used antisense oligonucleotides to knock down ApHTT transcripts in sensory-to-motor neuron cultures in which two sensory neurons make functional synaptic connections to one L7 motor neuron. For all the studies, we injected phosphothio-modified antisense oligonucleotides into one sensory neuron and the other sensory neuron received control oligonucleotides (sense oligonucleotides) or untreated. Microinjection of ApHTT antisense oligonucleotides (50 ng/μl) in presynaptic sensory neurons resulted in a 25±4% (Student's t test, p<0.01, n = 8) reduction in ApHTT mRNA level compared to the uninjected controls when cultures were fixed at 3 hours after the injections (Figure 5A). Sense oligonucleotides (50 ng/μl) injected

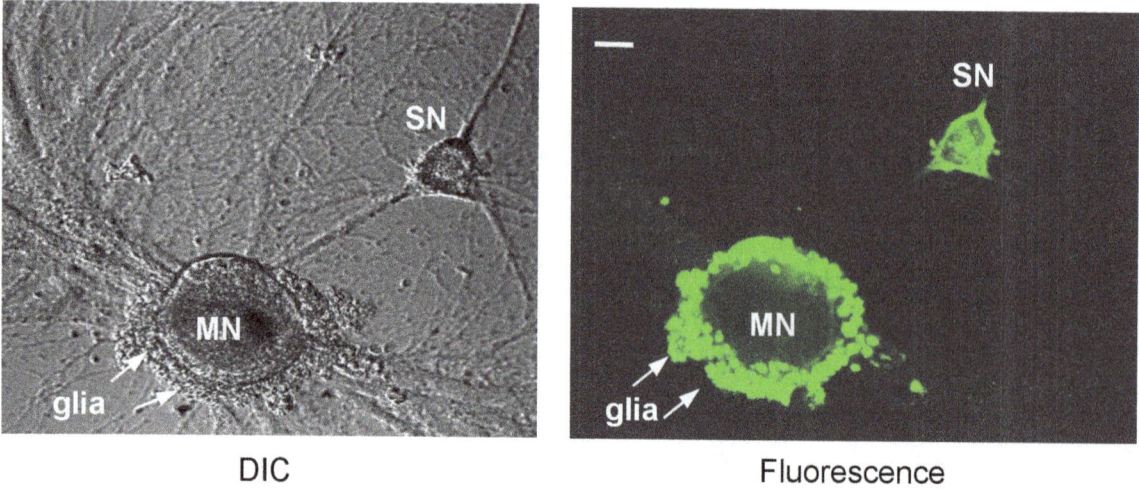

Figure 2. ApHTT mRNAs are expressed in *Aplysia* neurons. mRNA *in situ* analysis shows that ApHTT mRNAs are expression in *Aplysia* sensory neurons, motor neurons, and glial cells. Fluorescently labeled ribo probes were used to examine the distribution of ApHTT mRNAs. Confocal projection image is shown. The scale bar represents 20 μm.

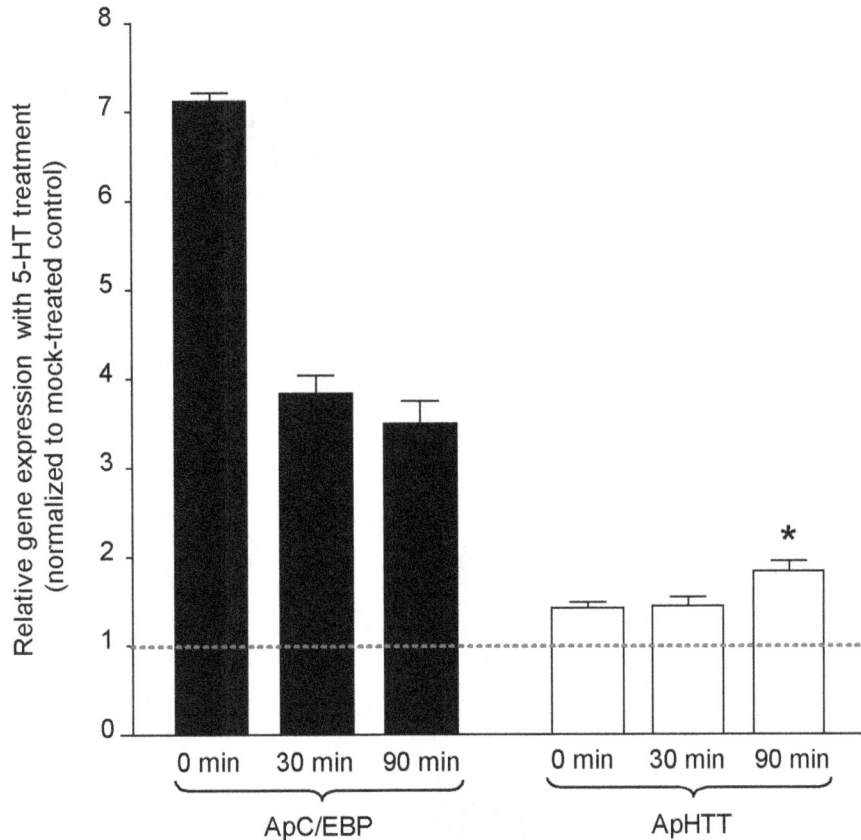

Figure 3. ApHTT mRNAs are induced by 5-HT. RNAs were isolated from pleural sensory neuron clusters at 0, 30 and 90 minutes after the end of five pulses of 5-HT treatment. qRTPCR analysis of RNA is shown in bar graphs. Data was first normalized to 18S rRNA levels. Each bar corresponds to gene expression ratio (5×5-HT treated/mock treated controls). ApC/EBP was used as a positive control. Error bars are SEM.

into the other sensory neuron in the co-culture as a control did not decrease the level of ApHTT mRNA.

Having established that antisense oligonucleotides are able to knock down ApHTT mRNA levels in sensory neurons, we examined whether the down regulation of ApHTT mRNA by antisense oligonucleotides in the presynaptic sensory neurons affects basal synaptic transmission in the sensory-motor neuron synapse by measuring excitatory postsynaptic potentials (EPSPs) at 24 hours after oligonucleotides injection (50 ng/µl) to the presynaptic sensory neurons. (Figure 5D; % change in EPSP amplitude: no injection -10.0 ± 6.0, n = 7; antisense oligo alone -3.4 ± 9.6, n = 7; sense oligo alone -10.2 ± 5.7, n = 8). One-way ANOVA (F = 0.28, p = 0.76, df = 21) revealed that a 25% reduction in ApHTT mRNA levels does not affect basal synaptic transmission.

We next studied the effect of ApHTT knock down on STF. At 3 hours after injection of the oligonucleotides into presynaptic sensory neurons, we treated cultures with one pulse of 5-HT (10 µM) for five minutes to induce STF. We measured the EPSPs again at 5 minutes after the 5-HT treatment (Figure 5B and C; % change in EPSP amplitude: no injection -13.2 ± 5.9, n = 8; antisense oligo alone -8.1 ± 4.9, n = 13; sense oligo alone -8.7 ± 5.1, n = 11; 5-HT 90.7 ± 17.8, n = 10; 5-HT + antisense 96.6 ± 20.0, n = 12; 5-HT + sense 95.8 ± 25.7, n = 9). One-way ANOVA revealed there were no significant differences among different 5-HT treated groups (F = 0.023, p = 0.98, df = 30). Thus, injection of the antisense oligonucleotides to ApHTT into the presynaptic sensory neuron did not block STF.

Injection of ApHTT anti-sense oligonucleotides into the presynaptic sensory neuron blocks LTF

We next evaluated the possible presynaptic role of ApHTT in LTF. At 3 hours after initial measurements of EPSPs and injection of the antisense oligonucleotides to ApHTT in the presynaptic sensory neuron, we treated cultures with five repeated pulses of 5-HT (10 µM, 5 minutes) and measured EPSPs again at 24 hours after 5-HT treatment. The injection of the antisense oligonucleotides to ApHTT into presynaptic sensory neurons led to a significant reduction of LTF at 24 hours, but the injection of sense oligonucleotides did not have any significant effect on LTF (Figure 5B and D; % change in EPSP amplitude: 5-HT 80.5 ± 20.8, n = 19; 5-HT + antisense 29.7 ± 6.5, n = 22, 5-HT + sense 85.7 ± 12.8, n = 19, one-way ANOVA: F = 5.10, p = 0.0092, df = 59, followed by Tukey HSD post-hoc test: p<0.05 for 5-HT versus 5-HT + antisense, no significance for 5-HT versus 5-HT + sense). These results, showing that depletion of ApHTT in the presynaptic sensory neuron blocks LTF, support the notion that ApHTT is an important regulatory component of long-term memory storage.

Injection of ApHTT anti-sense oligonucleotides into the postsynaptic motor neuron does not affect STF

We next examined the role of ApHTT in postsynaptic motor neurons as ApHTT mRNA is present in motor neurons as seen in Figure 2. We first tested whether knockdown of ApHTT mRNAs has any effect on STF. At 3 hours after oligonucleotides injections into the postsynaptic motor neurons, we measured basal EPSPs,

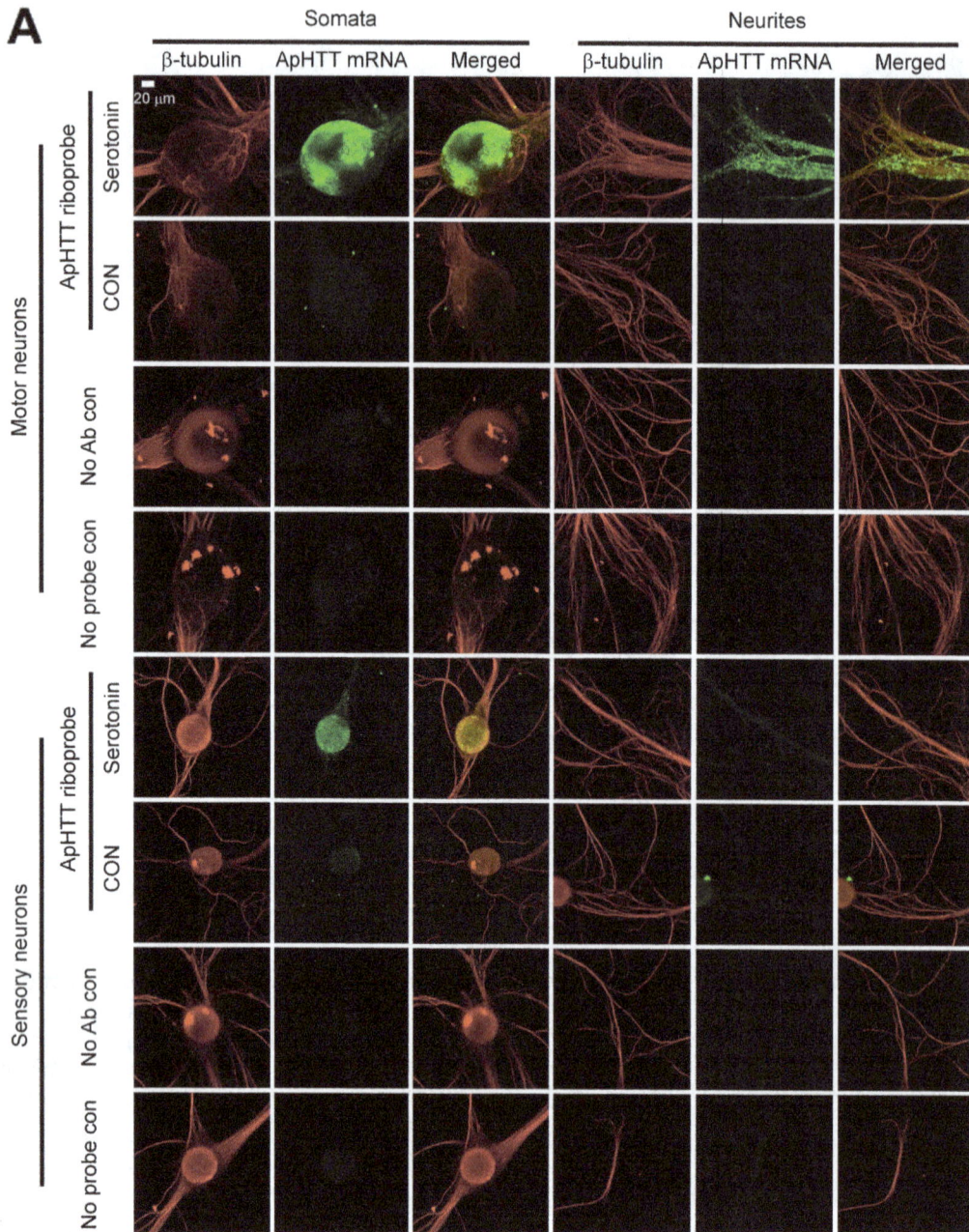

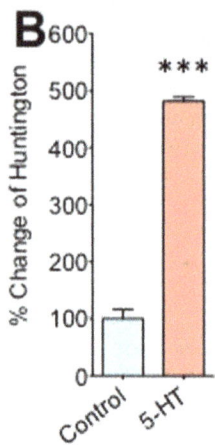

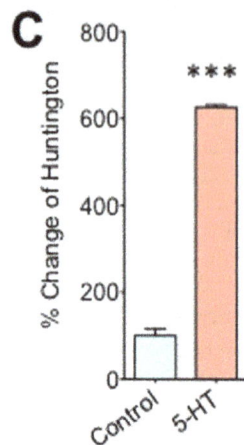

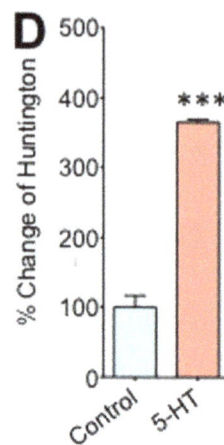

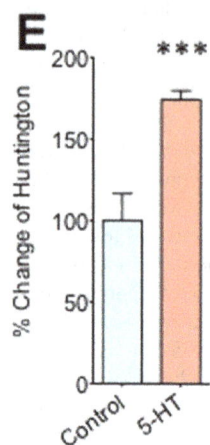

Motor neuron-Cell body   Motor neuron-Neurite   Sensory neuron-Cell body   Sensory neuron-Neurite

Figure 4. ApHTT mRNAs are induced both in presynaptic sensory neurons and in postsynaptic motor neurons by 5-HT. *Aplysia* sensory-to-motor neuron co-cultures were treated with 5×5-HT (10 μM, 5 minutes) and RNA *in situ* hyrbridization was carried out using riboprobes. A: Confocal projection images showing cell bodies and neurites of sensory neurons and motor neurons. Tubulin protein immunostaining was used visualizing major axon and neurites. No antibody (anti-DIG antibody) and no probe were used as controls for *in situ* hybridization. B, C, D and E: Quantitation of imaging data. % change in fluorescence compared to back ground are shown in bar graphs. Data was normalized to mock treated controls. Error bars are SEM.

then treated cultures with one pulse of 5-HT (10 μM) for five minutes, and again EPSPs were measured at 5 minutes after the 5-HT treatment (Figure 6A and B; % change in EPSP amplitude: no injection 0.8±9.0, n=6; antisense oligo alone −0.7±11.4, n=7; sense oligo alone −4.4±10.6, n=6; 5-HT 112.1±26.2, n=10; 5-HT + antisense 103.7±16.2, n=11; 5-HT + sense 129.0±26.6, n=9). One way ANOVA revealed there were no significant differences among different 5-HT treated groups (F=0.31, p=0.74, df=29). Thus, the injection of antisense oligonucleotides into postsynaptic motor neurons did not affect STF.

Injection of ApHTT anti-sense oligonucleotides into the postsynaptic motor neuron blocks LTF

Next, we examined whether ApHTT also plays a role in long-term synaptic plasticity in the postsynaptic neurons. At 3 hours after initial measurements of EPSPs and injection of the antisense oligonucleotides to ApHTT (50 ng/μl) in the postsynaptic motor neuron, we treated cultures with five pulses of 5-HT (10 μM) and measured EPSPs again at 24 hours after 5-HT treatment. Similar to our results in presynaptic sensory neurons, we find that basal synaptic transmission was not affected by the antisense oligonucleotides injections that knock down ApHTT mRNAs (Figure 6A

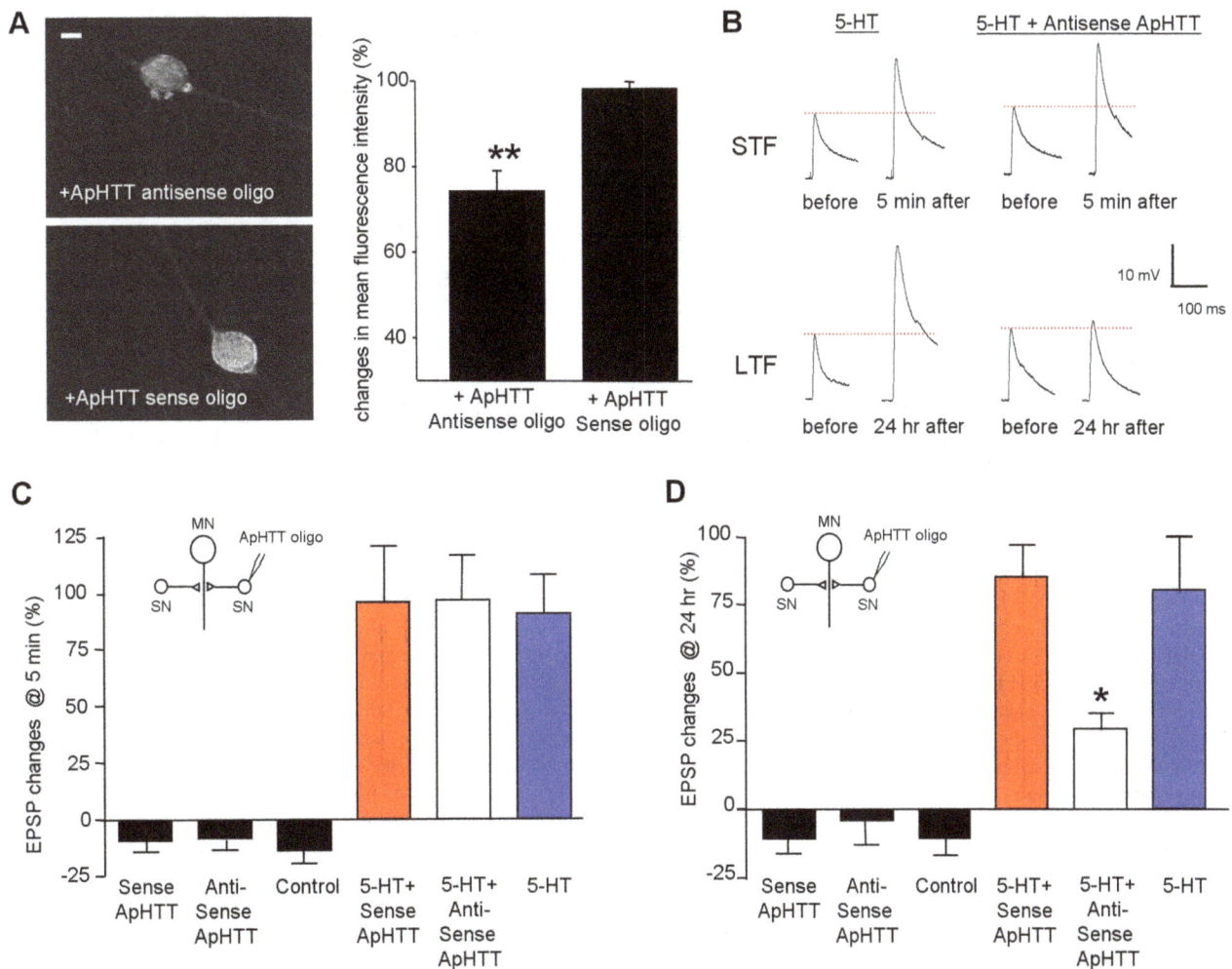

Figure 5. ApHTT in presynaptic sensory neurons is required for the initiation of LTF. A: RNA *in situ* hybridization at 3 hours after oligonucleotides injection. Injection of ApHTT anti-sense oligonucleotides into the presynaptic sensory neuron lead to a decrease in ApHTT mRNA level. Confocal projection images are shown. The scale bar represents 20 μm. The summary bar graph is on the right (N=8). B: Representative traces of EPSPs that were recorded from motor neurons in response to extracellular stimulation of sensory neurons before and 5 minutes after exposure to 1×5-HT (10 μM, 5 minutes) for STF or before and 24 hours after exposure to 5×5-HT (10 μM, 5 minutes) for LTF. C: Injection of ApHTT anti-sense oligonucleotides in the presynaptic sensory neuron has no effect on STF. D: Injection of ApHTT anti-sense oligonucleotides blocks LTF. Changes in EPSP amplitudes are shown in bar graphs. Error bars are SEM. SN: sensory neuron, MN: Motor neuron.

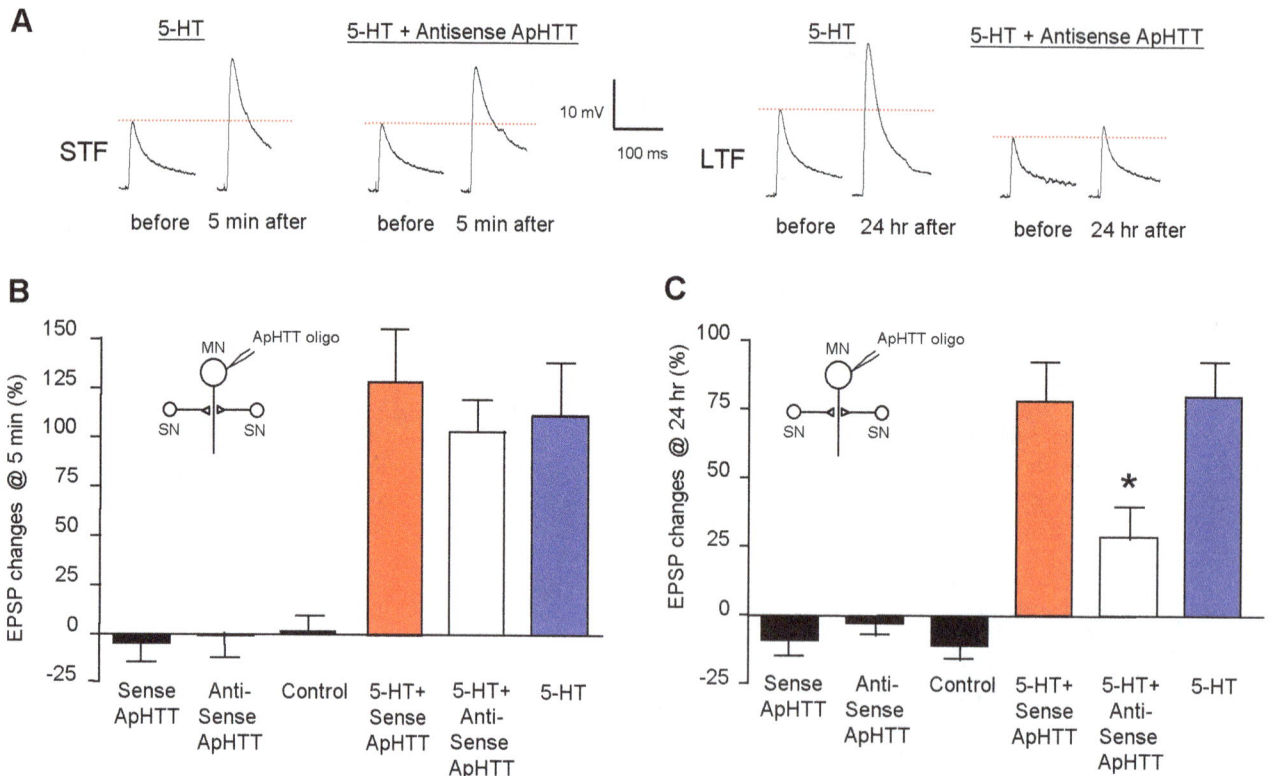

Figure 6. ApHTT in the postsynaptic motor neurons is required for the initiation of LTF. A: Representative traces of EPSPs that were recorded from motor neurons in response to extracellular stimulation of sensory neurons before and 5 minutes after exposure to 1×5-HT (10 μM, 5 minutes) for STF or before and 24 hours after exposure to 5×5-HT (10 μM, 5 minutes) for LTF. B: Injection of ApHTT anti-sense oligonucleotides in the postsynaptic motor neuron has no effect on STF. C: Injection of ApHTT anti-sense oligonucleotides blocks LTF. Changes in EPSP amplitudes are shown in bar graphs. Error bars are SEM. SN: sensory neuron, MN: Motor neuron.

and C; % change in EPSP amplitude: no injection -10.7 ± 4.9, n = 8; antisense oligo alone -2.8 ± 4.0, n = 9; sense oligo alone -8.9 ± 5.8, n = 8, one way ANOVA: F = 0.73, p = 0.49, df = 24). In contrast, injection of the antisense oligonucleotides to ApHTT leads to a significant reduction of LTF at 24 hours, but the injection of sense oligonucleotides did not have any significant effect on LTF (Figure 6A and C; % change in EPSP amplitude: 5-HT 80.1 ± 13.1, n = 15; 5-HT + sense 77.9 ± 14.8, n = 17; 5-HT + antisense 28.7 ± 11.7, n = 13, one way ANOVA: F = 4.22, p = 0.022, df = 44, followed by Tukey HSD post-hoc test, : p< 0.05 for 5-HT versus 5-HT + antisense, no significance for 5-HT versus 5-HT + sense). Taken together, these results show that the depletion of ApHTT in the postsynaptic motor neurons blocks the establishment of LTF whereas STF was unaffected by antisense oligonucleotides injections.

Discussion

Animal models such as *Drosophila* [43] zebrafish [44] and rodents [45] have been useful in obtaining important insights into HD. For example, mouse models of HD that express full-length human, or full-length mouse mutant huntingtin have been studied [46]. However, very few studies have examined regional- or temporal-specific knockdown of huntingtin or overexpression of mutant huntingtin. A study found that a knockdown of huntingtin expression using shRNAs in neuroepithelial cells of neocortex led to disturbed cell migration, reduced proliferation, and increased cell death in ways that are relatively specific to early neural development [47]. Interestingly, this study also found that

huntingtin knockdown results in cell death but not perturbed migration in the cerebellum, suggesting region-specific functions of huntingtin. In another study, reducing huntingtin mRNA levels transiently in a mouse model of HD using specific antisense oligonucleotides has reversed disease phenotypes such as cell death [48]. Even in these studies where a temporal control of knockdown is achieved, different neuronal populations including interneurons as well as non-neuronal cells such as glia are manipulated at the same time. Moreover, none of these earlier studies examined the selective role of huntingtin in pre- and postsynaptic compartments. As a result, we chose to study the sensory-to-motor neuron synapse of the *Aplysia* gill-withdrawal reflex reconstituted in culture in order to examine the function of normal huntingtin in memory storage. In *Aplysia*, selective manipulation of the presynaptic sensory neurons and postsynaptic motor neurons is readily manageable and addressing this issue seemed important because long-term memory storage is associated with specific and coordinated pre- and postsynaptic changes [35].

As the first step in investigating the role of huntingtin at the sensory-to-motor neuron synapse of *Aplysia* gill-withdrawal reflex, we identified the *Aplysia* homolog of huntingtin from the database. In wild type human huntingtin, the length of the N-terminal polyglutamine stretch is on average 18 amino acids and when the expansion of the polyglutamine stretch reaches to be greater than 37, it causes HD (The Huntington's Disease Collaborative Research Group, 1993). However, in mice huntingtin has seven glutamines, zebrafish huntingtin has only four glutamines, and *Drosophila* huntingtin has no glutamine stretch. Similar to *Drosophila* huntingtin, ApHTT does not have a polyglutamine stretch nor adjacent polyproline region. Thus, the polyglutamine stretch may not be required for the normal biological function of huntingtin [37]. Importantly ApHTT has high conservation in the region corresponding to the region of HEAT repeats clusters in the N-terminal of human huntingtin. Since HEAT repeats are important for normal huntingtin functions including cellular transport by mediating protein-protein interactions [40], ApHTT may have similar protein interacting partners as human huntingtin. In addition, consistent with data from huntingtin expression in other animals such as mouse and zebrafish, ApHTT mRNAs are ubiquitously expressed in presynaptic sensory neurons, postsynaptic motor neurons and glial cells.

During memory storage in *Aplysia,* transcription of several genes are upregulated in response to 5-HT exposure (Puthanveettil and Kandel, 2011). Most of the known genes that are transcriptionally upregulated by 5-HT are immediate early genes and the upregulation occurs within one hour of repeated 5-HT exposure. These genes include ApC/EBP [42], *Aplysia* kinesin heavy chain 1 (ApKHC1) and *Aplysia* kinesin light chain 2 (ApKLC2) [41]. Very few genes that are upregulated late in response to 5-HT treatment are known. For example, *Aplysia* eukaryotic translation elongation factor 1 alpha Ap (ApEF1 alpha) is upregulated by 4–6 hrs after 5-HT treatment [49]. Our qRTPCR data showed that there were no significant changes in ApHTT transcript levels immediately or at 30 minutes after 5-HT treatment. However, at 90 minutes after 5-HT treatment, we find significant upregulation of ApHTT. These results suggests that ApHTT mRNA levels are transcriptionally regulated as a late gene when compared to ApC/EBP and ApKHC1 during long-term memory storage. Furthermore our *in situ* hybridization analysis suggested that the transcriptional upregulation occurs both in presynaptic sensory neurons as well as postsynaptic motor neurons. This upregulation in both components of the the circuitry suggested a potential role in mediating long-term synaptic plasticity and memory storage.

To understand the role of ApHTT in long-term memory storage, we knocked down ApHTT mRNAs using specific phosphothio-modified antisense oligonucleotides. Injection of antisense oligonucleotides in either pre- or postsynaptic neurons inhibited LTF induced by 5 pulses of 5-HT without affecting basal synaptic transmission or STF. Interestingly, this phenotype is similar to what we observed previously that ApKHC1 knockdown in either pre- or postsynaptic neurons did not affect STF, but blocked the initiation of LTF [41]. Based on these results, we previously suggested that kinesin transport in the postsynatic motor neuron is important for the initiation of LTF and associated synaptic growth in both pre- and postsynaptic compartments and that these may be regulated by coordinated transynaptic signaling between the two compartments. In support of this idea, we have shown previously that transynaptic interaction of postsynaptic neuroligin with presynaptic neurexin is important for initiation of LTF and associated growth of new synaptic connection in the sensory-to-motor neuron synapse of the *Aplysia* gill-withdrawal reflex [50]. Both neurexin and neuroligins are protein cargos transported by ApKHC1 [41]. Since huntingtin may play a role in cellular trasnport [27] [28], hungtingtin along with kinesin motor may mediate one of critical pre and postsynpatic steps for the initiation of LTF.

Another possible mechanism that can explain the observed electrophysiological phenotype is the proposed role of huntingtin in BDNF production. Overexpression of wild type huntingtin increases BDNF protein levels *in vitro* and *in vivo* by regulating the BDNF gene transcription [25,26]. Moreover, huntingtin knockdown in zebrafish by antisense oligonucleotides leads to a reduction of BDNF expression [51]. Neurotrophins in general and

BDNF in particular, have important roles in neuronal survival and synaptic plasticity [52]. Indeed, BDNF has been shown to reverse LTP deficit in knock-in mouse model of HD [6]. We recently showed a neurotrophin and its receptor Trk (ApNT and ApTrk) are present in *Aplysia* and they are important for 5-HT induced LTF [53]. Huntingtin could also be involved in transcriptional regulation of genes other than BDNF important for long-term synaptic plasticity since it also interacts with transcription factors such as cAMP response-element binding protein (CREB)-binding protein (CBP) [54]. Knockdown of huntingtin may disrupt the transcription apparatus required for long-term synaptic plasticity.

Previously, an overexpression of the mutant human huntingtin N-terminal fragment containing 150 glutamine residues tagged with enhanced green fluorescent protein (Nhtt150Q-EGFP) in sensory neurons of the *Aplysia* sensory-to-neuron synapse impaired LTF indueced by repeated pulses of 5-HT without affecting basal synaptic transimssion or STF [36]. The same electrophysiological phenytypes observerd in our study using the knockdown of the ApHTT further support the idea that both the gain-of-function from the mutant huntington and the loss-of-function from the reduction of wild type huntingting may play a role in congnitive deficit in patients with HD.

One major limitation of our study is that we were not able to characterize endogenous ApHTT because of a lack of antibodies against ApHTT. Adlhough the half-life of ApHTT protein is not known, given the robust electrophysiooglical phyenotyes we observed with antisense oligonucleotide injections, we have made the assumption that a 25% decrease in mRNA at 3 hours post injection would be expected to reduce protein levels. Certainly, further investigations including generation of antibody against ApHTT are needed to delineate the full cadre of molecular mechanisms of ApHTT's role in long-term synaptic plasticity including the aforementioned possibilities. In conclusion, we find that ApHTT is induced following 5 pulses of 5-HT treatment that leads to LTF, a cellular correlate of behavioral sensitization of the *Aplysia* gill-withdrawal reflex and that learning-related regulation of mRNA levels of ApHTT in both presynaptic sensory neurons and postsynaptic motor neurons is important for long-term memory storage.

Materials and Methods

Ethics statement

The Institutional Biosafety Committee of The Scripps Research Institute (TSRI) has approved all of the experimental protocols (IBC Protocol 2010-019R1) described in this manuscript. There are no ethical approvals required for the research using invertebrate animals, such as the marine snail *Aplysia*. We have discussed the details of the experiments with the Institutional Animal Care and Use Committee of TSRI and Columbia University Medical Center, and every effort was made to lessen any distress of *Aplysia*.

mRNA *in situ* hybridization and imaging

A 400 base pair fragment from the start site of the ApHTT ORF was cloned into the EcoRI/XhoI site of the PCR TOPO II vector, linearized with EcoR1 and transcribed with T7 RNA polymerase (Roche, Basel, Switzerland) in the presence of digoxigenin (DIG) RNA labeling mix following the manufacturer's instructions to make an ApHTT antisense probe. For the sense probe, ApHTT-PCR TOPO II was linearized with Xho I and transcribed with SP6 RNA polymerase. After DNAse I treatment, the sense and antisense probes were used for *in situ* hybridization. A small aliquot (2 μl) was run on 1.5% agarose gel to confirm the integrity of RNA probes. About 1 ng of labeled RNA per μl of hybridization solution was used per culture dish. Sensory-to-motor neuron co-cultures were washed with artificial seawater and fixed for 10 minutes at room temperature with 2 ml of 4% paraformaldehyde in artificial seawater and washed three times in PBS. The *in situ* hybridization was followed as described in Giustetto et al (2003). After hybridization the sense and antisense RNAs were visualized using a Fluorescent Antibody Enhancer kit (Roche, Basel, Switzerland) for DIG detection. Images were acquired using a Zeiss LSM 780 confocal microscope system with 10X/63X objective. Mean fluorescence intensities were measured using NIH IMAGE J and corresponding background signal was subtracted from each mean fluorescence intensities. For the neurite analyses, we randomly selected regions that are minimum of 100 μm away from the initial segment. Percentage change of fluorescence intensity between the control and 5-HT treated neurons were calculated. In all the figures, only projection images are shown.

Gene expression analysis

Following five pulses of 5-HT treatment (0 minute, 30 minutes and 90 minutes after 5-HT treatment), total RNA was isolated from sensory neuron clusters of *Aplysia* pleural ganglia using the Trizol-chloroform method. The RNA pellet was resuspended in nuclease-free water. RNA concentration and quality was measured using Nanodrop (Thermo Scientific, Waltham, MA). cDNA was generated by reverse transcription from 1 μg of RNA using Quanta cDNA supermix (Quanta Biosciences) according to the manufacturer's instructions. All qRTPCR primers were synthesized by Integrated DNA technologies. The following primers were used for ApHTT: Ap-Htt-F2 5′-TGGACACTCAGAC-CACCAGT-3′ and Ap-Htt-R2 5′-CTCTAATAACGCTG-CACGGA-3′; for ApC/EBP: ApC/EBP-F1 5′-AGTAT-CATCCTGTGCCCTCACT-3′ and ApC/EBP-R1 5′-CTGCCTGTGGATGAAACTGTAG-3′; and for 18S rRNA control: Ap18S-F 5′-GTTCACTGCCCGTATCTCCT-3′ and Ap18S-R 5′-AGGCCTGCTTTGAACACTCT-3′. The expressions of ApHTT were first studied by qRTPCR with Power using SYBR green PCR master mix (Applied Biosystems Carlsbad, CA) and then used for the quantification of transcripts. All of the qRTPCR amplifications were performed in a total volume of 10 μl containing 2 μl of H_2O, 2 μl of cDNA, 5 μl of 2X Master Mix, 1.0 μl each of forward and reverse primers (10 μM) designed based on the ApHTT sequence available at NCBI (http://www.ncbi.nlm.nih.gov/). The qRTPCR reaction was carried out in a 7900 HT Fast Real-Time PCR System (Applied Biosystems) under the following conditions: 95°C for 10 minutes, followed by 40 cycles of 95°C for 15 seconds, 60°C for 1 minutes. Quantification of the target transcripts was normalized to the *Aplysia* 18S rRNA reference gene.

Microinjection of oligonucleotides to *Aplysia* neurons

Oligonucleotides were synthesized by Integrated DNA Technologies and were gel purified. The following oligonucleotides were used: ApHTT antisense: 5′ g*c*g* tct tca tct cct aaa a*g*a* g 3′, ApHTT sense: 5′ c*t*c* ttt tag gag atg aag a*c*g* c 3′. Both antisense and sense oligonucleotides were phosphothio-modified (indicated by "*" sign) to enhance their stability in the cell. We dissolved oligonucleotides (50 ng/μl) in a buffer containing 0.1% fast green, 10 mM Tris-Cl (pH 7.3), and 250 mM KCl. They were injected under visual guidance into the cytoplasm of *Aplysia* neurons by applying positive air pressure through a picospritzer.

Electrophysiological assessment of LTF and STF in sensory-to-motor neuron co-cultures

We prepared *Aplysia* sensory-to-motor neuron co-cultures and measured excitatory postsynaptic potentials (EPSPs) as previously described [33]. We evoked the EPSP in L7 motor neuron by stimulating the sensory neuron with a brief depolarizing stimulus using an extracellular electrode. The motor neuron was held at a potential of −30 mV below its resting potential to prevent eliciting action potentials. The synapses with initial EPSPs less than 4 mV were not used for analysis. To induce LTF, we treated cultures with five 5 minutes pulses of 5-HT (10 μM) at 20 minutes intervals. Then, the cultures were maintained at 18°C and the EPSPs were again measured at 24 hours after the initial EPSP measurement. To induce STF, we treated cultures with one 5 minutes pulse of 5-HT (10 μM) after the initial EPSP measurement. EPSP was measured again at 5 minutes after 5-HT treatment.

Statistical Analysis

Results are denoted as means ± SEM. We used a paired or unpaired Student's t test to determine statistical significance between two data sets, and one-way ANOVA followed by Tukey HSD post-hoc test to determine statistical significance for multiple comparisons using Graphpad Prism. The statistical significance was indicated by $*p<0.05$, $**p<0.01$, or $***p<0.001$.

Acknowledgments

We thank Huixiang "Vivian" Zhu and Edward Konstantinov for *Aplysia* culture preparation and Alexandra Kaye for help with standardization of the qRTPCR to quantify huntingtin expression. Craig H. Bailey provided critical reading and suggestions.

Author Contributions

Conceived and designed the experiments: SVP YBC ERK. Analyzed the data: YBC SVP. Contributed reagents/materials/analysis tools: SVP YBC BMK. Wrote the paper: YBC SVP ERK. Carried out all the electrophysiology experiments: YBC. Carried out 5-HT treatments and qRTPCRs: SVP BMK KA. Carried out in situ hybridization and imaging analyses: BMK XAL.

References

1. Ross CA, Tabrizi SJ (2011) Huntington's disease: from molecular pathogenesis to clinical treatment. Lancet neurology 10: 83–98.
2. Paulsen JS (2011) Cognitive impairment in Huntington disease: diagnosis and treatment. Current neurology and neuroscience reports 11: 474–483.
3. Giralt A, Puigdellivol M, Carreton O, Paoletti P, Valero J, et al. (2012) Long-term memory deficits in Huntington's disease are associated with reduced CBP histone acetylase activity. Human molecular genetics 21: 1203–1216.
4. Orth M, European Huntington's Disease N, Handley OJ, Schwenke C, Dunnett S, et al. (2011) Observing Huntington's disease: the European Huntington's Disease Network's REGISTRY. Journal of neurology, neurosurgery, and psychiatry 82: 1409–1412.

5. Schippling S, Schneider SA, Bhatia KP, Munchau A, Rothwell JC, et al. (2009) Abnormal motor cortex excitability in preclinical and very early Huntington's disease. Biological psychiatry 65: 959–965.
6. Lynch G, Kramar EA, Rex CS, Jia Y, Chappas D, et al. (2007) Brain-derived neurotrophic factor restores synaptic plasticity in a knock-in mouse model of Huntington's disease. The Journal of neuroscience: the official journal of the Society for Neuroscience 27: 4424–4434.
7. Murphy KP, Carter RJ, Lione LA, Mangiarini L, Mahal A, et al. (2000) Abnormal synaptic plasticity and impaired spatial cognition in mice transgenic for exon 1 of the human Huntington's disease mutation. The Journal of neuroscience: the official journal of the Society for Neuroscience 20: 5115–5123.

8. Usdin MT, Shelbourne PF, Myers RM, Madison DV (1999) Impaired synaptic plasticity in mice carrying the Huntington's disease mutation. Human molecular genetics 8: 839–846.

9. Milnerwood AJ, Cummings DM, Dallerac GM, Brown JY, Vatsavayai SC, et al. (2006) Early development of aberrant synaptic plasticity in a mouse model of Huntington's disease. Human molecular genetics 15: 1690–1703.

10. Cattaneo E, Rigamonti D, Goffredo D, Zuccato C, Squitieri F, et al. (2001) Loss of normal huntingtin function: new developments in Huntington's disease research. Trends in neurosciences 24: 182–188.

11. Harjes P, Wanker EE (2003) The hunt for huntingtin function: interaction partners tell many different stories. Trends in biochemical sciences 28: 425–433.

12. Cattaneo E, Zuccato C, Tartari M (2005) Normal huntingtin function: an alternative approach to Huntington's disease. Nature reviews Neuroscience 6: 919–930.

13. Rigamonti D, Bauer JH, De-Fraja C, Conti L, Sipione S, et al. (2000) Wild-type huntingtin protects from apoptosis upstream of caspase-3. The Journal of neuroscience: the official journal of the Society for Neuroscience 20: 3705–3713.

14. Leavitt BR, Guttman JA, Hodgson JG, Kimel GH, Singaraja R, et al. (2001) Wild-type huntingtin reduces the cellular toxicity of mutant huntingtin in vivo. American journal of human genetics 68: 313–324.

15. Zhang Y, Li M, Drozda M, Chen M, Ren S, et al. (2003) Depletion of wild-type huntingtin in mouse models of neurologic diseases. Journal of neurochemistry 87: 101–106.

16. Dragatsis I, Levine MS, Zeitlin S (2000) Inactivation of Hdh in the brain and testis results in progressive neurodegeneration and sterility in mice. Nature genetics 26: 300–306.

17. Nasir J, Floresco SB, O'Kusky JR, Diewert VM, Richman JM, et al. (1995) Targeted disruption of the Huntington's disease gene results in embryonic lethality and behavioral and morphological changes in heterozygotes. Cell 81: 811–823.

18. Duyao MP, Auerbach AB, Ryan A, Persichetti F, Barnes GT, et al. (1995) Inactivation of the mouse Huntington's disease gene homolog Hdh. Science 269: 407–410.

19. Zeitlin S, Liu JP, Chapman DL, Papaioannou VE, Efstratiadis A (1995) Increased apoptosis and early embryonic lethality in mice nullizygous for the Huntington's disease gene homologue. Nature genetics 11: 155–163.

20. MacDonald ME (2003) Huntingtin: alive and well and working in middle management. Science's STKE: signal transduction knowledge environment 2003: pe48.

21. Sun Y, Savanenin A, Reddy PH, Liu YF (2001) Polyglutamine-expanded huntingtin promotes sensitization of N-methyl-D-aspartate receptors via post-synaptic density 95. The Journal of biological chemistry 276: 24713–24718.

22. DiFiglia M, Sapp E, Chase K, Schwarz C, Meloni A, et al. (1995) Huntingtin is a cytoplasmic protein associated with vesicles in human and rat brain neurons. Neuron 14: 1075–1081.

23. Velier J, Kim M, Schwarz C, Kim TW, Sapp E, et al. (1998) Wild-type and mutant huntingtins function in vesicle trafficking in the secretory and endocytic pathways. Experimental neurology 152: 34–40.

24. Hilditch-Maguire P, Trettel F, Passani LA, Auerbach A, Persichetti F, et al. (2000) Huntingtin: an iron-regulated protein essential for normal nuclear and perinuclear organelles. Human molecular genetics 9: 2789–2797.

25. Zuccato C, Ciammola A, Rigamonti D, Leavitt BR, Goffredo D, et al. (2001) Loss of huntingtin-mediated BDNF gene transcription in Huntington's disease. Science 293: 493–498.

26. Zuccato C, Tartari M, Crotti A, Goffredo D, Valenza M, et al. (2003) Huntingtin interacts with REST/NRSF to modulate the transcription of NRSE-controlled neuronal genes. Nature genetics 35: 76–83.

27. Gauthier LR, Charrin BC, Borrell-Pages M, Dompierre JP, Rangone H, et al. (2004) Huntingtin controls neurotrophic support and survival of neurons by enhancing BDNF vesicular transport along microtubules. Cell 118: 127–138.

28. Gunawardena S, Her LS, Brusch RG, Laymon RA, Niesman IR, et al. (2003) Disruption of axonal transport by loss of huntingtin or expression of pathogenic polyQ proteins in Drosophila. Neuron 40: 25–40.

29. Gunawardena S, Goldstein LS (2001) Disruption of axonal transport and neuronal viability by amyloid precursor protein mutations in Drosophila. Neuron 32: 389–401.

30. Bowman AB, Kamal A, Ritchings BW, Philp AV, McGrail M, et al. (2000) Kinesin-dependent axonal transport is mediated by the sunday driver (SYD) protein. Cell 103: 583–594.

31. McGuire JR, Rong J, Li SH, Li XJ (2006) Interaction of Huntingtin-associated protein-1 with kinesin light chain: implications in intracellular trafficking in neurons. The Journal of biological chemistry 281: 3552–3559.

32. Marinesco S, Wickremasinghe N, Carew TJ (2006) Regulation of behavioral and synaptic plasticity by serotonin release within local modulatory fields in the CNS of Aplysia. The Journal of neuroscience: the official journal of the Society for Neuroscience 26: 12682–12693.

33. Montarolo PG, Goelet P, Castellucci VF, Morgan J, Kandel ER, et al. (1986) A critical period for macromolecular synthesis in long-term heterosynaptic facilitation in Aplysia. Science 234: 1249–1254.

34. Bailey CH, Chen M (1988) Long-term memory in Aplysia modulates the total number of varicosities of single identified sensory neurons. Proceedings of the National Academy of Sciences of the United States of America 85: 2373–2377.

35. Kandel ER (2001) The molecular biology of memory storage: a dialogue between genes and synapses. Science 294: 1030–1038.

36. Lee JA, Lim CS, Lee SH, Kim H, Nukina N, et al. (2003) Aggregate formation and the impairment of long-term synaptic facilitation by ectopic expression of mutant huntingtin in Aplysia neurons. Journal of neurochemistry 85: 160–169.

37. Li Z, Karlovich CA, Fish MP, Scott MP, Myers RM (1999) A putative Drosophila homolog of the Huntington's disease gene. Human molecular genetics 8: 1807–1815.

38. Karlovich CA, John RM, Ramirez L, Stainier DY, Myers RM (1998) Characterization of the Huntington's disease (HD) gene homologue in the zebrafish Danio rerio. Gene 217: 117–125.

39. Rockabrand E, Slepko N, Pantalone A, Nukala VN, Kazantsev A, et al. (2007) The first 17 amino acids of Huntingtin modulate its sub-cellular localization, aggregation and effects on calcium homeostasis. Human molecular genetics 16: 61–77.

40. Andrade MA, Bork P (1995) HEAT repeats in the Huntington's disease protein. Nature genetics 11: 115–116.

41. Puthanveettil SV, Monje FJ, Miniaci MC, Choi YB, Karl KA, et al. (2008) A new component in synaptic plasticity: upregulation of kinesin in the neurons of the gill-withdrawal reflex. Cell 135: 960–973.

42. Alberini CM, Ghirardi M, Metz R, Kandel ER (1994) C/EBP is an immediate-early gene required for the consolidation of long-term facilitation in Aplysia. Cell 76: 1099–1114.

43. Marsh JL, Pallos J, Thompson LM (2003) Fly models of Huntington's disease. Human molecular genetics 12 Spec No 2: R187–193.

44. Flinn L, Bretaud S, Lo C, Ingham PW, Bandmann O (2008) Zebrafish as a new animal model for movement disorders. Journal of neurochemistry 106: 1991–1997.

45. Pouladi MA, Morton AJ, Hayden MR (2013) Choosing an animal model for the study of Huntington's disease. Nature reviews Neuroscience 14: 708–721.

46. Ehrnhoefer DE, Butland SL, Pouladi MA, Hayden MR (2009) Mouse models of Huntington disease: variations on a theme. Disease models & mechanisms 2: 123–129.

47. Tong Y, Ha TJ, Liu L, Nishimoto A, Reiner A, et al. (2011) Spatial and temporal requirements for huntingtin (Htt) in neuronal migration and survival during brain development. The Journal of neuroscience: the official journal of the Society for Neuroscience 31: 14794–14799.

48. Kordasiewicz HB, Stanek LM, Wancewicz EV, Mazur C, McAlonis MM, et al. (2012) Sustained therapeutic reversal of Huntington's disease by transient repression of huntingtin synthesis. Neuron 74: 1031–1044.

49. Giustetto M, Hegde AN, Si K, Casadio A, Inokuchi K, et al. (2003) Axonal transport of eukaryotic translation elongation factor 1alpha mRNA couples transcription in the nucleus to long-term facilitation at the synapse. Proceedings of the National Academy of Sciences of the United States of America 100: 13680–13685.

50. Choi YB, Li HL, Kassabov SR, Jin I, Puthanveettil SV, et al. (2011) Neurexin-neuroligin transsynaptic interaction mediates learning-related synaptic remodeling and long-term facilitation in aplysia. Neuron 70: 468–481.

51. Diekmann H, Anichtchik O, Fleming A, Futter M, Goldsmith P, et al. (2009) Decreased BDNF levels are a major contributor to the embryonic phenotype of huntingtin knockdown zebrafish. The Journal of neuroscience: the official journal of the Society for Neuroscience 29: 1343–1349.

52. Chao MV (2003) Neurotrophins and their receptors: a convergence point for many signalling pathways. Nature reviews Neuroscience 4: 299–309.

53. Kassabov SR, Choi YB, Karl KA, Vishwasrao HD, Bailey CH, et al. (2013) A single Aplysia neurotrophin mediates synaptic facilitation via differentially processed isoforms. Cell reports 3: 1213–1227.

54. Steffan JS, Kazantsev A, Spasic-Boskovic O, Greenwald M, Zhu YZ, et al. (2000) The Huntington's disease protein interacts with p53 and CREB-binding protein and represses transcription. Proceedings of the National Academy of Sciences of the United States of America 97: 6763–6768.

3

Identification of Binding Sites in Huntingtin for the Huntingtin Interacting Proteins HIP14 and HIP14L

Shaun S. Sanders, Katherine K. N. Mui, Liza M. Sutton, Michael R. Hayden*

Department of Medical Genetics and Centre for Molecular Medicine and Therapeutics, Child and Family Research Institute, University of British Columbia, Vancouver, British Columbia, Canada

Abstract

Huntington disease is an adult onset neurodegenerative disease characterized by motor, cognitive, and psychiatric dysfunction, caused by a CAG expansion in the *HTT* gene. Huntingtin Interacting Protein 14 (HIP14) and Huntingtin Interacting Protein 14-like (HIP14L) are palmitoyl acyltransferases (PATs), enzymes that mediate the post-translational addition of long chain fatty acids to proteins in a process called palmitoylation. HIP14 and HIP14L interact with and palmitoylate HTT and are unique among PATs as they are the only two that have an ankyrin repeat domain, which mediates the interaction between HIP14 and HTT. These enzymes show reduced interaction with and palmitoylation of mutant HTT, leading to increased mutant HTT inclusion formation and toxicity. The interaction between HIP14 and HTT goes beyond that of only an enzyme–substrate interaction as HTT is essential for the full enzymatic activity of HIP14. It is important to further understand and characterize the interactions of HTT with HIP14 and HIP14L to guide future efforts to target and enhance this interaction and increase enzyme activity to remediate palmitoylation of HTT and their substrates, as well as to understand the relationship between the three proteins. HIP14 and HIP14L have been previously shown to interact with HTT amino acids 1–548. Here the interaction of HIP14 and HIP14L with N- and C-terminal HTT 1–548 deletion mutations was assessed. We show that HTT amino acids 1–548 were sufficient for full interaction of HTT with HIP14 and HIP14L, but partial interaction was also possible with HTT 1–427 and HTT 224–548. To further characterize the binding domain we assessed the interaction of HIP14-GFP and HIP14L-GFP with 15Q HTT 1-548Δ257-315. Both enzymes showed reduced but not abolished interaction with 15Q HTT 1-548Δ257-315. This suggests that two potential binding domains exist, one around residues 224 and the other around 427, for the PAT enzymes HIP14 and HIP14L.

Editor: Hiroyoshi Ariga, Hokkaido University, Japan

Funding: This work was supported by the CHDI Foundation, Inc. (chdifoundation.org operating grant to MRH). SSS is funded by the Canadian Institutes for Health Research (CIHR; www.cihr-irsc.gc.ca; Doctoral Research Award) and the Michael Smith Foundation for Health Research (MSFHR; www.msfhr.org; Junior Graduate Scholarship). LMS was funded by the Ripples of Hope Pfizer 2011 Trainee Award in Rare Diseases (http://www.cmmt.ubc.ca/getinvolved/trainees/funding/Ripples-of-Hope). MRH is a University Killam Professor and the Canada Research Chair in Human Genetics and Molecular Medicine. The funders had no role in study design and analysis, decision to publish or preparation of the manuscript.

Competing Interests: The authors have declared that no competing interests exist.

* E-mail: mrh@cmmt.ubc.ca

Introduction

Huntington disease (HD) is an autosomal dominant neurodegenerative disease characterized by motor, cognitive, and psychiatric dysfunction with onset in mid-life and death following, on average, 20 years later [1,2]. The striatum is the brain region to first undergo neurodegeneration with more widespread pathology occurring at later stages of the disease [1,2]. HD is caused by a CAG expansion in exon 1 of the *HTT* gene that results in a poly-Q expansion in the HTT protein (NP_002102) [3].

One approach that has been taken to determine the functions of the HTT protein and to understand the pathogenesis of HD is to identify and characterize HTT interacting proteins and to determine how these interactions are altered in the presence of the HD mutation. Huntingtin Interacting Protein 14 (HIP14; ZDHHC17; NP_056151) was first identified as a HTT interactor in a yeast 2-hybrid screen. HIP14 was further shown to interact with HTT in mammalian systems and to interact less with mutant HTT (mHTT) [4,5]. The HIP14 homolog Huntingtin Interacting Protein 14-like (HIP14L; ZDHHC13; NP_061901) was first identified based on its high amino acid sequence similarity to HIP14 and was later shown to also be a *bona fide* HTT interactor that also interacts less with mHTT [5,6].

HIP14 and HIP14L both belong to the 23 member family of DHHC (Asp-His-His-Cys) cysteine-rich (DHHC-CR) domain-containing palmitoyl acyltransferases (PATs) [7,8]. DHHC-CR PATs are a family of enzymes that mediate post-translational S-acylation of proteins, involving the addition of long chain fatty acids to proteins at cysteine residues via a thioester bond. S-acylation is commonly referred to as palmitoylation because palmitate is the most common long chain fatty acid in the cell [9,10]. Many proteins, including HTT, are dynamically palmitoylated and palmitoylation modulates membrane localization, function, protein-protein interactions, and other post-translational modifications of palmitoyl-proteins [11]. HIP14 and HIP14L are unique among the DHHC-CR PATs as they are the only two that have six transmembrane domains (TMDs) and seven ankyrin

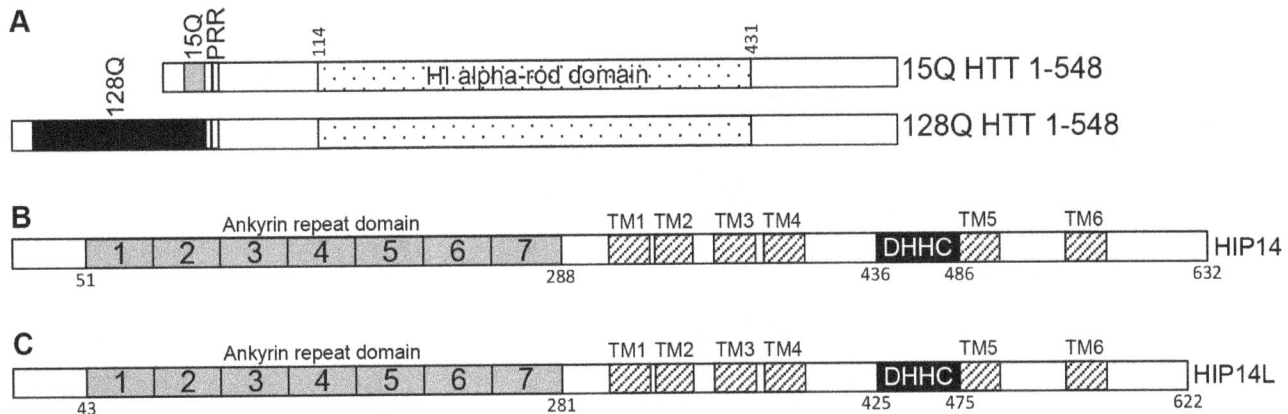

Figure 1. Overview schematics of the domain organization of HTT (A), HIP14 (B), and HIP14L (C). The domain organization of HTT is shown in (**A**) with the poly-glutamine domains of WT (15Q) and mutant (128Q) HTT (NP_002102) are shown in grey and black rectangles, respectively, the proline rich repeat is shown in a hatched rectangle, and the H1 alpha-rod domain is shown in a dotted rectangle with the amino acids indicated above. (**B**) The domain organization of HIP14 (NP_056151) is shown in (**B**) and of HIP14L (NP_061901) in (**C**) with the 7 ankyrin repeats making up the ankyrin repeat domain shown in numbered solid grey rectangles, the transmembrane domains shown in hatched rectangles labeled TM1-6, and the DHHC cysteine-rich domain shown in solid black rectangles labeled DHHC. The amino acids corresponding to the appropriate domains are indicated below.

repeats (Figure 1B and C). The ankyrin repeat domain is believed to mediate the interaction between HIP14 and HTT [11,12].

HIP14 and HIP14L are not only HTT interactors but they are also the primary PATs for HTT [12]. These PATs show reduced interaction and palmitoylation of mHTT leading to increased mHTT inclusion formation and toxicity [13]. Interestingly, both the *Hip14-* and *Hip14l*-deficient mouse models recapitulate many HD-like phenotypes suggesting that both proteins may play a role in the pathogenesis of HD [6,14]. Indeed, HIP14 has been shown to be dysfunctional in the presence of the HD mutation or upon loss of wild type HTT, making it unable to effectively palmitoylate its substrates SNAP25 and GluR1 [12,14]. These data suggest that the interaction between HIP14 and HTT goes beyond that of only a enzyme-substrate interaction and that HTT is essential for the full enzymatic activity of HIP14 [12,14]. HIP14L is structurally very similar to HIP14, containing all the same domains in the same orientation; thus it is possible that HTT also modulates the function of HIP14L.

It is important to further understand and characterize the interactions of HTT with HIP14 and HIP14L to guide future efforts to target and enhance this interaction to increase enzyme activity and remediate palmitoylation of HTT and their substrates. It is important to know if HIP14 and HIP14L interact with the same domain of HTT and, if so, if they compete for binding. A shared binding site would provide further support for the hypothesis that these two PATs are able to compensate for each other in palmitoylating HTT and that HTT may also modulate the activity of HIP14L. If they were to compete for binding, this would need to be taken into consideration when taking efforts to increase the interaction between HTT and one PAT or the other at the risk of decreasing the interaction with the other PAT. HIP14 has been previously shown to interact with HTT amino acids 1–548 (HTT 1–548) [12]. Here, amino (N)- and carboxy (C)-terminal deletions of HTT 1–548 were generated and their interaction with HIP14 and HIP14L was assessed to determine the location of the binding site.

Materials and Methods

Plasmids and Cloning

The generation of HIP14-GFP (NM_015336) and HIP14L-GFP (NM_001001483), 15Q and 128Q HTT 1–548 (15Q and 128Q 1955; NM_002111), and HTT 1–427 (1597) and HTT 1–224 (989) was described previously [6,7,15,16]. The C-terminal deletion mutants were generated by PCR cloning using the indicated primers in Table 1. The primers (Integrated DNA technologies) had EcoRI and NotI restriction enzyme sites added on the 5′ and 3′ sides of the PCR product respectively and the forward primers also had a start codon added. This allowed the PCR products to be digested and ligated into the EcoRI and NotI sites of pCI-neo (enzymes from New England Biolabs; pCI-neo from Promega). 15Q HTT 1-548Δ257-315 was generated by insertion of a *HTT* gBlock gene fragment into the BlpI and Bsu36I restriction enzyme sites following digestion with the same enzymes such that amino acids 257–315 were deleted. All clones were confirmed by sequencing.

Table 1. Cloning primers used to generate the HTT 1–548 N-terminal deletion mutants.

Primer name	Sequence
HTT N-term reverse	tcccatctgaccctgccatg**tga**gcggccgctactgctatg
HTT 427–548 forward	tcgtacttat*gaattc***atg**ggaggggggttcctcatgcag
HTT 224–548 forward	tcgtacttatgaattc**atg**tcagtccaggagaccttggc
HTT 151–548 forward	tcgtacttat*gaattc***atg**tgcctcaacaaagttatcaa
HTT 88–548 forward	tcgtacttat*gaattc***atg**cgaccaaagaaagaactttc

*Restriction enzyme sites are in italics (EcoRI in forward primers and NotI in the reverse), the start and stop codons are in bold, and the primer binding sequence is underlined.

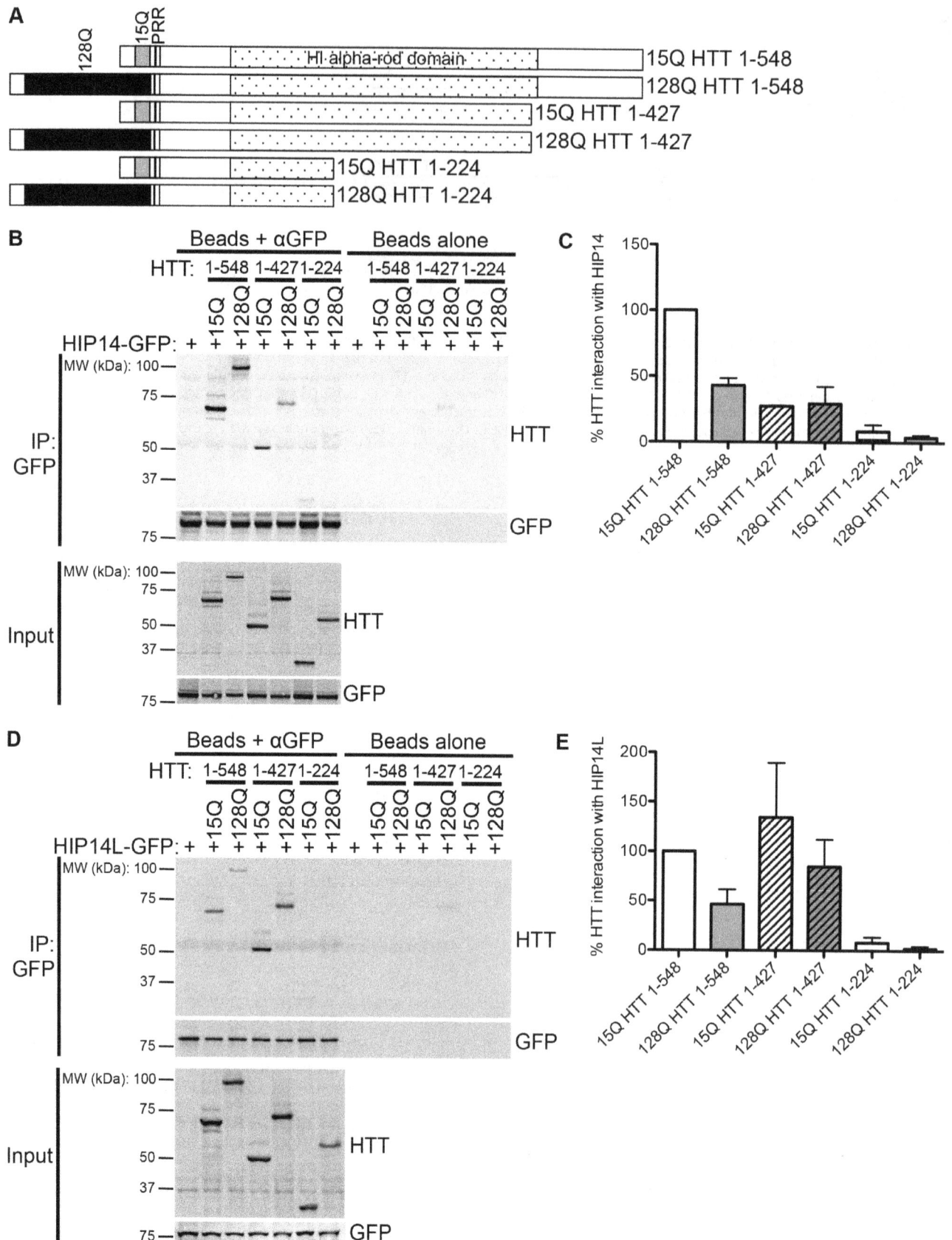

Figure 2. HIP14 and HIP14L interaction with C-terminal deletion mutants of HTT 1-548. (**A**) A schematic diagram of the HTT 1–548 C-terminal deletion mutants used in co-immunoprecipitation experiments with HIP14-GFP and HIP14L-GFP showing the 15Q or 128Q poly-Q domains, the proline rich region (PRR), and the H1 alpha-rod domain. (**B**) A representative image (top two panels) of the co-immunoprecipitation between

these C-terminal deletion mutants and HIP14-GFP where GFP was immunoprecipitated and the resulting blots were probed for HTT (top panel) and GFP (bottom panel) showing less 15Q and 128Q HTT 1–427 co-immunoprecipitated with HIP14-GFP. On the right is a beads alone (no antibody) control showing no non-specific binding of the proteins to the beads. The bottom two images show the expression of the HTT deletion mutants (top panel) and of HIP14-GFP (bottom panel). (C) Quantification of three independent co-immunoprecipitation experiments where the % HTT interaction with HIP14 is the indicated HTT band intensity as a percentage of the HIP14-GFP band intensity from the same sample, normalized to 15Q HTT 1–548. (D) A representative image (top two panels) of the co-immunoprecipitation between the HTT 1–548 C-terminal deletion mutants and HIP14L-GFP where GFP was immunoprecipitated and the resulting blots were probed for HTT (top panel) and GFP (bottom panel). Less 15Q and 128Q HTT 1–427 co-immunoprecipitated with HIP14L-GFP. On the right is a beads alone (no antibody) control showing no non-specific binding of the proteins to the beads. The bottom two panels show the expression of the HTT deletion mutants (top panel) and of HIP14L-GFP (bottom panel). (E) Quantification of three independent co-immunoprecipitation experiments where the % HTT interaction with HIP14L-GFP is the indicated HTT band intensity as a percentage of the HIP14L-GFP band intensity from the same sample, normalized to 15Q HTT 1–548.

Antibodies

The primary antibodies used were GFP goat polyclonal antibody (sc-5385, Santa Cruz Biotechnology, 1:50 for immuno-precipitation), HTT mouse monoclonal antibody (MAB2166, Millipore, 1:1000 for immunoblotting), HTT mouse monoclonal antibody (in-house BKP1, 1:100 for immunoblotting), and GFP rabbit polyclonal antibody (EU2, Eusera, 1:10000 for immuno-blotting). Fluorescently conjugated secondary antibodies for immunoblotting used were Alexa Fluor 680 goat anti-Rabbit (A21076, Molecular Probes, 1:10000) and IRDye 800CW goat anti-Mouse (610-131-121, Rockland, 1:2500).

Cell Culture and Transfection

Cells were cultured in DMEM with 10% fetal bovine serum, penicillin/streptomycin (1000 Units/mL Penicillin and 1000 ug/mL streptomycin), and 2 mM L-glutamine at 37°C in 5% CO_2 (Gibco). Constructs were transiently transfected in COS-7 cells (ATCC) with X-tremeGENE 9 DNA transfection reagent (Roche) according to the manufacturer's instructions. Cells were harvested after 24 h for co-immunoprecipitation experiments described below.

Cell Lysis and Co-immunoprecipitations

Cells were homogenized on ice for 5 min in one volume 1% SDS TEEN [TEEN: 1 M Tris pH 7.5, 0.5 M EDTA, 0.5 M EGTA, 3 M NaCl, 1 mM Complete protease inhibitor cocktail (Roche), 1 mM sodium vanadate, 1 mM phenylmethylsulfonyl fluoride and 5 µM zVAD-FMK] and subsequently diluted in four volumes 1% TritonX-100 TEEN for 5 min for further homogenization. Samples were sonicated at one time at 20% power for 5 seconds to shear DNA and the insoluble material was removed by centrifugation at 14000 revolutions per minute for 15 min. Samples were immunoprecipitated overnight with Dynabeads Protein G (Invitrogen) and antibody.

Western Blotting Analysis

Proteins in both the cell lysates and immunoprecipitates were heated at 70°C in 1×NuPAGE LDS sample buffer (Invitrogen) with 10 mM DTT before separation by SDS-PAGE. After transfer of the proteins onto nitrocellulose membrane, immunoblots were blocked in 5% milk TBS (TBS: 50 mM Tris pH 7.5, 150 mM NaCl). Primary antibody dilutions of HTT mouse monoclonal antibody and GFP rabbit polyclonal antibody in 5%BSA PBST (Bovine Serum Albumin, Phosphate Buffered Saline with 5% Tween-20) were applied to the immunoblots at 4°C overnight. Corresponding secondary antibodies were applied in 5% BSA PBST for an hour. Fluorescence was scanned and quantified with Odyssey Infrared Imaging system (Li-COR Bioscience) and

quantified using the Li-COR software. All error bars are standard error of mean.

Results

Deletion of HTT Amino Acids 224–548 Abolishes the Interaction of HTT with HIP14 and HIP14L

HIP14 was previously shown to interact with HTT 1–548 [5]. The domain organization of HTT 1–548 15Q and 128Q is shown in Figure 1A with the poly-Q, the proline rich region, and the H1 alpha-rod domain indicated [17]. HIP14 was previously shown in a yeast 2-hybrid experiment to have reduced interaction with HTT 1–427 compared to its interaction with HTT 1–548 and no interaction with HTT 1–224, HTT 1–151, HTT 1–88, and HTT 1–40 [12]. However, as this interaction analysis was performed in yeast it was repeated here in a mammalian system using the mammalian expression versions of the constructs used in the yeast 2-hybrid experiments [12,16]. Conveniently, these truncation spots remove the C-terminal region upstream of the H1 alpha-rod domain (HTT 1–427) or this C-terminal region and half of the H1 alpha-rod domain (HTT 1–224) (Figure 2A). HTT 1–548 and two C-terminal deletion mutants, 15Q or 128Q HTT 1–427 and 15Q or 128Q HTT 1–224 (Figure 2A), were transiently co-expressed with HIP14-GFP or HIP14L-GFP expressing constructs in COS-7 cells. GFP was immunoprecipitated and resulting blots were probed with antibodies to detect GFP and HTT. As previously shown, 57% less mutant HTT 1–548 (128Q HTT 1–548) co-immunoprecipitated with HIP14-GFP than WT HTT 1–548 (15Q HTT 1–548), indicating reduced interaction in the presence of the HD mutation (Figure 2B and C; n = 3). Both 15Q and 128Q HTT 1–427 exhibited decreased, but not abolished, interaction with HIP14-GFP while both 15Q and 128Q HTT 1–224 interacted very little or not at all with HIP14-GFP (Figure 2B and C; n = 3). The same interaction pattern was observed with a HIP14-FLAG tagged construct and HTT 1–548 did not interact with GFP alone (data not shown). All further experiments were performed using the GFP tagged constructs as they express better in COS cells. These data indicate that HTT 1-427 is required for full interaction with HIP14 and the interaction is abolished with deletion of amino acids 224–548 in the HTT 1–224 truncation protein. No interaction between HIP14-GFP and HTT 1–151, HTT 1–88, or HTT 1–40 was observed (data not shown).

As the domain of HTT that interacts with HIP14L has never been determined, the same co-immunoprecipitation experiment between HIP14L-GFP and the above-mentioned HTT C-terminal deletion mutants, 15Q or 128Q HTT 1–427 and 15Q or 128Q HTT 1–224 was performed. Similar to the results obtained with HIP14, 128Q HTT 1–548 interacted much less with HIP14L-GFP than did 15Q HTT 1–548, indicating reduced interaction with mutant HTT (54% decrease; Figure 2D and E; n = 3).

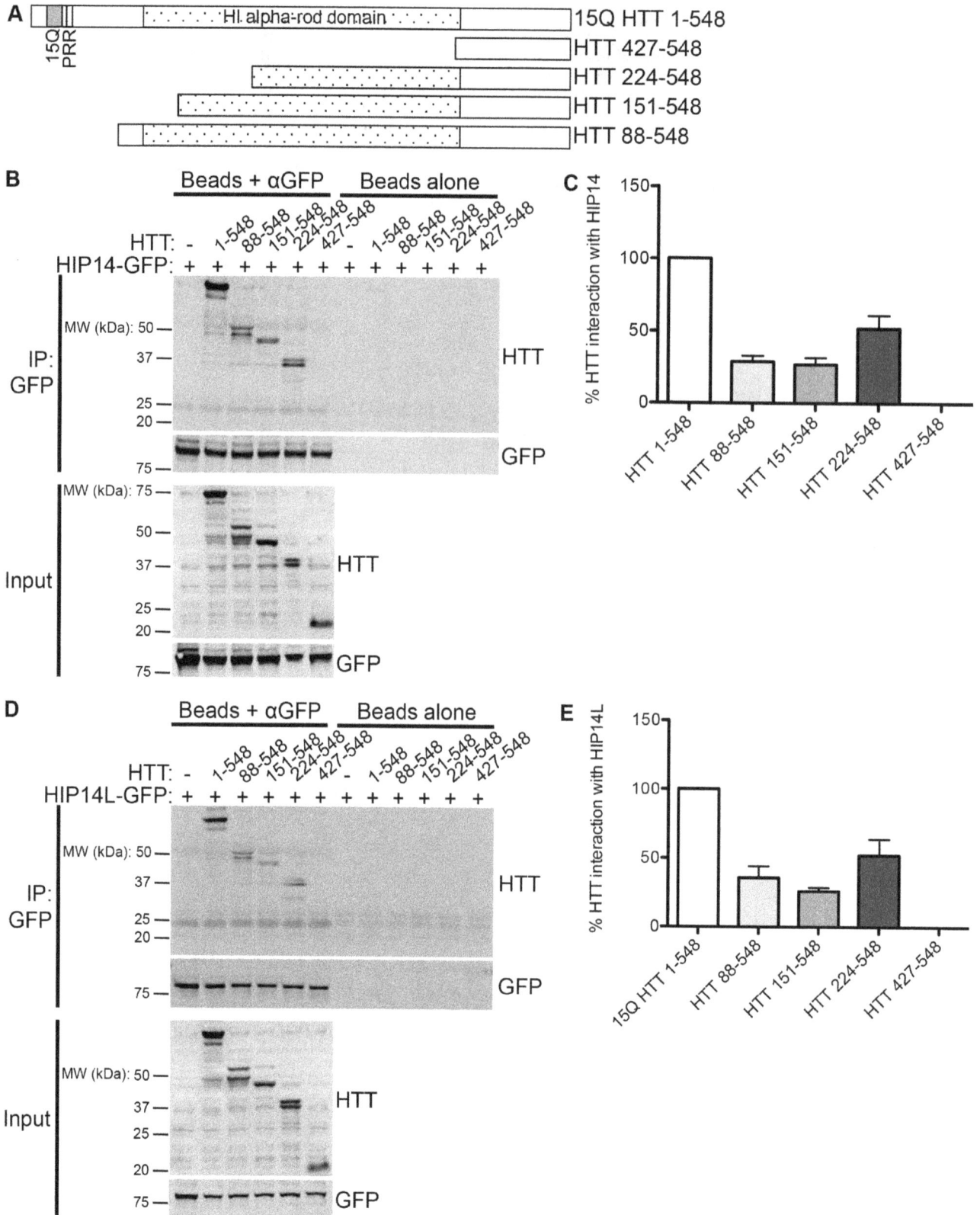

Figure 3. HIP14 and HIP14L interaction with N-terminal deletion mutants of HTT 1–548. (**A**) A diagram of the HTT 1–548 N-terminal deletion mutants used in co-immunoprecipitation experiments with HIP14-GFP and HIP14L-GFP showing the 15Q poly-Q domains, the proline rich region (PRR), and the H1 alpha-rod domain. (**B**) A representative image (top two panels) of the co-immunoprecipitation between these N-terminal deletion mutants and HIP14-GFP where GFP was immunoprecipitated and the resulting blots were probed for HTT (top panel) and GFP (bottom

panel) showing less HTT 88–548, HTT 151–548, and HTT 224–548 co-immunoprecipitated with HIP14-GFP and no HTT 427–548 was co-immunoprecipitated with HIP14. On the right is a beads alone control showing no non-specific binding of the proteins to the beads. The bottom two images show the expression of the HTT deletion mutants (top panel) and of HIP14-GFP (bottom panel). (**C**) Quantification of three co-immunoprecipitation experiments where the % HTT interaction with HIP14 is the indicated HTT band intensity as a percentage of the HIP14-GFP band intensity from the same sample, normalized to 15Q HTT 1–548. (**D**) A representative image (top two panels) of the co-immunoprecipitation between the HTT 1–548 N-terminal deletion mutants and HIP14L-GFP where GFP was immunoprecipitated and the resulting blots were probed for HTT (top panel) and GFP (bottom panel). Less HTT 88–548, HTT 151–548, and HTT 224–548 and no HTT 427–548 was co-immunoprecipitated with HIP14L-GFP. On the right is a beads alone control showing no non-specific binding of the proteins to the beads. The bottom two panels show the expression of the HTT deletion mutants (top panel) and of HIP14L-GFP (bottom panel). (**E**) Quantification of three co-immunoprecipitation experiments where the % HTT interaction with HIP14L-GFP is the indicated HTT band intensity as a percentage of the HIP14L-GFP band intensity from the same sample, normalized to 15Q HTT 1–548.

However, no change in interaction of HIP14L with the 15Q and 128Q HTT 1–427 deletion mutants was observed in co-immunoprecipitation experiments (Figure 2D and E; n = 4). The HTT 1–224 deletion mutant did not interact with HIP14L (Figure 2D and E; n = 3). No interaction between HIP14L-GFP and HTT 1–151, HTT 1–88, or HTT 1–40 was observed (data not shown). These data indicate that HTT 1–427 is sufficient for interaction with HIP14L and the interaction is abolished with deletion of amino acids 224–548 in the HTT 1–224 truncation protein.

Deletion of HTT Amino Acids 1–427 Abolishes the Interaction of HTT with HIP14 and HIP14L

To further characterize the domain of interaction of HTT with HIP14 or HIP14L, N-terminal deletion mutants complementary to the C-terminal deletion mutants were generated; HTT 88–548, HTT 151–548, HTT 224–548, and HTT 427–548 (Figure 3A). These deletion mutants were transiently co-expressed with HIP14-GFP or HIP14L-GFP in COS-7 cells. Reduced interaction of HTT with HIP14-GFP was observed with HTT 88–548, HTT 151–548, and HTT 224–548 and the interaction was abolished upon the deletion of amino acids 1–427 in the HTT 427–548 deletion mutant (Figure 3B and C; n = 3). These data indicate that HTT amino acids 224 to 548 are sufficient for partial interaction with HIP14.

A similar effect was observed between the interaction of HIP14L and the HTT C-terminal deletion mutants as with HIP14. Reduced interaction of HTT 88–548, HTT 151–548, and HTT 224–548 with HIP14L-GFP was observed in similar co-immunoprecipitation experiments and again complete loss of interaction was observed with the HTT 427–548 deletion mutant (Figure 3D and E; n = 3). These data also indicate that HTT amino acids 224 to 548 are sufficient for partial interaction with HIP14L and, along with the data discussed above, suggests that there may be a HIP14/HIP14L binding domain between amino acids 224–427 of HTT.

Deletion of Amino Acids 257–315 of HTT does not Abolish the Interaction with HIP14 and HIP14L

One potential mechanism of binding of HIP14 and HIP14L to HTT within amino acids 224–427 is a putatively methylated lysine at K262 within a LKS motif (in human HTT NP_002102). Gao *et al* determined the crystal structure of the HIP14 ankyrin repeat domain and found that it forms a surface aromatic cage that may bind methylated lysines, much like the ankyrin repeat domains of the G9a and G9a-like protein histone lysine methyltransferases [18]. The K262 of the LKS motif within residues 224–427 of HTT is the only lysine in this region that contains an adjacent

serine or threonine like that of the methylated lysine of the histone H3 tail sequence, making it a potential site of methylation [18]. To determine if this is a potential binding domain, a HTT deletion protein with amino acids 257–315 deleted, including the LKS motif, was generated (Figure 4A). This deletion mutant was transiently co-expressed with HIP14-GFP or HIP14L-GFP in COS-7 cells. Reduced but not abolished interaction of 15Q HTT 1–548Δ257-315 with HIP14-GFP and HIP14L-GFP was observed (Figure 4B and C for HIP14 and D and E for HIP14L; n = 3). These data indicate that the HIP14/HIP14L binding domain in HTT is not within these amino acids.

Discussion

HIP14 and HIP14L are HTT interacting and palmitoylating proteins and their interaction and palmitoylation of HTT are decreased in the presence of mHTT [5,6,13]. Interestingly, it appears that the interaction between HIP14 and HTT goes beyond that of only an enzyme-substrate interaction and that HTT actually modulates the enzymatic activity of HIP14 [12,14]. To further understand and characterize the interactions of HTT with HIP14 and HIP14L it is important to identify the domains of interaction to guide future efforts to target and enhance this interaction to increase enzyme activity and remediate palmitoylation of HTT and their substrates. It is necessary to know if HIP14 and HIP14L interact with the same domain of HTT and, if so, if they compete for binding.

HIP14 was previously shown to interact with HTT 1–548 [12]. Here the interaction between HIP14 and HIP14L with N- and C-terminal HTT 1–548 deletion mutants was characterized. HTT amino acids 1–548 are sufficient for the full interaction of HTT with HIP14 and partial interaction is achieved with amino acids 1–427 and 224–548. Full interaction between HTT and HIP14L was achieved with HTT amino acids 1–548 and 1–427 and partial interaction with 224–427. Amino acids 1–224 or 427–548 of HTT were not sufficient for interaction with HIP14 and HIP14L, indicating that a binding domain is likely to exist between amino acids 224–427. To further characterize this binding region a HTT deletion protein with amino acids 257–315 deleted was generated. Reduced but not abolished interaction of 15Q HTT 1–548Δ257-315 with HIP14-GFP and HIP14L-GFP was observed. These data indicate that the HIP14/HIP14L binding domain in HTT is not within these amino acids but that these amino acids are required for the structural integrity of the actual binding domain.

A larger region of HTT, amino acids 1–548, is required to achieve full interaction, possibly to achieve correct folding and structural stability of the binding domain or because other sequences outside of this region also contribute to the interaction.

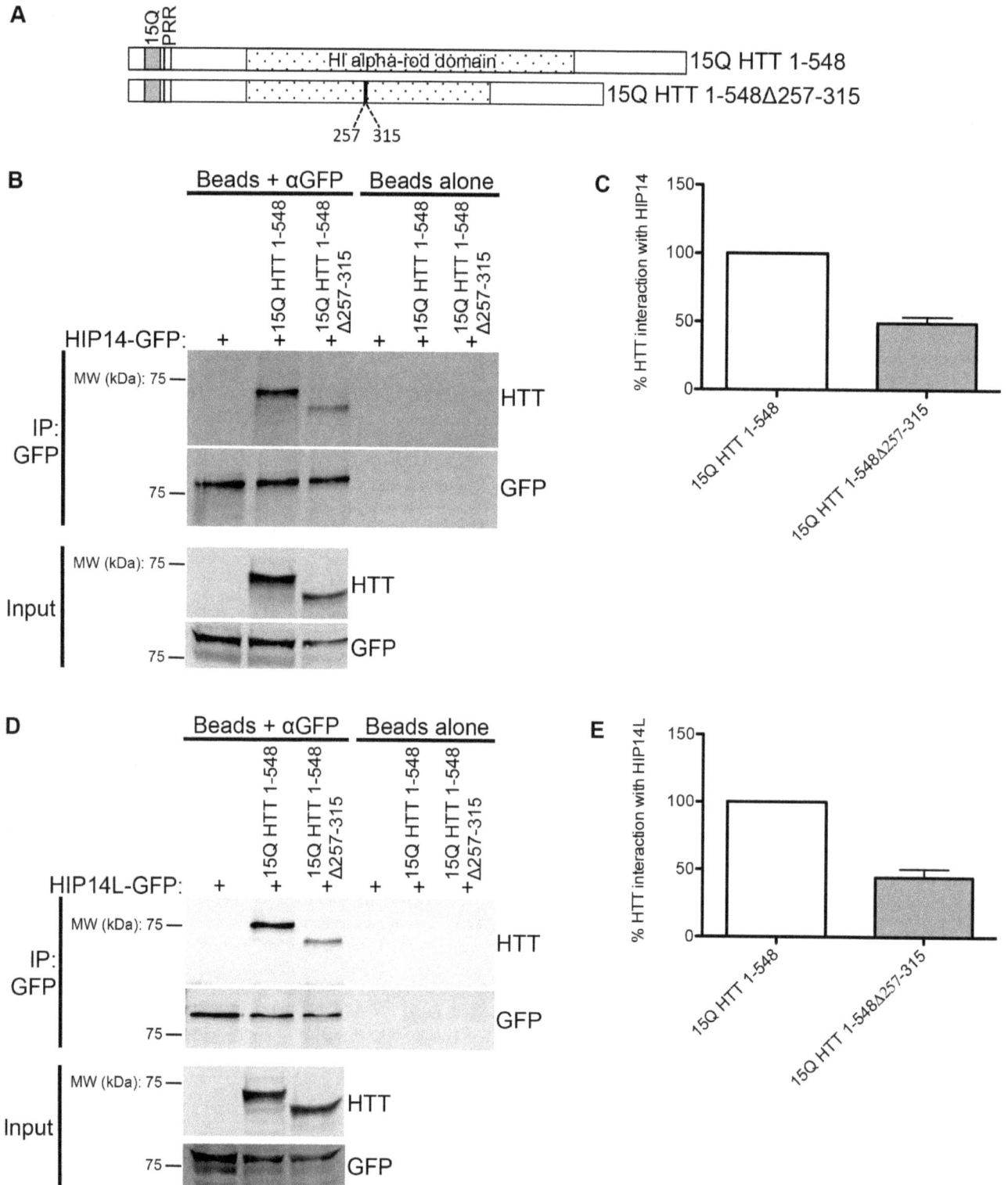

Figure 4. HIP14 and HIP14L interaction with 15Q HTT 1-548Δ257-315. (**A**) A diagram of the 15Q HTT 1-548Δ257-315 deletion mutant used in co-immunoprecipitation experiments with HIP14-GFP and HIP14L-GFP showing the 15Q poly-Q domains, the proline rich region (PRR), and the H1 alpha-rod domain. (**B**) A representative image (top two panels) of the co-immunoprecipitation between 15Q HTT 1-548Δ257-315 deletion mutant and HIP14-GFP where GFP was immunoprecipitated and the resulting blots were probed for HTT (top panel) and GFP (bottom panel) showing less of the 15Q HTT 1-548Δ257-315 deletion mutant co-immunoprecipitated with HIP14-GFP and compared to 15Q HTT 1–548. On the right is a beads alone (no antibody) control showing no non-specific binding of the proteins to the beads. The bottom two images show the expression of the 15Q HTT 1-548Δ257-315 deletion mutant (top panel) and of HIP14-GFP (bottom panel). (**C**) Quantification of three independent co-immunoprecipitation experiments where the % HTT interaction with HIP14 is the indicated HTT band intensity as a percentage of the HIP14-GFP band intensity from the

same sample, normalized to 15Q HTT 1–548. (**D**) A representative image (top two panels) of the co-immunoprecipitation between the 15Q HTT 1-548Δ257-315 deletion mutant and HIP14L-GFP where GFP was immunoprecipitated and the resulting blots were probed for HTT (top panel) and GFP (bottom panel). Less 15Q HTT 1-548Δ257-315 deletion mutant was co-immunoprecipitated with HIP14L-GFP. On the right is a beads alone (no antibody) control showing no non-specific binding of the proteins to the beads. The bottom two panels show the expression of the 15Q HTT 1-548Δ257-315 deletion mutant (top panel) and of HIP14L-GFP (bottom panel). (**E**) Quantification of three independent co-immunoprecipitation experiments where the % HTT interaction with HIP14L-GFP is the indicated HTT band intensity as a percentage of the HIP14L-GFP band intensity from the same sample, normalized to 15Q HTT 1–548.

The full 1–548 amino acids are required for structural integrity and the correct interaction conformation of HTT likely requires interactions between 1–548 N- and C-terminal parts of HTT to form a compact structure. Based on these data, it is likely that there are actually multiple binding sites, one around amino acid 224 and another around amino acid 427, and that both are required for full interaction and all of the amino acids from 1–548 are required for the structural integrity and confirmation of these binding sites (Figure 5; dashed lines).

Interestingly, in the hypothetical 3D structure of HTT proposed by Palidwor et al. HTT has 3 alpha-rod domains (H1-3) that fold back on and interact with each other and interact with HTT interacting proteins (Figure 1A) [17]. The two potential binding domains around residues 224 and 427 are contained within a single structural element of HTT, the H1 alpha-rod domain (resides within amino acids 114–431; Figure 1A). It would be logical that the PAT binding domain would be contained within a single structural element such as the H1 domain thus favoring our model that the PAT binding domains are fully contained within this structural element (Figure 5) [17]. This is consistent with the data presented here where the full 1–548 HTT protein is required for the correct confirmation of this large structural domain and of the two binding sites contained within.

This study identified two potential binding domains around residues 224 and 427 for the PAT enzymes HIP14 and HIP14L. Further characterization of the interactions of HTT with HIP14 and HIP14L is important, as this interaction is believed to go beyond that of a simple enzyme-substrate interaction where HTT actually modulates their function and facilitates palmitoylation of HIP14 substrates.

A common binding domain in HTT for HIP14 and HIP14L along with the fact that HIP14L's domain structure is virtually identical to HIP14, with all the same domains in the same orientation suggests that HTT may also modulate the enzymatic activity of HIP14L [11]. HTT may modulate the function of these enzymes in several ways. First, HTT is an α–solenoid protein made up of HEAT (Huntingtin, Elongation factor 3, protein phosphatase 2A, TOR1) repeats suitable for its function as a scaffolding protein with many protein-protein interactions [12,17,19–21]. It is possible that HTT may act as a scaffolding protein to bring substrates into close proximity with HIP14 and HIP14L, acting as an essential linker between PATs and their other substrates. Second, HTT may act as an allosteric activator of HIP14 by affecting the conformational structure of HIP14 thereby allowing substrates to access the DHHC active site [12]. Third, as HTT has been shown to be involved in trafficking of organelles along the cytoskeleton, interacting with multiple motor and motor-associated proteins, HTT may be important for trafficking HIP14 and/or HIP14L to particular subcellular locations allowing it to interact with and palmitoylate its substrates [12,22].

As the interactions between HTT and HIP14 or HIP14L are reduced in HD and these PATs are implicated in the pathogenesis of HD, understanding the nature of their interactions with HTT may guide future efforts to target and enhance this interaction to increase enzyme activity and remediate palmitoylation of HTT and its substrates. These data indicate that HIP14 and HIP14L share a binding site, providing evidence that these two PATs may compensate for each other in palmitoylating HTT and may compete for binding to HTT and other substrates. This needs to be considered when taking efforts to increase the interaction between HTT and HIP14 at the risk of decreasing the interaction with the other, which may have detrimental effects. If HTT acts as an allosteric activator of HIP14 and HIP14L, binding of a small HTT peptide, including the two binding sites, may enhance HIP14 and HIP14L activity in the disease state, which would likely have a beneficial effect by restoring palmitoylation of HTT and other proteins. This would not be possible without knowing which motifs of HTT bind HIP14 and HIP14L and this study brings us much closer to this goal.

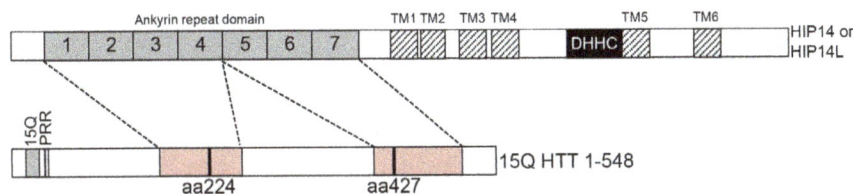

Figure 5. A schematic diagram of the two hypothetical binding scenarios of HTT with HIP14 or HIP14L. In both (**A**) and (**B**) for HIP14 or HIP14L the numbered, solid grey boxes are the seven ankyrin repeats that make up the ankyrin repeat domain, the six TMDs are in hatched boxes labeled TM1–TM6, and the DHHC-CR domain is a black box labeled DHHC. (**A**) In this first scenario, the HIP14 and HIP14L HTT binding site (solid pink box) is between amino acids 224–427 and this binding site interacts with the ankyrin repeat domain of HIP14 or HIP14L. (**B**) In an alternate scenario there are two binding sites (solid pink boxes), one between amino acids 1–427 and the other between amino acids 224–548, that both interact with the ankyrin repeat domain.

Acknowledgments

The authors would like to thank Dr. Elizabeth Conibear, Dr. Dale Martin, and Stefanie Butland for their input on experiment design and interpretation and for advice on the manuscript (Centre for Molecular Medicine and Therapeutics).

Author Contributions

Conceived and designed the experiments: SS LS MH. Performed the experiments: SS LS KM. Analyzed the data: SS LS KM. Wrote the paper: SS.

References

1. Roos RA (2010) Huntington's disease: a clinical review. Orphanet Journal of Rare Diseases 5: 40. doi:10.1186/1750-1172-5-40.

2. Sturrock A, Leavitt BR (2010) The Clinical and Genetic Features of Huntington Disease. Journal of Geriatric Psychiatry and Neurology 23: 243–259. doi:10.1177/0891988710383573.

3. The Huntington's disease collaborative research group (1993) A novel gene containing a trinucleotide repeat that is expanded and unstable on Huntington's disease chromosomes. Cell 72: 971–983.

4. Kalchman MA, Graham RK, Xia G, Koide HB, Hodgson JG, et al. (1996) Huntingtin is ubiquitinated and interacts with a specific ubiquitin-conjugating enzyme. J Biol Chem 271: 19385–19394.

5. Singaraja RR, Hadano S, Metzler M, Givan S, Wellington CL, et al. (2002) HIP14, a novel ankyrin domain-containing protein, links huntingtin to intracellular trafficking and endocytosis. Human Molecular Genetics 11: 2815–2828.

6. Sutton LM, Sanders SS, Butland SL, Singaraja RR, Franciosi S, et al. (2013) Hip14l-deficient mice develop neuropathological and behavioural features of Huntington disease. Human Molecular Genetics 22: 452–465. doi:10.1093/hmg/dds441.

7. Huang K, Yanai A, Kang R, Arstikaitis P, Singaraja RR, et al. (2004) Huntingtin-interacting protein HIP14 is a palmitoyl transferase involved in palmitoylation and trafficking of multiple neuronal proteins. Neuron 44: 977–986. doi:10.1016/j.neuron.2004.11.027.

8. Ohno Y, Kihara A, Sano T, Igarashi Y (2006) Intracellular localization and tissue-specific distribution of human and yeast DHHC cysteine-rich domain-containing proteins. Biochimica et Biophysica Acta (BBA) - Molecular and Cell Biology of Lipids 1761: 474–483. doi:10.1016/j.bbalip.2006.03.010.

9. Hallak H, Muszbek L, Laposata M, Belmonte E, Brass LF, et al. (1994) Covalent binding of arachidonate to G protein alpha subunits of human platelets. J Biol Chem 269: 4713–4716.

10. Smotrys JE, Linder ME (2004) Palmitoylation of Intracellular Signaling Proteins: Regulation and Function. Annu Rev Biochem 73: 559–587. doi:10.1146/annurev.biochem.73.011303.073954.

11. Young FB, Butland SL, Sanders SS, Sutton LM, Hayden MR (2012) Putting proteins in their place: palmitoylation in Huntington disease and other neuropsychiatric diseases. Progress in Neurobiology 97: 220–238. doi:10.1016/j.pneurobio.2011.11.002.

12. Huang K, Sanders SS, Kang R, Carroll JB, Sutton L, et al. (2011) Wild-type HTT modulates the enzymatic activity of the neuronal palmitoyl transferase HIP14. Human Molecular Genetics 20: 3356–3365. doi:10.1093/hmg/ddr242.

13. Yanai A, Huang K, Kang R, Singaraja RR, Arstikaitis P, et al. (2006) Palmitoylation of huntingtin by HIP14 is essential for its trafficking and function. Nat Neurosci 9: 824–831. doi:10.1038/nn1702.

14. Singaraja RR, Huang K, Sanders SS, Milnerwood AJ, Hines R, et al. (2011) Altered palmitoylation and neuropathological deficits in mice lacking HIP14. Human Molecular Genetics 20: 3899–3909. doi:10.1093/hmg/ddr308.

15. Wellington CL, Ellerby LM, Hackam AS, Margolis RL, Trifiro MA, et al. (1998) Caspase cleavage of gene products associated with triplet expansion disorders generates truncated fragments containing the polyglutamine tract. J Biol Chem 273: 9158–9167.

16. Hackam AS, Singaraja R, Wellington CL, Metzler M, McCutcheon K, et al. (1998) The influence of huntingtin protein size on nuclear localization and cellular toxicity. The Journal of Cell Biology 141: 1097–1105.

17. Palidwor GA, Shcherbinin S, Huska MR, Rasko T, Stelzl U, et al. (2009) Detection of alpha-rod protein repeats using a neural network and application to huntingtin. PLoS Comput Biol 5: e1000304. doi:10.1371/journal.pcbi.1000304.

18. Gao T, Collins RE, Horton JR, Zhang X, Zhang R, et al. (2009) The ankyrin repeat domain of Huntingtin interacting protein 14 contains a surface aromatic cage, a potential site for methyl-lysine binding. Proteins 76: 772–777. doi:10.1002/prot.22452.

19. Takano H, Gusella JF (2002) The predominantly HEAT-like motif structure of huntingtin and its association and coincident nuclear entry with dorsal, an NF-kB/Rel/dorsal family transcription factor. BMC Neurosci 3: 15.

20. Seong IS, Woda JM, Song J-J, Lloret A, Abeyrathne PD, et al. (2010) Huntingtin facilitates polycomb repressive complex 2. Human Molecular Genetics 19: 573–583. doi:10.1093/hmg/ddp524.

21. Li W, Serpell LC, Carter WJ, Rubinsztein DC, Huntington JA (2006) Expression and characterization of full-length human huntingtin, an elongated HEAT repeat protein. J Biol Chem 281: 15916–15922. doi:10.1074/jbc.M511007200.

22. Caviston JP, Holzbaur ELF (2009) Huntingtin as an essential integrator of intracellular vesicular trafficking. Trends in Cell Biology 19: 147–155. doi:10.1016/j.tcb.2009.01.005.

4

HD CAGnome: A Search Tool for Huntingtin CAG Repeat Length-Correlated Genes

Ekaterina I. Galkina[1⦿], Aram Shin[1⦿], Kathryn R. Coser[2], Toshi Shioda[2], Isaac S. Kohane[3,4,5], Ihn Sik Seong[1], Vanessa C. Wheeler[1], James F. Gusella[1], Marcy E. MacDonald[1], Jong-Min Lee[1]*

1 Center for Human Genetic Research, Massachusetts General Hospital, Boston, Massachusetts, United States of America, 2 Massachusetts General Hospital Cancer Center, Charlestown, Massachusetts, United States of America, 3 Children's Hospital Informatics program, Children's Hospital, Boston, Massachusetts, United States of America, 4 Center for Biomedical Informatics, Harvard Medical School, Boston, Massachusetts, United States of America, 5 i2b2 National center for Biomedical Computing, Boston, Massachusetts, United States of America

Abstract

Background: The length of the huntingtin (*HTT*) CAG repeat is strongly correlated with both age at onset of Huntington's disease (HD) symptoms and age at death of HD patients. Dichotomous analysis comparing HD to controls is widely used to study the effects of *HTT* CAG repeat expansion. However, a potentially more powerful approach is a continuous analysis strategy that takes advantage of all of the different CAG lengths, to capture effects that are expected to be critical to HD pathogenesis.

Methodology/Principal Findings: We used continuous and dichotomous approaches to analyze microarray gene expression data from 107 human control and HD lymphoblastoid cell lines. Of all probes found to be significant in a continuous analysis by CAG length, only 21.4% were so identified by a dichotomous comparison of HD versus controls. Moreover, of probes significant by dichotomous analysis, only 33.2% were also significant in the continuous analysis. Simulations revealed that the dichotomous approach would require substantially more than 107 samples to either detect 80% of the CAG-length correlated changes revealed by continuous analysis or to reduce the rate of significant differences that are not CAG length-correlated to 20% (n = 133 or n = 206, respectively). Given the superior power of the continuous approach, we calculated the correlation structure between *HTT* CAG repeat lengths and gene expression levels and created a freely available searchable website, "HD CAGnome," that allows users to examine continuous relationships between *HTT* CAG and expression levels of ~20,000 human genes.

Conclusions/Significance: Our results reveal limitations of dichotomous approaches compared to the power of continuous analysis to study a disease where human genotype-phenotype relationships strongly support a role for a continuum of CAG length-dependent changes. The compendium of *HTT* CAG length-gene expression level relationships found at the HD CAGnome now provides convenient routes for discovery of candidates influenced by the HD mutation.

Editor: David R. Borchelt, University of Florida, United States of America

Funding: This work was supported by grants from CHDI Foundation, Inc. and theNational Institutes of Health (NS16367, NINDS Massachusetts HD Center Without Walls (J.F.G.& M.E.M.), NS32765 (M.E.M.), NS049206 (V.C.W.), and LM008748 NLM i2b2 (I.S.K.)). The funders had no role in study design, data collection and analysis, decision to publish, or preparation of the manuscript.

Competing Interests: The authors have declared that no competing interests exist.

* E-mail: jlee51@mgh.harvard.edu

⦿ These authors contributed equally to this work.

Introduction

Huntington's disease (HD, OMIM # 143100) is an autosomal dominant neurodegenerative disorder caused by an expansion of a polymorphic CAG trinucleotide repeat in the first exon of huntingtin (*HTT*), the gene encoding huntingtin protein [1]. There is a strong inverse correlation of both age at onset of motor symptoms and age at death with the *HTT* CAG repeat length in HD subjects [1,2,3,4,5,6]. This continuous correlative relationship strongly supports a role for dominant CAG length-dependent mechanisms in determining the rate of disease processes that result in manifestation of neurological symptoms. In addition, the continuous relationships between *HTT* CAG repeat lengths and molecular energy phenotypes also extend across the range of

expanded disease alleles and into the normal *HTT* CAG repeat range (CAG<36), in a panel of blood-derived lymphoblastoid cell lines [7]. These suggested that the *HTT* CAG repeat is a functional polymorphism directly associated with an alteration of huntingtin function that leads eventually to disease phenotypes. These and other genotype-related phenotypes are also observed in induced pluripotent stem cell derived neuronal cell lines [8]. Thus, identifying biological processes that are influenced by the *HTT* CAG repeat in a length-dependent manner will significantly inform the molecular mechanisms underlying HD, and thereby, facilitate the development of effective treatments.

As a part of our ongoing efforts to comprehensively optimize the discovery of *HTT* CAG repeat length-dependent molecular changes, we undertook a global and unbiased approach to identify genes whose expression levels were continuously correlated with *HTT* CAG repeat lengths. We chose to study a panel of 107 human lymphoblastoid cell lines derived from HD subjects and normal controls, as there are currently many more such lines available than any other standardized cell types, making it possible to include samples to achieve a broad and continuous spectrum of CAG lengths. Although the effects of the *HTT* CAG repeat on gene expression in lymphoblastoid cells were relatively modest, a significant amount of variance in gene expression was attributable to the *HTT* CAG repeat length [9]. These findings indicated that: 1) *HTT* CAG repeat length-correlated gene expression changes exist, and 2) continuous analysis was able to identify *HTT* CAG repeat length-dependent molecular signals from other factors contributing noise, including genetic heterogeneity of the study subjects, thereby demonstrating the power of continuous analytical strategies. In addition, continuous analysis was able to detect modest but significant correlations between *HTT* CAG repeat lengths and genes that were not significant in a dichotomous analytical comparison, supporting the sensitivity of continuous analysis approaches. Taken together, these results demonstrated the power of continuous analysis strategies to capture *HTT* CAG length-correlated gene-expression signatures that conform to the criteria expected for effects of the mechanism that contribute to the HD disease process.

Despite their relevance to HD, continuous analysis approaches are not widely used in the HD field. Instead, dichotomous analysis methods comparing HD to normal controls are more widespread. We hypothesize that dichotomous analysis methods are not optimal for investigating HD where *HTT* CAG repeat length-correlated alterations are strongly implicated in playing an important role in HD pathogenesis. Thus, we performed a continuous analysis and a dichotomous analysis on the same data set comprising microarray gene expression data of 107 human lymphoblastoid cell lines derived from HD and normal controls. We then compared the results to evaluate the sensitivity and specificity of the dichotomous analysis method, relative to the continuous method based upon CAG length. In addition, based upon those results, we created a searchable internet website, HD CAGnome, where users can evaluate the relationships between genes of interest and *HTT* CAG repeat length in both continuous and dichotomous contexts.

Materials and Methods

Gene Expression Dataset

Gene expression profile data were generated from 107 Epstein–Barr virus-transformed human lymphoblastoid cell lines, which were maintained internally at the Massachusetts General Hospital. These cell lines were derived from 105 independent subjects, comprising 41 normal control samples (CAG<36) and 66 HD samples (CAG>35) [9]. The mean sizes of the longer and shorter alleles were 40.9 and 17.6 CAGs, respectively. The range of the longer alleles was 15–92. Cells were grown in RPMI-1640 media supplemented with 10% fetal bovine serum, 100 I.U./ml Penicillin, and 100 I.U./ml Streptomycin at 37°C. The *HTT* CAG repeat allele lengths for each sample were determined by a polymerase chain reaction assay, against sequenced allele size standards, as described previously [10]. For all analyses, only the longer CAG allele was utilized, as the shorter allele has been demonstrated not to contribute to HD age at onset [4]. For microarray gene expression profiling experiments, total RNA was extracted using TRIzol reagent (Invitrogen) and further purified using a RNeasy kit (Qiagen). All RNA samples passed quality

control by 260/280 ratio (NanoDrop) and 28S/18S ratio (Agilent Bioanalyzer assay). Total RNA (5 μg) was converted into cDNA using SuperScript II reverse transcriptase (Invitrogen) and labeled probe was synthesized by Single-Round RNA Amplification and Biotin Labeling System (Enzo). Labeled probe (25 μg) was hybridized to Affymetrix U133+2 arrays as recommended by the manufacturer. All microarray data were processed together for background correction and normalization using gcRMA (R, 2.11.1; gcrma, 2.20.0) followed by batch effect correction [11].

Statistical Analysis

We analyzed microarray expression data using two different approaches. For the continuous analysis approach, we performed 1) a Pearson's correlation test and 2) a Spearman's rank correlation test to evaluate the strength and significance of the continuous relationship between CAG repeat length and expression level of a given gene. Based on dominance in HD, we primarily used the length of longer CAG repeat in a given subject to calculate the strength of correlation with gene expression levels. In addition, due to the fact that the longer CAG repeat is highly correlated with the sum of two CAGs in our samples, we observed a high degree of similarity between two sets of correlation coefficients based on 1) the longer CAG or 2) the sum of CAGs. Therefore, we presented the results using the longer CAG repeat. The continuous analysis results are presented in a scatter plot and summary statistics of correlation tests in the HD CAGnome website. For the dichotomous analysis approach, we performed a Student's t-test, comparing HD (66 samples; CAG>35) to normal controls (41 samples, CAG<36) to determine whether the expression level of a gene in HD differs significantly from that in normal controls. Similarly, a box plot and a summary statistics table are presented in the HD CAGnome website. All computational and statistical analyses were performed using R (version 2.11.1).

Comparison of Continuous Analysis Results to those of Dichotomous Analysis

In order to estimate from dichotomous analysis 1) what percentage of CAG-length correlated probes were detected and 2) what percentage of probes predicted as significant were in fact not CAG-length correlated, we randomly selected variable numbers of HD and normal samples from our dataset and calculated the significance level of each probe using Student's t-test. These procedures were repeated 1,000 times for each sample size analysis. We varied the sample size from 3 to 41; for example, the first set of comparisons compared 3 randomly selected HD samples to 3 randomly selected normal samples (n = 3), the second set of comparisons compared 4 randomly selected HD samples to 4 randomly selected normal samples (n = 4), and so on. Since our dataset had 41 normal control samples but 66 HD samples, we compared up to 41 HD and 41 normal samples (n = 41). In each iteration, p-values of nominally significant probes were recorded and compared to p-values of the same probes obtained from continuous analysis by CAG length of all samples using the Pearson's correlation test. We calculated 1) the fraction of all probes significant in the continuous analysis that were also significant by dichotomous analysis (i.e., continuous dichotomous shared), 2) the fraction of all probes significant in the continuous analysis that were not significant by dichotomous analysis (i.e., continuous specific), and 3) the fraction of all probes significant in the dichotomous analysis that were not significant in the continuous analysis (i.e., dichotomous specific). Based on these results, statistical models were constructed in order to understand relationships between parameters and to predict the sample sizes that allow dichotomous analysis to detect 80% of the positives from continuous analysis and to reduce the rate of predicting differences that are not significant in the continuous analysis to 20%. Although relationships may not be linear, linear models were used because parametric models provide convenient tools for extrapolation, and linear models generated model fits with high R-squared values.

Website Construction

For each gene, the gene name, official HUGO symbol, and Affymetrix probe set ID are dynamically generated via Perl CGI scripts and presented. Pre-computed summary statistics and plots are presented upon user's input and selection. All raw data and normalized data are available at Gene Expression Omnibus (GSE34721). In addition, normalized data with summary statistics are available for download from HD CAGnome.

Results

We performed continuous analysis and dichotomous analysis, respectively, to identify genes whose expression levels were correlated with *HTT* CAG repeat length (Pearson's correlation test) or whose expression levels were significantly different between HD (CAG>35) and controls (CAG<36) (Student's t-test). Figure 1 summarizes characteristics of overall test statistics from continuous analysis (Fig. 1A and 1B) and dichotomous analysis (Fig. 1C and 1D). The range of Pearson's correlation coefficients in the continuous analysis was -0.431 to 0.396 (Fig. 1A), and the p-value of the most significantly correlated probe was 0.00000358 (Fig. 1B). In the dichotomous analysis, the range of fold-change was -2.33 to 2.39 (Fig. 1C), and the most significant p-value was 0.0000536 (Fig. 1D). Comparison of observed p-values to expected p-values based on the uniform distribution revealed that the overall test statistics were not inflated in either the continuous analysis (Fig. 2A) or the dichotomous analysis (Fig. 2B). Comparison of Pearson's correlation coefficients in the continuous analysis to fold-changes in the dichotomous analysis showed that 77% of microarray probes showed the same direction of change (Fig. 3A; top-right and bottom-left quadrants), and 23% of microarray probes showed an opposite direction of change (Fig. 3A; top-left and bottom-right quadrants). In addition, significance levels for probes in the continuous analysis showed a modest correlation with those in the dichotomous analysis (Fig. 3B), suggesting overall similarity between the continuous analysis results and the dichotomous analysis results.

Next, we compared significant probes. Nominal p-value of 0.01 was used to identify significant genes in each analysis. 718 microarray probes were significantly correlated with *HTT* CAG repeat length in the continuous analysis (315 probes with positive correlation and 403 probes with negative correlation). 464 probes were significant in the dichotomous analysis (175 increase in HD and 289 decrease in HD). Between significant probes in continuous analysis and those in dichotomous analysis, 154 probes were shared as shown in Fig. 4A. Probes significant in both analyses showed consistent direction of change (Fig. 4B). For example, 52 probes that showed nominally significant positive correlation with *HTT* CAG repeat length were significantly increased in HD compared to normal controls; 102 probes that were negatively correlated with *HTT* CAG repeat length also showed decreased expression levels in HD (Fig. 4B). Considering that truly correlated genes must necessarily show differences in dichotomous analysis, these observations indicate that statistics from correlation analysis and dichotomous analysis for commonly

significant genes were not significantly affected by a subset of influential data points.

Next, we evaluated potential limitations of the dichotomous analysis strategy in HD where the importance of continuous changes is strongly supported by human genotype-phenotype relationships. We calculated two metrics of dichotomous analysis: 1) the percentage of the probes significant in continuous CAG-length analysis that were also significant in dichotomous analysis, 21.4% (and by subtraction, the percentage not detected) and 2) the percentage of probes that were significant in the dichotomous analysis but not in the continuous analysis, 66.8%. Thus, the dichotomous analysis failed to identify 78.6% of the significant differences detected by continuous analysis, and only 33.2% of the genes detected by dichotomous analysis actually showed significant correlation with CAG length.

We predicted that dichotomous analysis may show even poorer performance when the sample size is small. To test this prediction, we performed simulation experiments employing dichotomous analyses on variable numbers of randomly selected samples, and determined the effect of sample size on the above metrics. For each random sampling, we performed dichotomous analysis utilizing Student's t-test and calculated the metrics by comparing to the results of all sample correlation analysis. For each sample size, starting with n = 3 (i.e., 3 HD vs. 3 controls) and ending with n = 41 (i.e., 41 HD vs. 41 controls), the dichotomous analysis and comparison to the all sample continuous analysis were repeated 1,000 times. Figure 5 shows variation in the two metrics with sample size, where the frequency of the percentages is represented as smoothed color density in which darker color represents higher frequency. For a given sample size, the outcomes were quite variable, but there was a clear trend for increased sample size in the dichotomous analysis to result in detection of a higher percentage of the significant differences from continuous analysis. Similarly, increasing sample size in the dichotomous analysis also resulted in a decrease in the percentage of genes seen to be significant in the dichotomous analysis but not the continuous analysis. Since we were interested in determining efficiency of dichotomous analysis approaches in capturing the continuous effects of *HTT* CAG repeat lengths on gene expression, we constructed regression models based on the simulation analysis (Fig. 5; red lines). Then we estimated the number of samples that would be required to achieve two arbitrarily selected performance criteria for the dichotomous analysis: 1) identification of 80% of the significant differences detected in continuous analysis and, 2) a yield of only 20% of differences predicted as significant that are actually non-significant by continuous analysis. By extrapolating models, we estimated that approximately 133 and 206 samples in each group would be required to achieve these respective limits, indicating that analysis in a dichotomous fashion requires significantly more samples than continuous analysis to capture the CAG-length correlated effects of the *HTT* repeat on gene expression (Fig. 5). Taken together, these results reveal potential limitations of dichotomous analytical approaches in studying the effects of a mutation/polymorphism with a continuum of lengths, reinforcing the importance of the use of appropriate analytical approaches in HD and potentially in other of the growing number of triplet repeat expansion disorders.

Finally, we created a searchable website (HD CAGnome) to encourage the application of continuous analysis approaches in HD by presenting correlation analysis results from our microarray gene expression data analysis. The web interface (Fig. 6) supports two options: 1) entering a human gene symbol in the search window or 2) browsing a list of genes. Selecting a gene using the search window and browse function retrieves identical informa-

A

B

C

D

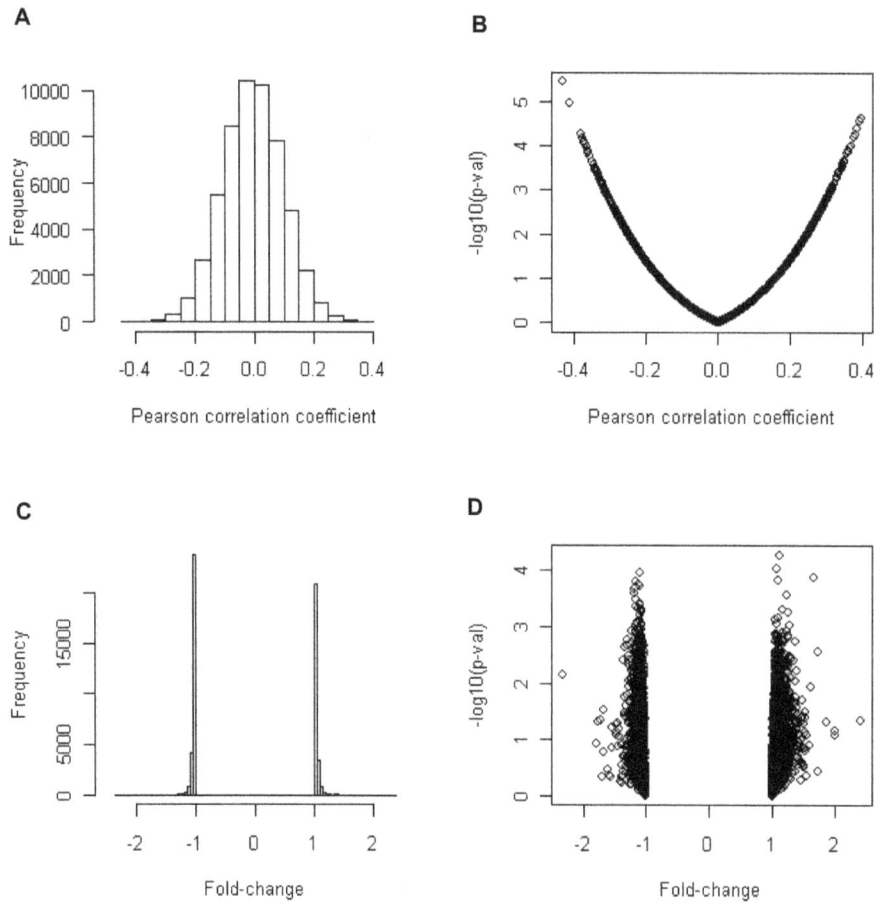

Figure 1. Overall characteristics of continuous and dichotomous analysis results. Pearson's correlation test was performed for continuous analysis. The distribution of correlation coefficient (A) and correlation coefficient vs. significance (i.e., −log10(p-value)) (B) were plotted. For dichotomous analysis, Student's-t test was used, and the distribution of fold-changes (C) and fold-change vs. significance (−log10(p-value)) (D) were plotted.

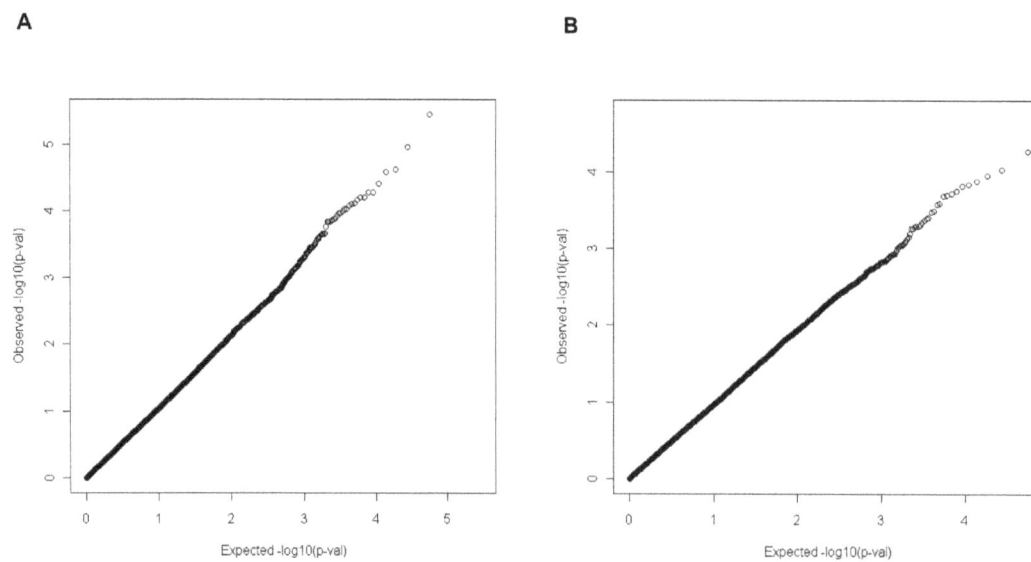

A

B

Figure 2. Quantile-quantile plot. Expected p-values assuming a uniform distribution (X-axis; expected −log10(p-value)) were compared to observed p-values (Y-axis; observed −log10(p-value)) in the continuous analysis (A) and dichotomous analysis (B) to evaluate the levels of inflation in test statistics. Expected p-values were calculated based on the uniform distribution assuming each test was independent of others.

A

B

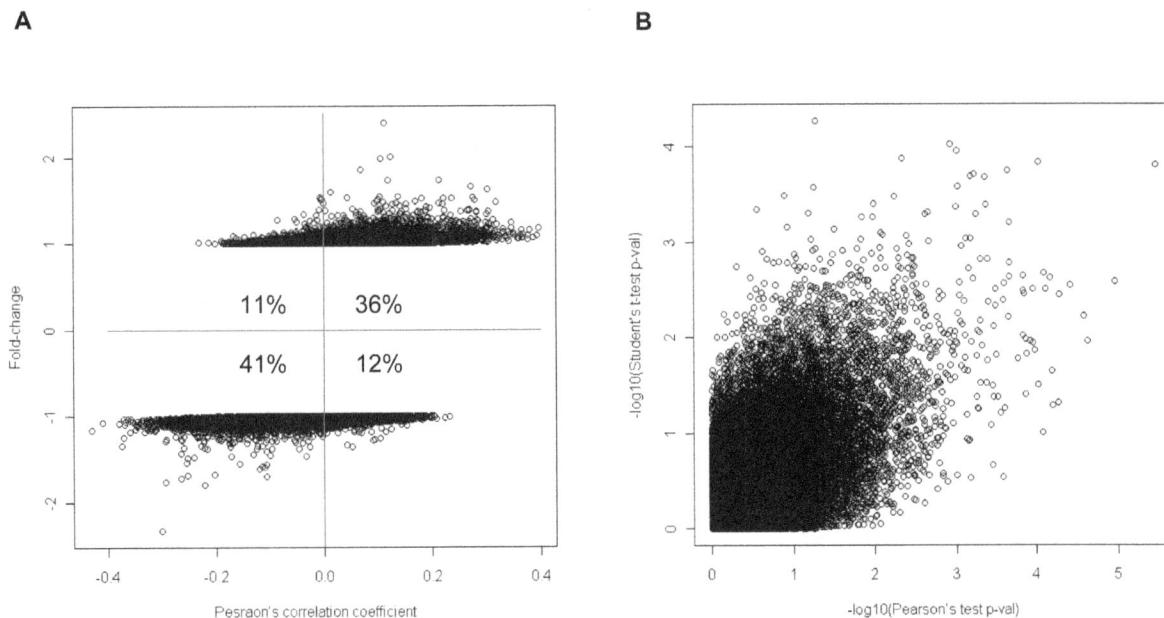

Figure 3. Comparison of test statistics. (A) Pearson's correlation coefficients in the continuous analysis were compared to fold-changes in the dichotomous analysis to evaluate overall similarity in direction of changes between two analytical methods. The number in each quadrant represents the percentage of probes relative to all probes analyzed. (B) Significance levels in the continuous analysis ($-\log10$(Pearson's test p-value); X-axis) were compared to those in the dichotomous analysis ($-\log10$(Student's t-test p-value); Y-axis) in order to evaluate overall similarity in significance between two analytical methods.

tion. The link to the HUGO Gene Nomenclature Committee (HGNC) is provided as a resource for obtaining the symbol of a gene of interest. The search results in HD CAGnome will show the full gene names, official gene symbols, Entrez IDs, and Affymetrix probe IDs. Primarily, HD CAGnome was designed to provide information concerning the correlation structure between gene expression levels and *HTT* CAG repeat length. The results (scatter plot) of the summary statistics from continuous analyses (Pearson's correlation analysis and Spearman's correlation analysis) are presented in the left side of the window. A box plot with summary

statistics of dichotomous analysis (Student's t-test) is also presented in the right side of window. HD CAGnome is freely available for online searching and downloading at http://chgr.partners.org/cagnome.cgi.

Discussion

The strong negative correlation between age at onset of HD motor symptoms and *HTT* CAG repeat size supports a role for CAG length-dependent continuous mechanisms in determining

A

B

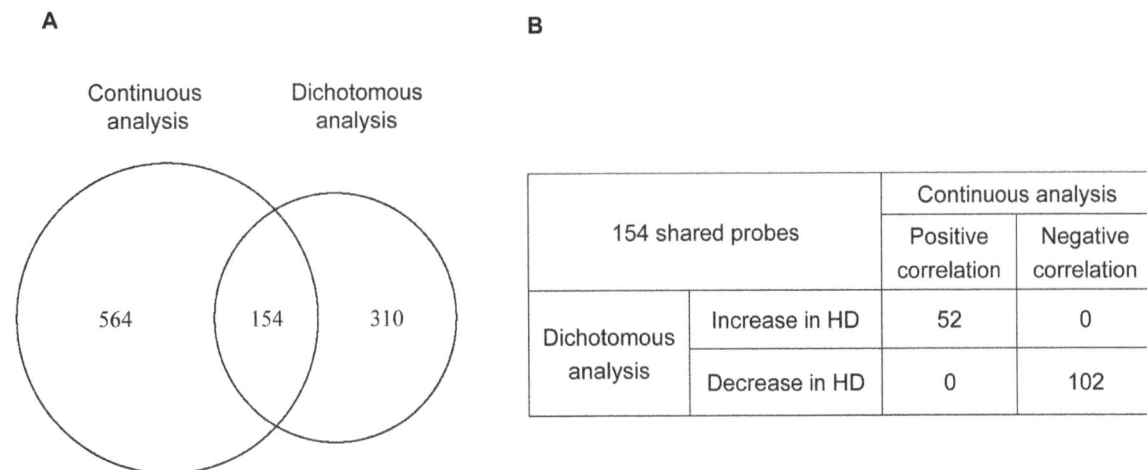

154 shared probes		Continuous analysis	
		Positive correlation	Negative correlation
Dichotomous analysis	Increase in HD	52	0
	Decrease in HD	0	102

Figure 4. Significant probes in continuous and dichotomous analysis. Pearson's correlation test and Student's-t test were used for continuous and dichotomous analysis, respectively. (A) From left to right, numbers in Venn diagram indicate the number of probes significant only in continuous analysis, probes significant in both continuous and dichotomous analysis, and probes significant only in dichotomous analysis by p-value cut-off of 0.01. We did not observe differences between shared genes and specific genes in terms of p-values, correlation coefficients, and fold-changes. (B) Probes significant in both analyses (154 probes) were further categorized based on the correlation coefficient and fold-change.

A

B

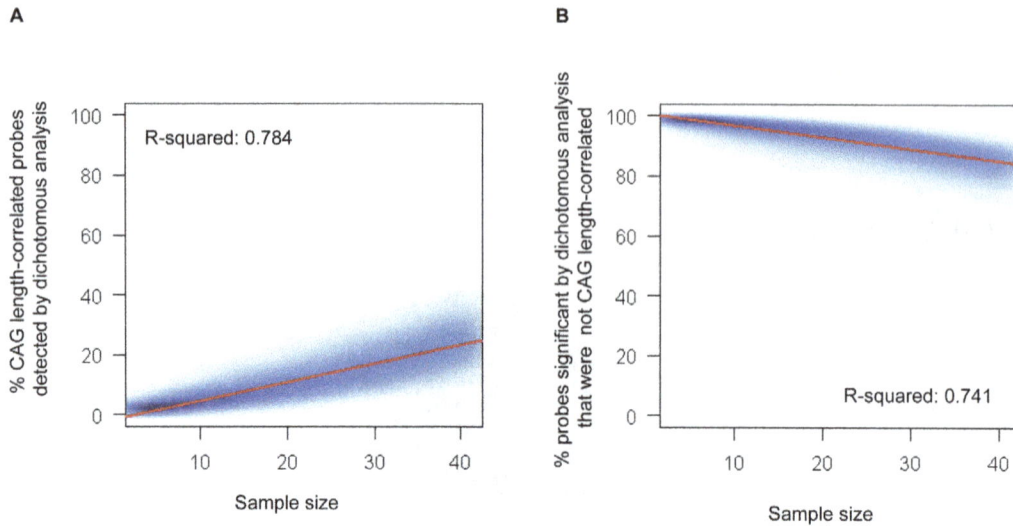

Figure 5. Efficiency of dichotomous analysis in capturing significantly correlated genes. From 107 samples, we randomly selected equal numbers (n = 3 to 41) of HD and controls to perform dichotomous analysis, repeating 1,000 times for each sample size, and compared to continuous CAG length analysis, as described in the text and methods, plotting the resulting percentages in scatter density plots. (A) Variation in the percentage of CAG-length correlated significant differences from continuous analysis that are detected by dichotomous analysis vs. sample size. (B) Variation in the percentage of differences judged significant by dichotomous analysis that are not CAG-length correlated by continuous analysis vs. sample size. Red lines represent linear regression models describing the relationship between sample size and the corresponding performance metric.

the rate of the underlying disease process in HD. However, dichotomous analysis comparing HD versus normal controls is a standard in the field, where differences in the *HTT* CAG repeat length between expanded alleles are rarely taken into account [12,13,14,15,16,17,18]. Based upon the knowledge that the rate-determining processes in pathogenesis leading to diagnostic onset are dependent on the *HTT* CAG repeat length, we predicted that dichotomous analytical methods have a lower sensitivity in identifying important biological changes that are relevant to HD compared to continuous analytical methods. To test this prediction, we compared a set of *HTT* CAG repeat length-correlated

genes to differentially expressed genes, and observed a minimal overlap between nominally significant genes in continuous and dichotomous analysis. As the *HTT* CAG repeat length-correlated genes fulfill the genetic criteria for being associated with the pathogenic process in HD, these findings suggested that dichotomous analysis likely generates results with significant false negatives and false positives that could confound further investigation. In addition, sample size directly influenced the levels of such false negative and false positive metrics in the dichotomous analysis, i.e., an increase of sample size by 10 (10 HD and 10 controls) had the effect of decreasing the corresponding metrics by

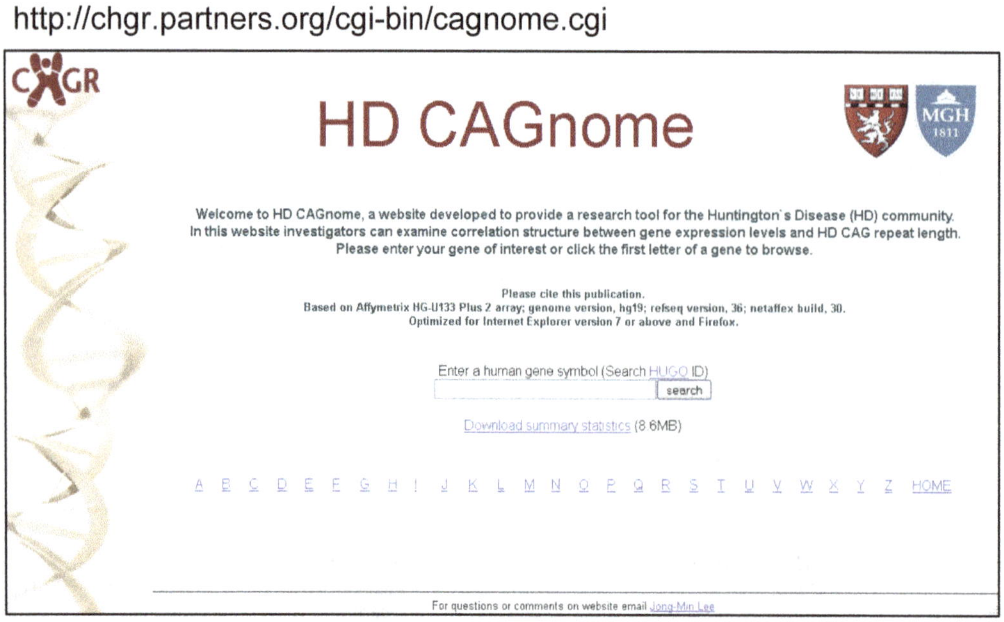

http://chgr.partners.org/cgi-bin/cagnome.cgi

Figure 6. HD CAGnome. HD CAGnome is accessible at http://chgr.partners.org/cgi-bin/cagnome.cgi.

6% and 4%, respectively. These observations imply that dichotomous analysis of HD will reveal *HTT* CAG repeat length-dependent changes only with significantly larger sample sizes.

Gene expression can be influenced by many factors, both genetic and environmental. We recently showed using a continuous analysis of microarray gene expression data that ~20% of variance in gene expression could be attributed to *HTT* CAG repeat length [9]. Together with the relative performance of dichotomous analysis in these experiments, the modest size of this CAG length effect suggests that most of the differences significant by dichotomous analysis are 'noise'. Pathway analysis, gene set enrichment analysis, and network analysis are popular in the field because the power and sensitivity would be increased if properly performed based on correct and unbiased gene level analysis results. However, we predict that such limitations of dichotomous analytical methods may result in elevated inaccuracy when genome-wide scale large data are analyzed by this approach since the inherent high rate of false positives would be compounded in subsequent pathway and molecular network analyses, reducing their reliability. Understanding how cells modulate the expression of genes in response to the expanded *HTT* CAG repeats is important as this can provide insights into underlying mechanisms and pathways of HD. In addition, genes with altered levels of expression are of great utility as HD biomarkers. As we described previously, the *HTT* CAG repeat length has a modest impact on the gene expression [9], indicating that analysis with insufficient power may generate significant numbers of false negatives. In addition, highly heterogeneous nature of human subjects poses a challenge to the discovery of genes whose expression levels are altered in blood and brains of HD subjects [12,13,17]. In this context, the use of CAG repeat length as a continuous variable may reduce false discoveries because influences of confounding factors on statistical models would be reduced in a continuous analysis.

In summary, our analysis reveals that there are potential limitations in using dichotomous analysis approaches when studying HD, especially when the number of samples may be constrained by the availability of a given tissue or cell type. Knowledge from direct comparisons between continuous and dichotomous analysis results is important as this will provide guidelines for molecular studies aiming at investigating the *HTT* CAG repeat length-dependent changes, for example in choosing samples that represent a full-spectrum of CAG repeat lengths. Motivated by these findings, we created a website, namely 'HD CAGnome' that can be used to examine the strength and direction of correlation between *HTT* CAG repeat length and expression levels of a given gene. We also provide a summary of dichotomous analysis results so users can compare two results. We believe that this novel resource will provide convenient ways of evaluating correlation structure of candidate genes and generating new hypotheses, that may be tested in other cell types, including neuronal cells, and tissue samples, for example studies with postmortem brain tissue. Therefore, our findings presented in HD CAGnome will facilitate the use of analytical approaches that are relevant to HD and contribute to identifying genes that can be used for therapeutic treatments and/or biomarkers.

Author Contributions

Conceived and designed the experiments: JML JFG MEM. Performed the experiments: KRC TS. Analyzed the data: EIG AS JML. Contributed reagents/materials/analysis tools: EIG JML. Wrote the paper: EIG AS ISK ISS VCW JFG MEM JML.

References

1. HDCRG (1993) A novel gene containing a trinucleotide repeat that is expanded and unstable on Huntington's disease chromosomes. The Huntington's Disease Collaborative Research Group. Cell 72: 971–983.
2. Andrew SE, Goldberg YP, Kremer B, Telenius H, Theilmann J, et al. (1993) The relationship between trinucleotide (CAG) repeat length and clinical features of Huntington's disease. Nat Genet 4: 398–403.
3. Duyao M, Ambrose C, Myers R, Novelletto A, Persichetti F, et al. (1993) Trinucleotide repeat length instability and age of onset in Huntington's disease. Nat Genet 4: 387–392.
4. Lee JM, Ramos EM, Lee JH, Gillis T, Mysore JS, et al. (2012) CAG repeat expansion in Huntington disease determines age at onset in a fully dominant fashion. Neurology 78: 690–695.
5. Persichetti F, Srinidhi J, Kanaley L, Ge P, Myers RH, et al. (1994) Huntington's disease CAG trinucleotide repeats in pathologically confirmed post-mortem brains. Neurobiol Dis 1: 159–166.
6. Snell RG, MacMillan JC, Cheadle JP, Fenton I, Lazarou LP, et al. (1993) Relationship between trinucleotide repeat expansion and phenotypic variation in Huntington's disease. Nat Genet 4: 393–397.
7. Seong IS, Ivanova E, Lee JM, Choo YS, Fossale E, et al. (2005) HD CAG repeat implicates a dominant property of huntingtin in mitochondrial energy metabolism. Hum Mol Genet 14: 2871–2880.
8. Consortium THi (2012) Induced pluripotent stem cells from patients with Huntington's disease show CAG-repeat-expansion-associated phenotypes. Cell Stem Cell 11: 264–278.
9. Lee JM, Galkina EI, Levantovsky RM, Fossale E, Anne Anderson M, et al. (2013) Dominant effects of the Huntington's disease HTT CAG repeat length are captured in gene-expression data sets by a continuous analysis mathematical modeling strategy. Hum Mol Genet 22: 3227–3238.
10. Perlis RH, Smoller JW, Mysore J, Sun M, Gillis T, et al. Prevalence of incompletely penetrant Huntington's disease alleles among individuals with major depressive disorder. Am J Psychiatry 167: 574–579.
11. Johnson WE, Li C, Rabinovic A (2007) Adjusting batch effects in microarray expression data using empirical Bayes methods. Biostatistics 8: 118–127.
12. Borovecki F, Lovrecic L, Zhou J, Jeong H, Then F, et al. (2005) Genome-wide expression profiling of human blood reveals biomarkers for Huntington's disease. Proc Natl Acad Sci U S A 102: 11023–11028.
13. Hodges A, Strand AD, Aragaki AK, Kuhn A, Sengstag T, et al. (2006) Regional and cellular gene expression changes in human Huntington's disease brain. Hum Mol Genet 15: 965–977.
14. Kuhn A, Goldstein DR, Hodges A, Strand AD, Sengstag T, et al. (2007) Mutant huntingtin's effects on striatal gene expression in mice recapitulate changes observed in human Huntington's disease brain and do not differ with mutant huntingtin length or wild-type huntingtin dosage. Hum Mol Genet 16: 1845–1861.
15. Luthi-Carter R, Hanson SA, Strand AD, Bergstrom DA, Chun W, et al. (2002) Dysregulation of gene expression in the R6/2 model of polyglutamine disease: parallel changes in muscle and brain. Hum Mol Genet 11: 1911–1926.
16. Luthi-Carter R, Strand AD, Hanson SA, Kooperberg C, Schilling G, et al. (2002) Polyglutamine and transcription: gene expression changes shared by DRPLA and Huntington's disease mouse models reveal context-independent effects. Hum Mol Genet 11: 1927–1937.
17. Runne H, Kuhn A, Wild EJ, Pratyaksha W, Kristiansen M, et al. (2007) Analysis of potential transcriptomic biomarkers for Huntington's disease in peripheral blood. Proc Natl Acad Sci U S A 104: 14424–14429.
18. Strand AD, Baquet ZC, Aragaki AK, Holmans P, Yang L, et al. (2007) Expression profiling of Huntington's disease models suggests that brain-derived neurotrophic factor depletion plays a major role in striatal degeneration. J Neurosci 27: 11758–11768.

5

Transplantation of Induced Pluripotent Stem Cells Improves Functional Recovery in Huntington's Disease Rat Model

Shuhua Mu[1,2◐], **Jiachuan Wang**[2◐], **Guangqian Zhou**[2], **Wenda Peng**[1], **Zhendan He**[2], **Zhenfu Zhao**[2], **CuiPing Mo**[2], **Junle Qu**[1]*, **Jian Zhang**[1,2]*

1 College of Optoelectronics Engineering, Shenzhen University, Shenzhen, China, **2** School of Medicine, Shenzhen University, Shenzhen, China

Abstract

The purpose of this study was to determine the functional recovery of the transplanted induced pluripotent stem cells in a rat model of Huntington's disease with use of ^{18}F-FDG microPET/CT imaging.

Methods: In a quinolinic acid-induced rat model of striatal degeneration, induced pluripotent stem cells were transplanted into the ipsilateral lateral ventricle ten days after the quinolinic acid injection. The response to the treatment was evaluated by serial ^{18}F-FDG PET/CT scans and Morris water maze test. Histological analyses and Western blotting were performed six weeks after stem cell transplantation.

Results: After induced pluripotent stem cells transplantation, higher ^{18}F-FDG accumulation in the injured striatum was observed during the 4 to 6-weeks period compared with the quinolinic acid-injected group, suggesting the metabolic recovery of injured striatum. The induced pluripotent stem cells transplantation improved learning and memory function (and striatal atrophy) of the rat in six week in the comparison with the quinolinic acid-treated controls. In addition, immunohistochemical analysis demonstrated that transplanted stem cells survived and migrated into the lesioned area in striatum, and most of the stem cells expressed protein markers of neurons and glial cells.

Conclusion: Our findings show that induced pluripotent stem cells can survive, differentiate to functional neurons and improve partial striatal function and metabolism after implantation in a rat Huntington's disease model.

Editor: Dinender K. Singla, University of Central Florida, United States of America

Funding: This research was supported by the National Science Foundation of China (No. 81301063), which URL is http://www.nsfc.gov.cn/. The funders played no role in study design, data collection and analysis, decision to publish, or preparation of the manuscript.

Competing Interests: The authors have declared that no competing interests exist.

* Email: jlqu70@gmail.com (JQ); jzhanghappy@163.com (JZ)

◐ These authors contributed equally to this work.

Introduction

Huntington's disease (HD) is characterized by the expansion of CAG repeats in the huntingtin gene and the loss of medium spiny neurons in the striatum, resulting in progressive cognitive impairment, neuropsychiatric symptoms, and involuntary choreiform movements [1]. The neuropathological changes in HD are selective and progressive degeneration of striatal GABAergic medium spiny projection neurons [2]. Intrastriatal injection of an excitotoxin such as quinolinic acid (QA) mimics some of the pathology of HD, including the loss of projection GABAergic neurons with a relative preservation of interneurons, and allows for the study of therapeutics, such as transplantation [3,4]. Currently, there is no proven medical therapy to alleviate the onset or progression of Huntington's disease [5].

The clinical uses of cell replacement therapy in neurodegenerative diseases have been investigated for the last 20 years. Although the procedures are theoretically feasible, some limitations of the therapy still give cause for concern [6]. The transplantation of fetal striatal tissue to the striatum to modify HD progression in humans has been investigated, and some favorable effects have been found [7,8], but it does not alter the toxic effects of mutant huntingtin and has difficulties in tissue availability and viability, high risk of rejection, ethical arguments and concerns about contamination and heterogeneity of the tissues [9].

One solution to above problems may be to use induced pluripotent stem cells (iPSCs). The projected use of iPSC derivative cell types in cell-based therapies offers unique advantages over the use of many adult stem cell types with respect to limited proliferation capacity and donor availability, and where patient matched cells may overcome the vexing issues of immune rejection associated with human cell transplantation treatments [6,10]. iPSCs can be generated by transduction of defined transcription factors from adult somatic cells through reprogram ming and have been differentiated in vitro into the early neural stem cell stage or the neural lineage, including neurons and glial cells [11]. More recently, iPSCs have been applied to a variety of nervous system disease, including stroke [11,12], spinal cord injury [13,14] and Parkinson disease [15,16]. However, to better understand the in vivo behavior and efficacy of iPSCs, a noninvasive, sensitive, and clinically applicable approach for tracking the transplanted iPSCs and monitoring the therapeutic response in living subjects needs to be developed.

PET is one of the best-suited modalities to evaluate stem cell therapy, since it can be used in patients clinically for both cell trafficking and monitoring the response to therapy [17,18]. PET studies of patients with HD demonstrate a dramatic loss of striatal glucose metabolism, even in presymptomatic stages [19,20]. PET can also be used to detect the subtle changes of glucose metabolism in vivo after stem cell therapy in various neurologic disease models, including traumatic brain injury [21], Parkinson disease [22], and Huntington disease [4]. To highly precise measurement of the FDG uptake in injured striatum, PET imaging in combination with contrast-enhanced CT was used in this study.

The aims of the present study were to investigate whether transplanted iPSC migrated and survived in QA-injured striatum of rats, improving functional and metabolic deficits of striatum, and whether ^{18}F-FDG PET imaging can monitor the improvement of cerebral energy metabolism in the striatum of rat model of HD.

Materials and Methods

1. Experimental design and animal groups

All animal procedures were performed according to the National Institutes of Health Guide for the Care and Use of Laboratory Animals and were approved by the Guangdong Medical Laboratory Animal Center Institutional Animal Care and Use Committee. Sprague-Dawley rats were housed with a 12-h light/dark cycle and *ad libitum* access to food and water. 24 adult Sprague-Dawley male rats (body weight, 250–280 g) were randomly assigned to one of the following three experimental groups (eitht per group): the iPSC transplantation group (rats received both QA injection and iPSC transplantation, QA+iPSC), the QA injection group (rats received both QA injection and PBS transplantation, QA+PBS), and the control group (rats received only saline injection). The stem cell transplantation or PBS injection was performed 10 d after QA lesions. The Morris water maze task was performed at 5 weeks after cell transplantation. ^{18}F-FDG small-animal PET/CT scans were performed before stem cell transplantation and at weeks 1, 2, 4, and 6 after cell transplantation. Animals were then sacrificed for histological, immunohistochemical (n = 4) and Western blot (n = 4) analysis.

2. Striatal quinolinic acid lesions

Unilateral lesions of the left striatum were achieved by intrastriatal injection of QA. Rats were anesthetized with a solution of ketamine (75 mg/kg) and xylazine (12.5 mg/kg). QA (Sigma) injections were made with the help of a Kopf stereotactic apparatus. Each rat was injected with 100 nmol of QA dissolved in 1 μl of saline into the left striatum at the following coordinates: 1.2 mm anterior, 2.5 mm lateral to bregma, and 5.0 mm below the dura surface. The control group received only vehicle. Injections were performed with a Hamilton syringe. The liquid was injected over a 5-min period, after which the needle was left in place for additional 15 min and then slowly removed. After surgery, rats were allowed to recover for at least 10 days before stem cell transplantation. There is no immune depressant being used during the experiment.

3. Stem Cell Preparation

Enhanced green fluorescent protein (EGFP)–labeled mouse iPSCs was bought from SiDan Sai Biotechnology Co., Ltd (China). The iPSCs was derived from the fibroblast of C57BL/6 mouse and was engineered to express green fluorescent protein (GFP) via stable transfection with a lentivirus construct containing EGFP gene under the control of the constitutive promoter from the elongation factor 1α. The iPSCs was cultured as described previously [10]. Briefly, mouse iPSCs was maintained on a mitotically inactivated mouse embryonic fibroblast feeder layer in knockout Dulbecco modified Eagle medium (Invitrogen) containing 10% fetal bovine serum (Invitrogen), 10% knockout serum replacement (Invitrogen), 2 mML-glutamine (Invitrogen), ×100 nonessential amino acids (Invitrogen), ×1000 β-2-mercaptoethanol (Invitrogen), 50 units of penicillin and a 50 mg/mL dose of streptomycin (Invitrogen), and mouse leukemia inhibitory factor (Invitrogen). Before stem cell transplantation, iPSC colonies were passaged up to 4 times without feeder cells on 60-mm culture dishes coated with 0.1% gelatin to eliminate contamination of the mouse embryonic fibroblasts.

4. Transplantation Procedure

Rats were anesthetized with a solution of ketamine (75 mg/kg) and xylazine (12.5 mg/kg) and placed in a stereotactic instrument. About 1.0×10^6 suspended iPSCs or PBS was stereotactically injected into the left lateral ventricle (0.92 mm anterior to the bregma, 1.2 mm lateral to the midline, and 3.1 mm beneath the dura) in a volume of 20 μl over 10 min with the use of a Hamilton microsyringe. The needle was left in place for an additional 10 min and then removed slowly. All surgical procedures were conducted under aseptic conditions. There is no immune depressant being used during the exprement.

5. Morris water maze task

As there is evidence that huntington's disease in rodents cause impairments when animals are tested in the Morris water maze [23], we used the Morris water maze for the current experiments. The Morris water maze task was performed according to our previous study [24] and the other [25]. Briefly, the rats were trained for 5 consecutive days, followed by the probe trial on day 6. The rats were let down in four random places (N, S, E, W) in the pool. The order of these was changed daily in a random manner. The rats were trained four times per day (120 sec/trial or until they found the platform). After the 120-sec swim, they were allowed to stay on the platform for 30 sec before the next swim trial. Single probe trials to test reference memory were conducted 1 day after the last training session. Rats were released at a random start position, and were allowed to swim during 120 sec in the absence of the platform. The tracks were recorded using video camera and Ethovision software (Noldus). Owing to different swim speeds in the different groups, the latencies of training days 1–5 were compared with the average latency for each day. For the analysis of the probe tests, the number of target annulus crossovers was compared.

6. MicroPET/CT scans and Image analysis

Lesion-induced deficits and changes after transplantation were assessed in vivo using microPET/CT scanning of [18F] fluorodeoxyglucose (^{18}F-FDG) uptake to image metabolic activity, as described previously [26]. Briefly, for the first set of animals, 10 days after striatal lesion as well as 1, 2, 4 and 6 weeks after transplantation, rats were injected with 450 μCi of ^{18}F-FDG in the tail vein, in a maximum volume of 0.5 ml of sterile saline. After injection, they were returned to their cages for a 45-min uptake period in a dark and quiet environment. After the uptake period each animal was anesthetized with a solution of ketamine (75 mg/kg) and xylazine (12.5 mg/kg). The PET data were acquired at 60 min after intravenous injection in 3-dimensional mode, with emission scans of 10 min per bed position. Imaging started with a low-dose CT scan (30 mA), immediately followed by a PET scan. The CT scan was used for attenuation correction and localization of the lesion site. The coronal, transaxial, and sagittal views of PET imaging and MIP (maximum intensity projection) of the model rats were obtained after image reconstruction with a slice thickness of two-micrometer. The average radioactivity concentration within the lesion area was obtained from the mean pixel values. The lesion-to-normal homologous contralateral ratio was used for semiquantitative analysis.

7. Histology and Immunohistochemistry

Animals were anesthetized with a solution of ketamine (75 mg/kg) and xylazine (12.5 mg/kg) and perfused first with 400 ml of saline and then 400 ml of 4% paraformaldehyde (in 0.1 M phosphate buffer, pH 7.4). Brains were then removed and postfixed in the same fixative, and then coronal sections (30 μm) were cut on a vibratome (VIBRATOME, #053746). Sections were stained with Nissl according to conventional staining methods.

For immunohistochemistry, sections were pretreated with 0.3% H_2O_2 in 0.01 M PBS at 37°C for 30 min. To carry out conventional single-label immunohistochemistry, separate series of sections were incubated overnight at 4°C in mouse anti-neuronal nuclei (NeuN) (1:1000, Millipore), rabbit anti-Dopamine- and cAMP-regulated neuronal phosphoprotein (Darpp32) (1:500, Millipore), mouse anti-glial fibrillary acidic protein (GFAP) (1:1000, Santa Cruz Biotechnology), and rabbit anti- ionized calcium binding adaptor molecule 1 (Iba-1) (1:1000, Millipore). Sections were then rinsed and incubated in anti-mouse IgG or anti-rabbit IgG (1:200, Sigma), followed by incubating in the appropriate mouse or rabbit PAP complex (1:200, Sigma) at room temperature for 2 h. The DAB-peroxidase reaction (0.05% in 0.01 M PBS, pH 7.4, Sigma) was carried out for 2–8 min and mounted onto gelatin-coated slides, dried, dehydrated, cleared with xylene, and covered with neutral balsam.

To follow up on the fate of the EGFP-labeled transplanted stem cells, immunofluorescent detection was performed. NeuN was used as a mature neuronal marker, Darpp32 as the medium-sized striatal projection neurons marker, GFAP as the mature astrocyte marker, and Iba-1 as the microglia marker. Sections were blocked and incubated overnight at 4°C with primary antibodies as mentioned above. After washing in PBS, sections were incubated with fluorescence-conjugated secondary antibodies (Alexa Fluor 594, 1:500; Invitrogen) for 2 h at room temperature. Sections were washed and counterstained with the nuclear dye hoechst33258 (1:1000, Sigma) for 15 min. Fluorescence-labeled sections were viewed and images captured with a confocal microscope (Olympus).

8. Western blot

Western blotting was carried out for the marker proteins for each cell type examined. Rats were killed by decapitation after being anesthetized, and the striatum was extracted and homogenized in a lysis buffer to which protease inhibitors had been freshly added. The homogenate was centrifuged at 1500 g for 25 min, and protein concentration was determined by using a Bio-Rad DC protein assay (Bio-Rad, Hercules, CA). Samples were separated by sodium dodecyl sulfate-polyacrylamide gel electrophoresis (1% SDS-PAGE) and transferred to PVDF membranes (Millipore). Membranes were incubated in blocking buffer (5% skim milk in TBST), then with mouse anti- NeuN (1:2000, Millipore), rabbit anti- Darpp32 (1:1000, Millipore), mouse anti-GFAP (1:2000, Santa Cruz Biotechnology), and rabbit anti- Iba-1 (1:2000, Millipore), or rabbit anti -β-actin (1:2000, Millipore) in TBST overnight at 48°C. Incubated membranes were then treated with secondary antibody conjugated with horseradish peroxidase in TBST for 2 hr at 37°C. Blots were developed by enhanced chemiluminescence and digitally scanned. The optical density of each resulting labeled band was measured in an image analysis program (Image pro-Plus 6.0).

9. Data collection and statistical analysis

Histologic analysis of rat-brain volumes was performed as previously described [27]. Continuous 50 μm coronal brain sections were taken from levels corresponding approximately to the interaural plane from 10.70 to 8.74 mm [according to the atlas of [28]] and were used for volumetric analysis. The areas of the striatum as determined by Nissl staining were calculated from each continuous section and total volumes were measured by integrating each section area and depth using Image-Pro Plus 6.0 software.

For immunohistochemistry analysis, eight sections for each rat were analyzed per neuron type. Quantitative analysis of the number of positively stained cells with NeuN, Darpp32, GFAP and Iba-1 was performed on adjacent coronal sections of the striatum. For NeuN and Darpp32, the number of labeled perikarya was counted in six randomly selected areas (0.01 mm^2 for each) in striatum for each section. For GFAP and Iba-1, the integral optical density (IOD) of positive cells in six randomly selected areas (0.01 mm^2 for each) in striatum was measured with an image analysis program (Image pro-Plus 6.0).

Comparisons were performed using one-way ANOVA and unpaired t-test. Data are presented as mean±SD, and differences considered significant at $p < 0.05$.

Results

1. Transplantation of iPSC improves recovery of learning and memory deficits induced by QA

In the Morris water maze task, the QA treated rats moved more along the wall of the pool and were significantly slower than controls in locating the hidden platform. However, in the iPSC-transplanted group, the animals could find the platform more quickly than the QA-treated rats (Fig. 1A). On the first day of testing, most of the animals in these three groups could not find the platform. After the initial trial, QA-treated rats showed consistently longer latencies in locating the hidden platform during the 5 days of testing, but, compared with the first day of testing, the iPSC-transplanted animals showed to find the platform sooner on Day 2 to Day 5. Analyses of the escape latency for hidden platform trials showed a significant difference among the three groups (compared between control and QA-treated groups on Day 2 to Day 5, $p < 0.05$; compared between QA-treated and iPSC-transplanted groups on Day 4 to Day 5, $p < 0.05$; compared between control and iPSC-transplanted groups on Day 2 to Day 5, $p < 0.05$, Fig. 1B, Table S1A in File S1).

On the following probe test without the platform, the control rats spent more time in the target quadrant, and the number of the animals crossing the target annulus was nearly 8; whereas the QA treated rats swam mainly in the periphery of the pool, and the mean crossover was only 2. In the iPSC-transplanted group,

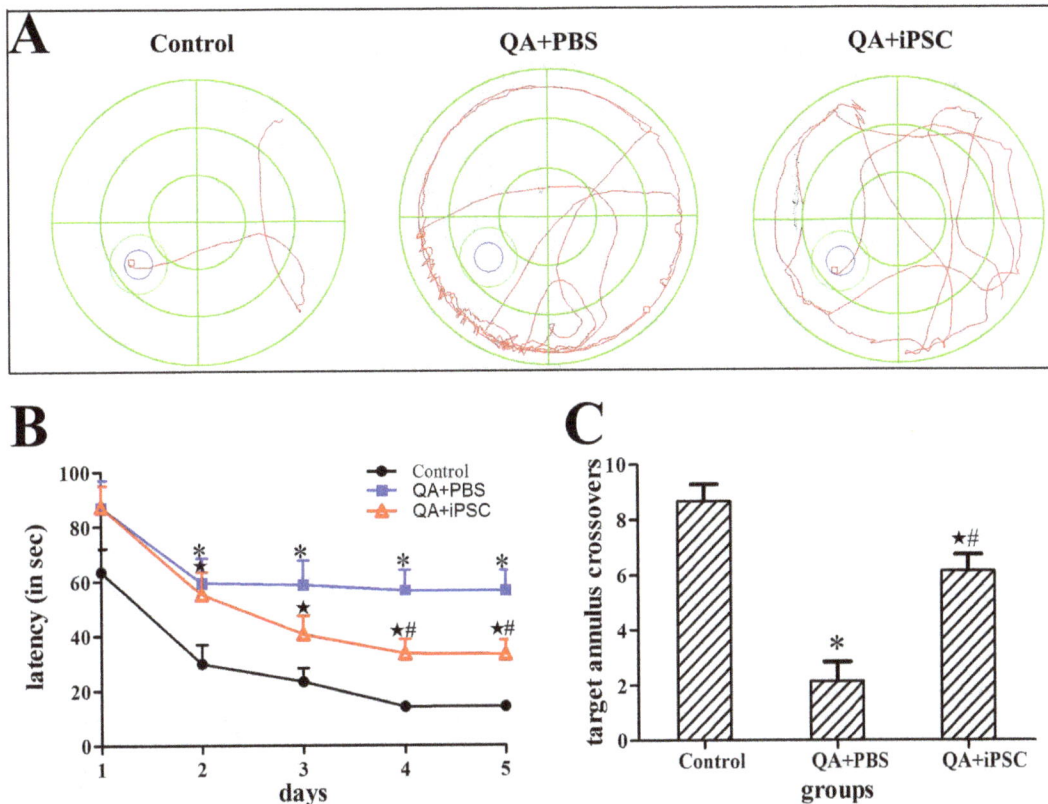

Figure 1. Transplanted iPSC improved functional recovery by Morris water maze testing. (A) The swim tracks of the rats during Morris water maze testing. The QA+iPSC rat obviously spent less time searching for the platform than the QA+PBS rat. (B) Comparison of the latency to find the platform among the three groups in Morris water maze testing. (C) Comparison of the crossovers among the three groups in probe test of Morris water maze testing. The 3 groups are presented as control (saline injection), QA+PBS (QA injection with PBS transplantation); and QA+iPSC (QA injection with iPSC transplantation) groups. Error bars represent SD, and * $P<0.05$, compared between control and QA+PBS groups; ★ $P<0.05$, compared between control and QA+iPSC groups; # $P<0.05$, compared between QA+PBS and QA+iPSC groups.

the mean crossovers could be up to 6 times. Statistical analysis showed a significant difference of the crossovers among the three groups (compared between the control and QA-treated groups, $p<0.001$; compared between QA-treated and iPSC-transplanted groups, $p<0.001$; compared between the control and iPSC-transplanted groups, $p<0.05$, Fig. 1C, Table S1B in File S1).

2. iPSC transplantation results in enhanced glucose metabolism of the lesioned striatum

To document that the iPSC implant corresponds to enhanced glucose metabolic activity, ^{18}F-FDG small-animal PET/CT scans were performed sequentially at 0, 1, 2, 4 and 6 weeks after iPSC transplantation. The ^{18}F-FDG PET/CT scans allowed the visualization and quantification of glucose metabolism throughout the brain at each time point (Fig. 2). For the animals included in this study, the lesion-to-normal homologous contralateral radioactivity ratio was used for semiquantitative analysis. In rats that were injected with QA into the left striatum and imaged 10 days later, there was a marked asymmetry of FDG uptake in the striatum, compared to the non-lesioned right hemisphere (Fig. 2A). From 1 week to 6 weeks after transplantation, glucose metabolism in the striatum of QA-treated animals remained unchanged. In contrast, the glucose metabolism in iPSC-transplanted rats showed a slight increase, resulting in a growth of the radioactivity ratio (Figs. 2A, 2B). This growth persisted through

the four-week scan, suggesting that the transplant protected the ipsilateral striatum from metabolic decline. Analysis of the radioactivity ratios demonstrated no significant differences between the QA-treated and iPSC-transplanted groups at either 1 or 2 weeks after transplantation ($p>0.05$, Fig. 2B). However, the radioactivity ratios were significantly increased in the iPSC-transplanted group at both 4 and 6 weeks after stem cell transplantation ($p<0.001$, Fig. 2B, Table S2 in File S1), indicating that transplantation of iPSC increased glucose metabolism in the lesioned area.

In addition, there was no focal abnormal increase in glucose metabolism in the cerebral lesioned area, thus indicating no tumor or teratoma formation at 6 weeks after stem cell transplantation.

3. iPSC transplantation improves striatum volume after QA-induced excitotoxicity

At 10th day after injection of QA, the striatal atrophy and lateral veniricle dilation were severe in the QA-injection side compared with the contra-lateral side. Nissl staining showed that a clear lesion was located in the striatum and neuronal loss was observed in the lesion area. Striatum volumes were calculated by Nissl staining to evaluate the effects of iPSC transplantation. Six weeks after surgery, striatum volumes were not changed in the control group, but were obviously decreased in the QA-lesioned and iPSC-transplanted groups (Fig. 2C). However, striatum volumes in iPSC-transplanted group were partially

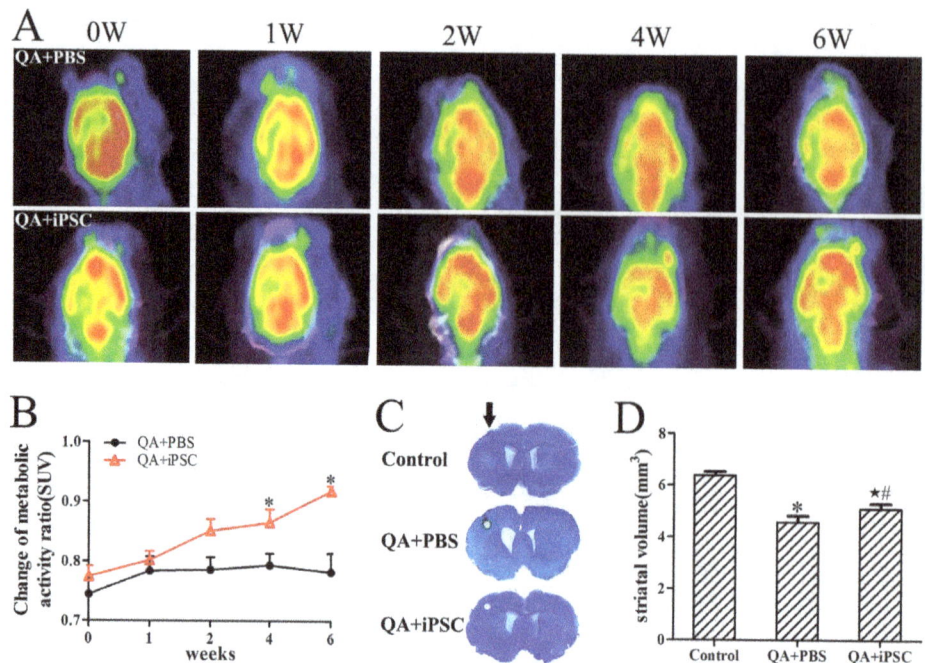

Figure 2. Enhanced glucose metabolism and decreased striatal atrophy following iPSC transplantation. (A) Serial PET images demonstrating metabolism recovery after stem cell treatment for QA-treated rats. Images are shown in axial view. Scale was set according to signal intensity. (B) Semiquantitative analysis of variance of glucose metabolism after stem cell transplantation in each group. (C) Photomicrographs show the difference in striatal volumes in unilateral lesion rat. There was no striatal atrophy in the control group, but the striatal volumes in the lesion side of QA+PBS and QA+iPSC groups were significantly decreased compared with the contralateral side. Arrow indicates surgery sites in each group. (D) Quantification of striatal volumes show increased volumes in the QA+iPSC group. The 3 groups are presented as control (saline injection), QA+PBS (QA injection with PBS transplantation); and QA+iPSC (QA injection with iPSC transplantation) groups. Error bars represent SD, and * $P<0.05$, compared between control and QA+PBS groups; ★ $P<0.05$, compared between control and QA+iPSC groups; # $P<0.05$, compared between QA+PBS and QA+iPSC groups.

recovered in comparison with QA-lesioned group (Fig. 2D). The striatum volume of the control group was approximately 6.37 ± 0.15 mm^3, while in the QA-lesioned and iPSC-transplanted groups striatum volume was 4.57 ± 0.25 mm^3 and 5.10 ± 0.20 mm^3, respectively. The statistical analysis showed a significant difference among these three groups ($P<0.001$ for control and QA groups, $P<0.05$ for QA and iPSC-transplanted groups, $P<0.05$ for control and iPSC-transplanted groups, Fig. 2D, Table S3 in File S1).

4. Histological confirmation of neural protection after iPSC transplantation

4.1 Neural loss and gliosis induced by QA injection. To evaluate QA-induced striatal lesion, immunohistochemical (NeuN, Darpp32, GFAP and Iba-1) methods were used. NeuN was used as a mature neuronal marker, and Darpp32 as the medium-sized striatal projection neurons marker. In QA-treated rats, a clear lesion area was obviously located in the striatum. NeuN and Darpp32 immunolabeling confirmed a serious loss of neurons in the lesion core (Fig. 3B, 3D). Quantitative data showed that the number of striatal neurons in the QA group was $93.5\pm10.4/0.01$ mm^2 (NeuN) and $74.9\pm8.6/0.01$ mm^2 (Darpp32), respectively, corresponding to $170.2\pm3.9/0.01$ mm^2 (NeuN) and $149.5\pm7.8/0.01$ mm^2 (Darpp32) in the control. The statistical analysis showed a significant difference between the two groups ($P<0.001$ for NeuN, $P<0.001$ for Darpp32, Fig. 3I, Table S4 in File S1). Furthermore, histological detection in astrocyte and microglia were carried out using GFAP and Iba-1 immunohistochemistry. In the control group, astrocyte

and microglia were scattered in striatum uniformly. After QA treatment, there were numerous glial cell proliferations in the lesion core (Fig. 3F, 3H). Statistical analysis showed that in the QA group, the optical density of GFAP and Iba-1 in striatum was $27045\pm1093/0.01$ mm^2 and $25137\pm1359/0.01$ mm^2, respectively, which showed a significant difference compared with the controls for Iba-1 ($19456\pm1453/0.01$ mm^2, $P<0.05$) but not for GFAP ($24560\pm1203/0.01$ mm^2, $P>0.05$, Fig. 3J, Table S5 in File S1).

4.2 Transplanted cells survive and differentiate into neurons and astrocytes in lesioned striatum. We next investigated the distribution and differentiation of the transplanted iPSC in QA-lesioned striatum. As labeled by EGFP, transplanted iPSC could be identified under fluorescence microscope. A number of transplanted iPSC appeared to have migrated from lateral ventricle to the lesioned striatum, and the cells spread out into the lesioned area (Fig. 4). While, there is no EGFP-marked cell can be detected in contra-lateral side.

Furthermore, we determined the cell types of differentiated iPSC surviving in the QA impaired striatum. Confocal microscope images showed a larger number of GFP-labeled cells in the QA-lesioned striatum co-expressing NeuN (Fig. 5A), Darpp32 (Fig. 5B), GFAP (Fig. 5C) and Iba-1 (Fig. 5D). Then, we counted the number of NeuN- and Darpp32-expressing cell in striatum. In the iPSC-transplanted animals, the number of NeuN-positive cells was significantly higher than that in the QA-injected group ($119.8\pm9.3/0.01$ mm^2 vs $93.5\pm10.4/0.01$ mm^2; $P<0.05$, Fig. 3I). The number of Darpp32-expressing cells in the iPSC-transplanted group was more than that in

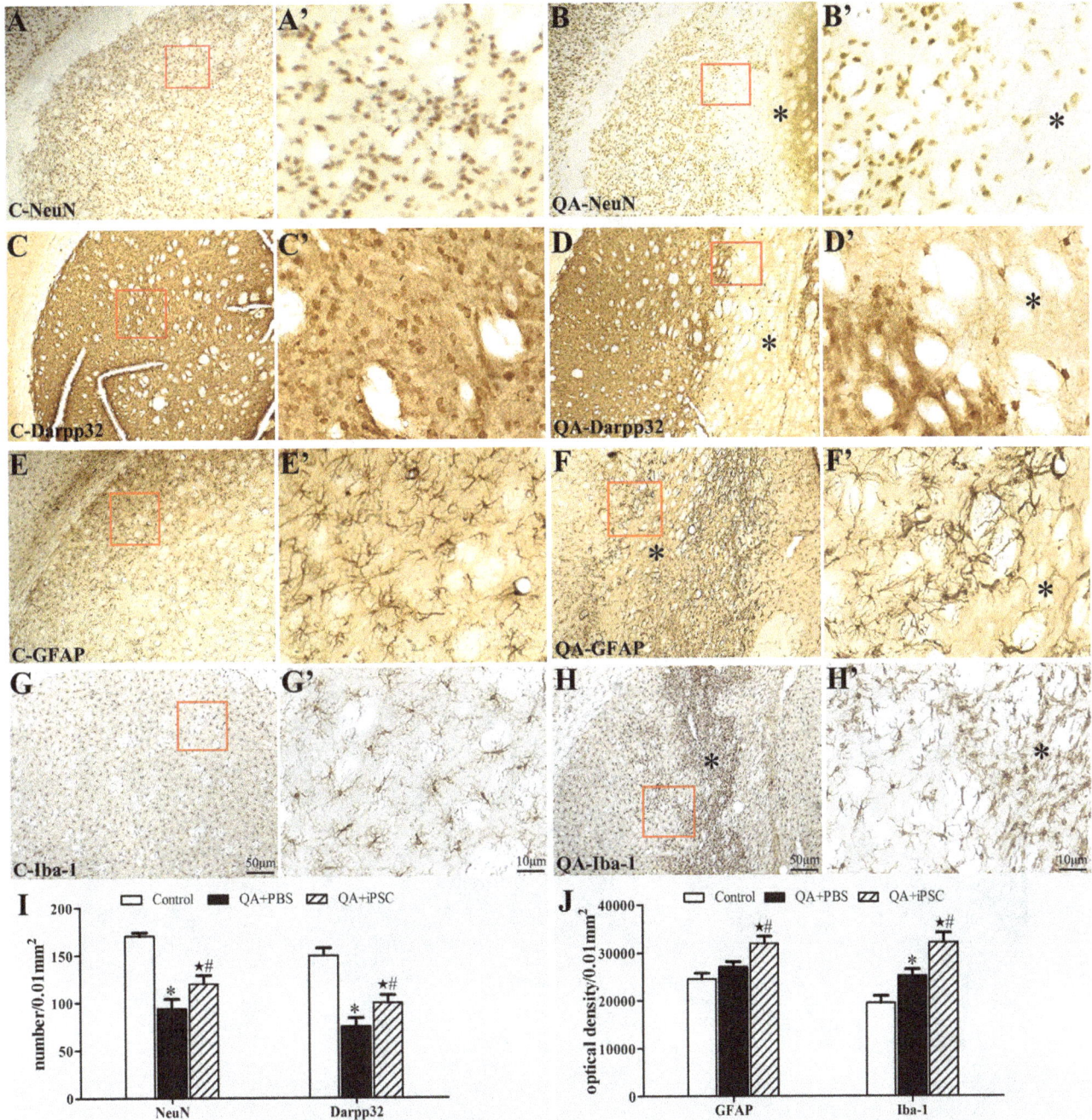

Figure 3. Neuronal loss and gliosis in striatum induced by QA injection. (A, C, E, G and A', C', E', G') Immunohistochemical staining for NeuN (A–A'), Darpp32 (B–B'), GFAP (C–C'), Iba-1 (D–D') in striatum in the control rats. (B, D, F, H and B', D', F', H') Immunohistochemical staining for NeuN (B–B'), Darpp32 (D–D'), GFAP (F–F'), Iba-1 (H–H') in striatum in the QA-treated rats, which showed the loss of NeuN- and Darpp32-positive neurons and proliferations of astrocyte and microglia in the lesion area. A–H were the same magnification; A'–H' were the same magnification; A'–H' were the higher magnification views of the red box in A–H. (I) Comparison of the number of NeuN- and Darpp32-positive neurons in striatum among the three groups. (J) Comparison of the optical density of GFAP- and Iba-1-positive glial cells in striatum among the three groups. The 3 groups are presented as control (saline injection), QA+PBS (QA injection with PBS transplantation); and QA+iPSC (QA injection with iPSC transplantation) groups. Error bars represent SD, and * $P<0.05$, compared between control and QA+PBS groups; ★ $P<0.05$, compared between control and QA+iPSC groups; # $P<0.05$, compared between QA+PBS and QA+iPSC groups.

the QA-treated group ($99.4\pm8.3/0.01$ mm^2 vs $74.9\pm8.6/0.01$ mm^2) and there was statistically significant difference between the two groups ($P<0.05$, Fig. 3I, Fig. 3J). The IOD of GFAP and Iba-1 in striatum was also quantified. Expression of GFAP in the iPSC-transplanted striatum was significantly higher than that in the QA-treated group ($31934\pm1493/$ 0.01 mm^2 vs $27045\pm1093/0.01$ mm^2; $P<0.05$). Meanwhile, the IOD of Iba-1 in the iPSC-transplanted group was significantly higher than that of the QA-injected group ($332143\pm2019/0.01$ mm^2 vs $25137\pm1359/0.01$ mm^2; $P<0.001$, Fig. 3J). Analyses of the four cell types between the control and iPSC-transplanted groups also showed a significant

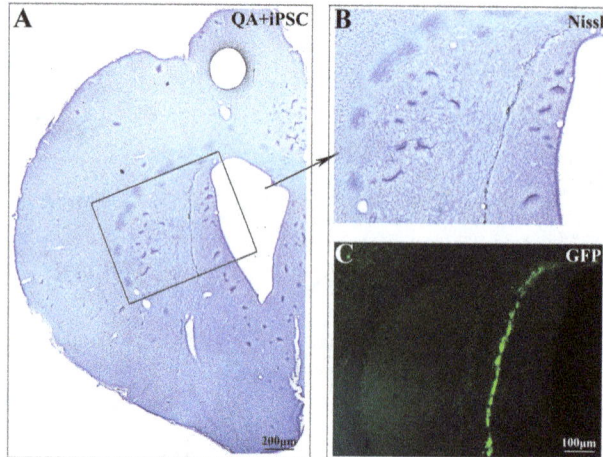

Figure 4. Transplanted iPSC migrated into the lesioned striatum after QA injection. (A, B) Nissl staining of striatum after iPSC transplantation. B was the higher magnification views of the black box in A. (C) Migration and distribution of the transplanted iPSC in QA-lesioned striatum were observed under fluorescence microscope. B and C were the same magnification.

difference ($P<0.05$ for NeuN and Darpp32, $P<0.001$ for GFAP and Iba-1, Fig. 3I, Fig. 3J, Table S4 and S5 in File S1).

5. Changes of protein marker in striatal neuron and gliocyte after iPSC transplantation

We then examined the protein expression of NeuN, Darpp32, GFAP and Iba-1 in striatum after iPSC transplanted for six weeks. Western blotting revealed that treated with QA significantly decreased NeuN and Darpp32 protein in rat striatum, but iPSC-transplanted rat had higher levels of these molecules than the QA-treated rat ($p<0.05$; Fig. 6). QA-treated rat expressed increased levels of both GFAP and Iba-1 in striatum compared with the control animals, and iPSC transplantation could enhance their expression more significantly than the QA-treated rats ($p<0.05$; Fig. 6), indicating that iPSC activated the proliferation of gliocyte. Statistical analysis also showed a significant difference between the control and iPSC-transplanted groups for NeuN, GFAP and Iba-1, but not Darpp32 ($p<0.05$ for NeuN; $p<0.001$ for GFAP and Iba-1; $p>0.05$ for Darpp32, Fig. 6, Table S6 in File S1).

Discussion

In the present study, we found that transplantation of iPSCs reduced learning and memory dysfunction in QA-lesioned rat, as determined by Morris water maze. Within the damaged striatum, a large number of iPSCs could migrate into the damaged striatal region and underwent differentiation, as shown by the expression

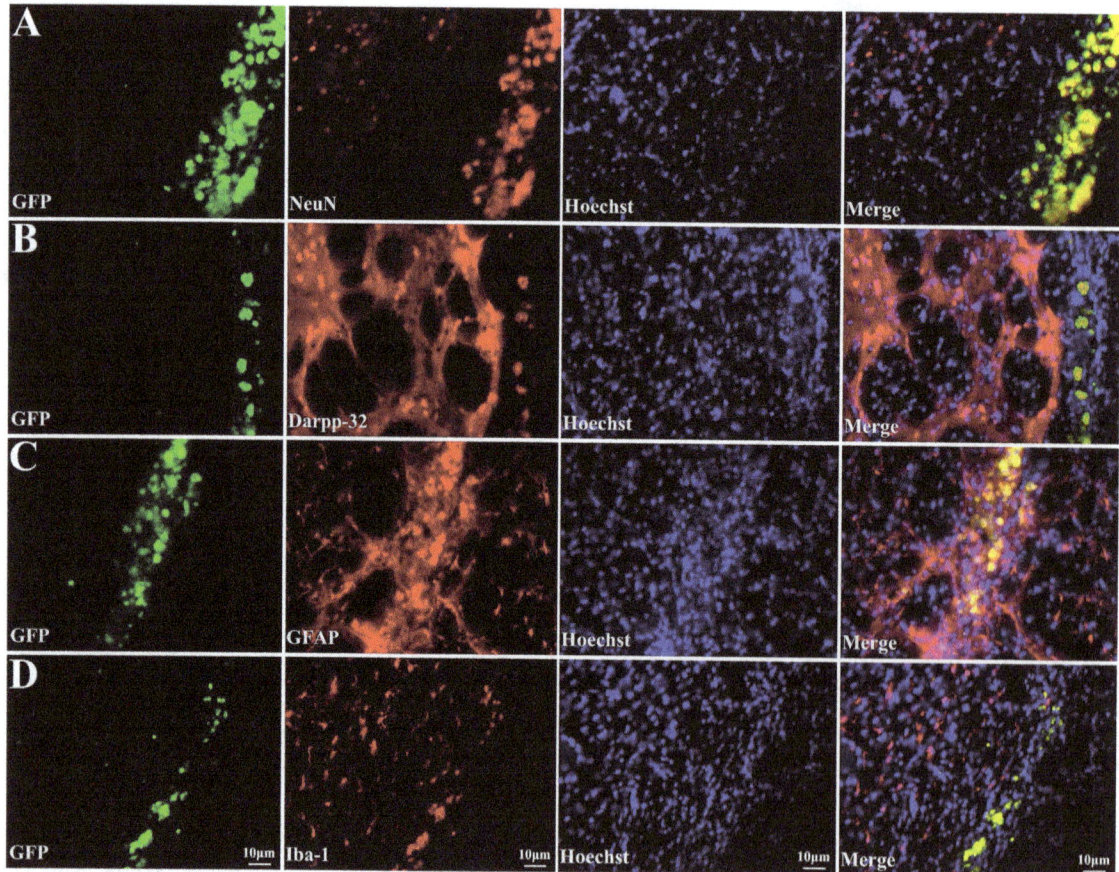

Figure 5. Transplanted cells differentiate into neurons and astrocytes in lesioned striatum. Transplanted iPSCs show green fluorescence; immunostaining with antibodies against NeuN (A), Darpp32 (B), GFAP (C) and Iba-1 (D) show red fluorescence; nuclei stained with Hoechst 33258 show blue fluorescence; and merged images show that engrafted iPSC express neuron, projection neuron, astrocyte, or microglia features.

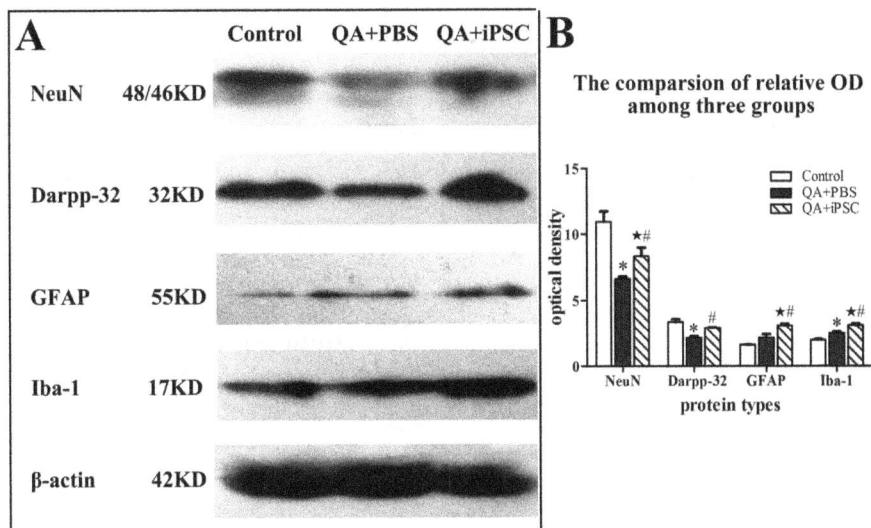

Figure 6. Increased protein expression of neurons and glia cell in striatum after iPSC transplantation. (B) was the semiquantitative analysis of (A) expressed as relative optical density, which showed that the levels of NeuN, Darpp32, GFAP and Iba-1 proteins increased after iPSC transplantation. The 3 groups are presented as control (saline injection), QA+PBS (QA injection with PBS transplantation); and QA+iPSC (QA injection with iPSC transplantation) groups. Error bars represent SD, and *$P<0.05$, compared between control and QA+PBS groups; ★ $P<0.05$, compared between control and QA+iPSC groups; # $P<0.05$, compared between QA+PBS and QA+iPSC groups.

markers for mature neurons, striatal medium spiny projection neurons, astrocytes and microglia. Moreover, the potential therapeutic effect of iPSCs was evaluated by serial ^{18}F-FDG PET/CT scans.

Elevated cerebral glucose uptake reflects a higher synaptic activity in the brain if no inflammatory or malignant process is present [29]. Reduction of the cerebral glucose metabolism, observed by PET imaging, is confirmed a well-known feature in symptomatic HD and the preclinical gene carrier state [30]. Therefore, monitoring glucose utilization in animal models of HD, and also in patients, can provide useful information about neuronal functional deficit before and after therapeutic interventions. It has reported that cystamine-induced neuroprotection in R6/2 transgenic mice can be monitored by micro PET-[^{18}F] FDG in the striatum, cortex and cerebellum [31]. Here, we used micro ^{18}F-FDG PET imaging to investigate whether iPSC transplantation can ameliorate the cerebral energy metabolism in the striatum of rat model of HD. The similar study has been verified in the cerebral ischemia. Wang et al reported that serial ^{18}F-FDG small-animal PET demonstrated metabolic recovery after iPSC and ESC transplantation in a rat model of cerebral ischemia [12]. Clinically, a previous study demonstrated enhanced glucose metabolism in some patients that had undergone transplantation of fetal striatum. Although the sample size was small, the metabolic rates, observed by PET appeared to correlate with improved clinical status [7]. In the present study, by using a rat model of Huntington's disease, we were able to find increased glucose metabolic activity in the striatum-lesioned area during the 6-wk period after iPSC transplantation under serial ^{18}F-FDG PET scans. Thus, PET seems likely to be one of the best-suited modalities to evaluate stem cell therapy, and it can be used in patients clinically for both cells trafficking and monitoring the response to therapy.

In the injured brain, some upregulated environmental elements may account for the migration of endogenous neural stem cells or transplanted immortalized, neonate-derived neural precursor cells to the lesioned region and their differentiation into neurons [32].

In previous studies, brain injury induced neurogenesis and enhanced neuronal migration to the lesioned region to enhance proliferation of correct cell types, such as Dcx-expressing neuroblasts, to reconstruct the damaged cell architecture, as seen after stroke [33] and HD [34]. In the present study, immunohistochemical analyses indicated that many transplanted cells survived and integrated close to the injured striatum and that most of the cells expressed protein markers for parenchymal cells such as neurons and astrocytes. What are the mechanisms or factors that promote reduced deficits with iPSC transplantation after HD? One possibility is that the transplanted stem cells integrate into the tissue, replace damaged cells, and reconstruct the neural circuitry. Previous reports demonstrated that human induced PSC-derived dopaminergic neurons have been shown to survive and improve behavioural impairments after intrastriatal transplantation in an animal model of Parkinson's disease [16]. Another reasonable explanation is that changes in the microenvironment may contribute to tissue protection and repair [35] or that the interaction of grafted stem cells with the host brain may lead to production of trophic factors [36]. For example, increased neurogenesis and neuroprotection by neurotrophic or growth factors, and new synapse formation with reorganization, have been suggested by stroke models [37]. The decreased striatal atrophy, the increased glucose metabolic activity and the improved functional recovery of the HD model in our study also suggest that iPSC transplantation protects the host brain from further destruction.

Recently, the role of glial cells in integrity of the central nervous system had been well elucidated, and accumulating evidence suggested that glial cells were critical to neuronal survival [38,39]. Gliocyte populations in different brain regions have been shown to have important roles in neurogenic support [40]. A recent report revealed a surprising outcome where SVZ-mediated astrogenesis may be beneficial over neurogenesis in a period after cortical injury, in agreement with potentially protective roles for astrocytes during recovery process in the spinal cord [41]. In both cultured astrocytes and HD mouse brains, mutant huntingtin reduces glial glutamate uptake and glial cells protected neurons against mutant htt-mediated neurotoxicity [42], suggesting that dysfunction of glial cell may critically contribute to neuronal excitotoxicity in HD. In addition, in injured striatum, mutant huntingtin may affect the production of chemokines and neurotrophic factors such as tumor necrosis factor alpha (TNF-a) [43], glial-derived neuro-trophic factor (GDNF) [44] and nerve growth factor (NGF) [45] from glial cells. In our present study, a large number of iPSCs that differentiated into astrocyte and microglia may contribute to chemokine secretion and iPSCs transplantation may provide a beneficial environment that attracts glial cell activation and proliferation. Once the numbers of activated glial cells are boosted, their trophic support will slow the excitotoxic damage to GABAergic neurons in the striatum.

Conclusion

In summary, we have demonstrated that iPSCs survive, migrate into injured striatum and differentiate into neurons and glial cells after transplantation in the QA-induced HD model, accompany with the decreased striatal atrophy, the increased glucose metabolic activity and the improved functional recovery. Further-more, we have demonstrated that ^{18}F-FDG PET scan seems likely to be a feasible modality to evaluate stem cell therapy in HD. Collectively, this study demonstrates the therapeutic potential of

iPSCs for cell replacement therapy and indicates that iPSCs may provide an alternative cell source for transplantation therapy in the treatment of HD and other neurodegenerative diseases.

Supporting Information

File S1 This file contains Tables S1–S6. Table S1–S6 showed the raw data of this study. Table S1 showed the raw data of Morris water maze testing, A is the latency and B is the target annulus crossovers. Table S2 showed the raw data of SUV of PET/CT. Table S3 showed the raw data of the striatal volume (mm^3). Table S4 showed the raw data of the number of NeuN and Darpp32/0.01 mm^2 in striatum. Table S5 showed the raw data of the optical density of GFAP and Iba-1/0.01 mm^2 in striatum. Table S6 showed the raw data of the optical density of Western blot.

Author Contributions

Conceived and designed the experiments: SHM GQZ JLQ JZ. Performed the experiments: SHM JCW CPM. Analyzed the data: SHM WDP. Contributed reagents/materials/analysis tools: SHM ZDH ZFZ. Contrib-uted to the writing of the manuscript: SHM JZ.

References

1. Landles C, Bates GP (2004) Huntingtin and the molecular pathogenesis of Huntington's disease. Fourth in molecular medicine review series. EMBO Rep, 5(10): p. 958–63.
2. Vonsattel JP, Myers RH, Stevens TJ, Ferrante RJ, Bird ED, et al. (1985) Neuropathological classification of Huntington's disease. J Neuropathol Exp Neurol, 44(6): p. 559–77.
3. Freeman TB, Hauser RA, Sanberg PR, Saporta S (2000) Neural transplantation for the treatment of Huntington's disease. Prog Brain Res, 127: p. 405–11.
4. Visnyei K, Tatsukawa KJ, Erickson RI, Simonian S, Oknaian N, et al. (2006) Neural progenitor implantation restores metabolic deficits in the brain following striatal quinolinic acid lesion. Exp Neurol, 197(2): p. 465–74.
5. Ramaswamy S, Shannon KM, Kordower JH (2007) Huntington's disease: pathological mechanisms and therapeutic strategies. Cell Transplant, 16(3): p. 301–12.
6. Payne NL, Sylvain A, O'Brien C, Herszfeld D, Sun G, et al. (2014) Application of human induced pluripotent stem cells for modeling and treating neurode-generative diseases. N Biotechnol.
7. Bachoud-Levi AC, Remy P, Nguyen JP, Brugieres P, Lefaucheur JP, et al. (2000) Motor and cognitive improvements in patients with Huntington's disease after neural transplantation. Lancet, 356(9246): p. 1975–9.
8. Keene CD, Sonnen JA, Swanson PD, Kopyov O, Leverenz JB, et al. (2007) Neural transplantation in Huntington disease: long-term grafts in two patients. Neurology, 68(24): p. 2093–8.
9. Bjorklund A (1993) Neurobiology. Better cells for brain repair. Nature, 362(6419): p. 414–5.
10. Takahashi K, Yamanaka S (2006) Induction of pluripotent stem cells from mouse embryonic and adult fibroblast cultures by defined factors. Cell, 126(4): p. 663–76.
11. Tornero D, Wattananit S, Gronning Madsen M, Koch P, Wood J, et al. (2013) Human induced pluripotent stem cell-derived cortical neurons integrate in stroke-injured cortex and improve functional recovery. Brain.
12. Wang J, Chao F, Han F, Zhang G, Xi Q, et al. (2013) PET demonstrates functional recovery after transplantation of induced pluripotent stem cells in a rat model of cerebral ischemic injury. J Nucl Med, 54(5): p. 785–92.
13. Tsuji O, Miura K, Okada Y, Fujiyoshi K, Mukaino M, et al. (2010) Therapeutic potential of appropriately evaluated safe-induced pluripotent stem cells for spinal cord injury. Proc Natl Acad Sci U S A, 107(28): p. 12704–9.
14. Nori S, Okada Y, Yasuda A, Tsuji O, Takahashi Y, et al. (2011) Grafted human-induced pluripotent stem-cell-derived neurospheres promote motor functional recovery after spinal cord injury in mice. Proc Natl Acad Sci U S A, 108(40): p. 16825–30.
15. Sundberg M, Bogetofte H, Lawson T, Jansson J, Smith G, et al. (2013) Improved cell therapy protocols for Parkinson's disease based on differentiation efficiency and safety of hESC-, hiPSC-, and non-human primate iPSC-derived dopaminergic neurons. Stem Cells, 31(8): p. 1548–62.
16. Hargus G, Cooper O, Deleidi M, Levy A, Lee K, et al. (2010) Differentiated Parkinson patient-derived induced pluripotent stem cells grow in the adult rodent brain and reduce motor asymmetry in Parkinsonian rats. Proc Natl Acad Sci U S A, 107(36): p. 15921–6.
17. Zhang Y, Ruel M, Beanlands RS, deKemp RA, Suuronen EJ, et al. (2008) Tracking stem cell therapy in the myocardium: applications of positron emission tomography. Curr Pharm Des, 14(36): p. 3835–53.
18. Jiang H, Cheng Z, Tian M, Zhang H (2011) In vivo imaging of embryonic stem cell therapy. Eur J Nucl Med Mol Imaging, 38(4): p. 774–84.
19. Kuwert T, Lange HW, Langen KJ, Herzog H, Aulich A, et al. (1990) Cortical and subcortical glucose consumption measured by PET in patients with Huntington's disease. Brain, 113 (Pt 5): p. 1405–23.
20. Antonini A, Leenders KL, Spiegel R, Meier D, Vontobel P, et al. (1996) Striatal glucose metabolism and dopamine D2 receptor binding in asymptomatic gene carriers and patients with Huntington's disease. Brain, 119 (Pt 6): p. 2085–95.
21. Zhang H, Zheng X, Yang X, Fang S, Shen G, et al. (2008) 11C-NMSP/18F-FDG microPET to monitor neural stem cell transplantation in a rat model of traumatic brain injury. Eur J Nucl Med Mol Imaging, 35(9): p. 1699–708.
22. Shyu WC, Li KW, Peng HF, Lin SZ, Liu RS, et al. (2009) Induction of GAP-43 modulates neuroplasticity in PBSC (CD34+) implanted-Parkinson's model. J Neurosci Res, 87(9): p. 2020–33.
23. Lione LA, Carter RJ, Hunt MJ, Bates GP, Morton AJ, et al. (1999) Selective discrimination learning impairments in mice expressing the human Huntington's disease mutation. J Neurosci, 19(23): p. 10428–37.
24. Mu S, OuYang L, Liu B, Zhu Y, Li K, et al. (2011) Preferential interneuron survival in the transition zone of 3-NP-induced striatal injury in rats. J Neurosci Res, 89(5): p. 744–54.
25. Vorhees CV, Williams MT (2006) Morris water maze: procedures for assessing spatial and related forms of learning and memory. Nat Protoc, 1(2): p. 848–58.
26. Araujo DM, Cherry SR, Tatsukawa KJ, Toyokuni T, Kornblum HI (2000) Deficits in striatal dopamine D(2) receptors and energy metabolism detected by in vivo microPET imaging in a rat model of Huntington's disease. Exp Neurol, 166(2): p. 287–97.
27. Lee ST, Chu K, Jung KH, Im WS, Park JE, et al. (2009) Slowed progression in models of Huntington disease by adipose stem cell transplantation. Ann Neurol, 66(5): p. 671–81.
28. Paxinos G, Watson (1986) The Rat Brain in Stereotaxic Coordinates.
29. Jueptner M, Weiller C (1995) Review: does measurement of regional cerebral blood flow reflect synaptic activity? Implications for PET and fMRI. Neuro-image, 2(2): p. 148–56.
30. Feigin A, Leenders KL, Moeller JR, Missimer J, Kuenig G, et al. (2001) Metabolic network abnormalities in early Huntington's disease: an [(18)F]FDG PET study. J Nucl Med, 42(11): p. 1591–5.
31. Wang X, Sarkar A, Cicchetti F, Yu M, Zhu A, et al. (2005) Cerebral PET imaging and histological evidence of transglutaminase inhibitor cystamine induced neuroprotection in transgenic R6/2 mouse model of Huntington's disease. J Neurol Sci, 231(1–2): p. 57–66.
32. Gaura V, Bachoud-Levi AC, Ribeiro MJ, Nguyen JP, Frouin V, et al. (2004) Striatal neural grafting improves cortical metabolism in Huntington's disease patients. Brain, 127(Pt 1): p. 65–72.

33. Arvidsson A, Collin T, Kirik D, Kokaia Z, Lindvall O (2002) Neuronal replacement from endogenous precursors in the adult brain after stroke. Nat Med, 8(9): p. 963–70.

34. Lin YT, Chern Y, Shen CK, Wen HL, Chang YC, et al. (2011) Human mesenchymal stem cells prolong survival and ameliorate motor deficit through trophic support in Huntington's disease mouse models. PLoS One, 6(8): p. e22924.

35. Feng M, Zhu H, Zhu Z, Wei J, Lu S, et al. (2011) Serial 18F-FDG PET demonstrates benefit of human mesenchymal stem cells in treatment of intracerebral hematoma: a translational study in a primate model. J Nucl Med, 52(1): p. 90–7.

36. Sadan O, Shemesh N, Barzilay R, Dadon-Nahum M, Blumenfeld-Katzir T, et al. (2012) Mesenchymal stem cells induced to secrete neurotrophic factors attenuate quinolinic acid toxicity: a potential therapy for Huntington's disease. Exp Neurol, 234(2): p. 417–27.

37. Emerich DF, Thanos CG, Goddard M, Skinner SJ, Geany MS, et al. (2006) Extensive neuroprotection by choroid plexus transplants in excitotoxin lesioned monkeys. Neurobiol Dis, 23(2): p. 471–80.

38. Chung WS, Clarke LE, Wang GX, Stafford BK, Sher A, et al. (2013) Astrocytes mediate synapse elimination through MEGF10 and MERTK pathways. Nature, 504(7480): p. 394–400.

39. Borlongan CV, Yamamoto M, Takei N, Kumazaki M, Ungsuparkorn C, et al. (2000) Glial cell survival is enhanced during melatonin-induced neuroprotection against cerebral ischemia. Faseb J, 14(10): p. 1307–17.

40. Dusart I, Marty S, Peschanski M (1991) Glial changes following an excitotoxic lesion in the CNS – II. Astrocytes. Neuroscience, 45(3): p. 541–9.

41. Benner EJ, Luciano D, Jo R, Abdi K, Paez-Gonzalez P, et al. (2013) Protective astrogenesis from the SVZ niche after injury is controlled by Notch modulator Thbs4. Nature, 497(7449): p. 369–73.

42. Shin JY, Fang ZH, Yu ZX, Wang CE, Li SH, et al. (2005) Expression of mutant huntingtin in glial cells contributes to neuronal excitotoxicity. J Cell Biol, 171(6): p. 1001–12.

43. Acarin L, Gonzalez B, Castellano B (2000) Neuronal, astroglial and microglial cytokine expression after an excitotoxic lesion in the immature rat brain. Eur J Neurosci, 12(10): p. 3505–20.

44. Marco S, Canudas AM, Canals JM, Gavalda N, Perez-Navarro E, et al. (2002) Excitatory amino acids differentially regulate the expression of GDNF, neurturin, and their receptors in the adult rat striatum. Exp Neurol, 174(2): p. 243–52.

45. Strauss S, Otten U, Joggerst B, Pluss K, Volk B (1994) Increased levels of nerve growth factor (NGF) protein and mRNA and reactive gliosis following kainic acid injection into the rat striatum. Neurosci Lett, 168(1–2): p. 193–6.

6

Effectiveness of Anti-Psychotics and Related Drugs in the Huntington French-Speaking Group Cohort

Gaëlle Désaméricq[1,2,3,4], **Guillaume Dolbeau**[1,2,5], **Christophe Verny**[6,7], **Perrine Charles**[8,9], **Alexandra Durr**[8], **Katia Youssov**[1,2,4,8], **Clémence Simonin**[10,11,12], **Jean-Philippe Azulay**[13], **Christine Tranchant**[14,15], **Cyril Goizet**[16], **Philippe Damier**[17], **Emmanuel Broussolle**[18,19,20], **Jean-François Demonet**[21], **Graca Morgado**[2,22,23], **Laurent Cleret de Langavant**[1,2,4,8], **Isabelle Macquin-Mavier**[2,3], **Anne-Catherine Bachoud-Lévi**[1,2,4,8,9], **Patrick Maison**[1,2,4,8*,9]

1 Equipe 01, U955, Inserm, Créteil, France, 2 Faculté de médecine, Université Paris Est, Créteil, France, 3 Service de Pharmacologie Clinique, Hôpital H. Mondor – A. Chenevier, AP-HP, Créteil, France, 4 Département d'Etudes Cognitives, Ecole Normale Supérieure, Paris, France, 5 Unité de recherche clinique, Hôpital H. Mondor – A. Chenevier, AP-HP, Créteil, France, 6 Centre de référence des maladies neurogénétiques, service de neurologie, CHU d'Angers, Angers, France, 7 UMR CNRS 6214 - INSERM U1083, Angers, France, 8 Centre de référence Maladie de Huntington, Hôpital H. Mondor – A. Chenevier, AP-HP, Créteil, France, 9 Département de génétique, Hôpital de la salpêtrière, AP-HP, Paris, France, 10 Departement of Neurology and Movement Disorders, CHRU Lille, Lille, France, 11 UMR837 INSERM – JPArc Team 6, Lille, France, 12 University Lille 2/Law & Health, Lille, France, 13 Service de Neurologie et pathologie du mouvement, Hôpital de la Timone, Marseille, France, 14 Service de Neurologie, CHU Hautepierre, Strasbourg, France, 15 Université de Strasbourg, Strasbourg, France, 16 Université Bordeaux Segalen, Laboratoire Maladies Rares: Génétique et Métabolisme (MRGM), EA4576, CHU Bordeaux, Service de Génétique médicale, Bordeaux, France, 17 Centre d'Investigation Clinique 004, Inserm, Nantes, France, 18 Faculté de Médecine et de Maïeutique Lyon Sud Charles Mérieux, Université Lyon I, Lyon, France, 19 Service de Neurologie C, Hôpital Neurologique Pierre Wertheimer, Hospices Civils de Lyon, Lyon, France, 20 Centre de Neurosciences Cognitives, UMR5229, CNRS, Bron, France, 21 Centre Leenaards de la Mémoire, Département des Neurosciences Cliniques, CHUV, Lausanne, Switzerland, 22 Centre d'Investigation Clinique 006, Inserm, Créteil, France, 23 Pôle Recherche clinique Santé Publique, Hôpital H. Mondor – A. Chenevier, AP-HP, Créteil, France

Abstract

Purpose: Huntington's disease is a rare condition. Patients are commonly treated with antipsychotics and tetrabenazine. The evidence of their effect on disease progression is limited and no comparative study between these drugs has been conducted. We therefore compared the effectiveness of antipsychotics on disease progression.

Methods: 956 patients from the Huntington French Speaking Group were followed for up to 8 years between 2002 and 2010. The effectiveness of treatments was assessed using Unified Huntington's Disease Rating Scale (UHDRS) scores and then compared using a mixed model adjusted on a multiple propensity score.

Results: 63% of patients were treated with antipsychotics during the survey period. The most commonly prescribed medications were dibenzodiazepines (38%), risperidone (13%), tetrabenazine (12%) and benzamides (12%). There was no difference between treatments on the motor and behavioural declines observed, after taking the patient profiles at the start of the drug prescription into account. In contrast, the functional decline was lower in the dibenzodiazepine group than the other antipsychotic groups (Total Functional Capacity: 0.41 ± 0.17 units per year *vs.* risperidone and 0.54 ± 0.19 *vs.* tetrabenazine, both $p<0.05$). Benzamides were less effective than other antipsychotics on cognitive evolution (Stroop interference, Stroop color and Literal fluency: $p<0.05$).

Conclusions: Antipsychotics are widely used to treat patients with Huntington's disease. Although differences in motor or behavioural profiles between patients according to the antipsychotics used were small, there were differences in drug effectiveness on the evolution of functional and cognitive scores.

Editor: Josef Priller, Charité-Universitätsmedizin Berlin, Germany

Funding: This work was supported by cooperative contracts between the Institut National de la Santé et la recherche Médicale (INSERM), the Association Française contre les Myopathies (AFM), the Association Huntington France (AHF), and the Groupement d'Interêt Scientifique (GIS) - Institut des Maladies Rares et l'AP-HP (DRCD). The team received a grant (about 5000 euro) from EUSA Pharma but EUSA Pharma did not fund directly this study. They wish only data on the use of tetrabenazine, not any result about effectiveness and comparisons. The funders had no role in study design, data collection and analysis, decision to publish, or preparation of the manuscript.

Competing Interests: PM has received grant/research support from EUSA Pharma.

* E-mail: patrick.maison@hmn.aphp.fr

9 These authors contributed equally to this work.

Introduction

Drug prescription is a complex process that takes into account many factors: primary clinical data, patient preferences, the prescriber's clinical and personal experience, external rules and constraints and scientific evidence [1]. Randomised controlled trials (RCTs) are considered the best practice methodology (the gold standard) to provide evidence about drug efficacy. However, RCTs have important limitations for informing clinical practice and policy decisions about treatments. In particular, it is unclear whether findings can be applied to patients seen in routine practice and RCTs do not make comparisons between several prescription options. Recent statistical tools [2] can now help address these issues by allowing multiple comparisons through cohort studies in "real-world" conditions. Such comparisons are particularly useful when studying rare diseases, as the number of patients can be low and may limit the feasibility of clinical trials.

Huntington's disease (HD) is a rare, autosomal dominant, neurodegenerative disorder resulting from expansion of a CAG repeat within the IT15 huntingtin (*HTT*) gene on chromosome 4p [3]. It is characterised by choreiform movements and progressive dementia, and, in 33% to 76% of cases, psychiatric manifestations (for example depression, apathy or irritability)[4]. Recent reviews of available drug trials and case reports [5–7] conclude that the management of HD is poorly documented. Antipsychotics and related drugs (for example tetrabenazine) are most commonly used for the treatment of chorea [8]. The use of antipsychotics and related drugs (APRs) differs between countries: olanzapine is widely prescribed in France and in the United-Kingdom, tiapride in Germany, and haloperidol is more common in Italy [9]. In France, only tetrabenazine and tiapride are approved for chorea. Little is known about the differences between the effects of different antipsychotics on motor abilities, cognitive disorders, psychiatric disturbances or metabolic impairments.

We aimed to describe APR use in HD patients in conditions of routine practice and compare their effectiveness using disease progression scores.

Materials and Methods

The study, carried out between 2002 and 2010, was based on the cohort from the Huntington French Speaking Network (HFSG, http://www.hdnetwork.org).

Patients

Patients were recruited at 13 centres in France and Belgium (Angers, Bordeaux, Bruxelles, Caen, Creteil, Lille, Lyon, Marseille, Nantes, Paris, Rennes, Strasbourg, and Toulouse); 956 patients, all genetically confirmed (CAG ≥37 repeats), completed at least one Unified Huntington's Disease Rating Scale (UHDRS) assessment. Patients were followed for up to 8 years between 2002 and 2010; the mean follow-up was 28.2 months (Table 1). For more than half of the patients, motor symptoms were the initial symptom of the disease. At the time of their first admission in the Huntington French-Speaking Network, 408 of the HD patients (44%) were in Stage 1, 276 (30%) were in Stage 2, 182 (19%) were in Stage 3, 53 (6%) were in Stage 4, and 12 (1%) were in Stage 5 (the final stage) of the disease as characterised by their Total Functional Capacity (TFC) [10].

Assessments

Patient demographics, age at onset of HD, expanded CAG repeat and body mass index were recorded. The motor, cognitive, behavioural and functional capabilities of each patient were assessed annually using the UHDRS [11]. The motor score quantified 15 different motor signs, with higher scores indicating more severely impaired motor function. The cognitive assessment was composed of three standardised tests: the Stroop interference test, Symbol Digit Modalities Test (SDMT), and the verbal fluency test. The behaviour score measured 11 characteristics; the frequency and severity of each of these were multiplied to give a single score for each characteristic and then added together to give the total behaviour score. The functional assessment tested common daily tasks using three measures: the Total Functional Capacity (TFC), the Independence Scale and the Functional Assessment Scale. All medications and indications for their use were recorded each time the patient was assessed, as well as the time since last evaluation. The average time between first visit and prescription of a drug was 13 months. We focused on antipsychotics (N05A) and the related drug tetrabenazine (N07XX06) as classified according to the Anatomical Therapeutic Chemical (ATC) Classification System [12]. These were chosen as they were the most commonly prescribed APRs within the cohort. The period of exposure to a drug was defined as the time between the date of prescription and the acknowledged end of prescription. All data were collected from electronic case report forms.

Statistical methods

Descriptive statistics are presented as means and standard deviation (for quantitative variables) or frequency counts by category (for qualitative variables).

We describe the baseline characteristics of the patient at the time of the first prescription of the drug. These were compared by univariate analysis using Chi^2 tests or Fisher's exact tests (for qualitative variables) and Kruskal-Wallis tests (for quantitative variables). If a patient received more than one drug at the same time or during follow-up, each period of drug prescription was taken into account independently.

We used a mixed model, adjusted with a multiple propensity score, to compare the effects of treatments on UHDRS scores [13]. Mixed models allow data from subjects tested once and data from those who participated in multiple evaluations to be evaluated together. Thus, any bias due to missing data, although not completely eliminated, is minimized. Multiple propensity scores take into account the lack of randomisation; this lack of randomisation is inherent in the observational data due to differences in treatment assignment by physicians and the conditional probability of being treated based on patient profile at the time of the first prescription. Firstly, multiple propensity scores were estimated for each subject and each drug using a multinomial regression model. Baseline characteristics were included if they had an independent association with the prescription of a drug ($P<0.25$). The size of centre (either fewer or more than 100 participants) was also included. Secondly, we estimated causal effects. These included: fixed effects of treatment levels, time from the start of the treatment until the next UHDRS score was taken, the treatment x time interaction and propensity score, and a random effect for the subject/treatment-specific intercepts. We calculated the overall change in UHDRS score over time and compared the effectiveness of treatments.

Analyses were performed using SAS 9.00 (SAS Institute Inc, Cary, North Carolina). All P values were two-tailed, and statistical significance was defined as $P<0.05$ for all tests.

Ethics statement

All patients, whose data are included in the database of the Huntington French-speaking Group cohort, carefully read an information sheet that present the goal of the network and provide

Table 1. Characteristics and evolution of the overall cohort and the groups of patients taking antipsychotics and related drugs.

	Overall			Subjects with anti-psychotics and related drugs			Subjects having never taking anti-psychotics and related drugs		
	n	Baseline	Change per year	n	Baseline	Change per year	n	Baseline	Change per year
Age at HD onset, years	850	43.8±12.0		518	44.7±12.0		283	42.2±12.3	
Male	951	51		546	55		351	45	
CAG repeat length	956	44.8±4.1		548	44.7±4.0		354	45.1±4.4	
Motor score	890	35.1±22.4	4.4±0.2	524	43.5±22.2	4.8±0.2	319	28.4±23.4	3.1±0.4
Chorea	889	8.4±6.1	0.4±0.1	524	9.9±6.3	0.5±0.1	319	7.0±6.3	0.6±0.1
Dystonia	887	3.1±3.6	0.7±0.1	524	4.2±4.2	0.9±0.1	318	2.7±4.0	0.5±0.1
Behavioural score	885	16.7±11.7	−0.1±0.1	524	18.8±12.0	−0.2±0.2	332	12.9±10.4	−0.3±0.2
Functional scores									
Functional assessment scale	927	30.8±6.2	1.5±0.1	538	33.4±6.4	1.8±0.1	337	28.8±5.5	0.8±0.1
Independence scale	928	81.3±16.8	−3.7±0.2	536	73.9±16.8	−4.2±0.3	338	86.8±15.4	−2.0±0.3
Total functional capacity	931	8.9±3.6	−0.8±0.0	539	7.2±3.5	−0.7±0.3	342	10.1±3.3	−0.4±0.1
Cognitive score									
Literacy fluency	623	20.4±13.1	−0.7±0.1	341	16.5±11.6	−1.0±0.1	254	24.9±14.4	0.6±0.3
SDMT	590	23.8±14.3	−2.0±0.1	315	17.0±10.9	−1.9±0.1	246	29.6±14.8	−1.3±0.3
Stroop colour	651	44.0±18.3	−2.6±0.2	345	36.5±16.5	−2.7±0.2	257	50.6±19.8	−1.8±0.3
Stroop word	649	60.7±24.0	−4.1±0.2	344	50.3±22.6	−4.2±0.3	256	67.7±24.7	−2.9±0.4
Stroop interference	644	23.5±13.0	−1.4±0.1	339	18.7±11.2	−1.5±0.1	254	28.1±14.4	−0.8±0.2

HD Huntington' disease; SDMT Symbol digit modality test.
n: available data; Baseline: Mean ± SD; Change per year: Mean ± SE.

their verbal consent to participate the day at the first evaluation. In France, as the study was observational and no biological sample was collected, the data do not justify specific patient consent. The study was approved by the local ethics committee (Comité de Protection des Personnes Ile-de-France IX, Créteil, France).

Results

Prescription of APRs

During the study period, 602 patients (63% of the overall HD population) received APRs. The most commonly prescribed medications were dibenzodiazepines (38%, mainly olanzapine), risperidone (13%), tetrabenazine (12%) and benzamides (12%, mainly tiapride). Sixty-four percent of these patients were using APRs because of chorea and the others for behavioural disorders such as irritability, aggressiveness or agitation. Figure 1 shows the percentage of prescriptions for each class of drug between 2002 and 2010. As only a small number of patients were treated with aripiprazole, this medication was not taken into account in the following analyses.

Characteristics of the treated population at the first prescription

A total of 347 patients treated with APRs were evaluated just before the beginning of their treatment. Patients treated with dibenzodiazepines had a shorter history of HD at baseline whereas neither age nor age at disease onset differed between patients treated with the other APRs (Table 2). Approximately half of all patients were also treated with an antidepressant. At the initiation of APR treatment, patients taking dibenzodiazepines tended to have less severe motor impairments than those taking other treatment ($P = 0.05$); there was no significant difference in motor score, except in eye movement scores for which $P = 0.006$. Behavioural scores were similar between APR groups. Scores on the Functional Assessment Scale (FAS), Independence Scale (IS) and Total Functional Capacity (TFC) differed between the four treatment groups. Patients taking dibenzodiazepines were less disabled than others; they had lower FAS scores (32.4±6.3) and the highest IS (75.7±17.2) and TFC (7.8±3.4) scores. The four

APR treatment groups performed differently in the verbal fluency test ($p<0.05$) and the Stroop interference test ($p<0.05$). Dibenzodiazepines were prescribed to patients with less impairment as defined by these tests.

Impact of these APRs on disease evolution

No significant differences were observed between treatments in terms of motor or behavioural scores (table 3). There was no significant difference between treatment groups for changes in score for chorea (dibenzodiazepines: 0.3±0.2 units per year, risperidone: 0.4±0.4 units per year, tetrabenazine: 0.8±0.5 units per year, benzamides: 0.2±0.5 units per year), and for dystonia impairment (dibenzodiazepines: 0.8±0.1 units per year, risperidone: 0.9±0.3 units per year, tetrabenazine: 1.0±0.4 units per year, benzamides: 1.1±0.3 units per year) but for total motor score minus involuntary movement scores, dibenzodiazepines and risperidone performed better than tetrabenazine (dibenzodiazepines: 2.2±0.2 units per year, risperidone: 2.4±0.4 units per year, tetrabenazine: 4.0±0.6 units per year, benzamides: 3.3±0.5 units per year). There was no significant difference between treatment groups for changes in score for apathy (dibenzodiazepines: 0.4±0.2 units per year, risperidone: 0.5±0.3 units per year, tetrabenazine: 1.0±0.4 units per year, benzamides: 0.4±0.4 units per year), obsessive-compulsive symptoms (dibenzodiazepines: 0.6±0.2 units per year, risperidone: 0.6±0.5 units per year, tetrabenazine: 0.0±0.6 units per year, benzamides: 0.0±0.6 units per year), symptoms of depression (dibenzodiazepines: −0.7±0.4 units per year, risperidone: −0.7±0.8 units per year, tetrabenazine: −0.7±0.9 units per year, benzamides: −0.5±0.9 units per year) or psychosis (dibenzodiazepines: 0.0±0.1 units per year, risperidone: 0.0±0.1 units per year, tetrabenazine: 0.1±0.1 units per year, benzamides: 0.0±0.1 units per year). For irritability and aggression, dibenzodiazepines and tetrabenazine performed better than risperidone (dibenzodiazepines: −0.5±0.2 units per year, risperidone: 0.6±0.4 units per year, tetrabenazine: −0.9±0.5 units per year, benzamides: −0.6±0.5 units per year). An adjustment on multiple propensity score and antidepressant use over time did not modify the results for behavioral scores.

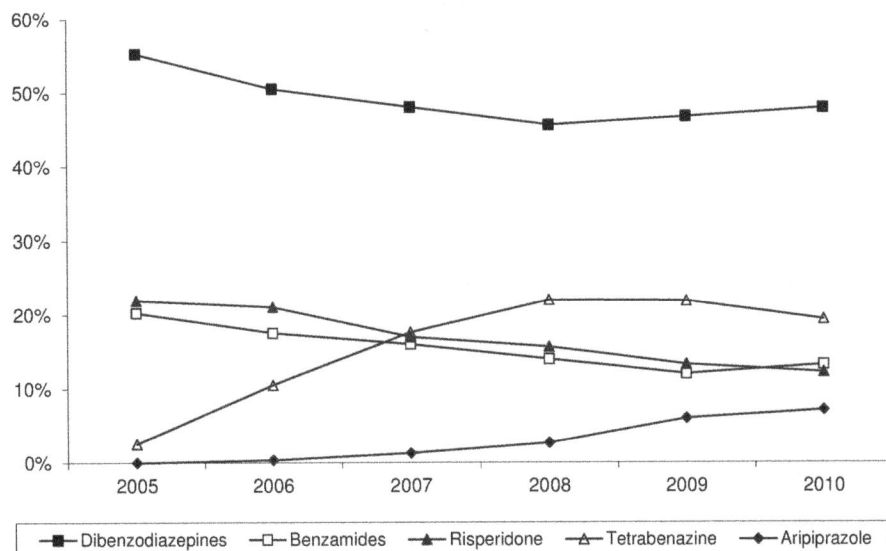

Figure 1. Percentage of prescriptions made for each class of antipsychotic and related drugs (2002–2010). Aripiprazole and tetrabenazine obtained market authorisation in 2004 and 2005, respectively.

Table 2. Baseline patient profile on the day of first prescription of an anti-psychotic or related drug.

		Dibenzodiazepines		Risperidone		Tetrabenazine		Benzamides	p
Age (year)	187	49.6±11.6	60	52.1±10.1	63	53.1±12.4	56	49.7±10.5	NS
Age at HD onset (year)	179	42.9±12.0	55	44.0±10.1	61	44.9±12.3	52	42.0±10.4	NS
Males (%)	186	52.2	60	48.3	63	49.2	56	60.7	NS
Study year	175	11.6±3.4	54	10.8±3.2	58	11.6±3.3	54	11.9±3.4	NS
Duration of HD (year)	179	6.9±5.5	55	8.5±5.0	61	8.5±4.7	52	8.0±4.6	0.002
CAG repeat length	187	45.3±4.1	60	44.0±3.4	63	44.5±3.3	56	45.6±4.2	0.05
Antidepressant use (%)	187	49.2	60	53.3	63	65.1	56	44.6	NS
BMI	153	22.8±3.7	51	23.2±4.5	44	22.2±3.5	45	23.2±3.7	NS
Motor score	177	44.3±21.7	58	45.9±20.6	57	50.6±22.0	51	52.3±24.0	0.05
Behavioural score	176	20.0±11.9	56	22.5±10.3	59	18.0±12.6	50	20.9±11.7	NS
Functional scores									
Functional Assessment Scale	182	32.4±6.3	59	34.7±6.5	61	34.8±7.2	54	36.4±7.5	0.0005
Independence scale	181	75.6±17.2	59	70.6±16.3	60	69.0±18.6	53	66.5±18.9	0.0003
Total Functional Capacity	182	7.8±3.4	59	6.6±3.2	62	6.8±3.3	55	6.2±3.8	0.004
Cognitive scores									
Literacy fluency 1mn	113	18.9±11.3	39	14.1±11.0	42	16.8±12.1	39	13.9±8.1	0.01
SDMT	108	18.7±10.7	33	13.4±8.9	40	15.5±11.6	38	15.7±9.8	NS
Stroop colour	112	38.6±15.8	38	31.2±16.6	42	32.4±15.6	40	32.1±14.0	NS
Stroop word	112	51.7±20.7	38	44.7±23.0	42	47.3±20.5	40	43.5±21.2	NS
Stroop interference	112	20.5±11.1	37	14.3±10.0	42	15.9±12.0	40	16.0±11.5	0.007

SDMT: Symbol digit modality test, BMI: body mass index.
Mean ± SD.

There were, however, significant differences for functional impairment: patients taking dibenzodiazepine showed a greater change in TFC score than patients receiving risperidone or tetrabenazine (p<0.05).

Overall, cognitive abilities decreased to a greater extent with benzamide treatment than with dibenzodiazepine, risperidone or tetrabenazine treatments (p<0.05). The impairment in cognition was greater with benzamides than with dibenzodiazepines as assessed with the symbol digit modality test, Stroop colour and interference measures (p<0.05). Significant differences in the literacy fluency (1 minute timing), Stroop colour and interference measures were observed between the benzamide group and the tetrabenazine group (p<0.05). Performance in the symbol digit modality test was also significantly poorer in the benzamide group of patients than in the risperidone group (p<0.05).

The change in body mass index (BMI) over time depended on the APR used. BMI change was significantly less with benzamides (−0.9±0.3 kg/m² per year) than with dibenzodiazepines (0.2±0.1 kg/m² per year) or risperidone (0.0±0.2 kg/m² per year).

There was no significant difference between treatments when analysing tiapride as single drug (n = 43 out of 56 benzamide), except for the results of some of the functional and cognitive assessments. Deterioration was less marked in the Functional Assessment Scale for patients on dibenzodiazepines than for those on tiapride (p<0.05) as well as in the Total Functional Capacity in patients on dibenzodiazepines comparing with patients on tiapride (p<0.05). Decline in the Stroop interference score was greater in patients on tiapride than those on dibenzodiazepines or tetrabenazine (p<0.05).

Changes in control and treatment groups

In a set of secondary analyses, the group, who had never received an APR, was less severely affected than the groups administered antipsychotics, and the propensity scores failed to correct the differences observed at baseline for motor impairments, some of the behavioural items (dystonia, apathy, obsessive-compulsive symptoms and psychosis), the functional assessment scale and the total functional capacity, and some cognitive assessments (literacy fluency and symbol digit modality test). For chorea, behaviour and symptoms of depression, the patterns of changes through time did not differ between the groups. Irritability and aggression progressed faster in the risperidone group than in the controls (0.8±0.4 units per year, p<0.05). There were significant differences for the independence scale: deterioration was less marked for controls than patients. Decline was greater in the benzamide than controls groups at all Stroop scores (p<0.05) and also at Stroop word and interference (p<0.05) in the dibenzodiazepine group. There were significant differences in the changes in BMI between the control group (−0.1±0.1 kg/m² per year) and the dibenzodiazepine group, where the BMI increased, and benzamide group, where the BMI decreased.

Discussion

We followed 956 patients from 2002 to 2010; of these, 63% were treated with antipsychotics and related drugs (APRs). Dibenzodiazepines were given to patients with relatively less disability on functional and cognitive scales (literal fluency and Stroop interference) at the time of the first prescription. Patient profiles did not differ in other UHDRS components. Taking into account existing differences in patient profiles at the beginning of

Table 3. Pairwise comparisons of effectiveness during the treatment period.

		Dibenzodiazepinessesses	Risperidone	Tetrabenazine
Motor score (n = 305)	Risperidone	0.05±1.06		
	Tetrabenazine	−2.15±1.29	−2.21±1.53	
	Benzamides	−1.77±1.21	−1.82±1.46	0.39±1.64
Behavioural score (n = 305)	Risperidone	−0.65±0.93		
	Tetrabenazine	−1.10±1.04	0.55±1.26	
	Benzamides	0.52±1.06	1.17±1.28	0.62±1.36
Functional scores				
Functional Assessment Scale (n = 301)	Risperidone	−0.55±0.33		
	Tetrabenazine	−0.09±0.38	0.45±0.46	
	Benzamides	−0.61±0.36	−0.06±0.44	−0.51±0.48
Independence scale (n = 297)	Risperidone	−0.16±0.85		
	Tetrabenazine	−1.10±0.97	−0.93±1.18	
	Benzamides	−0.17±0.92	0.00±1.14	0.93±1.23
Total Functional Capacity (n = 301)	Risperidone	−0.41±0.17 * †		
	Tetrabenazine	−0.54±0.19 *	−0.13±0.24	
	Benzamides	−0.31±0.19	0.10±0.23	0.23±0.25
Cognitive scores				
Literacy fluency 1 mn (n = 210)	Risperidone	0.34±0.74		
	Tetrabenazine	1.19±0.74	0.84±0.95	
	Benzamides	−0.79±0.74	−1.13±0.95	−1.97±0.94 *
SDMT (n = 201)	Risperidone	0.67±0.57		
	Tetrabenazine	0.06±0.55	−0.61±0.72	
	Benzamides	−1.02±0.49 *	−1.70±0.68 *	−1.08±0.67
Stroop colour (n = 201)	Risperidone	0.22±0.93		
	Tetrabenazine	0.47±0.92	0.24±1.20	
	Benzamides	−1.99±0.85 *	−2.21±1.15	−2.46±1.14 *
Stroop word (n = 206)	Risperidone	0.49±1.38		
	Tetrabenazine	0.84±1.36	0.35±1.78	
	Benzamides	−1.80±1.27	−2.29±1.70	−2.63±1.69
Stroop interference (n = 205)	Risperidone	0.03±0.73		
	Tetrabenazine	0.63±0.71	0.60±0.94	
	Benzamides	−1.42±0.66 *	−1.45±0.90	−2.05±0.88 *

Adjusted difference (line minus column) in mean change per year ± standard error.
SDMT: Symbol digit modality test.
*P<0.05.
† Scores were reversed if necessary (change under risperidone minus the change under dibenzodiazepines = −0.41); the mean evolution of TFC was greater with dibenzodiazepines than with risperidone.

the treatment as well as antidepressant undertaken, there was no difference in the changes in motor and behavioural symptoms between the patients on different treatments. The decline in functional score was less severe with dibenzodiazepines than with other APRs. Benzamides were associated with more rapid cognitive decline than the other antipsychotics.

The rate of decline of these patients was similar to that seen in other cohorts (TFC: 0.80±0.00 *vs.* 0.63±0.75 units per year for 129 patients [14], 1.4±0.1 units per year for 92 patients with average follow-up of 3.7 years [15], 0.68±1.39 units per year for 42 patients with average follow-up of 1.9 years [16]; motor capacity: 4.40±0.20 *vs.* 4.42±7.30 units per year [16]). This suggests that our results on effectiveness could be generalised to stages 1 to 3 of the disease. Although our study addressed a rare disease, the number of patients and the length of the study provided sufficient statistical power to obtain significant results. The study is novel in that it provides a comparison of different APRs used in treating HD. We were also able to follow patients for much longer than the relatively short follow-up times of clinical trials (4–12 weeks in clinical trials for antipsychotic drugs [5] *vs.* more than two years in our study).

A secondary goal of this study was to compare disease progression in the four groups of treated patients with that in non-medicated patients. Because, never-treated patients were less severely affected, the value of this group for comparisons provided limited information (even if we use multiple propensity score). A further sub-analysis was performed with patients who received APRs after 2006. This was due to possible changes in prescription habits for tetrabenazine, following the new marketing authorisation in 2005. The results support the same conclusions as the full data sample. The mean time lag between first visit and prescription was 13 months. It is possible that a patient's health could deteriorate during this period and that the administration of APRs could have been started without a visit to a participating centre. We conducted a sub-analysis of the patients for who this delay was only six months or less. The findings were consistent with those for the complete data set (data not shown). Drugs within one class could have a different effect and side effect profile, more patients are needed to analyse each drugs separately. Finally, the side effect profile of APRs depends to a large extent on the dose prescribed. Unfortunately, medicated doses were not available in our study.

In our cohort, tetrabenazine and benzamides tended to be given to patients with a more impaired motor score at the time of first prescription. This may be because they are the only APRs to have market authorisation in France for treatment of motor disability and, in particular, chorea. However, there was no difference in motor decline between patients treated with tetrabenazine and those treated with other APRs (0.8 ± 0.5 units per year). This result contrasts with previous studies showing an improvement in chorea under tetrabenazine by a mean of 5.0 units on the UHDRS after 12 weeks [17] and by 4.6 units after 80 weeks in an open-label continuation study [18]. Tetrabenazine might be less effective against motor symptom progression in the long term, and this would explain the discordance between our and previous studies. Less evidence is available for olanzapine: only one open-label study has shown improvement of the motor scale [19] whereas in two other open-label studies, the statistical tests indicated no significant differences [20,21]. Two trials with tiapride (the most commonly used benzamide) produced contradictory results and used reduced movement count rather than the UHDRS score to assess motor features [22]. To our knowledge, no clinical trials have assessed risperidone in HD.

Our functional assessments with the TFC scale revealed differences between APR groups. In a multicentre, double-blind, controlled trial (TETRA-HD), 84 ambulatory patients with HD were randomised to receive either tetrabenazine (n = 54) or a placebo (n = 30) for 12 weeks. Tetrebenazine was found to have a deleterious effect on functional capacity [17]. A mild improvement in the disability scale score was observed in case studies with risperidone [23] and olanzapine [24]. A small-scale trial comparing tiapride treatment to a placebo found no difference in functional scores [25].

Antipsychotics may act on multiple psychiatric symptoms. The summary of product characteristics for tetrabenazine states that it is not advisable to initiate this treatment for patients suffering from symptoms of depression. Depressed mood, low self-esteem, anxiety and suicidal ideation as assessed with the UHDRS at baseline did not differ between treatment groups. This suggests that tetrabenazine was not only used in patients with less severe depressive symptoms. Our study shows no difference in behavioural scores between patients on different APRs. It provides no evidence for a deleterious effect of tetrabenazine, or a beneficial effect of dibenzodiazepines, on psychiatric symptoms. In contrast with our results, two small open-pilot studies showed a significant improvement in some UHDRS psychiatric sub-scores (depression, anxiety, irritability and obsessions) after olanzapine treatment and in the short term [21][20]. There are also case reports of successful risperidone use in aggressive HD patients [26].

Although APRs are commonly used in Huntington's disease, only the TETRA-HD study has reported the effect of tetrabenazine on cognition. Stroop word-reading scores were worse in the tetrabenazine than the placebo group [17]. In our study, tetrabenazine was more effective than benzamides on Stroop colour, Stroop interference and verbal fluency tests. As observed in schizophrenia [27], the decline in digit symbol test scores is smaller with dibenzodiazepines than with benzamides. Thus, the effect of APRs on cognition should be considered when prescribing an antipsychotic for patients with HD.

Weight loss is a common feature in Huntington's disease [28]; the impact of APRs on changes in body mass index over time is well known. As expected, patients under benzodiazepines or risperidone did not loss weight. However, these drugs are associated with weight gain in schizophrenia [29].

In conclusion, we observed similar changes in motor and behavioural scores. Patients taking dibenzodiazapine presented fewer declines in functional scores than patients receiving risperidone and tetrabenazine. Benzamides tended to be associated with the greatest cognitive decline. These differences may be explained by differential pharmacological mechanisms. Tetrabenazine is chemically related to antipsychotic drugs but works as a dopamine depletor by inhibiting the central vesicular monoamine transporter [30]. Benzamides are selective for dopaminergic D2 receptors, dibenzodiazepine and risperidone are less selective for dopaminergic receptors and are antagonists of serotoninergic and alpha-adrenergic receptors. The findings of this observational study, which may have been affected by unmeasured or unaccounted factors, need to be confirmed by further controlled studies. Consequently, we have now initiated a multicentre randomised controlled study (Neuro-HD) comparing olanzapine, tetrabenazine and tiapride. The results are expected in three years.

Author Contributions

Conceived and designed the experiments: G. Désaméricq ACBL MP. Performed the experiments: G. Dolbeau CV CP AD KY CS JPA CT CG PD EB FJ GM LCDL IMM. Analyzed the data: G. Désaméricq G. Dolbeau ACBL MP. Wrote the paper: G. Désaméricq CV CP AD KY CS JPA CT CG PD EB FJ ACBL MP.

References

1. Mulrow CD, Cook DJ, Davidoff F (1997) Systematic reviews: critical links in the great chain of evidence. Ann Intern Med 126: 389–391.

2. Schneeweiss S (2007) Developments in post-marketing comparative effectiveness research. Clin Pharmacol Ther 82: 143–156. doi:10.1038/sj.clpt.6100249.

3. (1993) A novel gene containing a trinucleotide repeat that is expanded and unstable on Huntington's disease chromosomes. The Huntington's Disease Collaborative Research Group. Cell 72: 971–983.

4. Van Duijn E, Kingma EM, Van der Mast RC (2007) Psychopathology in verified Huntington's disease gene carriers. J Neuropsychiatry Clin Neurosci 19: 441–448. doi:10.1176/appi.neuropsych.19.4.441.

5. Mestre T, Ferreira J, Coelho MM, Rosa M, Sampaio C (2009) Therapeutic interventions for symptomatic treatment in Huntington's disease. Cochrane Database Syst Rev: CD006456. doi:10.1002/14651858.CD006456.pub2.

6. Ross CA, Tabrizi SJ (2011) Huntington's disease: from molecular pathogenesis to clinical treatment. Lancet Neurol 10: 83–98. doi:10.1016/S1474-4422(10)70245-3.

7. Venuto CS, McGarry A, Ma Q, Kieburtz K (2012) Pharmacologic approaches to the treatment of Huntington's disease. Mov Disord 27: 31–41. doi:10.1002/mds.23953.

8. Orth M, Handley OJ, Schwenke C, Dunnett SB, Craufurd D, et al. (2010) Observing Huntington's Disease: the European Huntington's Disease Network's REGISTRY. PLoS Curr 2. Available:http://www.ncbi.nlm.nih.gov/pubmed/20890398. Accessed 21 February 2012.

9. Priller J, Ecker D, Landwehrmeyer B, Craufurd D (2008) A Europe-wide assessment of current medication choices in Huntington's disease. Mov Disord 23: 1788. doi:10.1002/mds.22188.

10. Shoulson I (1981) Huntington disease. Neurology 31: 1333–1333.

11. Unified Huntington's Disease Rating Scale: reliability and consistency. Huntington Study Group (1996). Mov Disord 11: 136–142. doi:10.1002/mds.870110204.

12. WHO collaborating centre for drug statistics methodology (n.d.) WHOCC - ATC/DDD Index. Available:http://www.whocc.no/atc_ddd_index/. Accessed 21 February 2012.

13. Spreeuwenberg MD, Bartak A, Croon MA, Hagenaars JA, Busschbach JJV, et al. (2010) The multiple propensity score as control for bias in the comparison of more than two treatment arms: an introduction from a case study in mental health. Med Care 48: 166–174. doi:10.1097/MLR.0b013e3181c1328f.

14. Feigin A, Kieburtz K, Bordwell K, Como P, Steinberg K, et al. (1995) Functional decline in Huntington's disease. Mov Disord 10: 211–214. doi:10.1002/mds.870100213.

15. Penney JB Jr, Young AB, Shoulson I, Starosta-Rubenstein S, Snodgrass SR, et al. (1990) Huntington's disease in Venezuela: 7 years of follow-up on symptomatic and asymptomatic individuals. Mov Disord 5: 93–99. doi:10.1002/mds.870050202.

16. Van Vugt JPP, Piet KKE, Vink IJ, Siesling S, Zwinderman AH, et al. (2004) Objective assessment of motor slowness in Huntington's disease: clinical correlates and 2-year follow-up. Mov Disord 19: 285–297. doi:10.1002/mds.10718.

17. Tetrabenazine as antichorea therapy in Huntington disease: a randomized controlled trial (2006). Neurology 66: 366–372. doi:10.1212/01.wnl.0000198586.85250.13.

18. Frank S (2009) Tetrabenazine as anti-chorea therapy in Huntington disease: an open-label continuation study. Huntington Study Group/TETRA-HD Investigators. BMC Neurol 9: 62. doi:10.1186/1471-2377-9-62.

19. Bonelli RM, Mahnert FA, Niederwieser G (2002) Olanzapine for Huntington's disease: an open label study. Clin Neuropharmacol 25: 263–265.

20. Squitieri F, Cannella M, Piorcellini A, Brusa L, Simonelli M, et al. (2001) Short-term effects of olanzapine in Huntington disease. Neuropsychiatry Neuropsychol Behav Neurol 14: 69–72.

21. Paleacu D, Anca M, Giladi N (2002) Olanzapine in Huntington's disease. Acta Neurol Scand 105: 441–444.

22. Bonelli RM, Wenning GK (2006) Pharmacological management of Huntington's disease: an evidence-based review. Curr Pharm Des 12: 2701–2720.

23. Erdemoglu AK, Boratav C (2002) Risperidone in chorea and psychosis of Huntington's disease. Eur J Neurol 9: 182–183.

24. Laks J, Rocha M, Capitão C, Domingues RC, Ladeia G, et al. (2004) Functional and motor response to low dose olanzapine in Huntington's disease: case report. Arq Neuropsiquiatr 62: 1092–1094. doi:/S0004-282X2004000600030.

25. Quinn N, Marsden CD (1985) Tiapride in 12 Huntington's disease patients. J Neurol Neurosurg Psychiatr 48: 292.

26. Bonelli RM, Wenning GK, Kapfhammer HP (2004) Huntington's disease: present treatments and future therapeutic modalities. Int Clin Psychopharmacol 19: 51–62.

27. Guo X, Zhai J, Wei Q, Twamley EW, Jin H, et al. (2011) Neurocognitive effects of first- and second-generation antipsychotic drugs in early-stage schizophrenia: a naturalistic 12-month follow-up study. Neurosci Lett 503: 141–146. doi:10.1016/j.neulet.2011.08.027.

28. Nance MA, Sanders G (1996) Characteristics of individuals with Huntington disease in long-term care. Movement Disorders 11: 542–548. doi:10.1002/mds.870110509.

29. Rummel-Kluge C, Komossa K, Schwarz S, Hunger H, Schmid F, et al. (2010) Head-to-head comparisons of metabolic side effects of second generation antipsychotics in the treatment of schizophrenia: a systematic review and meta-analysis. Schizophr Res 123: 225–233. doi:10.1016/j.schres.2010.07.012.

30. Jankovic J, Beach J (1997) Long-term effects of tetrabenazine in hyperkinetic movement disorders. Neurology 48: 358–362.

7

Two-Point Magnitude MRI for Rapid Mapping of Brown Adipose Tissue and its Application to the R6/2 Mouse Model of Huntington Disease

Katrin S. Lindenberg[1]Ꙩ, Patrick Weydt[1]Ꙩ, Hans-Peter Müller[1], Axel Bornstedt[2], Albert C. Ludolph[1], G. Bernhard Landwehrmeyer[1], Wolfgang Rottbauer[2], Jan Kassubek[1], Volker Rasche[2,3]*

1 Department of Neurology, Ulm University, Ulm, Germany, 2 Department of Internal Medicine II, Ulm University, Ulm, Germany, 3 Core Facility Small Animal Imaging, Ulm University, Ulm, Germany

Abstract

The recent discovery of active brown fat in human adults has led to renewed interest in the role of this key metabolic tissue. This is particularly true for neurodegenerative conditions like Huntington disease (HD), an adult-onset heritable disorder with a prominent energy deficit phenotype. Current methods for imaging brown adipose tissue (BAT) are in limited use because they are equipment-wise demanding and often prohibitively expensive. This prompted us to explore how a standard MRI set-up can be modified to visualize BAT *in situ* by taking advantage of its characteristic fat/water content ratio to differentiate it from surrounding white fat. We present a modified MRI protocol for use on an 11.7 T small animal MRI scanner to visualize and quantify BAT in wild-type and disease model laboratory mice. In this application study using the R6/2 transgenic mouse model of HD we demonstrate a significantly reduced BAT volume in HD mice vs. matched controls (n = 5 per group). This finding provides a plausible structural explanation for the previously described temperature phenotype of HD mice and underscores the significance of peripheral tissue pathology for the HD phenotype. On a more general level, the results demonstrate the feasibility of MR-based BAT imaging in rodents and open the path towards transferring this imaging approach to human patients. Future studies are needed to determine if this method can be used to track disease progression in HD and other disease entities associated with BAT abnormalities, including metabolic conditions such as obesity, cachexia, and diabetes.

Editor: Marià Alemany, Faculty of Biology, Spain

Funding: Funding provided by European Huntington's Disease Network (EHDN) seed fund 414, http://www.eurohd.net/html/network. The funders had no role in study design, data collection and analysis, decision to publish, or preparation of the manuscript.

* Email: volker.rasche@uni-ulm.de

Ꙩ These authors contributed equally to this work.

Introduction

Brown adipose tissue (BAT) is a key tissue for the regulation of whole-body energy metabolism [1]. Through the expression of mitochondrial uncoupling protein 1 (UCP-1), which allows proton leakage across the inner mitochondrial membrane, BAT is capable of dissipating energy in the form of heat. BAT is thus the principal effector tissue of adaptive, non-shivering thermogenesis. A series of breakthrough positron emission tomography (PET) and computed tomography (CT) imaging studies has recently shown BAT deposits even in adult humans [2–5]. This resulted in a renewed interest in the role of BAT especially for metabolic conditions such as obesity and cachexia, thereby creating the need for appropriate imaging technologies [6]. Large-scale studies aiming at the structural and functional characterization of BAT by PET/CT in human adults are still scarce [4,6,7]. Factors contributing to this limitation include the high costs for the required tracers, safety concerns about the radiation involved, and the required activation

of BAT either via cold-exposure or pharmacologically.

Huntington disease (HD), an autosomal dominant adult-onset neurodegenerative disease caused by the abnormal expansion of the CAG-repeat tract in the huntingtin gene, represents an area of research where these new developments are of particular interest [8]. In addition to the classic triad of neuro-psychiatric symptoms, i.e. movement disorder, cognitive decline and psychiatric abnormalities, HD patients display a progressive energy deficit that is of high clinical and scientific relevance [9]. This energy deficit is recapitulated in transgenic mouse models of HD and this led to the implication of brown fat dysfunction in HD pathogenesis, even before BAT-activity in human adults was discovered [10,11]. Selected transgenic mouse models of HD therefore provide a useful model system to study disease-related BAT dysfunction *in vivo*.

Hamilton and colleagues performed an in-depth analysis of the magnetic resonance (MR) signatures of BAT and white adipose tissue (WAT) [12]. They reported several key MR properties that are different between BAT and WAT, including fat fraction, changes in the T1 relaxation rate of the water-bond protons, and the degree of lipid saturation. The use of the histological and physiological properties of BAT has the major advantage of not requiring prior stimulation and has been applied for fat characterization by means of magnetic resonance spectroscopy (MRS) and chemical-shift imaging (CSI) [13–15].

With the exception of intermolecular zero-quantum coherences spectroscopy aiming for assessment of the intravoxel distribution of fat and water spins [16] and blood oxygen level dependent MRI [17], the majority of published fat fraction imaging methods by MRI relies on direct fat/water quantification as initially introduced by Dixon and colleagues in 1984 [18]. Based on the original publication, several modifications of the technique have been proposed [19]. Although in principle off-resonance contributions can be compensated by the multi-point techniques, additional non-static phase errors and the need for phase unwrapping quite frequently introduce errors in the resulting fat/water maps and may cause exclusion of data [15] especially at ultrahigh field strength.

The goal of this work was to establish and validate a simplified two-point technique for direct visualization of BAT, using the difference between the magnitude of images obtained with in-phase and opposed-phase condition. The applicability of the proposed technique was tested pre-clinically in an HD disease model (R6/2 transgenic mouse). HD appears of special interest since brown fat abnormalities are of emerging interest in the investigation of the HD energy deficit, and the clear genetic pathogenesis of HD provides an excellent basis for future mechanistic studies in transgenic model systems and facilitates validation in human patients and translational approaches.

Results

All scans could be completed successfully in the investigated cohorts. Automatic thresholding applying the Otsu method was effective in full suppression of background signal as well as pixels with low signal intensities as e.g. present in the lung and cortical bone. **Figure 1** shows a direct *in vivo* comparison of the 2PM approach with the conventional 3PD method. The image intensity in the 2PM approach is linearly related to the fat-water fraction with a maximum at equal magnetization of fat- and water spins. Since BAT is expected to show an almost equal magnetization of fat- and water spins, BAT presents as bright signal intensity in the final 2PM images. Water- and fat-only voxels show a clearly reduced intensity. The signal in the fat fraction images derived from the 3PD method scales linearly with the fat fraction in the magnetization. Water-only voxels appear dark, fat-only voxels appear bright, and BAT voxels present with intermediate signal intensity. The direct comparison shows an excellent resemblance of the resulting BAT distribution between the two approaches. The interscapular fat deposits (Figure 1, arrows) can be clearly appreciated as well as some smaller pads of BAT extending anteriorly and bilaterally around a large vessel (Figure 1, arrowheads). Note that both methods show a similar sensitivity to partial volume effects.

An overview of the BAT pattern for the wild-type and transgenic R6/2 mice is provided in **Figure 2** for a slice centered at the location of the prominent interscapular BAT. As expected and as described previously [20,21], the reduced body size and general organ atrophy of R6/2 mice vs. wild-type controls is immediately evident.

Even though the spatial resolution was lowered for reduction of the acquisition time, the BAT distribution can be readily retrieved from the resulting 2PM images. Semi-automatic quantification of the BAT volumes showed a highly significant positive correlation of the 2PM and the conventional 3PD method ($R = 0.976$, $p < 0.01$, Spearmans's rho). Further analysis allowed for direct and quantitative comparison of BAT volumes in the region of interest between HD mice and matched wild-type controls. As shown in **Figure 3a**, R6/2 mice have a greatly reduced BAT volume ($P < 0.01$) of 18.46 µl (min: 14.18 µl, max: 23.85 µl) ml vs. 36.82 µl (min: 32.34 µl, max 45.40 µl) in controls. The difference is blunted but still manifest and statistically significant ($P < 0.05$) when normalization to total body volume as a correction for the different body sizes is introduced (**Figure 3b**).

Discussion

The study evaluates a non-invasive method, which allows for *in vivo* and *ex vivo* BAT volume quantification from magnitude images. The intrinsic insensitivity of the technique to any kind of phase errors introduced by system imperfections should cause an at least similar reproducibility of 2PM as the more established fat-fraction methods [14,22,23]. Since the approach is based on a conventional FLASH technique, it can be readily used on any conventional MRI scanner without further modification of acquisition methods. In comparison to other MRI-based BAT-imaging techniques, the advantage of the 2PM method is the straightforward approach, which does not require any special expertise in advanced MRI techniques or image processing. The technique can be readily modified further to provide blood oxygen level dependent contrast. Khanna et al. [17] showed that T2* weighting times of about 2 ms are sufficient for the assessment of BAT activity. For magnetic field strengths between 1.5 and 11.7 T as used for clinical and pre-clinical imaging, one of the required in- and opposed-phase echo times can be chosen close to the suggested value. Furthermore, the 2PM method can also easily be adapted to the suggested asymmetric spin echo acquisition if the required echo times cannot be met due to gradient power constraints. In this context the possibility of intrinsic identification of the BAT location from the scans obtained at normal body temperature is advantageous. Compared to the more complex intermolecular zero-quantum MRI [16,24], 2PM is hampered by partial volume effects similar to the fat fraction methods. However, slightly higher spatial resolution can be realized without significant scan time penalties since images with only two different echo times are required for providing the BAT information.

By use of our MRI-based tissue analysis, we show that R6/2 mice have significantly reduced BAT, even when corrected for reduced overall body size. This finding provides a plausible structural explanation for the striking cold-sensitive phenotype of R6/2 mice and other HD models [10,11]. The results are also in accordance with earlier reports of structural BAT abnormalities in transgenic mouse models of HD, including the R6/2 strain, all of which were obtained through non-survival conventional tissue dissection [10,11,25,26]. Importantly, our MRI-method now provides a practical strategy for monitoring BAT structure *in vivo* and longitudinally in the same individual animal.

While we focused our present study on the R6/2 mice, other transgenic mouse strains with a cold-sensitive body temperature phenotype such as the N171-82Q model of HD [10] and the mutant SOD1 model of amyotrophic lateral sclerosis [27] should also be investigated with respect to BAT structure, distribution and function *in vivo*. We would like to emphasize that this approach can naturally be applied to other diseases, e.g. obesity and

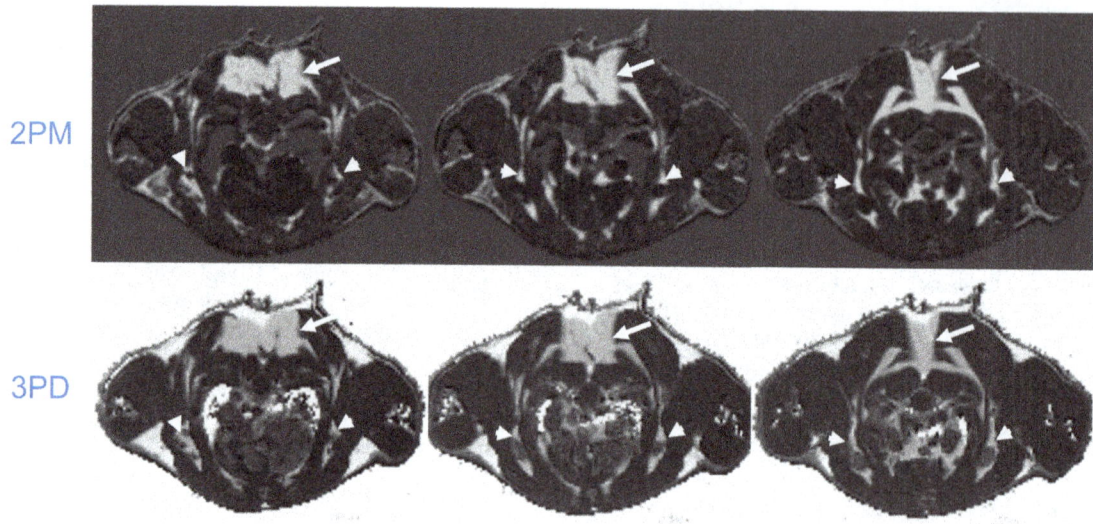

Figure 1. Direct comparison of the novel two-point magnitude method (2PM) and the conventional three-point phase-based Dixon method (3PD) in a wild-type mouse. Interscapular BAT deposits (arrows) as well as smaller pads of BAT (arrowheads) can be appreciated. Please note the excellent agreement between the two methods. Due to the suppression of pure fat and water voxels in the 2PM technique, a clear improvement of contrast between WAT and BAT areas can be appreciated with the 2PM technique.

diabetes. The results further suggest that this non-invasive methodology can be readily applied to human patients and control subjects. However, the different distribution of the BAT in humans especially in small pads as e.g. as in perivascular tissue may in general limit the direct BAT imaging approaches independent of the imaging technique used. In this context the improved scan efficiency of the proposed 2PM method may be beneficial due to better spatial resolution without sacrificing scan time compared to multi-point Dixon methods.

An important limitation of the data set presented here is the focus on a single fat pad in the interscapular region. We selected this region as it is recognized as the largest and most prominent BAT depot in rodents [28]. This choice permitted reliable anatomical localisation of the region of interest. It also allowed for direct comparison with the histological data from HD models, as to the best of our knowledge all the BAT tissue dissection studies in HD used interscapular BAT. This focus, however, did preclude characterisation of the BAT distribution patterns. As we know from imaging studies, fat distribution can vary in specific disease

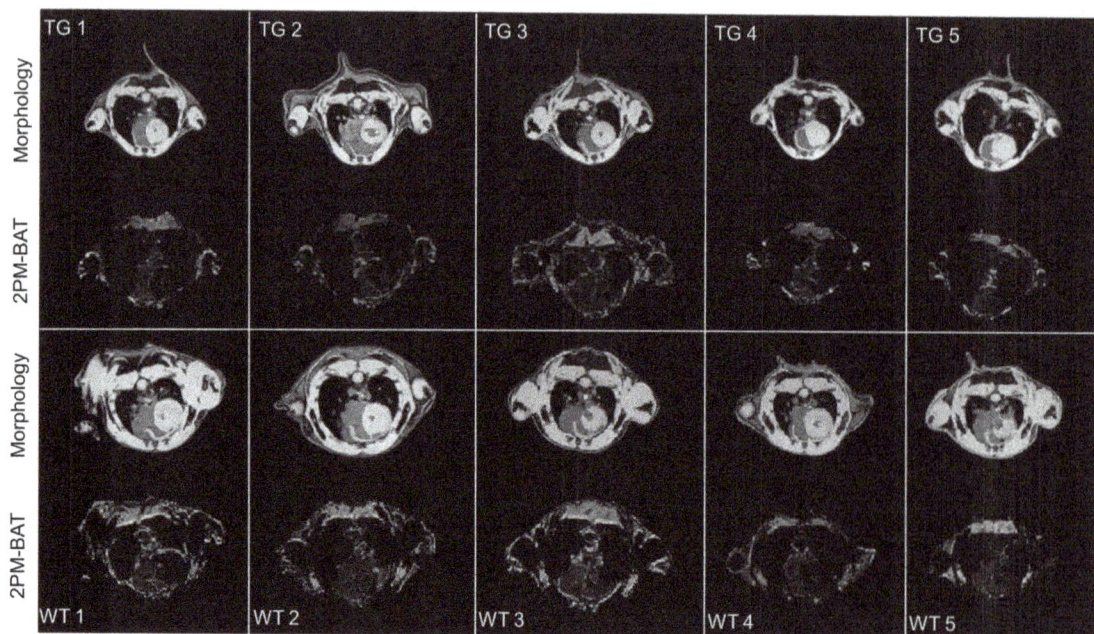

Figure 2. Comparison of morphological images and resulting BAT-weighed images from R6/2-transgenic (TG) and corresponding wild-type (WT) mice. Note the overall reduced tissue volume in the R6/2 mice. The slices were selected to comprise the shoulder region where the prominent interscapular BAT pad is located.

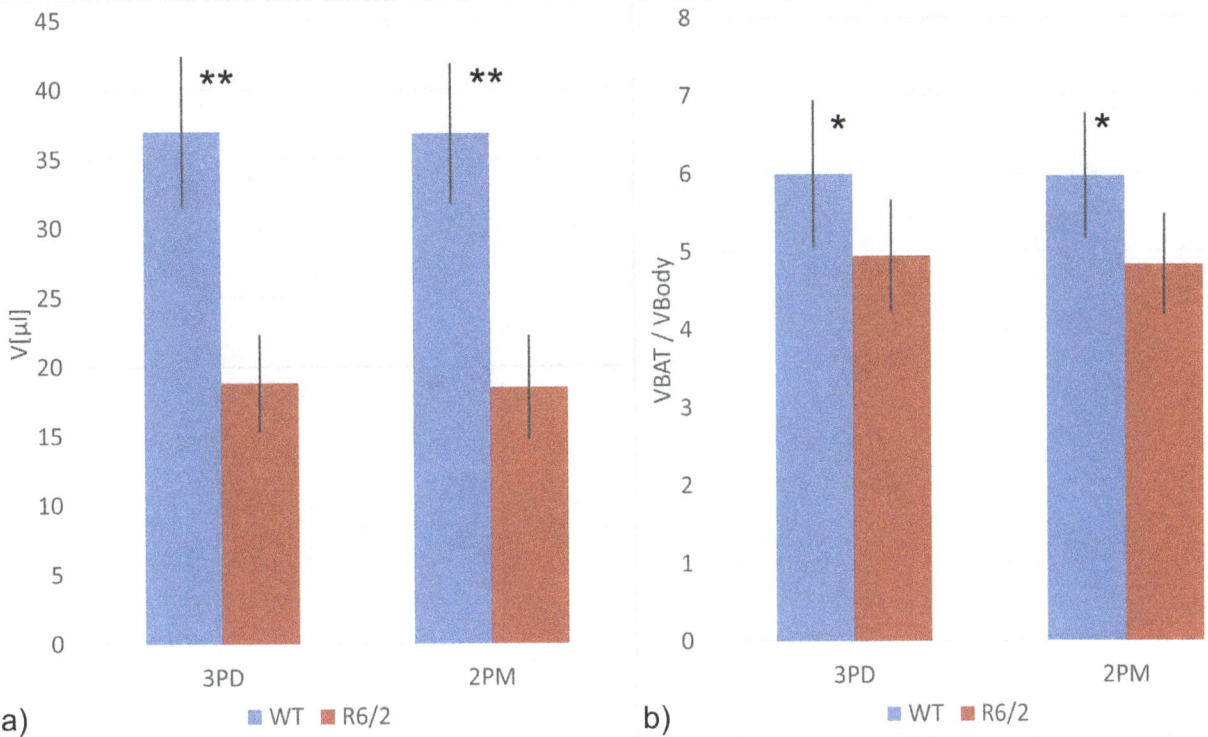

Figure 3. Total BAT volumes a) and BAT volumes normalized to total body volume b) for female HD-transgenic (R6/2) and matched wild-type control mice. (n = 5 per group; *P<0.05, **P<0.01; unrelated Wilcoxon Rank sum test; columns (error bars) represent means (standard deviation)).

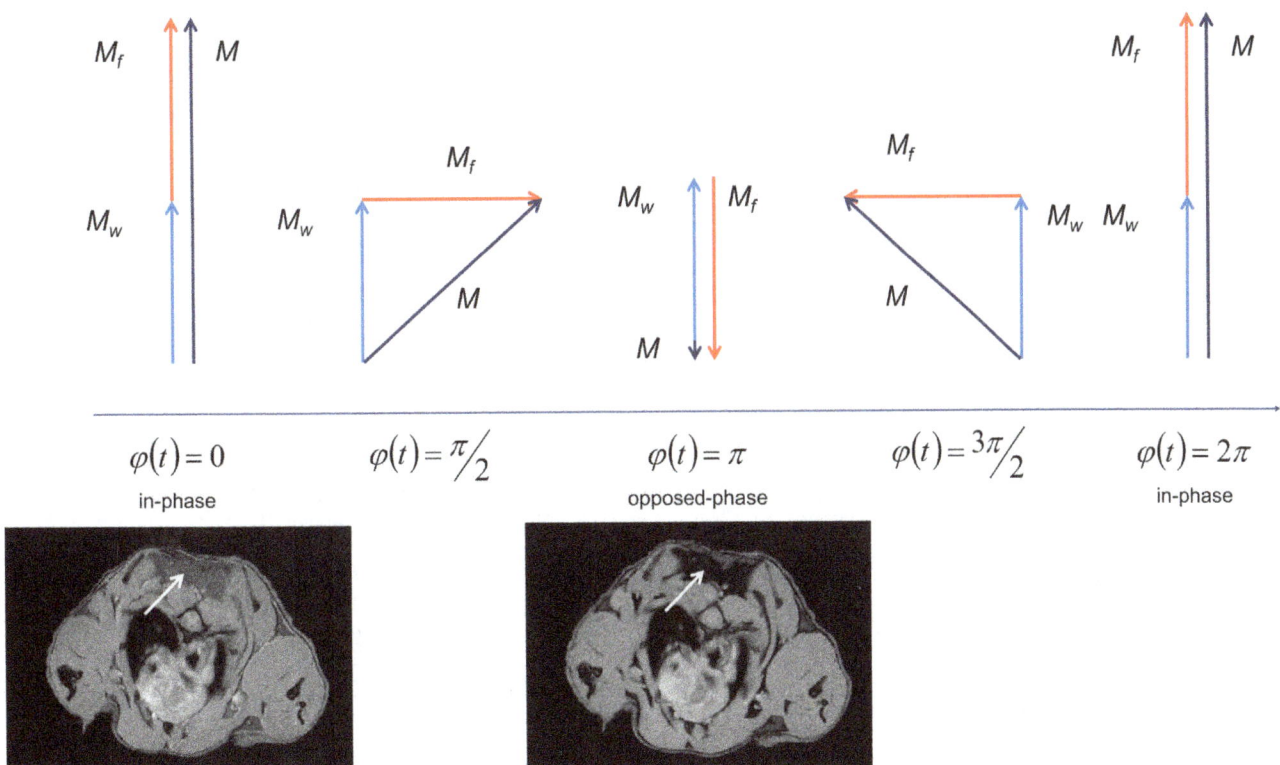

$$\varphi(t) = 0 \qquad \varphi(t) = \frac{\pi}{2} \qquad \varphi(t) = \pi \qquad \varphi(t) = \frac{3\pi}{2} \qquad \varphi(t) = 2\pi$$

in-phase opposed-phase in-phase

Figure 4. Resulting magnetization M (black) in a voxel containing almost equal concentration of water- (M_w, blue) and fat- (M_f, red) bond protons for different phase differences. Respective MR images of the mouse neck in axial orientation are exemplarily shown for in-phase (left) and opposed-phase (right) condition. The reduction of signal intensity in the interscapular BAT (arrows) is clearly appreciable.

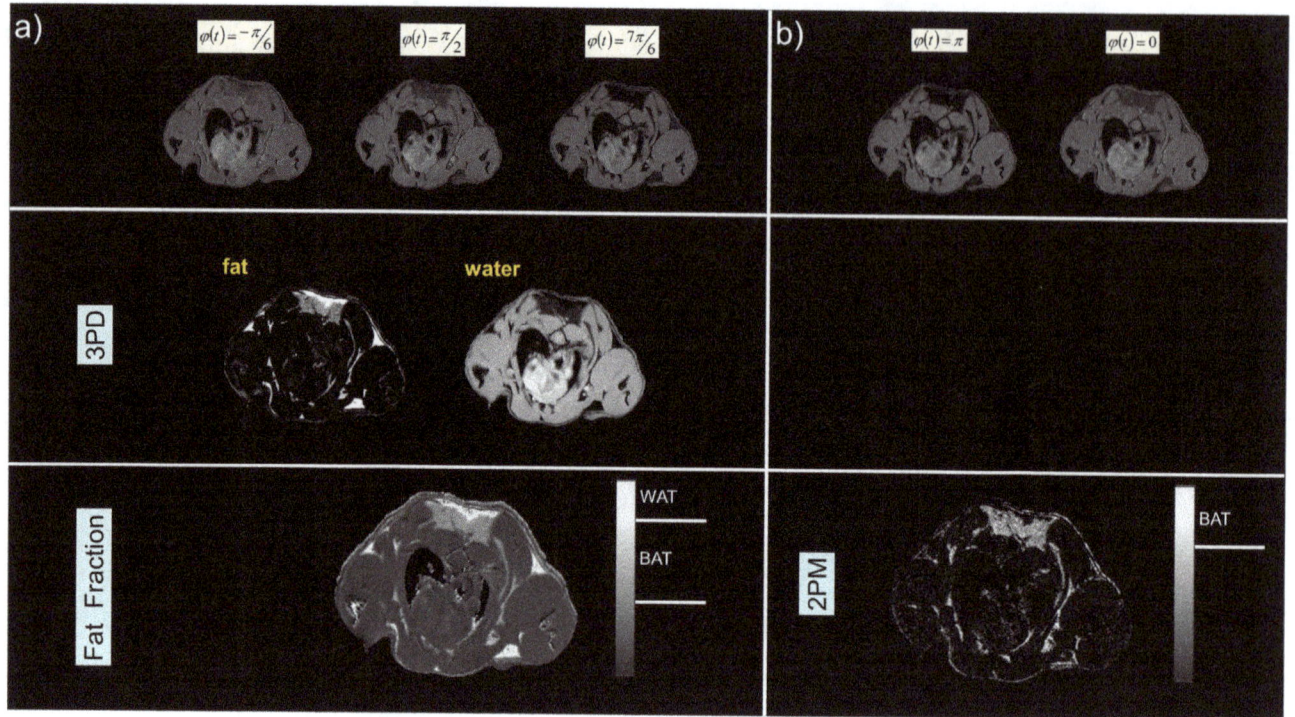

Figure 5. Comparison of the fat-fraction method based on a three-point Dixon approach (3PD, a), and the proposed two-point magnitude based method (2PM, b). The fat-fraction a) and BAT b) image are normalized from 0 to 1. The grey bars indicate the respective grey values used as threshold for WAT (>0.8, 3PD) and for BAT (>0.4 and <0.8, 3PD; >0.7, 2PM). WAT cannot be identified by the 2PM method, since signal from voxels containing only fat or water will be cancelled out during the involved subtraction.

states [29] and how such distribution changes play out in BAT pathology remains to be investigated. As a further limitation, our study was not designed to detect the so called beige or *brite* (*brown-in-white*) adipocytes [30] but in principle the presented tissue characterisation algorithm can be utilized to do so, if sufficient spatial resolution was achieved. Further in vivo studies with cold exposure have to be performed since the assessment of activated BAT has not been tested in this study. Also, since the method presented here relies on the characteristic relative fat/water content of BAT the use under conditions where the BAT composition is altered, e.g. starvation, require adjustments that were beyond the scope of this study.

In summary, we present a straightforward technique for assessing BAT structure with conventional MRI set-ups. Further research and development is necessary to integrate functional information, e.g. in the form of blood oxygen level dependent signal, into the MRI data acquisition protocol. The non-invasive *in vivo* character of the methodology allows longitudinal studies that were not previously possible. In a first application of the new methodology, we were able to show that symptomatic R6/2 mice have a reduced BAT volume. This finding provides insight into to the energy deficit in HD and highlights the importance of the peripheral tissue pathology for the understanding of the HD phenotype [31].

Materials and Methods

Theory

Depending on the environment, differently bond ^{1}H protons experience different resonance frequencies caused by the shielding effects of the electrons. This characteristic chemical shift can be utilized for tissue characterization and structural analysis by MRS

and is frequently applied to chemical analysis [32–34] in biomedical research. For ^{1}H proton spectroscopy, the reference with 0 ppm chemical shift is defined by tetramethysilane (TMS) and the chemical shift of different organic compounds is defined relative to TMS. Chemical shifts of fat bond ^{1}H protons range from 0.9 ppm $(-(CH_2)_n-CH_3)$ to 5.3 ppm $(-CH=CH-)$ and water (H_2O) showing a chemical shift of 4.7 ppm.

Hamilton et al. [12] investigated the MR properties of WAT and BAT. Important findings included alteration of endogenous biochemical characteristics as water – fat fraction $(wff = \frac{S_{water}}{S_{fat}}$, with S_{water} being the MR signal from water-bond protons and S_{fat} the respective MR signal from fat-bond protons), T1 relaxation times, and lipid saturation. From the investigated parameters wff showed the most pronounced difference between WAT $(wff < 0.2)$ and BAT $(wff\text{-}1)$. The higher amount of water in BAT has driven the application of fat fraction quantification to BAT quantification in mice [14] as well as in humans [15,22,35].

Fat fraction quantification demands accurate knowledge of the fat and water content in each voxel. Separation of water and fat can be achieved by Dixon techniques [18,23,36]. Dixon methods rely on the phase differences between MRI images obtained with different echo times (TE). The phase differences are introduced by the chemical shift of the different compounds. The MRI signal $S(t)$ from voxels containing different compounds results as

$$S(t) = \sum M_i(t) e^{i2\pi \Delta f_i^{CS} t} \qquad (1)$$

with $M_i(t)$ being the magnetization of the i-th component at time t and Δf_i^{CS} it's chemical shift. Although, different proton moieties are present, the fat contribution in BAT and WAT is dominated by the methylene protons (1.3 ppm), followed by methyl (0.9 ppm) and allylic protons (2.0 ppm). Considering water and methylene protons, only, Eq. 1 simplifies to

$$S(t) = M_w(t) + M_f(t)e^{i\varphi(t)}, \qquad (2)$$

with $\varphi(t) = 2\pi\Delta f_f^{CS} t$ being the phase between water and fat-bond protons. Theoretically, the fat (M_f) and water (M_w) image can be easily reconstructed from the sum (M_w) and the difference (M_f) of gradient echo images acquired in in-phase ($\varphi = 2n\pi$) and opposed-phase ($\varphi = (2n-1)\pi$) condition as suggested as the original two-point Dixon method [18]. A major limitation for the two-point Dixon method arises from local off-resonances, introducing an additional TE-dependent phase term and Eq. 2 must be rewritten as:

$$S(t) = \left(M_w(t) + M_f(t)e^{i\varphi(t)}\right)e^{i\Delta\varphi(t)}, \qquad (3)$$

with $\Delta\varphi(t) = 2\pi\Delta f^{\Delta B0} t$ being the off-resonance introduced phase error at time t. To compensate for the additional phase term, off-resonance maps and phase unwrapping techniques have to be used. Several techniques have been introduced so far for compensation of the off-resonance induced phase errors [36–38]. All techniques require additional measurements, which prolong the overall acquisition time. Off-resonance contributions can be compensated by the multi-point techniques, additional non-static phase errors and the need for phase unwrapping frequently introduce errors in the resulting fat/water maps especially at ultrahigh field strength.

In this study, a magnitude-based approach is introduced suggesting the use of the difference of the magnitude of two images acquired with echo times (TE) values for BAT volume quantification. The approach is based on the assumption that a major difference between WAT, normal biological tissue, and BAT results from the almost equal concentration of water- and fat-bond protons in BAT. The magnitude of $S(t)$ results from [Eq. 3] as

$$|S(t)| = |M_w(t) + M_f(t)e^{i\varphi(t)}|, \qquad (4)$$

where the phase $\varphi(t)$ between the water- and fat-bond protons cause an intensity modulation depending on the magnetization of the fat M_f and water M_w with almost complete signal cancellation at opposed phase condition in case of equal water and fat contributions as shown in **Figure 4**. For background suppression of voxels containing a single tissue, only, the final BAT signal is calculated according to:

$$S_{BAT} = |S_{in-phase}| - |S_{opposed-phase}| \qquad (5)$$

Animal groups

The suggested two-point magnitude (2PM) technique was initially evaluated in vivo in direct comparison with the three-point Dixon (3PD) technique in a group of three wild-type mice (C57/B6, 12 months, female). All in vivo data acquisition was carried out under isoflurane anesthesia (3% for induction and 1.5% for maintenance).

Applicability to cohort studies was evaluated in the R6/2 transgenic mouse model compared to sex-matched wild-type litter mates. The R6/2 mouse is among the most commonly used transgenic models of HD [20,39]. They display cold-intolerance highly suggestive of BAT dysfunction, and structural abnormalities

of white and brown adipose tissue are well-documented [10,25,40]. Female mice were used at 12 weeks, an age when this model is clearly symptomatic. Assuming a volume change in the order of 50% in the R6/2 group, to achieve a statistical power of 80% sample sizes of 5 animals per group were required. Power was calculated with nQuery (version 10). To exclude any impact of respiratory and cardiac motion artifacts in this feasibility study, the animals were sacrificed (CO_2 inhalation) immediately prior to the MRI investigation.

In vivo animal experiments were performed in accordance with German animal protection laws and had been approved by the national animal board (TVA 1001, "Etablierung Kleintierbildgebung an 3T und 11.7T", Regierungspräsidium Baden-Württemberg, Tübingen, Germany).

MRI protocol

The proposed two-point magnitude method (2PM) was implemented and evaluated against a 3PD method based on data acquired on a dedicated high-field 11.7T small animal MRI system (BioSpec 117/16, Bruker, Germany, Ettlingen). All data were acquired applying a 4cm quadrature volume resonator.

For initial in vivo evaluation (C57/B6) of the 2PM methods, a high-spatial resolution spoiled fast low-angle shot gradient echo technique (HR-FLASH, $\Delta r = 100 \times 100 \times 500$ μm^3) was applied. Data were acquired at five different echo times (TE = 1.203 ms, 1.313 ms, 1.459 ms, 1.507 ms, 1.751 ms), yielding phase shifts of $-\pi/6$, $\pi/2$, $7\pi/6$, π, 2π respectively. The applicability to cohort studies (R6/2, wild-type) was tested with a reduced spatial resolution protocol (LR-FLASH, $\Delta r = 120 \times 200 \times 500$ μm^3) to ensure rapid quantification of the BAT volumes. In all animals, the complete neck area was covered by acquiring 9 slices of 500 μm slice thickness with 1 mm spacing. Acquisition time T_{ACQ} for the acquisition of a single TE resulted to $T_{ACQ} = 3$m: 50s (LR-FLASH) and $T_{ACQ} = 6$m 24s (HR-FLASH). Excitation angle α and repetition time TR were as $\alpha = 15°$ and TR = 75 ms.

Data processing

After acquisition, the data was transferred to an independent workstation and further processed for BAT quantification. Fat fraction images were derived from the images acquired with $-\pi/6$, $\pi/2$, $7\pi/6$ phase shifts applying a multi-point Dixon method. For ensuring high quality of the fat fraction maps, the "fat-water toolbox" (http://ismrm.org/workshops/FatWater12/data.htm) provided by the ISMRM was applied for all calculations. For evaluation of the suggested two-point magnitude technique, the difference of the magnitude of the images obtained with in-phase and opposed-phase condition was calculated. An overview of the two approaches is provided in **Figure 5**. For noise reduction prior to further analysis, a 3×3 point medium filter was applied. Background signal was removed by thresholding the input data. The respective threshold value was derived from the in-phase images according to the Otsu threshold algorithm [41].

Volume quantification of the BAT was performed using a semi-automatic segmentation tool (http://www.itksnap.org/,[42]). Regions of BAT were identified in a slice-by-slice fashion according to the mean normalized grey value $\bar{I}$ with $\bar{I} > 0.7$ for the 2PM method and $0.4 < \bar{I} < 0.8$ for the 3PD method. Falsely identified regions due to partial volume effects were removed manually for both approaches. The evaluation was performed by an experienced MRI scientist (VR, >15 yrs in research). Quantification was performed blinded for the two investigated approaches.

After semi-automated classification, resulting BAT volumes were compared between 2PM and 3PD as well as between the

HD-transgenic mice and the wild-type controls. Correlation of the volumes derived from the investigated methods was assessed applying a Spearman's rho test and the significance of BAT volume changes between the different groups was assessed by an unrelated Wilcoxon rank sum test. P-values below 0.05 were considered significant. All statistical analysis was performed with SPSS 21.0 (IBM Corp, Armonk, NY).

Author Contributions

Conceived and designed the experiments: VR KL PW JK WR AL BL. Performed the experiments: AB VR. Analyzed the data: AB VR HPM. Contributed reagents/materials/analysis tools: KL PW. Contributed to the writing of the manuscript: VR PW KL JW.

References

1. Lee P, Swarbrick MM, Ho KK (2013) Brown adipose tissue in adult humans: a metabolic renaissance. Endocr Rev 34: 413–438.
2. Nedergaard J, Bengtsson T, Cannon B (2007) Unexpected evidence for active brown adipose tissue in adult humans. Am J Physiol Endocrinol Metab 293: E444–452.
3. Cypess AM, Lehman S, Williams G, Tal I, Rodman D, et al. (2009) Identification and importance of brown adipose tissue in adult humans. N Engl J Med 360: 1509–1517.
4. van Marken Lichtenbelt WD, Vanhommerig JW, Smulders NM, Drossaerts JM, Kemerink GJ, et al. (2009) Cold-activated brown adipose tissue in healthy men. N Engl J Med 360: 1500–1508.
5. Virtanen KA, Lidell ME, Orava J, Heglind M, Westergren R, et al. (2009) Functional brown adipose tissue in healthy adults. N Engl J Med 360: 1518–1525.
6. Bauwens M, Wierts R, van Royen B, Bucerius J, Backes W, et al. (2014) Molecular imaging of brown adipose tissue in health and disease. Eur J Nucl Med Mol Imaging 41: 776–791.
7. Wijers SL, Saris WH, van Marken Lichtenbelt WD (2010) Cold-induced adaptive thermogenesis in lean and obese. Obesity (Silver Spring) 18: 1092–1099.
8. Rona-Voros K, Weydt P (2010) The role of PGC-1alpha in the pathogenesis of neurodegenerative disorders. Curr Drug Targets 11: 1262–1269.
9. Mochel F, Haller RG (2011) Energy deficit in Huntington disease: why it matters. J Clin Invest 121: 493–499.
10. Weydt P, Pineda VV, Torrence AE, Libby RT, Satterfield TF, et al. (2006) Thermoregulatory and metabolic defects in Huntington's disease transgenic mice implicate PGC-1alpha in Huntington's disease neurodegeneration. Cell Metab 4: 349–362.
11. Chaturvedi RK, Calingasan NY, Yang L, Hennessey T, Johri A, et al. (2010) Impairment of PGC-1alpha expression, neuropathology and hepatic steatosis in a transgenic mouse model of Huntington's disease following chronic energy deprivation. Hum Mol Genet 19: 3190–3205.
12. Hamilton G, Smith DL, Jr., Bydder M, Nayak KS, Hu HH (2011) MR properties of brown and white adipose tissues. J Magn Reson Imaging 34: 468–473.
13. Lunati E, Marzola P, Nicolato E, Fedrigo M, Villa M, et al. (1999) In vivo quantitative lipidic map of brown adipose tissue by chemical shift imaging at 4.7 Tesla. J Lipid Res 40: 1395–1400.
14. Hu HH, Smith DL Jr, Nayak KS, Goran MI, Nagy TR (2010) Identification of brown adipose tissue in mice with fat-water IDEAL-MRI. J Magn Reson Imaging 31: 1195–1202.
15. Rasmussen JM, Entringer S, Nguyen A, van Erp TG, Guijarro A, et al. (2013) Brown adipose tissue quantification in human neonates using water-fat separated MRI. PLoS One 8: e77907.
16. Branca RT, Warren WS (2011) In vivo brown adipose tissue detection and characterization using water-lipid intermolecular zero-quantum coherences. Magn Reson Med 65: 313–319.
17. Khanna A, Branca RT (2012) Detecting brown adipose tissue activity with BOLD MRI in mice. Magn Reson Med 68: 1285–1290.
18. Dixon WT (1984) Simple proton spectroscopic imaging. Radiology 153: 189–194.
19. Hu HH, Bornert P, Hernando D, Kellman P, Ma J, et al. (2012) ISMRM workshop on fat-water separation: insights, applications and progress in MRI. Magn Reson Med 68: 378–388.
20. Mangiarini L, Sathasivam K, Seller M, Cozens B, Harper A, et al. (1996) Exon 1 of the HD gene with an expanded CAG repeat is sufficient to cause a progressive neurological phenotype in transgenic mice. Cell 87: 493–506.

21. Sathasivam K, Hobbs C, Turmaine M, Mangiarini L, Mahal A, et al. (1999) Formation of polyglutamine inclusions in non-CNS tissue. Hum Mol Genet 8: 813–822.
22. Chen YI, Cypess AM, Sass CA, Brownell AL, Jokivarsi KT, et al. (2012) Anatomical and functional assessment of brown adipose tissue by magnetic resonance imaging. Obesity (Silver Spring) 20: 1519–1526.
23. Hu HH, Kan HE (2013) Quantitative proton MR techniques for measuring fat. NMR Biomed 26: 1609–1629.
24. Branca RT, Zhang L, Warren WS, Auerbach E, Khanna A, et al. (2013) In vivo noninvasive detection of Brown Adipose Tissue through intermolecular zero-quantum MRI. PLoS One 8: e74206.
25. Johri A, Calingasan NY, Hennessey TM, Sharma A, Yang L, et al. (2012) Pharmacologic activation of mitochondrial biogenesis exerts widespread beneficial effects in a transgenic mouse model of Huntington's disease. Hum Mol Genet 21: 1124–1137.
26. Ho DJ, Calingasan NY, Wille E, Dumont M, Beal MF (2010) Resveratrol protects against peripheral deficits in a mouse model of Huntington's disease. Exp Neurol 225: 74–84.
27. Dupuis L, Oudart H, Rene F, Gonzalez de Aguilar JL, Loeffler JP (2004) Evidence for defective energy homeostasis in amyotrophic lateral sclerosis: benefit of a high-energy diet in a transgenic mouse model. Proc Natl Acad Sci U S A 101: 11159–11164.
28. Cannon B, Nedergaard J (2004) Brown adipose tissue: function and physiological significance. Physiol Rev 84: 277–359.
29. Lindauer E, Dupuis L, Muller HP, Neumann H, Ludolph AC, et al. (2013) Adipose Tissue Distribution Predicts Survival in Amyotrophic Lateral Sclerosis. PLoS One 8: e67783.
30. Rosenwald M, Wolfrum C (2014) The origin and definition of brite versus white and classical brown adipocytes. Adipocyte 3: 4–9.
31. van der Burg JM, Bjorkqvist M, Brundin P (2009) Beyond the brain: widespread pathology in Huntington's disease. Lancet Neurol 8: 765–774.
32. Jahnke W, Widmer H (2004) Protein NMR in biomedical research. Cellular and Molecular Life Sciences 61: 580–599.
33. Pellecchia M, Sem DS, Wuthrich K (2002) NMR in drug discovery. Nat Rev Drug Discov 1: 211–219.
34. Marion D (2013) An introduction to biological NMR spectroscopy. Mol Cell Proteomics 12: 3006–3025.
35. Hu HH, Yin L, Aggabao PC, Perkins TG, Chia JM, et al. (2013) Comparison of brown and white adipose tissues in infants and children with chemical-shift-encoded water-fat MRI. J Magn Reson Imaging 38: 885–896.
36. Ma J (2008) Dixon techniques for water and fat imaging. J Magn Reson Imaging 28: 543–558.
37. Glover GH (1991) Multipoint Dixon technique for water and fat proton and susceptibility imaging. J Magn Reson Imaging 1: 521–530.
38. Bley TA, Wieben O, Francois CJ, Brittain JH, Reeder SB (2010) Fat and water magnetic resonance imaging. J Magn Reson Imaging 31: 4–18.
39. Pouladi MA, Morton AJ, Hayden MR (2013) Choosing an animal model for the study of Huntington's disease. Nat Rev Neurosci 14: 708–721.
40. Fain JN, Del Mar NA, Meade CA, Reiner A, Goldowitz D (2001) Abnormalities in the functioning of adipocytes from R6/2 mice that are transgenic for the Huntington's disease mutation. Hum Mol Genet 10: 145–152.
41. Otsu N (1979) Threshold Selection Method from Gray-Level Histograms. Ieee Transactions on Systems Man and Cybernetics 9: 62–66.
42. Yushkevich PA, Piven J, Hazlett HC, Smith RG, Ho S, et al. (2006) User-guided 3D active contour segmentation of anatomical structures: significantly improved efficiency and reliability. Neuroimage 31: 1116–1128.

8

Quantification Assays for Total and Polyglutamine-Expanded Huntingtin Proteins

Douglas Macdonald[1*9], Michela A. Tessari[29], Ivette Boogaard[4], Melanie Smith[3], Kristiina Pulli[2], Agnieszka Szynol[4], Faywell Albertus[4], Marieke B. A. C. Lamers[3], Sipke Dijkstra[4], Daniel Kordt[5], Wolfgang Reindl[5], Frank Herrmann[5], George McAllister[3], David F. Fischer[4¶], Ignacio Munoz-Sanjuan[1¶]

1 CHDI Management/CHDI Foundation, Los Angeles, California, United States of America, 2 Galapagos B.V., Leiden, The Netherlands, 3 BioFocus, a Charles River company, Saffron Walden, United Kingdom, 4 BioFocus, a Charles River company, Leiden, The Netherlands, 5 Evotec AG, Hamburg, Germany

Abstract

The expansion of a CAG trinucleotide repeat in the huntingtin gene, which produces huntingtin protein with an expanded polyglutamine tract, is the cause of Huntington's disease (HD). Recent studies have reported that RNAi suppression of polyglutamine-expanded huntingtin (mutant HTT) in HD animal models can ameliorate disease phenotypes. A key requirement for such preclinical studies, as well as eventual clinical trials, aimed to reduce mutant HTT exposure is a robust method to measure HTT protein levels in select tissues. We have developed several sensitive and selective assays that measure either total human HTT or polyglutamine-expanded human HTT proteins on the electrochemiluminescence Meso Scale Discovery detection platform with an increased dynamic range over other methods. In addition, we have developed an assay to detect endogenous mouse and rat HTT proteins in pre-clinical models of HD to monitor effects on the wild type protein of both allele selective and non-selective interventions. We demonstrate the application of these assays to measure HTT protein in several HD *in vitro* cellular and *in vivo* animal model systems as well as in HD patient biosamples. Furthermore, we used purified recombinant HTT proteins as standards to quantitate the absolute amount of HTT protein in such biosamples.

Editor: Yoshitaka Nagai, National Center of Neurology and Psychiatry, Japan

Funding: CHDI Foundation is a privately-funded not-for-profit biomedical research organization exclusively dedicated to discovering and developing therapeutics that slow the progression of Huntington's disease. CHDI Foundation conducts research in a number of different ways; for the purposes of this manuscript, research was conducted at the contract research organizations BioFocus, Galapagos B.V., and Evotec under fee-for-service agreements. The listed authors all contributed to the conception, planning, and direction of the research, including generation, analysis, and interpretation of the data.

Competing Interests: DM and IMS are employed by CHDI Management, Inc., as advisors to CHDI Foundation, Inc. MAT, IV, AS, FA, and SD are employed by Galapagos B.V. MS, KP, MBACL, GA, and DFF are employed by BioFocus, a Galapagos company. DK, WR, and FH are employed by Evotec. There are no patents, products in development, or marketed products to declare.

* E-mail: Douglas.Macdonald@chdifoundation.org

9 These authors contributed equally to this work.

¶ These authors also contributed equally to this work.

Introduction

The measurement of disease-causing mutant and/or misfolded proteins is essential for the successful development of disease-modifying therapies that target such pathogenic or pathologic proteins. Development of assays to detect these types of proteins is dependent on the availability of selective antibodies as well as a sensitive and robust platform for detection. To this end, we have characterized a set of novel antibodies and employed a unique assay platform for the detection of the huntingtin protein (HTT), the causative agent in Huntington's disease (HD).

HD is an autosomal dominant neurodegenerative movement and mood disorder caused by an expansion of a CAG trinucleotide repeat, to greater than 35 repeats, in exon-1 of the huntingtin gene [1]. The gene product is a ubiquitously-expressed 350 kDa HTT protein, with the greatest expression found in the central nervous system [2]. The mutant polyglutamine expanded form of HTT is cytotoxic leading to the hallmark pathology of HD, pronounced atrophy of the striatum as well as other brain regions [3].

Currently there are no disease-modifying therapies for HD, however, multiple investigators have recently reported efforts to develop therapeutic approaches that suppress huntingtin expression through RNA interference [4–10]. These approaches decrease the amount of mutant HTT in transgenic animals which has resulted in amelioration of HD phenotypes [11]. To enable such therapeutic programs it is crucial that the HTT protein be quantified in a reliable and robust manner to determine the pharmacodynamic effects of such potential therapeutics. To date, this has been difficult due to the structural complexity of the large HTT protein which exists in several conformers and states including soluble monomers, intermediate fibrils, insoluble aggregates, as well as several possible cleavage products [12,13].

Here, we have developed a panel of detection assays for soluble polyglutamine-expanded (mutant) and total (polyglutamine-independent) human HTT protein as well as the rodent HTT protein ortholog using the sensitive ELISA-based Meso Scale Discovery

(MSD) electrochemiluminescence assay platform [14]. We demonstrate that we are able to quantitate different forms of the polyglutamine-expanded and non-expanded HTT soluble proteins in cellular, animal, and HD patient biosamples. The MSD platform is based on the electrochemical properties of the ruthenium cation in conjunction with carbon electrode arrays held within microtiter plate footprints. A capture antibody is first non-specifically adsorbed onto the carbon surface of the plate and after analyte capture, a detection antibody labeled with the MSD SULFO-TAG ruthenium-based reagent (the electrochemiluminescent label) will generate a signal relative to the amount of analyte, such as HTT protein, present.

The advantages of this technology include high sensitivity and selectivity due to the use of two detecting antibodies, an increased dynamic range over other methods, and the ability to multiplex these assays in a high-throughput manner [15]. Alternative technologies have recently been used to quantify mutant HTT in biosamples [16–19]. However, each of these methods has limitations in their ability to detect some protein states; for example, one may be limited in the distance between the donor and acceptor antibody epitopes using Time-Resolved Fluorescence Resonance Energy Transfer (TR-FRET) and thus not be able to develop assays with antibody pairs that recognize the HTT protein at a considerable distance from each other; although this attribute may allow one to infer changes in conformational state which is not possible using the MSD platform. Nevertheless, this complication, along with the need to measure multiple states or species of HTT (e.g., total, expanded, and truncated) highlights the need for assays that detect HTT with antibodies that recognize different domains and are not subject to conformational effects. The MSD assays described here are amenable to detection of HTT proteins in complex fluids and tissues, which enables the implementation of multiplex measurements from single samples.

Importantly, in order to be able to quantitate the amount of HTT protein in various biosamples, we have expressed and purified both human and mouse recombinant HTT proteins with different polyglutamine lengths and have used them as reference standards in our detection assays. This has allowed us to quantitate the amount of soluble total, polyglutamine-expanded, or mouse HTT proteins in a variety of different biosamples.

We describe here three of our HTT quantification assays specific for: 1) human polyglutamine-expanded huntingtin, 2) human pan-huntingtin (polyglutamine length independent, expanded and non-expanded proteins), and 3) rodent wildtype huntingtin (endogenous mouse and rat proteins) using our novel anti-huntingtin antibodies. We show that these novel assays are able to selectively measure the amount of soluble HTT protein in a variety of biosamples including cellular, rodent, and HD patient tissues. Furthermore, we demonstrate that using our standard reference proteins, we are able to quantitatively compare the amount of HTT protein in a variety of samples which will provide guidance for dose selection and provide an ability to monitor the pharmacodynamic effects of molecular therapies and other approaches that modulation the levels of HTT protein, an important and critical step in the development of such targeted therapies.

Materials and Methods

Recombinant human and mouse huntingtin proteins

cDNA corresponding to the N-terminal 573 amino acid fragment of human HTT (relative to GenBank accession CAD38447.1) was amplified by PCR from full length human HTT cDNA in pcDNA3.1+ containing either 23 or 73 glutamine repeats. The polyglutamine tract was generated synthetically and is of a mixed codon (CAG/CAA) structure to reduce the risk of contraction or expansion during propagation and cloning. The N-terminal fragments were cloned into pPHNFLAG in frame with the N-terminal FLAG tag for expression of constructs either 571 amino acids in length (23Q) or 621 amino acids in length (73Q). The sequences of the constructs were confirmed by DNA sequencing before transfecting into Sf9 cells. Recombinant baculoviruses were generated [42], harvested, amplified, and used to infect Sf9 cells for protein production. Cells infected with HTT (1–573) Q23 were harvested at 72 h post infection whereas cells infected with HTT (1–573) Q73 were harvested at 48 h post infection due to a decrease in expression levels of HTT (1–573) Q73 after 48 h. Cell pellets were lysed by freeze/thaw in 50 mM Tris-HCl pH 7.4, 500 mM NaCl, 10% Glycerol, 1% CHAPS, 1 mM EDTA and protease inhibitors (Complete, EDTA-free; Roche Diagnostics). Clarification was carried out by centrifugation (22,500 rpm, 2 h, 4°C) and the soluble lysate was incubated with anti-FLAG M2 affinity gel (Sigma) overnight at 4°C on a rotator. FLAG-tagged HTT proteins were eluted with 0.4 mg/ml FLAG peptide in 50 mM Tris pH 7.4, 500 mM NaCl, 10% glycerol, 1% CHAPS, 1 mM EDTA and loaded onto a Superdex 200 16/60 column equilibrated with 50 mM Tris-HCl pH 7.4, 500 mM NaCl, 10% glycerol, 0.1% CHAPS and 1 mM EDTA. Peak fractions were analyzed by SDS-PAGE. Monomeric protein fractions were pooled and concentrated using a 5 kDa MWCO spin concentrator (Vivascience). HTT protein concentration was determined by Bradford assay. Purified HTT protein was aliquoted and stored at −80°C.

cDNA corresponding to the N-terminal 549 amino acid fragment of mouse HTT (relative to RefSeq accession number NM_010414) was amplified by PCR from full length mouse Htt cDNA in pPHNFLAG containing seven glutamine repeats. The N-terminal fragment was cloned into pPHNFLAG in frame with the N-terminal FLAG tag for expression of a 549 amino acid construct (7Q). The sequence of the construct was confirmed by DNA sequencing before transfecting into Sf9 cells. Recombinant baculovirus was harvested, amplified, and used to infect Sf9 cells for protein production. Cells infected with mouse Htt (1–549) Q7 were harvested at 72 h post infection. Cell pellets were lysed by freeze/thaw in 50 mM Tris-HCl pH 7.4, 500 mM NaCl, 10% Glycerol, 1% CHAPS, 1 mM EDTA and protease inhibitors (Complete, EDTA-free; Roche Diagnostics). Clarification was carried out by centrifugation (22,500 rpm, 2 h, 4°C) and the soluble lysate was incubated with anti-FLAG M2 affinity gel (Sigma) overnight at 4°C on a rotator. FLAG-tagged mouse HTT protein was eluted with 0.4 mg/ml FLAG peptide in 50 mM Tris-HCl pH 7.4, 150 mM NaCl and loaded onto a Superdex™ 200 16/60 column equilibrated with 50 mM Tris-HCl pH 7.4, 500 mM NaCl, 10% glycerol, 0.1% CHAPS and 1 mM EDTA. Peak fractions were analyzed by SDS-PAGE and monomeric fractions were pooled. Since the purity of the mouse HTT protein was not improved following size exclusion chromatography an ion exchange step was performed. The protein was loaded onto a MonoQ 5/50 column in a buffer containing 50 mM Tris pH 7.4, 5% glycerol, 0.1% CHAPS, 1 mM EDTA and eluted with a gradient to 500 mM NaCl over 30 column volumes. The mouse HTT protein eluted in two distinct peaks; each peak fraction was separately pooled and concentrated using a 5 kDa MWCO spin concentrator (Vivascience). Mouse HTT protein concentration was determined by Bradford assay. Purified mouse HTT protein was aliquoted and stored at −80°C.

Anti-HTT Antibodies

Rabbit polyclonal antibodies were generated and purified using epitope peptide exclusion chromatography by the CHDI Foundation at 21st Century Biochemical (Waltham, MA). Please note that, in this paper, the antibody epitope mapping is relative to GenBank accession CAD38447.1 (HTT protein carrying 25 glutamines). CHDI-90000137 (pAb137) was generated using an antigenic peptide corresponding to the HTT amino acids 4–19 (acetyl-LEKLMKAFESLKSFQQC-amide), CHDI-90000145 (pAb145) was generated using an antigenic peptide corresponding to the HTT amino acids 32–53 (acetyl-QQQQQQQQQQQQQPPPPPPPPPPP-Ahx-C-amide), CHDI-90000146 (pAb146) was generated using an antigenic peptide corresponding to the HTT amino acids 54–70 (human proline-rich region; acetyl-QLPQPPPQAQPLLPQPQC-amide), CHDI-90000147 (pAb147) was generated using an antigenic peptide corresponding to the HTT amino acids 37–53 of the mouse HTT (mouse proline-rich region; acetyl-pppQPPQPPPQGQPPPPC-amide) carrying seven CAG repeats (GenBank accession NP_034544), and CHDI-90000148 (pAb148) was generated using an antigenic peptide corresponding to the HTT amino acids 79–92 (acetyl-CPPGPAVAEEPLHRP-amide). The mouse monoclonal MW1 antibody against the expanded polyglutamine domain [20] was obtained from the Developmental Studies Hybridoma Bank. The mouse monoclonal MW8 antibody binding amino acid 83–90 (AEEPLHRP) near the C-terminus of exon-1 [20] was provided by the CHDI Foundation. The rabbit polyclonal BML-PW0595 antibody against amino acids 2–17 of the HTT protein was obtained from Enzo Life Science. The mouse monoclonal MAB2166 antibody, generated using a HTT fragment from amino acids 183 to 812 as a fusion protein, was obtained from Millipore. The epitope of the MAB2166 antibody has been then further mapped to a 15-amino acid region spanning from amino acid 445 to 459 of the human HTT protein [30]. A detailed overview of the antibody epitopes is reported in Table S1 in Text S1. The SULFO TAG labelling of the pAb137 antibody was performed using the MSD SULFO-TAG NHS-Ester reagent (Meso Scale Discovery, Gaithersburg, MD, USA) according to manufacturers' instructions. Preservatives in the pAb137 antibody storage buffer (e.g., sodium azide, EDTA) were removed prior to the conjugation reaction using the Zeba Spin desalting columns (Thermo Scientific) according to manufacturers' instructions. A challenge ratio of 1:7.5 (antibody:SULFO-TAG NHS-Ester reagent) was used for the labeling of the pAb137 antibody. The SULFO TAG-labeled pAb137 antibody was stored at −80°C in 30% glycerol.

HD patient-derived material

HD patient-derived lymphoblast cell line carrying an HTT 73Q HD mutant allele (GM-04282) and one age-, passage number- and sex-matched control lymphoblast cell line (GM-03354) were obtained from Coriell Institute for Medical Research (New Jersey, USA). Cell culturing was performed according to protocols provided by the Coriell Institute for Medical Research. The CAG length of each cell line was verified by Laragen, Inc. [21]. For analysis in the MSD assays, approximately 2×10^7 lymphoblast cells were lysed in 150 μl of MSD assay buffer 2 (50 mM Tris (pH 7.4), 120 mM NaCl, 1 mM EDTA, 1 mM DTT, 0.5% NP-40, 1 mM PMSF, protease inhibitors (Complete, EDTA-free; Roche Diagnostics) on ice for 15 min. Lysates were then cleared by centrifugation at 10,000× g for 15 min at 4°C and supernatants stored at −80°C until required. Total protein concentration was determined using a bicinchoninic acid assay (BCA, Thermo Scientific) according to standard procedure.

Human post mortem brain tissues including HD samples: HD-1 (Q46/17; cat# T-1991), HD-2 (Q43/19; cat# T-2019), HD-3 (Q43/17; cat# T-2476), HD-4 (Q45/16; cat# T-2959), and non-HD control samples: C-1 (cat# T-343), C-2 (cat# T-638), C-3 (cat# T-4518), were obtained from the New York Brain Bank at Columbia University (New York, USA).

Huntington's disease *in vivo* models

Fresh snap-frozen rodent brain tissues were obtained from several sources and stored at −80°C until homogenization. If not otherwise indicated, R6/2 [22] were supplied by Dr. G. Bates (KCL, United Kingdom). Hemizygous R6/2 mice were bred in Dr. G. Bates' laboratory by backcrossing R6/2 males to (CBA×C57Bl/6) F1 (CBF) females (B6CBAF1/OlaHsd, Harlan Olac) [18]. Alternatively, R6/2 B6CBA-Tg(HDexon1)62 Gpb/1 J snap frozen brain tissues were provided by the CHDI Foundation from their colony at The Jackson Laboratories (Bar Harbor, USA). BAC HD mice [23] were obtained from the CHDI Foundation colony at the University Medical Center Hamburg-Eppendorf (UKE) and were supplied by Evotec AG (Hamburg, Germany); zQ175 C57B/L6J knock-in mice, derived from a spontaneous expansion of the CAG copy number in the CAG 140 knock-in mice [24–26] were provided by Evotec AG (Hamburg, Germany). Wistar (RccHan:WIST, cat# 168) rat brain tissues were obtained from Harlan Laboratories (Horst, The Netherlands).

Immunoblot analysis of huntingtin proteins

For immunoblotting, 25 μg of brain homogenate or 5 ng of HTT recombinant protein were mixed with 4× Laemmli loading buffer, denatured at 100°C for 5 min and loaded on the 3–8% pre-cast Tris-Acetate gels (Bio-Rad). The electrophoresis was carried out at 30 mA for 5 h (full length HTT proteins) or for 1.5 h (exon-1 HTT proteins). During long run electrophoresis, the XT Tricine Running buffer (Bio-Rad) was replaced every 1–2 h to restore the ionic content and pH. After electrophoresis, proteins were transferred to nitrocellulose membrane (Hybond-C Extra; Amersham Biosciences) in 192 mM glycine, 25 mM Tris-HCl, 20% v/v methanol for approximately 3 h at 4°C. Membranes were blocked for 1 h in PBS-T (0.1% Tween-20 in PBS) containing 5% non-fat dried milk at room temperature, washed with PBS-T, and incubated for overnight at 4°C with primary anti-HTT antibodies (in PBS-T containing 5% non-fat dried milk). Blots were washed with PBS-T, probed with HRP-linked secondary antibodies (in PBS-T with 5% non-fat dried milk) for 1 h and washed again with PBS-T. Bound antibodies were visualized using the ChemiDoc XRS Molecular Imager (Bio-Rad) according to manufacturers' instructions. Primary antibodies and dilutions were: BML-PW0595 (Enzo Life Science) (1:3,000), pAb137, pAb147, and pAb146 (CHDI Foundation) (1:300), pAb145 (CHDI Foundation) (1:200), pAb148 (CHDI Foundation) (1:1,500), MW1 (Developmental Studies Hybridoma Bank, University of Iowa) (1:500), MAB2166 (Millipore) (1:10,000, if not otherwise stated), MW8 (CHDI Foundation) (1:5000), ATP5B (LSBio) (1:20,000). HRP-conjugated secondary antibodies were as follows: goat anti-rabbit (Millipore 1:2,000) and goat anti-mouse (Millipore 1:500).

MSD electrochemiluminescence assays

Dissected or whole brain human and rodent homogenates were generated using the FastPrep system (MP Biomedicals) by lysing the tissue 3×30 s in Lysing matrix tubes (Lysing matrix D; MP Biomedicals) in MSD assay buffer 1 (Tris lysis buffer (Meso Scale Discovery), Phosphatase inhibitor II 100× stock (Sigma), Phosphatase inhibitor III 100× stock (Sigma), PMSF 2 mM, protease inhibitors (Complete, EDTA-free; Roche Diagnostics), 10 mM NaF). Typically, approximately 100–150 mg of human frontal cortex and approximately 50 mg of rodent brain tissues were homogenized. Lysates were centrifuged for 20 min at 20,000× g at 4°C. Supernatant was collected, aliquoted, quickly frozen in dry ice, stored at −80°C, and used within 3–4 days to limit any detrimental effects of storage time on these samples (such as *in vitro* aggregation of HTT protein). Total protein concentration was determined using a bicinchoninic acid assay (BCA, Thermo Scientific) according to standard procedure. Besides the typical technical optimization required to develop a sensitive and robust ELISA-based assay (e.g., optimization of the antibody concentrations), the optimization of the following aspects was crucial in the development of the MSD electrochemiluminescence HTT detection assays: 1) anti-HTT antibody orientation (i.e., selection of capture and detection antibodies); 2) selection of the carbonate-bicarbonate buffer (15 mM Na_2CO_3/35 mM $NaHCO_3$, pH 9.6) as coating buffer; 3) establish the detergent concentration compatibility to the MSD assay (e.g., Tween-20 and NP-40 are both compatible to the MSD platform up to a concentration of 0.2% and 0.5%, respectively, however other detergents are not). MSD 96-well or 384-well plates (Meso Scale Discovery) were coated overnight at 4°C with the pAb146 polyclonal antibody (expanded polyglutamine and pan human HTT assays) at a concentration of 4 µg/ml or the pAb147 polyclonal antibody (mouse HTT-specific assay) at a concentration of 8 µg/ml in carbonate-bicarbonate coating buffer (15 mM Na_2CO_3/35 mM $NaHCO_3$, pH 9.6). Plates were then washed three times with wash buffer (0.2% Tween-20 in PBS) and blocked (2% probumin/0.2% Tween-20 in PBS) for 1 h at RT with rotational shaking and then washed three times with wash buffer. Because high detergent concentrations interfered with the ELISA, brain extracts were made up to the appropriate concentration by diluting them 5× in blocking buffer. Samples were transferred to an antibody-coated MSD plate and incubated with shaking for 1 h at RT. After removal of the lysates, the plate was washed three times with wash buffer and, depending on the assay, 25 µl (or 10 µl for 384-well plate format) MW1 (expanded polyglutamine human HTT assay) secondary antibody (diluted to 1.5 µg/ml in blocking buffer), pAb137-MSD SULFO TAG (exon-1 - pan human HTT assay), MAB2166 (pan human HTT assay) secondary antibody (diluted to 4.5 µg/ml or to 1:7,500 in blocking buffer, respectively), or MAB2166 (mouse HTT-specific assay) secondary antibody (1:7,500 in blocking buffer) was added to each well and incubated with shaking for 1 h at RT. In the expanded polyglutamine and in the pan human HTT assays and in the mouse HTT-specific assay, after three washes with wash buffer, 25 µl (or 10 µl for 384-well plate format) goat anti-mouse SULFO TAG detection antibody (Meso Scale Discovery) (1: 1,000 in blocking buffer) was added to each well and incubated with shaking for 1 h at RT. After washing three times with wash buffer, 150 µl (or 35 µl for 384-well plate format) of read buffer T with surfactant (Meso Scale Discovery) was added to each empty well and the plate was imaged on the SI 6000 imager (Meso Scale Discovery) according to manufacturers' instructions for 96- or 384-well plates.

Where it was necessary to use different lots of an antibody, the antibody concentration was re-optimized to generate a similar signal to background on recombinant HTT proteins as found previously (data not shown).

Total neuronal Tau protein levels were measured using a commercially available MSD ELISA-based assay kit (#K151DSA-3 Meso Scale Discovery, Gaithersburg, MD, USA) according to manufacturers' instructions.

Competition antibody binding assay

MSD-based competition binding assays were performed in 384-well format. Wells of a bare MSD Multi-Array 384-well plate (Meso Scale Discovery) were coated with 10 µl of 4 µg/ml pAb146 or pAb147 antibody in carbonate-bicarbonate coating buffer (15 mM Na_2CO_3/35 mM $NaHCO_3$, pH 9.6) overnight at 4°C. After washing with wash buffer (0.2% Tween-20 in PBS), wells were blocked with 35 µl of blocking buffer (2% probumin (Millipore)/0.2% Tween-20 in PBS) for 1 h at RT under shaking and washed again. Competition for binding was tested by mixing 0.1 fmol/µl human HTT (1–573) Q23 (for pAb146) or 0.1 fmol/µl mouse HTT (1–549) Q7 (for pAb147) with a concentration range from 0.001 ng/ml up to 10 µg/ml of the peptides CHDI-90000208 (acetyl-QLPQPPPQAQPLLPQPQC-amide; synthetic peptide corresponding to the proline-rich region of human HTT; epitope for pAb146 antibody), CHDI-9000209 (acetyl-PPPQPPQPPPQGQPPPPC-amide; synthetic peptide corresponding to the proline-rich region of mouse HTT; divergent from human protein sequence), and CHDI-90000210 (acetyl-CPPGPAVAEEPLHRP-amide; synthetic peptide corresponding to the C-terminus of the exon-1 region of HTT) in a mixture of 20% MSD assay buffer 2 (50 mM Tris pH 7.4, 120 mM NaCl, 1 mM EDTA, 1 mM DTT, 0.5% NP-40, 1 mM PMSF, protease inhibitors (Complete, EDTA-free; Roche Diagnostics) and 80% blocking buffer, and adding 10 µl per sample to the wells. Control wells without peptides or buffer only were included. After incubation for 1 h at RT under shaking, plates were washed and subsequently treated with 10 µl of the antibody MAB2166 (1:1,000; Millipore), followed by 10 µl of a SULFO-tagged anti mouse antibody (1:1,000; Meso Scale Discovery). Both antibodies were diluted in blocking buffer and in each case incubated in the wells for 1 h at RT under shaking followed by washing. After complete removal of buffer from the last wash step, 35 µl of Read Buffer T with surfactant (Meso Scale Discovery) were added to each well and plates were analyzed on a SI6000 Reader (Meso Scale Discovery) using the recommended settings for 384-well plates. Assays were performed in triplicate.

Recombinant AAV particles for neuronal transduction

Plasmids for expression of shRNAs were modified from the AAV vector pAAV-6P-SEWB [27]. For expression of shRNAs, transcriptional control units containing the H1 promoter followed by the DNA-encoded short hairpin constructs were inserted as XbaI-XhoI fragments into pAAV-6P-SEWB to build AAV vectors with bicistronic expression units. shRNA sequences: non-allele specific *HTT* targeting shRNA sh4 (AGCTTGTCCAGGTTTATGAA; [28] and scr6 (GGCTACCTTCGTGAGTGAT), an shRNA without known target sequence in the mouse. Primary neurons were isolated from the cortex of heterozygous zQ175 [25,26] mouse embryos (E16). The genotype of each embryo was individually determined by PCR (amplicon within transgenic neomycin cassette) and zQ175 positive cells were pooled. Typically, 2×10^5 cells per well were seeded in 1 ml of plating medium (Minimum Essential Medium (MEM; Gibco) supplemented with 10% fetal bovine serum (Sigma-Aldrich), 2 mM L-alanyl-L-glutamine dipeptide (GlutaMAX; Life Technologies), 100 U/ml Penicillin and 100 µg/ml Streptomycin (Gibco)) into poly-L-lysine coated 24-well plates and incubated at 37°C and 5% CO_2. 3 h after plating the medium was changed for 1 ml of culture medium (Neurobasal Medium (Gibco), 1×B27-Supplement (Invitrogen), 2 mM L-glutamine (PAA), 100 U/ml Penicillin and 100 µg/ml Streptomycin (Gibco)). Cells were cultivated for three days prior to infection with 1×10^8 virus particles of AAV-SEWB-scr6 or AAV-SEWB-mhtt-sh4. The multiplicity of infection

(MOI) based on the physical AAV titer (viral genome copies) was 500, leading to more than 90% transduced neurons which was monitored by a GFP reporter. Cells were subsequently harvested, lysed in 100 μl MSD assay buffer 2 per well (50 mM Tris pH 7.4, 120 mM NaCl, 1 mM EDTA, 1 mM DTT, 0.5% NP-40, 1 mM PMSF, protease inhibitors (Complete, EDTA-free; Roche Diagnostics), snap-frozen in liquid nitrogen, and stored at −80°C until further use.

Statistical analysis

Unless otherwise indicated, the data in the graphs represent averages with standard deviations of the mean. Significance was calculated using a two-tailed Student's t-test.

Statistical power analysis

The significance level (α) was set at 5% and the statistical power (π) at 90%. The effect of interest (difference in mean of control and test group, $\mu 0 - \mu 1$) was set at 25% or 50%. When the variance between the control and test groups was not significantly different (F-test), the pooled variance ($\sigma 0$) (mean of the %CV of the control group and the %CV of the test group) was set based on experimental observations. The size (N) of each group (assuming equal numbers of treated and control subjects) with one-sided testing was given by the formula: $N = (2*[(z\alpha - z\pi)/(\mu 1 - \mu 0/\sigma 0)^{\wedge}2]) + ((z\alpha)^{\wedge}2/4)$. However, when the variance between the control and test group was significantly different (F-test), the group size was calculated based on the control group variance only using the following formula: $N = ([1 + ((100 + (\mu 1 - \mu 0))/100)^{\wedge}2] * [(z\alpha - z\pi)/(\mu 1 - \mu 0/\sigma 0)^{\wedge}2]) + ((z\alpha)^{\wedge}2/4)$.

The values of z come from the standardized normal distribution, depending on the chosen significance level and power. For the analysis reported in this study, with $\alpha = 0.05$ and $\pi = 0.9$, zα is 1.645 and zπ is −1.282.

Results

Anti-huntingtin antibody characterization

We characterized a panel of anti-HTT antibodies raised to different epitopes of the HTT protein (Figure 1A and Table S1 in Text S1) by immunoblot using purified large fragment (HTT 1–573) recombinant HTT proteins with different CAG repeat lengths (Figure 1B) as well as brain homogenates obtained from 3 month-old BAC HD mice or wild type littermates (Figure 1C). BAC HD mice express full-length human mutant HTT with 97 glutamine repeats under the control of the endogenous *Htt* regulatory machinery [23]. This animal model recapitulates several key phenotypic features of HD (e.g. late onset, atrophy of the cortex and striatum).

Each of the antibodies tested, recognized proteins at the appropriate molecular weights in gels containing both purified large fragment recombinant HTT proteins, indicated as HTT (1–573) Q23 and HTT (1–573) Q73 (Figure 1B), and BAC HD mouse brain homogenates containing the endogenous mouse HTT protein, indicated as WT HTT, and the human mutant transgene, indicated as Tg mHTT (Figure 1C). As shown in Figure 1B, the BML-PW0595, the MAB2166 [30], the pAb137, pAb145, pAb146, pAb148, and the MW1 [20] antibodies recognized both HTT (1–573) Q23 and HTT (1–573) Q73 purified large fragment proteins. The MW1 antibody, which specifically recognizes the polyglutamine domain [20], showed a higher specificity for the HTT (1–573) Q73 compared to the HTT (1–573) Q23 purified large fragment protein. The pAb147 antibody was raised against an epitope (proline-rich region) derived from the HTT mouse protein sequence that is divergent

from the human HTT protein sequence and, therefore, it did not detect the human recombinant large fragment proteins. Because multiple proteins contain polyglutamine domains it was important to determine whether these antibodies bind other proteins in addition to HTT. Therefore, immunoblots of normal and transgenic mouse brain extracts were performed (Figure 1C). The antibodies tested displayed a very specific binding pattern, recognizing the HTT protein that is approximately 350 kD in size. The BML-PW0595, the MAB2166, and the pAb137 antibodies were able to detect both the lower molecular weight wild type and the higher molecular weight polyglutamine-expanded forms of HTT, whereas the pAb145, pAb146, pAb148, and the MW1 antibodies only recognized the expanded polyglutamine form present in transgenic BAC HD samples. The mouse HTT-specific pAb147 antibody only recognized, as expected, the lower molecular weight non-expanded, mouse wild type HTT endogenously expressed by both transgenic BAC HD mice and age-matched wild type littermates.

Electrochemiluminescence assays for human huntingtin protein detection

We utilized the MSD electrochemiluminescence platform to develop a detection assay for expanded polyglutamine human HTT and an assay for pan (wild type and mutant) human HTT proteins. The pAb146 antibody was used as capture antibody in both the expanded polyglutamine human HTT and the pan human HTT assays. This antibody binds to an epitope within the proline-rich region of the human HTT protein and ensures the detection of both N-terminal fragments and full length HTT. When used in combination with MW1, a polyglutamine binding antibody, the pAb146-MW1 antibody pair specifically detected HTT (1–573) Q23 and HTT (1–573) Q73 large fragment as well as full length wild type (17Q) and mutant (46Q) [29] recombinant proteins (Figure 2A). In this assay, we used a commercially available anti-mouse MSD SULFO-TAG antibody as labeled secondary detection reagent to generate the electrochemiluminescence signal in the assay. As shown in Figure 2A, the intensity of the signal was not only dependent on the protein concentration, but also on the polyglutamine length of the proteins tested. This was expected due to the number of theoretical epitopes for the MW1 detection antibody in an expanded polyglutamine stretch [32]. Therefore, an increase in the polyglutamine length can allow for either more MW1 molecules to bind to the protein or a cooperative binding of multiple antibodies when binding sites are present in close proximity [20]. We calculated an approximately 120-fold increase in the signal for HTT (1–573) Q73 compared with HTT (1–573) Q23 measured as the ratio between the slopes calculated from the linear portion of the two standard curves (Figure 2A). The observed signal increase between full length mutant (Q46) and wild type (Q17) was approximately 23-fold. With the same calculation, we estimated approximately an 8-fold signal increase when HTT (1–573) Q73 was compared with the full length mutant (Q46) protein. The limit of detection for the MSD assay performed with the pAb146 and MW1 antibodies was calculated to be between the low nM and high pM range depending on the protein tested (Table 1).

All together, these results demonstrated a specific detection of human HTT protein in a polyglutamine-dependent manner by using the antibody pair pAb146-MW1 in an electrochemiluminescence assay. Both large N-terminal fragments and full length polyglutamine-expanded HTT proteins were detected with a high sensitivity and specificity and across a broad dynamic range of concentrations.

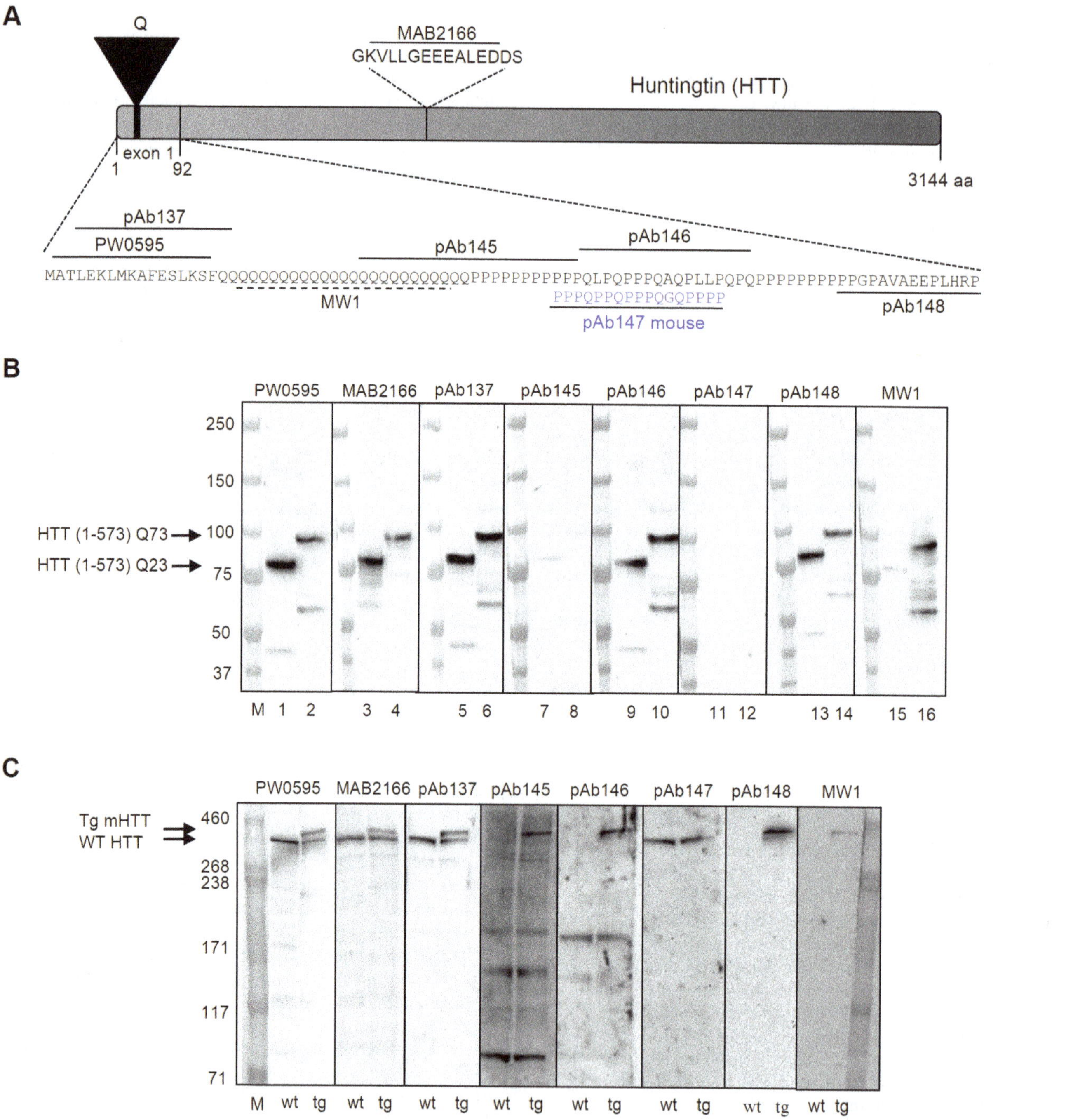

Figure 1. Anti-HTT antibody epitopes and analysis by immunoblot. (A) Diagram representing antibody epitopes on human HTT protein (relative to GenBank accession CAD38447.1). A stretch of glutamine (Q) residues near the N-terminus is expanded in individuals affected by Huntington's disease. Amino-acid 1-92 encoded by exon-1 are shown. Blue, pAb147 antibody epitope on mouse HTT protein (GenBank accession NP_034544). (B) Immunoblot analysis of human large fragment recombinant HTT proteins detected by the indicated anti-huntingtin antibodies. 5 ng of both HTT (1–573) Q23 (lanes 1, 3, 5, 7, 9, 11, 13 and 15) and HTT (1–573) Q73 (lanes 2, 4, 6, 8, 10, 12, 14, and 16) purified large fragment proteins were analyzed by SDS-PAGE. M, molecular weight marker (kDa). (C) Immunoblot analysis of wild type littermate and transgenic BAC HD mouse whole brain extracts. Mouse endogenous wild type and human transgenic polyglutamine-expanded HTT proteins were detected using the indicated anti-huntingtin antibodies. 25 μg of normal (wt) and transgenic (tg) mouse brain extracts were analyzed by SDS-PAGE as indicated. M, molecular weight marker (kDa). Tg mHTT, transgenic human polyglutamine-expanded HTT. WT HTT, endogenous mouse wild type HTT.

The specificity of the human mutant HTT signal detection by the pAb146-MW1 MSD assay was further confirmed in heterozygous zQ175 knock-in mouse primary neurons after adeno-associated virus (AAV) - mediated shRNA knockdown (Figure 3A). We detected a significant signal reduction in neurons transduced with the *HTT*-specific AAV-SEWB-sh4 [28], confirming the specificity of the human mutant HTT signal detected by the expanded polyglutamine human HTT MSD assay. When quantified as percentage of signal versus the control transduction (AAV-SEWB-scr6), the mutant human HTT signal in primary

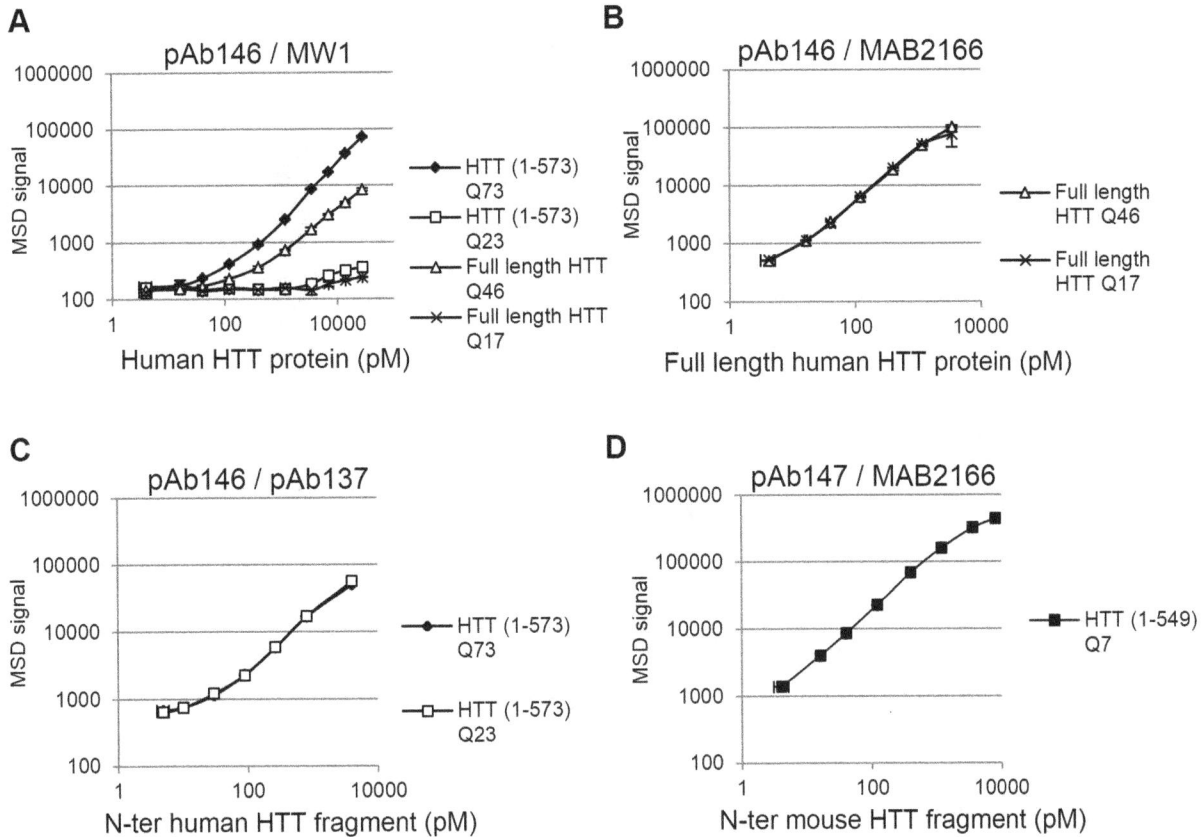

Figure 2. MSD assay performance with human and mouse HTT purified proteins. HTT (1–573) Q23 and HTT (1–573) Q73 large fragment and full length wild type (Q17) and mutant (Q46) recombinant human HTT proteins were spiked in the MSD assay buffer 1 at different concentrations and tested in the expanded polyglutamine human HTT MSD assay (antibody pair pAb146/MW1) (A), in the pan (antibody pair pAb146/MAB2166) (B), and in the exon-1 - pan (antibody pair pAb146/pAb137) (C) human HTT MSD assays. The HTT (1–549) Q7 mouse large fragment recombinant HTT protein was spiked in the MSD assay buffer 1 at different concentrations and tested in the mouse/rat HTT MSD assay (antibody pair pAb147/MAB2166) (D). Data are averages of n = 2 technical replicates with correspondent standard deviations.

neurons transduced with the *HTT*-specific AAV-SEWB-sh4 was estimated to be reduced by 84%. Detection of neuronal total tau in the same zQ175 primary neuron lysates, monitored using a commercially available MSD ELISA-based assay, was used as sample normalizer (Figure 3C). These results were also confirmed by immunoblot (Figure 3D).

The same MSD ELISA-based platform was used to develop the pan (expanded mutant and wild type), or "total" human HTT

Table 1. HTT MSD assay sensitivity and dynamic range.

HTT MSD assay	HTT purified protein	MSD assay lower detection limit	MSD assay dynamic range (log units)
Expanded polyQ human HTT (antibody pair: pAb146/MW1)	HTT (1-573) Q73	40 pM	2
	HTT (1-573) Q23	8 nM	N/A
	FL HTT Q46	120 pM	1.5
	FL HTT Q17	16 nM	N/A
Pan human HTT (antibody pair: pAb146/MAB2166)	FL HTT Q46	<4 pM	2
	FL HTT Q17	<4 pM	2
Exon-1 – pan human HTT (antibody pair: pAb146/pAb137)	HTT (1-573) Q73	~4 pM	1.5
	HTT (1-573) Q23	~4 pM	1.5
Mouse/Rat HTT (antibody pair: pAb147/MAB2166)	HTT (1-549) Q7	<4 pM	2.5

Note. Lower detection limit was determined from the calibration curve using the calculation of background mean +3× Standard deviation. Log units were defined by visual interpretation.
Antibody pairs are indicated as capture/detection antibody.

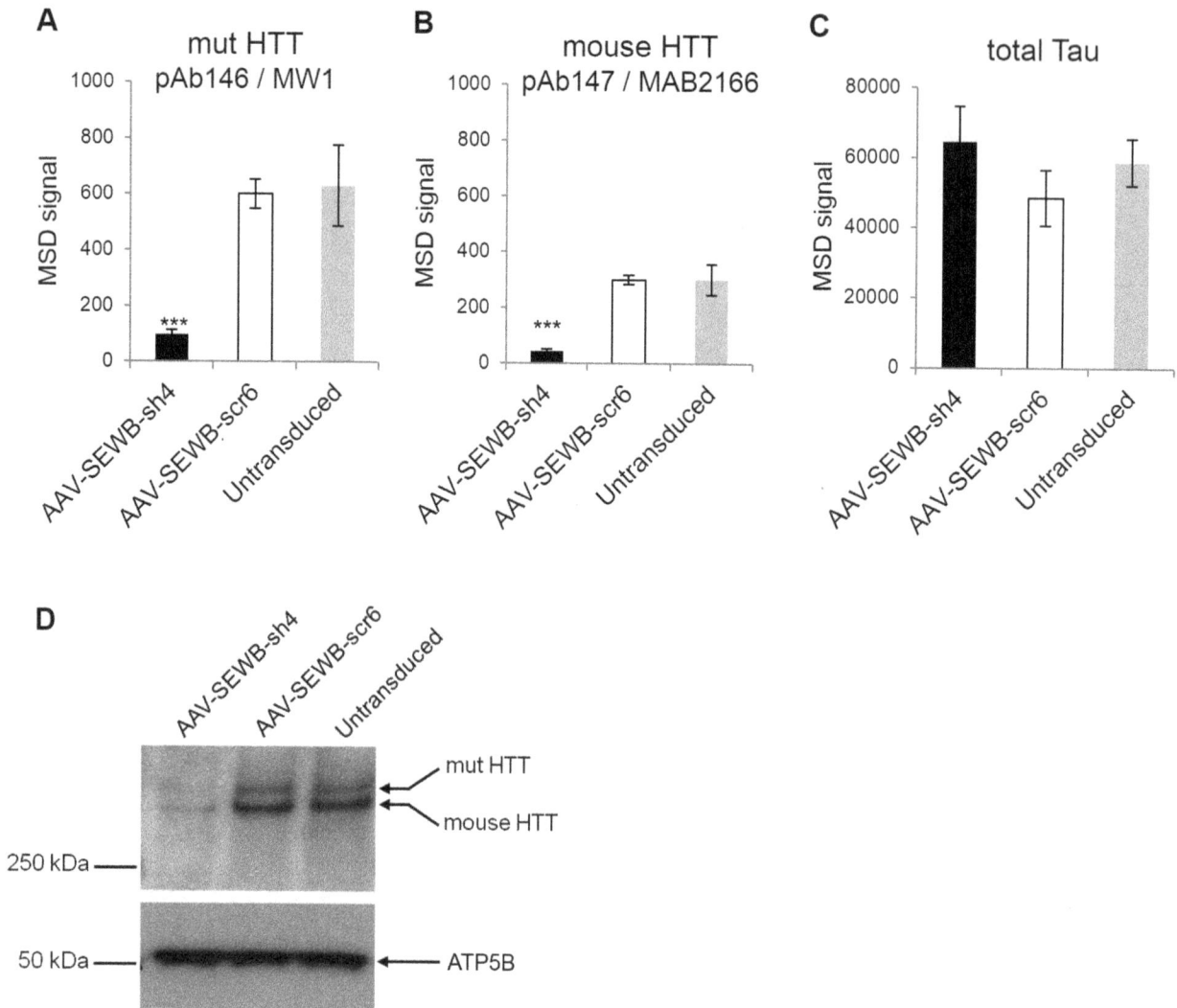

Figure 3. Specificity of human mutant and mouse HTT detection. The adeno-associated AAV-shRNA expression vector AAV-SEWB-sh4 was transduced into heterozygous zQ175 mouse primary neurons and humanized mutant (A) or endogenous mouse (B) HTT proteins were evaluated using the expanded polyglutamine human HTT MSD assay (antibody pair pAb146/MW1) or the mouse/rat HTT MSD assay (antibody pair pAb147/MAB2166), respectively. sh4, *HTT* targeting shRNA. scr6, scramble control shRNA. (C) Neuronal total tau protein levels measured using a commercially available MSD ELISA-based assay kit were monitored as loading control. Data are averages of n = 3 independent samples with correspondent standard deviations. ***, P<0.001. (D) Immunoblot confirming the AAV-mediated knockdown of humanized mutant (mut) and endogenous mouse HTT in transduced heterozygous zQ175 mouse primary neurons (AAV-SEWB-sh4: *HTT* targeting shRNA; AAV-SEWB-scr6: scrambled control shRNA). Immunoblot was probed for HTT (MAB2166, 1:1,000; Millipore) or ATP5B as loading control.

assay. For this assay, the polyclonal pAb146 antibody was again used as a capture antibody. This antibody was used in combination with the MAB2166, a mouse monoclonal antibody raised against a fusion protein encompassing the region from amino acid 183 to 812 of the HTT protein. The target epitope of this antibody has been subsequently narrowed down to a region spanning amino acid 445 to 459 of the human HTT protein [30]. The assay performed using the pAb146-MAB2166 antibody combination enables the detection of more full length wild type (Q17) and mutant (Q46) HTT proteins (Figure 2B) as defined by the distant antibody epitopes. As shown in Figure 2B, the very good overlap of the two standard curves indicated that this assay can detect human HTT proteins independently of the length of the polyglutamine tract of the proteins. This was expected because both capture and detection antibodies target epitopes located outside the polyglutamine region. The limit of detection of the

assay performed using the pAb146-MAB2166 antibodies was determined to be in the low pM range for both full length HTT proteins tested (Table 1).

The target epitope of the monoclonal MAB2166 antibody maps outside the HTT protein sequence encoded by the exon-1 of the HD gene and this makes the pan, polyglutamine length-independent, human HTT assay developed with the pAb146 and MAB2166 antibodies not suited for detection of HTT exon-1 protein fragments. Therefore, we developed an alternative version of the pan human HTT assay that allows for the detection of shorter HTT fragments. The MAB2166 detection antibody was replaced by pAb137, an antibody raised to an epitope in the N-terminal region (amino acid 4-19) of the HTT protein (Figure 1A) and pAb146 remained the capture antibody. To enable the use of two rabbit antibodies in the same assay, the pAb137 detection antibody was directly labeled using the SULFO-TAG NHS-ester labeling reagent available from Meso Scale Discovery. The assay performed using the pAb146-pAb137 antibody combination enables the specific detection of HTT (1–573) Q23 and HTT (1–573) Q73 large fragment HTT proteins (Figure 2C). Also in this version of the assay, the detection of the human large fragment HTT proteins appeared to be completely independent of the length of the polyglutamine tract. The signal detected using the pAb146-pAb137 antibodies was slightly lower compared to that seen when using the pAb146-MAB2166 antibody combination. Also of note is that the assay sensitivity appeared to be slightly lower, although still in the low pM range (Table 1).

For simplicity, in this paper we refer to the MSD assay developed using the pAb146-MAB2166 antibody combination as pan (i.e., polyQ-independent) human HTT assay and the MSD assay for which the pAb146-pAb137 antibody combination as exon-1 - pan human HTT assay.

Electrochemiluminescence assay for rodent huntingtin protein detection

The MSD electrochemiluminescence platform was also used to develop a detection assay for endogenously expressed mouse HTT protein. The mouse HTT-selective pAb147 antibody, which binds to an epitope within the proline-rich region of the mouse HTT protein, was used as capture antibody. The MAB2166 antibody was used as detection antibody. The epitope of this antibody maps to a 15-amino acid region spanning from amino acid 445 to 459, a conserved region between human and mouse HTT proteins [30]. In this assay, we used a commercially available anti-mouse MSD SULFO-TAG antibody as labeled secondary detection reagent to generate the electrochemiluminescence in the assay. The mouse HTT-specific assay functionality was confirmed using the purified mouse HTT (1–549) Q7 large fragment protein (Figure 2D) and sensitivity for this assay was estimated to be in the low pM range (Table 1).

To confirm the specificity of the mouse HTT signal detection by the pAb147-MAB2166 MSD assay, the endogenous mouse HTT protein was monitored in zQ175 mouse primary neurons after adeno-associated virus (AAV)-mediated shRNA knockdown (Figure 3B). The effect of the *HTT*-specific AAV-SEWB-sh4 [28] on the mouse HTT protein signal was clearly detected by the mouse HTT-specific ELISA-based MSD assay. When quantified as a percentage of signal versus control transduction (AAV-SEWB-scr6), the mouse HTT signal in heterozygous zQ175 primary neurons transduced with the *HTT*-specific AAV-SEWB-sh4 was found to be reduced by 86%. Detection of neuronal total tau in the zQ175 primary neuron lysates, monitored using a commercially available MSD ELISA-based assay, was used as sample normalizer (Figure 3C).

For an evaluation of potential species cross-reactivity effects of the used capture antibodies pAb146 and pAb147, competition binding assays between human HTT (1–573) Q23 or mouse HTT (1–549) Q7 large fragment proteins and various peptides were performed. The human peptide CHDI-90000208 represents the epitope for pAb146, CHDI-90000209 is the mouse equivalent of CHDI-90000208 which represents the epitope for pAb147, and CHDI-90000210 is a peptide corresponding to an unrelated region of human HTT. The competition binding assay showed that only the human peptide CHDI-90000208 competes with human HTT (1–573) Q23 protein for binding to the capture antibody pAb146, neither the mouse peptide CHDI-9000209 nor the unrelated peptide CHDI-90000210 showed any significant competitive effect (Figure S1A). Conversely, the mouse peptide CHDI-90000209 was the only peptide to compete for binding to pAb147 (Figure S1B); albeit the mouse peptide displayed a slight

10% inhibition of binding at the highest concentration tested (10 mM). These data demonstrate that the pAb146 and pAb147 antibodies are selective for the respective species with little to no cross-reactivity.

We also tested whether the MSD assay performed with the pAb147 and MAB2166 could be used to detect endogenous HTT in rat brain tissue as the target epitope of both antibodies is completely conserved between mouse and rat HTT proteins. Extracts generated from RccHan:WIST wild type rat brains were prepared and tested in the pAb147-MAB2166 HTT MSD assay and showed a significant signal over background (Figure S2), whereas human-derived cortical tissue extracts containing human HTT used as negative control showed a signal at background level, confirming that this MSD assay can be used to monitor both mouse and rat HTT proteins, but not human HTT.

Assessment of huntingtin levels in biological samples

Our ultimate goal is to develop assays that allow the detection and quantification of HTT proteins in biological samples. The added complexity of cell lysates and tissue homogenate extracts may influence antibody binding and affect the overall performance of the assay. In order to establish the effect of the biological sample matrix on the MSD assays, we performed a spike-and-recovery experiment. A constant amount (20 micrograms) of mouse brain homogenate generated from a (CBA×C57Bl/6) F1 (CBF) (B6CBAF1/OlaHsd, Harlan Olac) wild type mouse was spiked with increasing concentrations of recombinant human HTT (1–573) Q73 and HTT (1–573) Q23 proteins. The samples were tested in both the expanded polyglutamine and the exon-1 - pan human HTT MSD assays (Figure S3A and S3C, respectively). The effect of the biological sample matrix was also tested on the signal recovery of the purified full length human HTT Q46 and HTT Q17 proteins in the pan human HTT assay (Figure S3B). Because the developed assays are specific for human HTT we did not expect, nor did we observe, any interference by the endogenous mouse HTT protein present in the brain extract.

The same assessment was carried out for the mouse HTT-specific MSD assay but, in this case, the recombinant mouse HTT (1–549) Q7 protein was spiked in a brain homogenate obtained from a 3 month-old homozygous zQ175 mouse which carries two chimeric huntingtin alleles comprised of human exon-1 knocked into the mouse gene (Figure S3D). Because the sequence of the exon-1 polyproline domain of this chimeric HTT protein is derived from human HTT, we would not expect any detection by the mouse polyproline sequence-specific pAb147 antibody.

The performance of all samples in the different MSD assays was compared with that of recombinant HTT proteins spiked in assay buffer diluent. In order to accurately evaluate the effect of the sample biological matrix, the same lysis buffer (MSD assay buffer 1) used as diluent for the HTT recombinant proteins was also used to generate the mouse brain extracts. An alternative lysis buffer (MSD assay buffer 2) was also tested for the human HTT recombinant fragments (see Figure S4) and overall results obtained with the two different lysis buffers were found to be comparable. The influence of the sample biological matrix on all of the MSD assays was minimal. The limit of detection for all the MSD assays performed in brain lysates did not substantially differ from that calculated for the recombinant HTT proteins spiked in assay buffer and, in agreement with what was observed previously, was estimated to be in the pM range, independently from the presence of the sample biological matrix (Figure S3A–D).

Detection and quantification of soluble HTT in brain tissues of HD *in vivo* models

To establish whether the pAb146-MW1 MSD HTT detection assay is suitable to measure mutant HTT levels in tissue samples, we generated brain tissue homogenates from different transgenic and knock-in HD mouse models and tested them in the HTT MSD assays.

Brain tissue homogenates obtained from 4, 8 and 12 week-old R6/2 mice were analyzed using the expanded polyglutamine human HTT MSD assay. This transgenic mouse model contains a 1.9-kb fragment encompassing the human HTT promoter and exon-1 [22] bearing an expanded polyglutamine tract of 120 CAG repeats on average in the colony used. The R6/2 mice exhibit both early and severe behavioral and anatomical symptoms [19,22]. Significant signals were observed for all transgenic R6/2 tissue samples analyzed (Figure 4A). In addition, tissue homogenates showed a decreased signal with increased age of the R6/2 mice. We measured a 2-fold signal decrease for 8 week-old brains compared with 4 week-old R6/2 tissues, whereas no additional signal reduction was seen for 12 week-old R6/2 samples. This signal decrease is most likely caused by a shift of mutant HTT exon-1 fragment protein from a soluble to aggregated form as a function of disease progression as previously reported [36] and was also observed in immunoblot analysis of these tissues (Figure 4B). Similar results were seen when micro-dissected cortex, striatum and brain stem tissue homogenates obtained from 4, 8, 12, and 15 week-old R6/2 mice of a different colony (bearing an expanded polyglutamine tract of 206 CAG repeats on average) were analyzed using the expanded polyglutamine human HTT MSD assay (Figure S5). The overall signals observed for cortex and striatum samples were comparable, whereas those detected for the brain stem samples were lower, especially for the 4 and 8 week time-points, suggesting lower levels of HTT exon-1 expression in this tissue. The most significant signal decrease was observed up to 12 weeks where we we measured a 2.7-, 3-, and 2-fold signal decrease respectively for 12 week-old cortex, striatum, and brain stem tissues compared with 4 week-old R6/2 tissues. The signals detected for 12 and 15 week time-points were comparable for all tissues tested. These data demonstrated that the pAb146-MW1 MSD HTT assay is specific for predominantly soluble forms of mutant HTT.

The ability of the MSD HTT assays to detect mutant HTT levels in tissue samples was further assessed using whole brain homogenates obtained from several HD rodent models. Tissues obtained from 3 month-old BAC HD mice [23], 3 month-old heterozygous zQ175 knock-in mice [25,26] and their correspondent wild type littermates were homogenized and assessed in the MSD assay performed using the pAb146-MW1 antibody combination for specific detection of the mutant human HTT protein (Figure 5A). Hemispheres of 4 week-old R6/2 brain extracts were also included in the analysis and levels of transgenic HTT detection compared to those in age-match wild type controls (Figure 5A). Specific detection of mutant full length human HTT proteins were detected in the BAC-HD and z_Q175 mice as well as the human HTT exon-1 fragment protein in R6/2 mice when compared to wild type controls. An approximately 10-fold higher MSD signal was seen in both BAC HD and zQ175 mouse models compared to the correspondent age-matched control mice. A slightly lower signal increase was detected in the R6/2 mouse model (approximately 8-fold higher compared to age-matched control mice). This result confirmed the utility of this assay for detection of soluble full length and fragment forms of mutant HTT in different HD mouse models.

The brain tissue extracts generated from the different HD mouse models were also analyzed in the pan human HTT MSD assay (BAC HD and zQ175 mice) or in the exon-1 - pan human HTT MSD assay (R6/2 mice) (Figure 5B). Because these models express only mutant human HTT, the results showed the same pattern as that evidenced when samples were assessed in the expanded polyglutamine human HTT assay (see also Figure 5A). However, because the pan human HTT assays detect human HTT proteins independently of polyglutamine repeat-length, the use of these assays also allows an accurate quantification of the human mutant HTT protein expression levels in the samples. On the other hand, the availability of recombinant HTT proteins carrying a significantly different polyglutamine length compared to that of HTT proteins expressed by the HD mouse models makes the estimation of HTT concentration in the expanded polyglutamine human HTT MSD assay inaccurate without using a CAG repeat length correction factor. We therefore employed the exon-1 - pan human HTT assay and used the HTT (1–573) Q73 fragment to generate standard curves to quantify human mutant exon-1 HTT expression levels in R6/2 mice. The purified full length Q46 HTT protein was used as standard reference in the pan human HTT assay for the quantification of human mutant HTT in both BAC HD and zQ175 full length mouse models. Although the effect of the sample biological matrix on the pan human HTT assay signal recovery was previously shown to be minimal (see also Figure S3), the recombinant HTT proteins were spiked in mouse brain homogenate generated from wild type age-matched control mice to account for any effects, although minimal, of the sample biological matrix. Between the two mouse models expressing full length HTT, the transgenic BAC HD model, likely to carry multiple copies of the transgene, showed higher levels of mutant human HTT protein compared to heterozygous zQ175 knock-in mice, which only carry one chimeric mouse/human exon-1 allele (Figure 5C).

We also quantified the levels of endogenous mouse HTT in the different animal models using the pAb147-MAB2166 antibody combination for specific detection of the endogenous mouse HTT protein and used the purified mouse HTT (1–549) Q7 large fragment protein as the standard (Figure 5D). Both BAC HD and R6/2 transgenic animal models showed comparable levels of endogenous mouse HTT expression, which, as expected, were also found to be very similar to those detected in wild type age-matched control mice. A significant difference (approximately 50%) in endogenous mouse HTT expression was seen between heterozygous zQ175 mice and the correspondent wild type controls. This was expected because, as previously mentioned, the heterozygous zQ175 mice carry only one complete mouse *HTT* allele.

Detection of HTT protein in human samples

Because the sensitivity and specificity of the human HTT MSD assays were successfully demonstrated for human *HTT* transgenes in rodent brain tissues, we next focused on the detection of polyglutamine expanded and non-expanded HTT in a clinically relevant setting and analyzed human lymphoblast cell lines and post mortem cortex tissues obtained from HD and age-matched healthy control patients. These samples offered the opportunity to also evaluate the performance of the pan human HTT assay which was not possible to investigate in the animal samples not expressing wild type human HTT. HD (GM-04282 Q73/19) and non-HD control (GM-03354 Q23/19) lymphoblast samples analyzed in the pan human HTT assay showed comparable total (polyglutamine expanded and non-expanded) levels of HTT expression; 143.1 ± 41.2 and 155.9 ± 36.6 femtomoles HTT per

A

B

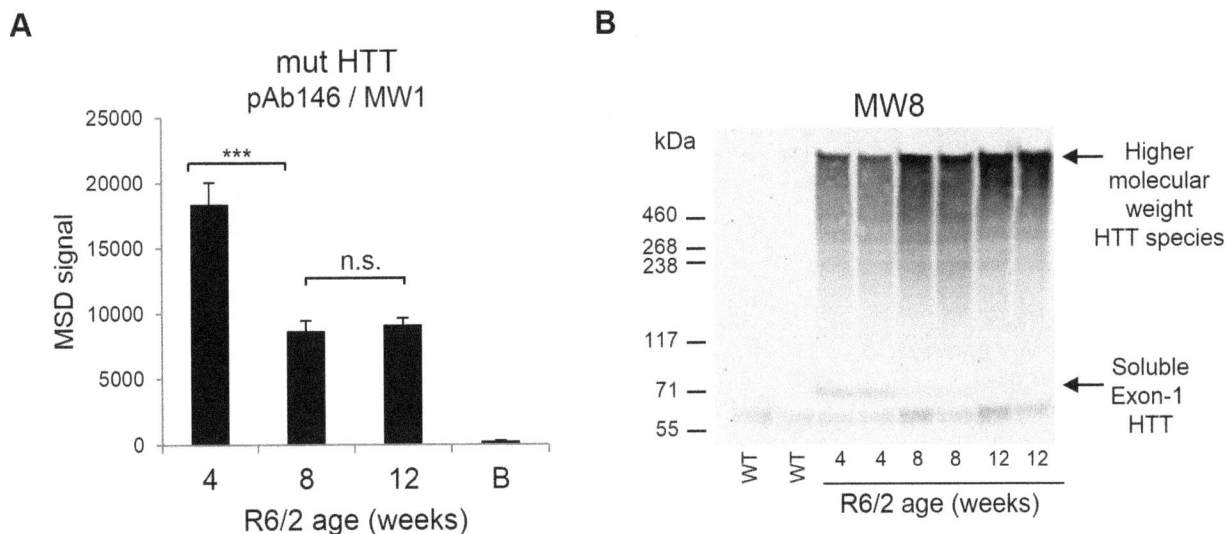

Figure 4. Decrease of soluble mutant HTT levels in R6/2 brain tissues is associated with increased age of the mice. (A) Homogenates from brains of R6/2 female mice obtained from The Jackson Laboratory (bearing an expanded polyglutamine tract of 120 CAG repeats on average) were analyzed for detection of soluble mutant human HTT at different ages (4, 8 and 12 weeks). Tissues analyzed showed significant signals in the expanded polyglutamine human HTT MSD assay (antibody pair pAb146/MW1) and a significant signal decrease between 4 and 8 weeks of age. Data are averages of n = 4 independent samples with correspondent standard deviations. B, assay background. ***, P<0.001. (B) SDS-PAGE and immunoblotting for HTT with the MW8 antibody reveals high molecular weight bands (presumably HTT aggregates) in R6/2 brain homogenates that increase with increasing age of the animals. Progressive decrease of soluble monomeric HTT fragments can be observed. WT, wild type (CBA×C57Bl/ 6) F1 (CBF) (B6CBAF1/OlaHsd, Harlan Olac) mice.

milligram total input protein, respectively (Figure 6A). Healthy control patient lymphoblasts showed, as expected, a signal close to background levels when tested in the expanded polyglutamine human HTT MSD assay, whereas mutant HTT expression level in HD patient lymphoblasts was found to be approximately 44% lower (63.0 ± 16.0 femtomoles mutant HTT per milligram total input protein) compared to the correspondent total HTT amount. Quantification of mutant HTT levels was performed using the purified human HTT (1–573) Q73 large fragment protein as standard reference. The estimation of mutant HTT expression levels is in this case accurate, because both standard and endogenously expressed mutant HTT proteins carry the same CAG repeat length. Post mortem cortex homogenates of HD patients (HD-1 (Q46/17), HD-2 (Q43/19), HD-3 (Q43/17), HD-4 (Q45/16)) and non-HD control donors (C-1, C-2, C-3) were tested and estimated amounts of HTT for each sample were calculated using standard curves of recombinant full length human mutant (Q46) HTT protein (Figure 6B). Also in this case, the estimation of mutant HTT expression levels is accurate because both standard and endogenously expressed mutant HTT proteins carry approximately the same CAG repeat length. Amounts of total HTT vary between 100 and 190 femtomoles per milligram total input protein across all tested samples, with average values of 171.2 ± 30.0 femtomoles HTT per milligram total input protein in non-HD control samples and 119.2 ± 17.5 femtomoles HTT per milligram total input protein in HD samples. Polyglutamine-expanded HTT could only be detected in the HD homogenates with an average value of 64.8 ± 17.1 femtomoles mutant HTT per milligram total input protein, which is equivalent to approximately 54% of the respective amount of total HTT.

An overview of the HD patient details and the corresponding estimated mutant and pan HTT amounts, based on data generated using the HTT MSD assays, is reported in Table 2.

Discussion

We have developed a panel of versatile and highly sensitive ELISA-based bioassays utilizing the MSD electrochemilumines-cence platform to quantify soluble polyglutamine-expanded and non-expanded human HTT protein in animal and human tissues. Additionally, we have developed an assay that specifically detects soluble mouse and rat HTT proteins. Importantly, we have generated both human and mouse recombinant huntingtin fragment proteins as references to estimate the quantity of human HTT and mouse HTT in biological samples. The use of the MSD technology, based on stable electrochemiluminescent labels, ensures that only labels near the electrode are excited and detected leading to precise and reproducible quantitation of HTT. In addition, the multiple excitation cycles of each label amplify the signal to enhance light levels and improve sensitivity; all assays described can detect HTT proteins in the low pM range. The assays are conducted in high-throughput 96- or 384-well plate format and, contrary to other assays using alternative technologies to measure HTT in biosamples [16,17,19,36], in principle they can be multiplexed to evaluate HTT levels with respect to other unrelated proteins. The assays are also relatively resistant to changes in biological matrix (e.g., whole brain homogenate) and thereby allows for the comparison of diverse preclinical samples.

We have successfully quantified HTT proteins in different rodent HD models using our bioassays. Of the two full-length HTT-expressing mouse models analyzed, the BAC HD mice showed higher levels of mutant HTT expression compared to the heterozygous zQ175 KI mice, in line with what one might expect from a mouse model carrying multiple transgenic copies of exogenously derived mutant HTT. In R6/2 mice, the level of soluble exon-1 mutant HTT in whole brains and different brain regions was significantly lower in older symptomatic mice than in younger pre-symptomatic mice. This has been attributed to a progressive shift from the soluble to aggregated form of HTT

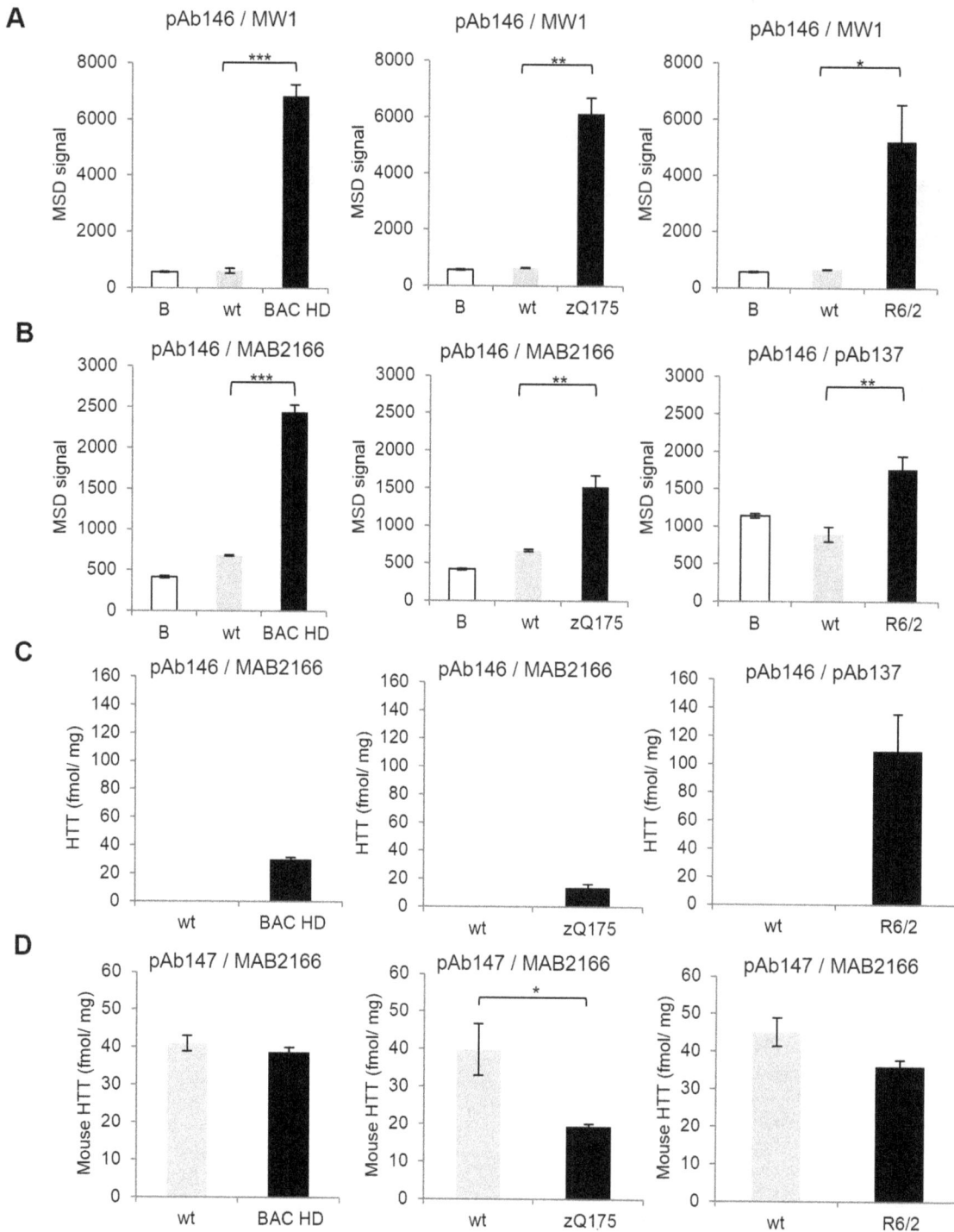

Figure 5. Quantification of mutant human HTT and endogenous mouse HTT detection in brain extracts derived from three different mouse HD models. Human mutant HTT proteins expressed in 3 month-old BAC HD, 4 week-old R6/2 and 3 month-old heterozygous zQ175 mouse models were detected using the expanded polyglutamine human HTT MSD assay (antibody pair pAb146/MW1) (A) and the pan human HTT MSD assay (antibody pair pAb146/MAB2166) for BAC HD and zQ175 mice or the exon-1 - pan human HTT MSD assay (antibody pair pAb146/pAb137) for R6/2 mice (B). A total of 20 μg of whole brain tissue homogenates were used for the analysis. Correspondent wild type age-matched control animals (wt) were included as negative controls. (C) Human mutant HTT proteins in the above mentioned HD mouse models were quantified using standard curves of large fragment (exon-1 - pan human HTT MSD assay) or full length HTT recombinant proteins (pan human HTT MSD assay) as standards. (D) The expression of mouse endogenous HTT was detected using the mouse/rat HTT MSD assay (antibody pair pAb147/MAB2166) and quantified using standard curves of purified HTT (1–549) large fragment mouse HTT protein. Quantified human HTT and mouse HTT proteins are expressed as femtomoles per milligrams of total brain extract input protein. Data are averages of n = 3 independent samples with correspondent standard deviations. B, assay background. *, P<0.05; **, P<0.01; ***, P<0.001.

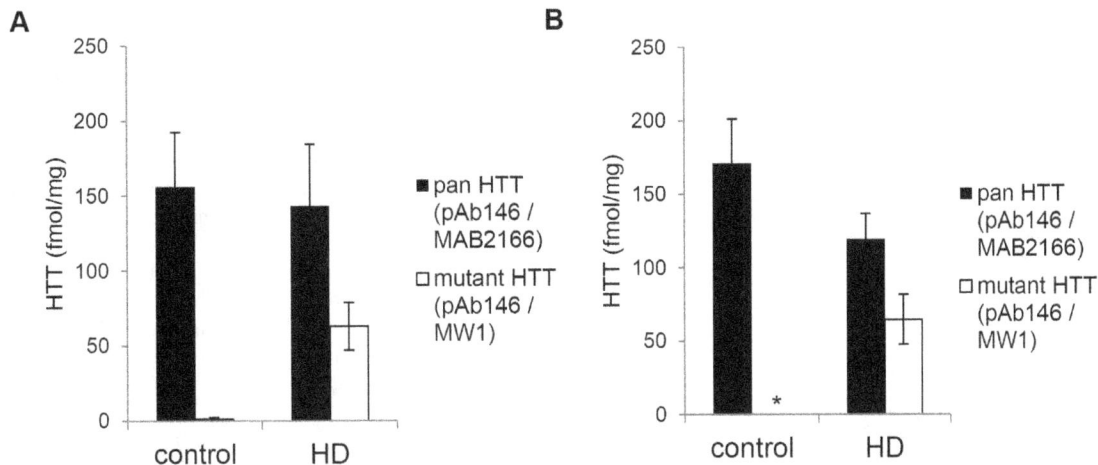

Figure 6. Detection of polyglutamine-expanded (antibody pair pAb146/MW1) and non-expanded (antibody pair pAb146/MAB2166) human HTT proteins in HD patient lymphoblast cell lines and human brain tissues. (A) Detection and quantification of human HTT proteins in HD and non-HD control patient lymphoblast lysates. Human HTT proteins were quantified using standard curves of HTT (1–573) Q73 recombinant protein. Technical triplicates with standard deviations are shown. 1 mg/ml of total protein lysates was tested. (B) Detection and quantification of human HTT proteins in post mortem frontal cortex homogenates of 4 HD patient and 3 non-HD control donors. Human HTT proteins were quantified using standard curves of human full length Q46 HTT recombinant protein. Data are presented as average values with correspondent standard deviations. Asterisk marks HTT levels below the limit of detection. 0.5 mg/ml of total protein homogenates was tested. For the analysis of the human brain extracts in the HTT MSD assays, the MW1 detection antibody was used at a concentration of 7.5 µg/ml and the MAB2166 detection antibody was used at a dilution of 1:1,000.

which correlates with disease progression [31]. This highlights the point that our assays detect soluble HTT and not higher molecular species of HTT such as aggregates. Therefore, when employing these assays one must keep in mind that the amounts measured do not include those higher molecular species.

The mouse monoclonal antibody MW1, used as detection antibody in our expanded polyglutamine HTT assay, binds to expanded polyglutamine tracts in a linear lattice model [32] and its epitope is rapidly lost upon aggregation [13]. In line with these findings, we concluded that our expanded polyglutamine-HTT MSD assay specifically detects soluble forms of HTT, which are progressively recruited into non-detectable insoluble species with the progression of the disease phenotype in the R6/2 HD mouse model. To specifically detect early aggregated species of HTT, alternative assays such as the Seprion assay [18] or the MW8/MW8 TR-FRET assay [33] are highly complementary to the assays described here. Absolute quantification with these assays will, however, be very challenging since the generation of an aggregated protein standard may prove difficult as this is a Q length-, time-, and concentration-dependent process *in vitro* [34].

The use of MW1 as a detection antibody has resulted in the MSD signals of the expanded polyglutamine human HTT MSD assay directly proportional to the CAG length of the HTT proteins analyzed. Data in this paper and our unpublished data from congenic animal models with different CAG expansions between 100 and 270 repeats suggest that the signal increase with CAG expansion remains linear throughout this range. This is in contrast to the HTT TR-FRET assay, which appears to demonstrate a plateau in CAG expansion-mediated signal increase around 60 repeats [35]. Since we have utilized recombinant HTT proteins with CAG-repeat length within the range of both human wild type (17Q and 23Q) and human expanded (46Q and 73Q) alleles, we were able to estimate the HTT concentration in human biosamples using our MSD assays. However, because the majority of the HD mouse models carry a far larger polyglutamine tract than the currently available purified standard proteins, HTT

quantification using the expanded-polyglutamine human HTT MSD bioassay leads to an inaccurate HTT protein estimation, even when the linear correction factor for CAG expansion is used. Therefore, we developed a polyglutamine-length-independent MSD assay (which should detect all soluble HTT conformers) in human biosamples which ensures accurate quantification of human mutant HTT protein expressed in HD mouse models. Importantly, we have optimized two different versions of this assay to quantify both full length and exon-1 human HTT proteins in respective HD models. Recent findings suggest that the HTT exon-1 fragment could also play a role in pathogenesis in HD patients [36] and assays able to measure this fragment could be important.

To ensure that pre-clinical efficacy studies (e.g., knock-down treatments of the mutant HTT protein in HD animal models) are adequately powered to detect the predicted change in expression levels using the expanded polyglutamine MSD assay, we have performed a statistical power analysis of the assay for BAC HD, zQ175 KI and R6/2 HD mouse models (Figure S6). The estimation of the group size was carried out for 25% and 50% reduction in mutant HTT levels. We found that a maximum sample size of three animals is required to have a 90% probability of measuring a significant effect (difference between treated and untreated groups), distributed around the 25% true difference, using the expanded polyglutamine human HTT assay. The group size is reduced to two animals for a 50% effect (Table S2 in Text S1). The group size was comparable among the various HD mouse models tested, independently from the expression of full-length (BAC HD and zQ175 KI) or exon-1 (R6/2) human mutant HTT protein (Table S2 in Text S1).

Endogenous mouse HTT protein was successfully quantified in HD mouse models using the mouse HTT purified standard protein in the mouse HTT-specific MSD assay. The availability of a mouse HTT-specific assay, allowing the analysis of endogenous mouse HTT protein, provides, for the first time, the opportunity to

Table 2. Human sample overview.

Sample	Age (yrs)	Gender	Diagnosis	CAG Repeats	Cold PMI	Frozen PMI	Mut HTT (fmol/mg)	Total HTT (fmol/mg)
C-1	62	male	No diagnostic abnormality recognized	n/a	04:16	08:16	N/A	188.8±38.3
C-2	78	male	No diagnostic abnormality recognized	n/a	05:20	08:00	N/A	136.6±2.3
C-3	56	male	Control	n/a	n/a	08:50	N/A	188.2±20.8
HD-1	53	male	Huntington's Disease, Vonsattel grade 3/4	46/17	06:45	11:17	77.0±18.0	125.8±5.4
HD-2	61	male	Huntington's Disease, Vonsattel grade 3/4	43/19	17:05	18:25	57.9±10.6	140.4±13.8
HD-3	60	male	Huntington's Disease, Vonsattel grade 3/4	43/17	00:00	22:55	43.9±10.0	109.6±10.0
HD-4	47	male	Huntington's Disease, Vonsattel grade 3/4	45/16	02:20	11:40	80.7±22.2	100.9±14.6
GM-04282	20	female	Huntington's Disease onset at age 14 yrs	73/19	N/A	N/A	63.0±16.0	143.1±41.2
GM-03354	25	female	Diabetes Mellitus, juvenile onset	23/19	N/A	N/A	N/A	155.9±36.6

Note. HTT amounts are intended per mg of total input protein in the homogenate.
Cold PMI: Post mortem interval calculated from the patients reported time of death to the time the patient was brought into the cold room.
Frozen PMI: Post mortem interval calculated from the patients reported time of death to the time the brain was processed.

accurately monitor the effects of therapeutic agents on wild type rodent HTT in pre-clinical studies.

Our human HTT bioassays allow an accurate detection of HTT in lysates obtained from human post mortem brain tissues as well as lymphoblast cell lines derived from both HD and non-HD control patients (Figure 6). Analysis of post mortem cortex homogenates of HD patients and non-HD control donors using the MSD assays for total and polyglutamine-expanded HTT showed comparable amounts of total HTT across all tested samples, with an approximate total average of 145 femtomoles HTT per milligram of total input protein. This suggests that total HTT levels are not affected by HD. Determined levels of both total and polyglutamine-expanded HTT are in accordance with previously published data using a HTT-specific TR-FRET assay [16]. Total and polyglutamine-expanded HTT protein levels in HD and non-HD control patients were also comparable between lymphoblast and brain tissue samples.

In addition, when tested in the expanded-polyglutamine HTT assay, HD patient-derived samples were clearly distinct from control patient samples, indicating that the HTT MSD assays have the potential to become a simple test to monitor the patients' response to novel HTT suppression therapeutics, making clinical development of such treatments more efficient. This also potentially enables phenotypic screening strategies for the discovery of novel approaches to allele-selective HTT lowering. The ability to measure HTT proteins in peripheral blood cells allows the incorporation of these endpoints in clinical trials aimed at lowering HTT via the modulation of cellular mechanisms implicated in disease pathogenesis, such as autophagy, the heat shock response, or the modulation of enzymes implicated in HTT post-translational modifications, which affect its turnover and degradation pathways.

It is also important to test these assays for their potential to monitor disease progression. We are currently testing the ability of these assays to monitor human HTT proteins in more accessible rodent and human tissue samples, such as whole blood and cerebrospinal fluid, in order to generate flexible assay protocols for HTT protein bioanalysis to aid pre-clinical and clinical drug development. Future assay development for HTT detection includes assays to monitor truncation or cleavage of HTT [37] and post-translational modifications as phosphorylation [38], sumoylation [39], ubiquitination [40] and acetylation [41], which have all been reported to modulate HTT-mediated neurotoxicity.

These MSD HTT protein quantitation bioassays represent an initial set of tools to define fundamental aspects of the biology of the HTT protein and a critical step forward for the field of HD research which will help facilitate the advancement of potential therapies for HD. Furthermore, we are committed to making these assays available to the wider HD research community as soon as is feasible.

Supporting Information

Figure S1 Determination of species-selectivity of MSD assays using species-specific peptides. Competition between the peptides CHDI-90000208 (antigenic peptide of the pAb146 antibody), CHDI-90000209 (antigenic peptide of the pAb147 antibody) and CHDI-90000210 (unrelated HTT peptide included as a negative control) and human HTT (1-573) Q23 or mouse HTT (1-549) Q7 for binding to the capture antibody demonstrated species-specificity of pAb146 (A) and pAb147 (B).

Figure S2 Detection of endogenous rat HTT protein. Endogenous rat HTT expressed in RccHan:WIST wild type rat whole brains was detected using the pAb147-MAB2166 antibody pair originally used to develop the mouse HTT MSD assay. The target epitope sequence of both antibodies used in this MSD assay is conserved between mouse and rat HTT proteins and rat endogenous HTT protein was, as expected, significantly detected. Homogenates generated from human-derived cortical tissue were included as a negative control and, as expected, showed signals at background level. Data are averages of n = 2 independent samples with correspondent standard deviations.

Figure S3   Effect of the biological sample matrix on the HTT MSD assays. A spiking-and-recovery experiment was performed and purified large fragment and full length HTT proteins were used to assess the effect of the biological sample matrix on the expanded polyglutamine human HTT MSD assay (antibody pair pAb146/MW1) (A), the pan (antibody pair pAb146/MAB2166) (B), and the exon-1 - pan (antibody pair pAb146/pAb137) (C) human HTT MSD assays. The effect of the sample biological matrix on signal recovery of the mouse HTT (1–549) Q7 protein in the mouse/rat HTT MSD assay (antibody pair pAb147/MAB2166) (D) was also tested. The indicated recombinant protein concentrations were spiked in 20 μg of (CBA×C57Bl/6) F1 (CBF) (B6CBAF1/OlaHsd, Harlan Olac) 'wild type' mouse brain homogenate (lysate) or in MSD assay buffer 1 (buffer). The mouse HTT (1–549) Q7 protein was spiked in 20 μg of a 3 month-old homozygous zQ175 mouse, carrying two chimeric mouse/human exon1 alleles. Mouse brain extracts were generated using the MSD assay buffer 1. Data are averages of n = 2 technical replicates with correspondent standard deviations.

Figure S4   MSD assay performance with HTT purified proteins spiked in MSD assay buffer 2. A (CBA×C57Bl/6) F1 (CBF) (B6CBAF1/OlaHsd, Harlan Olac) 'wild type' mouse brain homogenate was generated using an alternative lysis buffer (MSD assay buffer 2: 50 mM Tris, pH 7.4, 120 mM NaCl, 0.5% NP-40, 1 mM EDTA, 1 mM DTT, 1 mM PMSF, protease inhibitors (Complete, EDTA-free; Roche Diagnostics)) and used in a spike-and-recovery experiment with the HTT (1–573) Q23 and HTT (1–573) Q73 large fragment proteins. MSD signals obtained for the different HTT proteins spiked in 20 μg of wild type mouse brain homogenate (lysate) or in MSD assay buffer 2 (buffer) in the expanded polyglutamine human HTT MSD assay (antibody pair pAb146/MW1) (A) and in the exon-1 - pan human HTT MSD assay (antibody pair pAb146/pAb137) (B) are shown. Data are averages of n = 2 technical replicates with correspondent standard deviations.

Figure S5   Decrease of soluble mutant HTT levels in dissected R6/2 brain tissues is associated to increased age of the mice. Homogenates from cortical (A), striatal (B), and brain stem (C) regions from R6/2 female mice (bearing an expanded polyglutamine tract of 206 CAG repeats on average) were analyzed for detection of soluble mutant human HTT at different ages (4, 8, 12 and 15 weeks). All brain regions analyzed showed significant signals in the expanded polyglutamine human HTT MSD assay (antibody pair pAb146/MW1) and a progressive signal decrease over time. Data are averages of n = 3 independent samples with correspondent standard deviations. B, assay background. *, P<0.05; **, P<0.01; ***, P<0.001.

Figure S6   Group size estimation for sample analysis in the expanded polyglutamine human HTT MSD assay. Expanded polyglutamine human HTT MSD assay power analysis was performed for BAC HD (A), zQ175 KI (B) and R6/2 (C) HD mouse models. Brain extracts generated from different HD mice were mixed at different ratios with a brain homogenate generated from one correspondent wild type mouse (HD:WT ratios 100:0, 75:0 and 50:50). The so prepared samples were tested in the expanded polyglutamine human HTT MSD assay (antibody pair pAb146/MW1). Electrochemiluminescence signals obtained for each sample tested are represented by the different histograms. Tables show the inter-samples variability, the average residual MSD signal and the average MSD signal reduction for the different HD:WT ratios and for the different HD mouse models. Data are averages of n = 3 technical replicates with correspondent standard deviations. The coefficient of variation (CV) is defined as the ratio of the standard deviation to the mean.

Figure S7   Production of purified human HTT proteins. (A) SDS-PAGE of FLAG affinity purified HTT (1–573) Q23 and HTT (1–573) Q73 proteins. e1–e5 represent each 1 ml elution with the FLAG peptide. M, molecular weight marker (kDa). Additional proteins/truncated products are visible on the gel. (B) SDS-PAGE of Superdex 200 16/60 gel filtration column-purified HTT (1–573) Q23 and HTT (1–573) Q73 proteins. A dilution series from 1,600 ng to 100 ng of both HTT (1–573) Q23 (lane 1–5) and HTT (1–573) Q73 (lane 6–10) proteins was loaded on the gel. M, molecular weight marker (kDa). The concentrations of both proteins were determined by Bradford assay, in triplicate.

Figure S8   Determination of human HTT (1–573) Q23 and HTT (1–573) Q73 recombinant protein stability. (A) Native gel electrophoresis of purified proteins in 50 mM Tris pH 7.4, 500 mM NaCl, 10% glycerol, 0.1% CHAPS, 1 mM EDTA (lane 1) or in the same buffer with the following modifications: 50% glycerol (lane 2), 0.25% BSA (lane 3), 1 M sodium chloride (lane 4), 25% glycerol, 0.25% BSA and 1 M sodium chloride (lane 5) after 72 h or 57 days of storage at −80°C. Monomeric HTT (1–573) Q23 and HTT (1–573) Q73 are indicated by arrows. C, 0.25% BSA only. M, molecular weight marker (kDa). (B) Native gel analysis of purified HTT (1–573) Q23 and HTT (1–573) Q73 large fragment proteins stored in 50 mM Tris pH 7.4, 500 mM NaCl, 10% glycerol, 0.1% CHAPS, 1 mM EDTA after 386 days of storage at −80°C. Monomeric and higher molecular weight HTT (1–573) Q23 and HTT (1–573) Q73 are indicated by arrows. M, molecular weight marker (kDa).

Figure S9   Production of purified mouse HTT protein. (A) SDS-PAGE of FLAG affinity purified mouse HTT (1–549) Q7 protein. Cells from 3 L culture were lysed by freeze/thaw in a buffer containing 50 mM Tris pH 7.4, 500 mM NaCl, 10% glycerol, 1% CHAPS, 1 mM EDTA and Complete EDTA-free protease inhibitors. Soluble fractions following centrifugation were incubated with anti-FLAG M2 affinity gel overnight at 4°C before washing (w1–w3) and eluting with 5×1 ml of 0.4 mg/ml FLAG peptide in 50 mM Tris pH 7.4, 500 mM NaCl, 10% glycerol, 1% CHAPS, 1 mM EDTA (e1–e5). M, molecular weight marker (kDa). (B) SDS-PAGE of Superdex 200 16/60 purified mouse HTT (1–549) Q7 protein. M, molecular weight marker (kDa). Ld, sample loaded onto the column. (C) MonoQ 5/50 chromatogram showing ion exchange separation of mouse HTT (1–549) Q7 protein. The mouse HTT (1–549) Q7 protein eluted as two distinct peaks in the middle of the NaCl gradient. (D) SDS-PAGE

of MonoQ 5/50 ion exchange purified mouse HTT (1–549) Q7 protein. M, molecular weight marker (kDa). Ld, sample loaded onto the column. Protein contained in each peak was separately pooled and concentrated. Protein concentration was determined by Bradford assay, in triplicate.
(TIF)

Text S1

Acknowledgments

The authors would like to thank Myrna van West, Marlijn Steger-van Zutphen, Sandra Griffioen, Annelieke Strijbosch (BioFocus) and Dr. Andreas Ebneth (Evotec AG) for their input in this project. We thank Isabell Cardaun and Dr. Volker Mack for support with the primary neuron work. We thank Dr. Gillian Bates (King's College London) for supply of the R6/2 mouse samples as described in "Mangiarini L, Sathasivam K, Seller M, Cozens B, Harper A, Hetherington C, Lawton M, Trottier Y, Lehrach H, Davies SW, Bates GP (1996) Exon 1 of the HD gene with an expanded CAG repeat is sufficient to cause a progressive neurological phenotype in transgenic mice. Cell 87, 493–506.", Dr. X. William Yang (UCLA) for supply of the BAC HD mouse, Dr. Stefan Kochanek (University of Ulm, Germany) for the recombinant full length Q17 and Q46 HTT proteins, and Dr. David Corey (UT Southwestern Medical Center) for technical advice on immunoblot of HTT proteins.

Author Contributions

Conceived and designed the experiments: DM MAT IB MS KP AS FA MBACL SD DK WR FH GMcA DFF IMS. Performed the experiments: IB MS KP AS FA SD DK WR. Analyzed the data: DM MAT IB MS KP AS FA MBACL SD DK WR FH GMcA DFF IMS. Contributed reagents/materials/analysis tools: DM MS DFF IMS. Wrote the paper: DM MAT DFF IMS.

References

1. The Huntington's Disease Collaborative Research Group (1993) A novel gene containing a trinucleotide repeat that is expanded and unstable on Huntington's disease chromosomes. Cell 72: 971–983.
2. Sharp AH, Loev SJ, Schilling G, Li SH, Li XJ, et al. (1995) Widespread expression of Huntington's disease gene (IT15) protein product. Neuron 14: 1065–1074.
3. Tabrizi SJ, Langbehn DR, Leavitt BR, Roos RA, Durr A, et al. (2009) Biological and clinical manifestations of Huntington's disease in the longitudinal TRACK-HD study: cross-sectional analysis of baseline data. Lancet Neurol 8: 791–801.
4. Carroll JB, Warby SC, Southwell AL, Doty CN, Greenlee S, et al. (2011) Potent and selective antisense oligonucleotides targeting single-nucleotide polymorphisms in the huntington disease gene/allele-specific silencing of mutant huntingtin. Mol Ther 19: 2178–2185.
5. McBride JL, Pitzer MR, Boudreau RL, Dufour B, Hobbs T, et al. (2011) Preclinical Safety of RNAi-Mediated HTT Suppression in the Rhesus Macaque as a Potential Therapy for Huntington's Disease. Mol Ther 19: 2152–2162.
6. Sah DW, Aronin N (2011) Oligonucleotide therapeutic approaches for Huntington disease. J Clin Invest 121: 500–507.
7. Hu J, Matsui M, Gagnon KT, Schwartz JC, Gabillet S, et al. (2009) Allele-specific silencing of mutant huntingtin and ataxin-3 genes by targeting expanded CAG repeats in mRNAs. Nat Biotechnol 27: 478–484.
8. Harper SQ, Staber PD, He X, Eliason SL, Martins IH, et al. (2005) RNA interference improves motor and neuropathological abnormalities in a Huntington's disease mouse model. Proc Natl Acad Sci U S A 102: 5820–5825.
9. DiFiglia M, Sena-Esteves M, Chase K, Sapp E, Pfister E, et al. (2007) Therapeutic silencing of mutant huntingtin with siRNA attenuates striatal and cortical neuropathology and behavioral deficits. Proc Natl Acad Sci U S A 104: 17204–17209.
10. Kordasiewicz HB, Stanek LM, Wancewicz EV, Mazur C, McAlonis MM, et al. (2012) Sustained Therapeutic Reversal of Huntington's Disease by Transient Repression of Huntingtin Synthesis. Neuron 74: 1031–1044.
11. Stanek LM, Yang W, Angus S, Sardi PS, Hayden MR, et al. (2013) Antisense Oligonucleotide-Mediated Correction of Transcriptional Dysregulation is Correlated with Behavioral Benefits in the YAC128 Mouse Model of Huntington's Disease. J Huntington's Disease 2: 217–228.
12. DiFiglia M, Sapp E, Chase KO, Davies SW, Bates GP, et al. (1997) Aggregation of huntingtin in neuronal intranuclear inclusions and dystrophic neurites in brain. Science 277: 1990–1993.
13. Miller J, Arrasate M, Brooks E, Libeu CP, Legleiter J, et al. (2011) Identifying polyglutamine protein species in situ that best predict neurodegeneration. Nat Chem Biol 7: 925–934.
14. Pyati R, Richter MM (2007) ECL–Electrochemical luminescence. Annu Rep Prog Chem, Sect C 103: 12–78.
15. Fu Q, Zhu J, Van Eyk JE (2010) Comparison of multiplex immunoassay platforms. Clin Chem 56: 314–318.
16. Weiss A, Abramowski D, Bibel M, Bodner R, Chopra V, et al. (2009) Single-step detection of mutant huntingtin in animal and human tissues: A bioassay for Huntington's disease. Anal Biochem 395: 8–15.
17. Paganetti P, Weiss A, Trapp M, Hammerl I, Bleckmann D, et al. (2009) Development of a method for the high-throughput quantification of cellular proteins. Chembiochem 10: 1678–1688.
18. Sathasivam K, Lane A, Legleiter J, Warley A, Woodman B, et al. (2010) Identical oligomeric and fibrillar structures captured from the brains of R6/2 and knock-in mouse models of Huntington's disease. Hum Mol Genet 19: 65–78.
19. Davies SW, Sathasivam K, Hobbs C, Doherty P, Mangiarini L, et al. (1999) Detection of polyglutamine aggregation in mouse models. Methods Enzymol 309: 687–701.
20. Ko J, Ou S, Patterson PH (2001) New anti-huntingtin monoclonal antibodies: implications for huntingtin conformation and its binding proteins. Brain Res Bull 56: 319–329.
21. Duzdevich D, Li J, Whang J, Takahashi H, Takeyasu K, et al. (2011) Unusual Structures Are Present in DNA Fragments Containing Super-Long Huntingtin CAG Repeats. PLoS ONE 6: e17119.
22. Mangiarini L, Sathasivam K, Seller M, Cozens B, Harper A, et al. (1996) Exon 1 of the HD gene with an expanded CAG repeat is sufficient to cause a progressive neurological phenotype in transgenic mice. Cell 87: 493–506.
23. Gray M, Shirasaki DI, Cepeda C, Andre VM, Wilburn B, et al. (2008) Full-length human mutant huntingtin with a stable polyglutamine repeat can elicit progressive and selective neuropathogenesis in BACHD mice. J Neurosci 28: 6182–6195.
24. Menalled LB, Sison JD, Dragatsis I, Zeitlin S, Chesselet MF (2003) Time course of early motor and neuropathological anomalies in a knock-in mouse model of Huntington's disease with 140 CAG repeats. J Comp Neurol 465: 11–26.
25. Heikkinen T, Lehtimaki K, Vartiainen N, Puolivali J, Hendricks SJ, et al. (2012) Characterization of neurophysiological and behavioral changes, MRI brain volumetry and 1H MRS in zQ175 knock-in mouse model of Huntington's disease. PLoS One 7: e50717.
26. Menalled LB, Kudwa AE, Miller S, Fitzpatrick J, Watson-Johnson J, et al. (2012) Comprehensive behavioral and molecular characterization of a new knock-in mouse model of Huntington's disease: zQ175. PLoS One 7: e49838.
27. Kügler S, Lingor P, Scholl U, Zolotukhin S, Bahr M (2003) Differential transgene expression in brain cells in vivo and in vitro from AAV-2 vectors with small transcriptional control units. Virology 311: 89–95.
28. McBride JL, Boudreau RL, Harper SQ, Staber PD, Monteys AM, et al. (2008) Artificial miRNAs mitigate shRNA-mediated toxicity in the brain: implications for the therapeutic development of RNAi. Proc Natl Acad Sci U S A 105: 5868–5873.
29. Huang B, Schiefer J, Sass C, Kosinski CM, Kochanek S (2008) Inducing huntingtin inclusion formation in primary neuronal cell culture and in vivo by high-capacity adenoviral vectors expressing truncated and full-length huntingtin with polyglutamine expansion. J Gene Med 10: 269–279.
30. Cong SY, Pepers BA, Roos RA, Van Ommen GJ, Dorsman JC (2005) Epitope mapping of monoclonal antibody 4C8 recognizing the protein huntingtin. Hybridoma (Larchmt) 24: 231–235.
31. Bates G (2003) Huntingtin aggregation and toxicity in Huntington's disease. Lancet 361: 1642–1644.
32. Li P, Huey-Tubman KE, Gao T, Li X, West AP Jr, et al. (2007) The structure of a polyQ-anti-polyQ complex reveals binding according to a linear lattice model. Nat Struct Mol Biol 14: 381–387.
33. Baldo B, Paganetti P, Grueninger S, Marcellin D, Kaltenbach LS, et al. (2012) TR-FRET-Based Duplex Immunoassay Reveals an Inverse Correlation of Soluble and Aggregated Mutant huntingtin in Huntington's Disease. Chem Biol 19: 264–275.
34. Scherzinger E, Sittler A, Schweiger K, Heiser V, Lurz R, et al. (1999) Self-assembly of polyglutamine-containing huntingtin fragments into amyloid-like fibrils: Implications for Huntington's disease pathology. Proc Natl Acad Sci USA 96: 4604–4609.
35. Weiss A, Trager U, Wild EJ, Grueninger S, Farmer R, et al. (2012) Mutant huntingtin fragmentation in immune cells tracks Huntington's disease progression. J Clin Invest 122: 3731–3736.
36. Sathasivam K, Neueder A, Gipson TA, Landles C, Benjamin AC, et al. (2013) Aberrant splicing of HTT generates the pathogenic exon 1 protein in Huntington disease. Proc Natl Acad Sci U S A 110: 2366–2370.
37. Graham RK, Deng Y, Slow EJ, Haigh B, Bissada N, et al. (2006) Cleavage at the caspase-6 site is required for neuronal dysfunction and degeneration due to

mutant huntingtin. Cell 125: 1179–1191.

38. Pardo R, Colin E, Regulier E, Aebischer P, Deglon N, et al. (2006) Inhibition of calcineurin by FK506 protects against polyglutamine-huntingtin toxicity through an increase of huntingtin phosphorylation at S421. J Neurosci 26: 1635–1645.

39. Steffan JS, Agrawal N, Pallos J, Rockabrand E, Trotman LC, et al. (2004) SUMO modification of Huntingtin and Huntington's disease pathology. Science 304: 100–104.

40. Kalchman MA, Graham RK, Xia G, Koide HB, Hodgson JG, et al. (1996) Huntingtin is ubiquitinated and interacts with a specific ubiquitin- conjugating enzyme. J Biol Chem 271: 19385–19394.

41. Jeong H, Then F, Melia TJ Jr, Mazzulli JR, Cui L, et al. (2009) Acetylation targets mutant huntingtin to autophagosomes for degradation. Cell 137: 60–72.

42. Zhao Y, Chapman DA, Jones IM (2003) Improving baculovirus recombination. Nucleic Acids Res. 31(2):E6–6.

9

Reducing *Igf-1r* Levels Leads to Paradoxical and Sexually Dimorphic Effects in HD Mice

Silvia Corrochano[1], Maurizio Renna[2], Georgina Osborne[3], Sarah Carter[1], Michelle Stewart[1], Joel May[1], Gillian P. Bates[3], Steve D. M. Brown[1], David C. Rubinsztein[2], Abraham Acevedo-Arozena[1]*

1 MRC Mammalian Genetics Unit, Harwell, Oxfordshire, United Kingdom, **2** Department of Medical Genetics, Cambridge Institute for Medical Research, University of Cambridge, Wellcome/MRC Building, Addenbrooke's Hospital, Cambridge, United Kingdom, **3** Department of Medical and Molecular Genetics, King's College London, London, United Kingdom

Abstract

Many of the neurodegenerative diseases that afflict people in later life are associated with the formation of protein aggregates. These so-called "proteinopathies" include Alzheimer's disease (AD) and Huntington's disease (HD). The insulin/insulin-like growth factor signalling (IIS) pathway has been proposed to modulate such diseases in model organisms, as well as the general ageing process. In this pathway, insulin-like growth factor binds to insulin-like growth factor receptors, such as the insulin-like growth factor 1 receptor (IGF-1R). Heterozygous deletion of *Igf-1r* has been shown to lead to increased lifespan in mice. Reducing the activity of this pathway had benefits in a HD *C. elegans* model, and some of these may be attributed to the expected inhibition of mTOR activity resulting in an increase in autophagy, which would enhance mutant huntingtin clearance. Thus, we tested if heterozygous deletion of *Igf-1r* would lead to benefits in HD related phenotypes in the mouse. Surprisingly, reducing *Igf-1r* levels led to some beneficial effects in HD females, but also led to some detrimental effects in HD males. Interestingly, *Igf-1r* deficiency had no discernible effects on downstream mTOR signalling in HD mice. These results do not support a broad beneficial effect of diminishing the IIS pathway in HD pathology in a mammalian system.

Editor: Sandrine Humbert, Institut Curie, France

Funding: We are grateful for a Wellcome Trust Principal Fellowship in Clinical Science (DCR), an M.R.C. Programme Grant (DCR and SB), and the CHDI Foundation (GPB). The funders had no role in study design, data collection and analysis, decision to publish, or preparation of the manuscript.

Competing Interests: The authors have declared that no competing interests exist.

* Email: a.acevedo@har.mrc.ac.uk

Introduction

Huntington's disease (HD) is an autosomal dominant, progressive, fatal, neurodegenerative disorder caused by an expanded CAG tract (polyglutamine or PolyQ) in exon one of the huntingtin gene [1]. The length of the polyQ tract is directly associated with the age-of onset signs of disease [2]. The major symptoms that characterize the disease are motor (chorea) and cognitive (behavioural mood changes, memory lapses and depression). There are no current treatment to cure Huntington's disease [3].

The huntingtin protein is ubiquitously expressed, and appears to function in a variety of cellular processes from transport to apoptosis [4]. The mutation confers a toxic gain of function on the protein, which becomes aggregate-prone, leading to intracellular aggregates that are the hallmark of the disease [5]. A possible loss of function component is also associated with HD pathology [6]. Many of the neurodegenerative diseases that afflict people in later life are associated with the formation of intraneuronal or extraneuronal protein aggregates. These proteinopathies include Alzheimer's disease (AD), Parkinson's disease and conditions caused by polyglutamine tract expansion mutations, like HD. While the pathological hallmark of these proteinopathies is the presence of large protein aggregates, the most toxic species may be oligomers, with the aggregation process itself being an important factor [7]. A range of possible strategies for tackling proteino-pathies have been proposed. On the one hand, one can try to decrease the levels of the toxic protein. This could be achieved by enhancing the degradation of cytoplasmic aggregate-prone proteins by for example inducing autophagy [8–10]. Indeed, autophagy-inducing drugs and genes can alleviate the toxicity of mutant huntingtin in a range of models [9,11]. Another strategy may be to decrease the rate of protein aggregation. This may be possible by up-regulating chaperones like HSP70 via the HSF-1 transcription factor, to enhance productive and non-toxic protein folding [12], although the ability of HSF1 to up regulate this pathway has been shown to decrease with disease progression in HD mice [13].

One pathway that has attracted considerable attention for its ability to modulate proteotoxicity is the insulin/insulin-like growth factor signalling pathway (IIS). In this pathway, insulin-like growth factor (IGF-1) binds to insulin-like growth factor receptors, such as the insulin-like growth factor 1 receptor (IGF-1R), resulting in their activation. The tyrosine kinase activities of these receptors phosphorylate signalling molecules, including important effectors such as the insulin receptor substrate (IRS) protein family. Once phosphorylated, the IRS proteins act as molecular adaptors to facilitate downstream signalling pathways via protein kinase B or AKT (PKB/AKT), which serves as a major downstream effector of IIS signalling.

IIS has been shown to be altered in several neurodegenerative disorders [14–16]. The phosphorylation of AKT is found to be upregulated in many neurodegenerative diseases which could indicate a compensatory response to maximize IGF-1 signalling in these disorders [17]. On the other hand, a prolonged activation of IIS may also lead to a maladaptive response in HD [18]. AKT levels have also been found to be reduced in a rat model of HD and HD patients [19]. Activated AKT can have beneficial effects in neurodegeneration by activating anti-apoptotic pathways. Indeed, stimulation of IGF-1/AKT has been shown to be neuroprotective in HD through direct phosphorylation of huntingtin [17,20] and arfaptin 2 [21], leading to amelioration of HD toxicity in cellular [22] and animal models [23]. Moreover, IGF-1 treatment (stimulating IIS) prevented age-related body weight loss in a HD mouse model, with no differences in motor behaviour, but restoring blood insulin levels [24].

In the opposite direction, IIS inhibition has been shown to ameliorate the proteotoxicity of different aggregate-prone proteins in *C elegans* models, including mutant huntingtin and beta-Amyloid (Abeta) [25,26]. This protection was recently confirmed in AD mouse models [27,28]. Cohen et al found that the heterozygous deletion of *Igf-1r* reduced Abeta induced behavioural impairment in mice, while correlating with the formation of denser soluble amyloid oligomers. One potential mechanism to explain this protection may be by the induction of autophagy due to diminished mTOR activation via AKT. Indeed, numerous studies have suggested that IGF-1 blocks autophagy via mTOR complex 1 (mTORC1) [29–31]. However, in a recent study we have shown that in the long term IGF-1R inhibition leads *in vitro* and *in vivo* to diminished autophagy by reducing the rate of autophagosome precursor formation at the plasma membrane in an mTORC2- and endocytosis-dependent manner [32].

Hence, based on previous data from different model organisms, reducing IIS may lead to both beneficial and deleterious consequences in HD. We thus tested the consequences of the heterozygous deletion of *Igf-1r* in a HD mouse model. We felt this was an important scenario to investigate, since the excess amyloid beta in AD is predominantly extracellular, while in HD, mutant huntingtin is intracellular. We considered that decreased *Igf-1r* levels in heterozygous null mice would be more relevant to potential therapeutic scenarios, given the lethality of a complete *Igf-1r* null background. Interestingly, the behavioural and pathological consequences of reducing IIS in HD mice were equivocal.

Results

Heterozygous deletion of IGF-1R has paradoxical effects in HD mice

Our initial experiments examined whether reduction of *Igf-1r* affected the classical phenotypes of an HD mouse model expressing the mutant fragment of the human huntingtin gene with 82 expanded polyglutamine repeats (hemizygous N171-82Q). We examined heterozygous Knock Out (KO) *Igf-1r* mice, since adult mice with complete deletion of this gene are not viable [33]. To produce all relevant genotypes in one generation, we crossed congenic C57BL6/J N171-82Q HD mice with C57BL6/J *Igf-1r*+/− mice. In order to examine not only the age at the onset of the symptoms, but also the disease progression, we carried out a battery of behavioural test every two weeks, (modified SHIRPA analysis, see methods), together with motor testing via rotarod and grip-strength and weight measurements. We started at 8 weeks of age, before the onset of the symptoms, and stopped the phenotyping at 22 weeks, after which we left mice to reach their

humane end-points to analyse survival. As different HD endophenotypes are differentially affected by sex in mice [34,35], we separated data from males and females.

The development of tremors is a progressive endophenotype that appears in all HD mouse models. We measured tremor onset as part of the SHIRPA analysis in HD mice (non-HD mice have no tremors). In females, tremor onset was delayed in heterozygous *Igf-1r* HD mice (HD; *Igf-1r*+/−) when compared to controls (HD; *Igf-1r*+/+ mice) (Figure 1A; p = 0.002). The average tremor age at onset in females was 16.3 weeks for HD; *Igf-1r*+/− versus 14.1 weeks for controls. However, tremor onset was not significantly different between control and *Igf-1r* deficient HD males (Figure 1B; p = 0.278). Thus, *Igf-1r* deficiency has no significant effect in HD males, but significantly delays the onset of this critical HD endophenotype in HD females. Previous data shows that heterozygous *Igf-1r* null female mice (*Igf-1r*+/−) live longer than littermate controls, while no significant lifespan differences were seen in males [33,36]. When fed *ad libitum* on a standard diet and maintained in regular housing until reaching their humane end-points, *Igf-1r* deficiency did not significantly affect survival defined as time to reach the humane end-points for either male or female HD mice (Figure 1C, D).

In our C57BL/6J background, we found no significant differences in body weight between Non-HD; *Igf-1r*+/+ and Non-HD; *Igf-1r*+/− males or females from 12 weeks of age (Figure 2A, B). However, in HD male mice, *Igf-1r* deficiency resulted in significantly reduced body weight in HD; *Igf-1r*+/− when compared to HD controls (Figure 2B; from 9 weeks of age onwards, p<0.05). Interestingly, *Igf-1r* deficiency did not significantly affect the weights of HD female mice at any stage (Figure 2A). Thus, *Igf-1r* deficiency has only a significant deleterious effect on the weight of HD males.

In agreement with the body weight phenotypes, *Igf-1r* deficiency significantly impaired rotarod performance on HD male mice, but had no significant effects on HD females (Figures 2C, 2D); no significant effects were present when comparing *Igf-1r* deficient Non-HD male or female mice (data not shown). When both sexes are combined, the overall differences between HD genotypes are significant for both weight and rotarod performance (Table S1). Grip strength was also assessed, but no significant differences were found in neither male nor female HD mice (Figure S1A, S1B).

Overall, *Igf-1r* deficiency had no significant effects on lifespan or grip-strength in HD mice, but on affected endophenotypes had opposite effects in male and female mice: In HD females, *Igf-1r* deficiency was neutral (rotarod, weight) or beneficial (delayed tremor onset), whereas in HD males had neutral (tremor onset) or detrimental effects (worsened rotarod performance and weight loss).

Circulating levels of IGF-1 are differentially regulated in HD males and females at 12 weeks of age

A possible explanation for the paradoxical effect observed above could be that males and females present different circulating levels of IGF-1. As a consequence of having less IGF-1 receptor, mice tend to compensate by increasing the levels of circulating IGF-1 [33]. We measured IGF-1 levels in blood and found no significant differences between Non-HD mice at 12 weeks of age (Figure 3A, 3B). For HD mice, we again found sexual dimorphism in the levels of circulating IGF-1. In females, IGF-1 levels were higher in HD mice compared to Non-HD controls (Figure 3A, p = 0.02), but *Igf-1r* deficiency had no effect and thus HD; *Igf-1r*+/+ and HD; *Igf-1r*+/− females had similar amounts of circulating IGF-1. However, in males, the HD transgene alone could not significantly

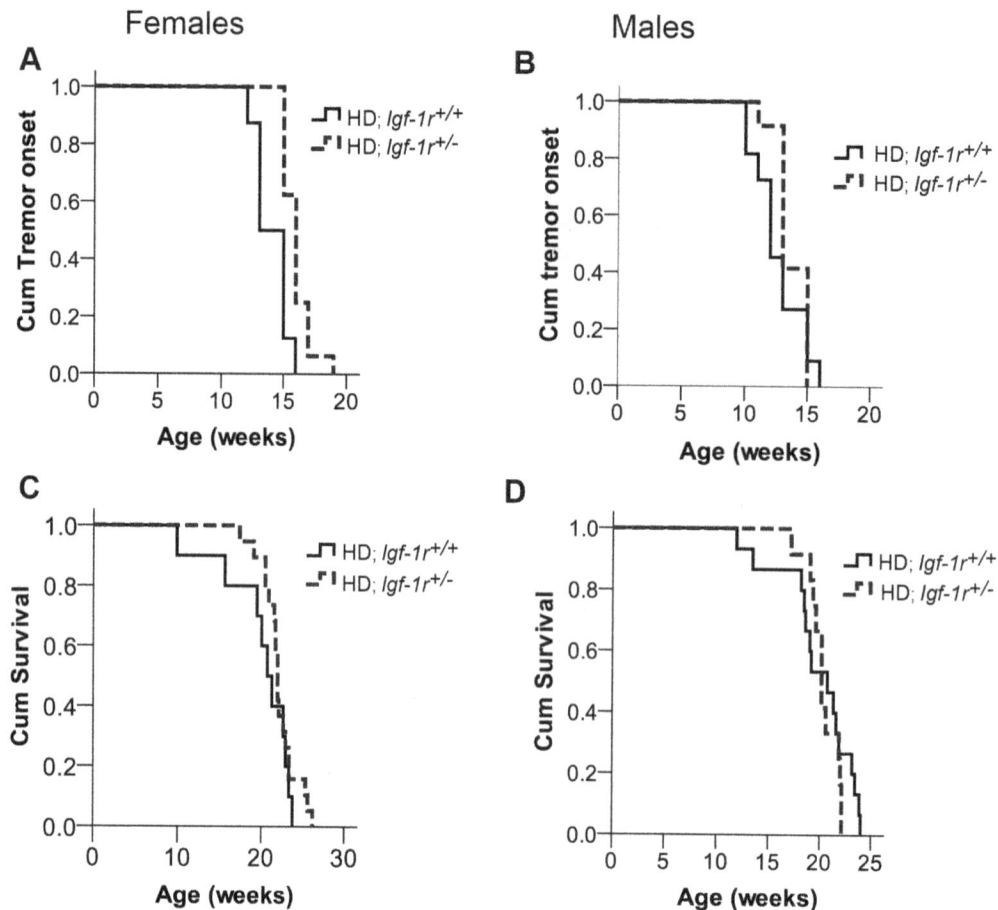

Figure 1. *Igf-1r* deficiency delays tremor onset in HD females without significantly affecting HD males or overall survival. A–B. Tremor onset was estimated via SHIRPA analysis on at least 8 mice per genotype per sex and time point. Tremor onset is significantly reduced in females (**A**) (average onset HD; *Igf-1r*$^{+/-}$: 16.3 weeks compared HD; *Igf-1r*$^{+/+}$: 14.1 weeks, p(Log-rank) = 0.002), but not in males (**B**) HD; *Igf-1r*$^{+/-}$: 13.6 weeks compared HD; *Igf-1r*$^{+/+}$: 12.6 weeks, p(Log-rank) = 0.278). **C–D.** Time to reach end-stage (survival) of the N171-82Q HD mice is not modified by *Igf-1r* status. Survival was measured on at least 10 mice per sex and genotype. No significant differences were observed when comparing survival between HD; *Igf-1r*$^{+/+}$ and HD; *Igf-1r*$^{+/-}$ in female (**C,** n = 10 and 19 respectively, p (Log-rank) = 0.26) or males (**D,** n = 15 and 12 respectively, p(Log-rank) = 0.48), or when both sexes were combined p(Log-rank) = 0.79.

elevate IGF-1 levels; upregulation of circulating IGF-1 levels was found only in *Igf-1r* deficient HD males (Figure 3B, p = 0.002 comparing HD; *Igf-1r*$^{+/+}$ to HD; *Igf-1r*$^{+/-}$). Remarkably, glucose levels in serum have a tendency to correlate with the IGF-1 levels (Figure S2A, S2B). Thus, circulating IGF-1 levels are differentially regulated in HD males and females at 12 weeks of age, with *Igf-1r* deficiency only significantly affecting IGF-1 levels in HD males. These differences in circulating IGF-1 levels paralleled the sexual behavioural differences and may contribute towards the opposite effects of *Igf-1r* deficiency in HD males and females.

IGF-1R deficiency does not affect mutant huntingtin protein levels or overall aggregate numbers but modulate aggregate size

Igf-1r deficiency has been shown to affect mutant huntingtin aggregation in multiple models. One of our initial hypotheses was that loss of one copy of *Igf-1r* gene would result in decreased mTORC1 activity, which would increase autophagy and enhance removal of mutant huntingtin, as previously showed when inhibiting mTOR with rapamycin treatment [11,37].

We thus evaluated both, the levels of mutant huntingtin protein in brain homogenates and the inclusion depositions in brain slices

from HD females, as the slight beneficial phenotypical effects were only observed in mice of this gender. We first compared soluble huntingtin levels in the HD; *Igf-1r*$^{+/-}$ mice with that in controls by western blots from whole brain lysates at 12 weeks of age, but no differences were found (Figure 4A, p = 0.6). In the N171-82Q HD mouse model, inclusions are much more abundant in the cerebellum than in the cortex or striatum. We then measured mutant huntingtin in cerebellum using quantitative ELISA [38] in both male and female HD controls and *Igf-1r* deficient mice, and found no significant differences (Figure 4B, p = 0.29 for females and p = 0.69 for males).

We then quantified the number of inclusions formed in the piriform cortex and cerebellum of these mice. The chosen time point criteria was dictated by the age of onset of tremors in the HD; *Igf-1r*$^{+/+}$ group of females, which was around 13.5 weeks of age. In the piriform cortex at 13 weeks of age, compared to HD controls, the number of huntingtin inclusions had a trend towards being lower in *Igf-1r* deficient females (Figure 4C, p = 0.06). We thus counted overall inclusion numbers and also classified the inclusions according to size in cerebellum slices from HD females using a commercial automated analysing system (as detailed in the methods section). The total number of aggregates was significantly

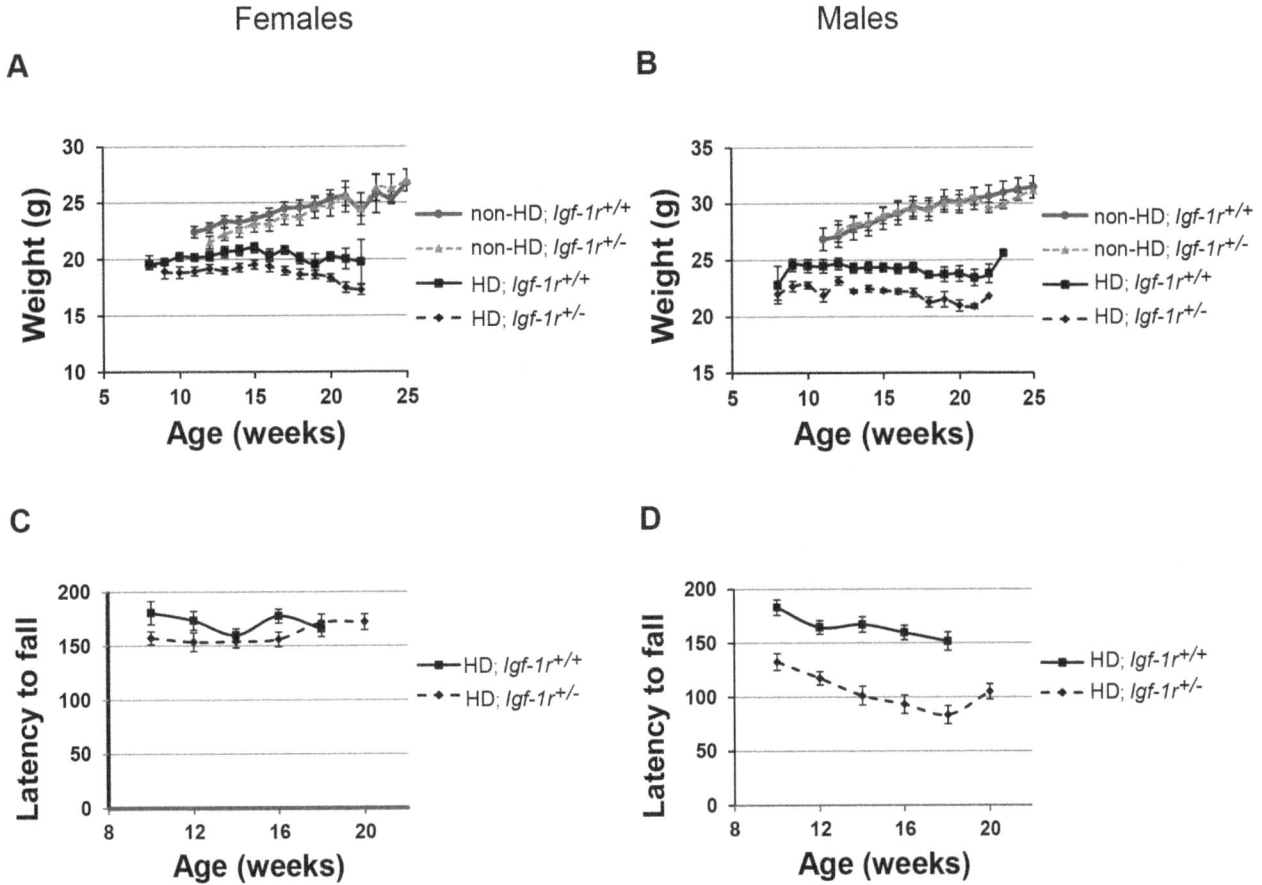

Figure 2. *Igf-1r* hemizygosity differentially affects body weight and rotarod performance in HD males and females. A, B. Body weights of at least 8 mice per genotype per sex and time point were scored. There were no significant weight differences between HD; *Igf-1r*$^{+/+}$ and HD; *Igf-1r*$^{+/-}$ female mice (**A**), except the 13 week time point. Male HD; *Igf-1r*$^{+/-}$ mice showed a significantly reduced body weight from the 9 week time point onwards (**B**). No differences between Non-HD; *Igf-1r*$^{+/+}$ and Non-HD; *Igf-1r*$^{+/-}$ mice. **C, D.** A reduced Rotarod performance was observed in HD; *Igf-1r*$^{+/-}$ compared to HD; *Igf-1r*$^{+/+}$ males (**C**), whereas no significant differences were observed in the female groups (**D**). No differences were observed between Non-HD; *Igf-1r*$^{+/+}$ and *Igf-1r*$^{+/-}$ mice (data not shown). Error bars represent 1×s.e.m (standard error of the mean).

diminished in HD; *Igf-1r*$^{+/-}$ females when compared to littermate controls (Figure 4D, p = 0.019). Aggregates were then classified as small (in the range of 0 to 0.31 μm^2), medium (0.32 to 0.9 μm^2), large (0.91 to 1.8 μm^2) and larger (1.81 to 4.5 μm^2). Overall, small

and medium inclusions are the major species in the cerebellum at this stage (13 weeks of age). Represented as percentage of total inclusions, big inclusions (large and larger) were similar between the genotypes. However, when compared to controls, the

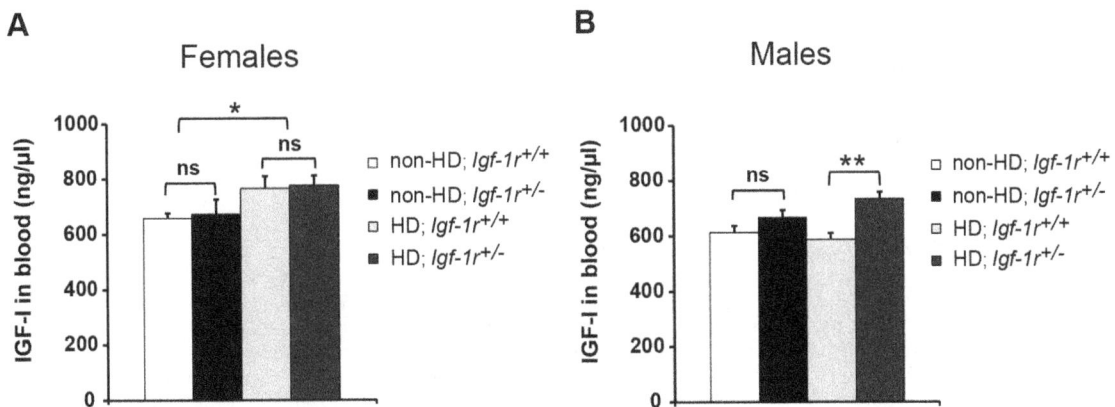

Figure 3. Serum levels of Igf-1 and glucose differ between male and female HD mice. A, B. Blood serum from fasted mice at 12 weeks of age (more than 4 mice per group). IGF-1 circulating levels measured by ELISA in females (**A**) and males (**B**) comparing the four possible genotypes. Error bars represent 1×s.e.m. *P<0.05; **P<0.01. ns = non-significant.

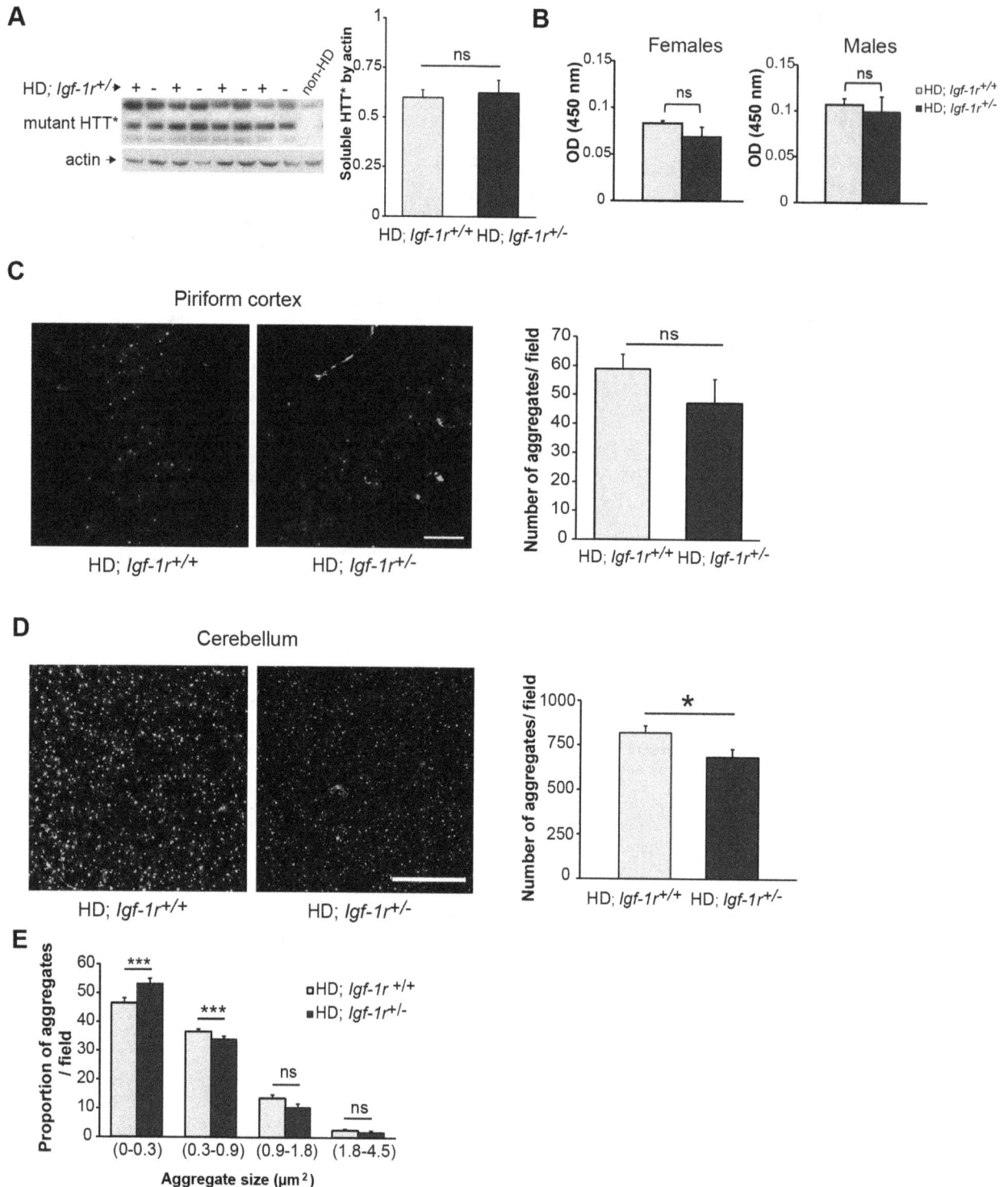

Figure 4. *Igf-1r* hemizygosity has minimal effect on the levels of mutant huntingtin protein. A. Female half-brain homogenates at 12 weeks of age of the indicated genotypes were subject to western blot analysis to measure soluble mutant huntingtin levels (HTT*). The corresponding graph represents the comparison of the densitometry analysis of HTT* levels relative to actin between HD; *Igf-1r*$^{+/+}$ and HD; *Igf-1r*$^{+/-}$ groups (n = 4 per genotype; p = 0.67). B. Using Microsens Aggregate Purification ELISA we measured the mutant HTT aggregates in homogenised cerebellums of 12 weeks old male and female HD mice (n = 4 per group and gender). No significant differences were found between female HD (p = 0.29) or male HD mice (p = 0.69). C. Quantification of huntingtin inclusions in the piriform cortex. Brain slices obtained from 13 weeks old female mice of the indicated genotypes were stained to detect the mutant huntingtin aggregates. Confocal images of the piriform cortex were obtained and analysed as detailed in the methods section. (n = 4 per HD group; p = 0.06). Scale bar represents 25 μm D. Quantification of huntingtin inclusions in the cerebellum of HD female mice. Representative images of confocal projections from the granular layer of cerebellum containing mutant huntingtin aggregates. The quantification of the total number of mutant huntingtin inclusions in the cerebellum shows a modest decreased in the number of inclusions found in the HD; *Igf-1r*$^{+/-}$ group compared to the HD; *Igf-1r*$^{+/+}$ (n = 6 per HD group; p = 0.019). Scale bar represents 50 μm. E. Automated quantification of images from D according to aggregate size reveal an increase in the percentage of small-size aggregates (0–0.3 μm^2)

coupled with a decreased in the percentage of medium-sized aggregates (0.3–0.9 μm²) in HD; *Igf-1r*⁺/⁻ cerebellum compared to controls (p<0.001). Data are expressed as mean ± 1×s.e.m. *P<0.05; **P<0.01; ***P<0.001. ns = non-significant.

percentage of small aggregates in *Igf1-r* deficient HD females was significantly increased (Figure 4E, p = 0.001). This, taken together with a lower number of medium aggregates in HD; *Igf-1r*⁺/⁻ than in controls (p<0.001) suggest that *Igf-1r* deficiency may have an effect on the formation and growth of cerebellar huntingtin aggregates.

In this context, it is possible to speculate that *Igf-1r* levels might influence huntingtin oligomerization and/or aggregation kinetics, as previously proposed for the Alzheimer's disease-linked human peptide, Abeta [27]. For instance, this decrease in inclusion numbers, observed at 13 weeks of age, coincides with the delay in tremor onset seen in HD; *Igf-1r*⁺/⁻ females, although it has no discernible effect on survival or other motor phenotypes assessed in HD mice.

IGF-1R inhibition does not modulate mTOR signalling or autophagosome numbers in HD brains

Our data above suggest that *Igf-1r* deficiency is not sufficient to affect mutant huntingtin levels in brain or cerebellum, although it may have an effect on cerebellar inclusions in females. We thus decided to explore how *Igf-1r* deficiency affected downstream AKT and mTOR activation just before the age of phenotypic onset in female mice (12 weeks of age). *Igf-1r* would result in decreased mTOR activity, which would increase autophagy and enhance removal of mutant hungtingtin. The slight effect observed on the removal of mutant protein by *Igf-1r* deficiency in female brains could indicate that the expected mTORC1 activity, or downstream mTOR signalling, might not be as initially expected.

We first confirmed that *Igf-1r* heterozygosis leads to decreased levels of the receptor (Figure 5A). However, this was not associated with any obvious change in the phosphorylation of AKT at T308 (which correlates with its activation activity [39], nor any change in the phosphorylation of the mTORC1 substrate p70S6K in mouse brains between any of the genotypes (Figure 5A). We then tested whether *Igf-1r* deficiency affected autophagosome numbers at this early age by measuring LC3-II levels (as a function of actin). We could not detect any significant changes in the levels of LC3-II in the brains of non-HD or HD mice regardless of their *Igf-1r* levels, although this may be due in part to mouse-to-mouse variability (Figure 5B). We found similar results with the male brains at 12 weeks (Figure S3A) and female lysates at a later time point (18 weeks, Figure S3B). Phosphorylation of AKT at serine 473 (S473), which correlates with mTORC2 activity [39] was not significantly affected in *Igf-1r* deficient females at 12 weeks of age despite having low levels of IGF-1R protein. Indeed, AKT phosphorylation at S473 has a tendency to be diminished (as ratio with total AKT) in Non-HD *Igf-1r*⁺/⁻ females at 18 weeks and in *Igf-1r*⁺/⁻ males at 12 weeks of age (Figure S3A, B). Interestingly, at both time points, no differences were found in AKT phosphorylation at S473 in the HD context regardless of their *Igf-1r* levels, suggesting that HD pathology affects AKT activation independent of *Igf-1r* status. Collectively, these observations suggest that the contribution of IGF-1R to the modulation of the downstream signalling pathways *in vivo* is influenced by multiple factors, such as age and sex, and can be influenced by the HD background.

Discussion

Based on the current literature, there are data supporting both protective and deleterious effects of diminishing IIS pathway in HD models. Thus, perhaps not surprisingly, we found that heterozygous deletion of *Igr-1r* lead to complex behavioural effects in HD mice, with opposite effects in male and female HD mice that did not lead to an overall modification of survival. This was accompanied by unchanged levels of AKT activation and mTOR signalling in the HD mice, leading to no effects in autophagy. Thus, modulating IIS pathway via *Igf-1r* deficiency leads to paradoxical effects in the onset and progression of HD in male and female mice.

Igf-1r deficient mice have previously shown sexually dimorphic phenotypes, such as lifespan extension, which is only significant in *Igf-1r*⁺/⁻ females [33,36]. This lifespan extension is accompanied with resistance to acute oxidative stress after paraquat injections that are present in *Igf-1r*⁺/⁻ females but not *Igf-1r*⁺/⁻ males. This is interesting, as here the only beneficial effects of *Igf-1r* deficiency are seen in HD females. However, this model is not generally applicable, because no sexual dimorphism was reported upon *Igf-1r*⁺/⁻ mice 1-methyl-4-phenyl-1,2,3,6-tetrahydropyridine (MPTP) treatment [40] or when crossed to AD mouse models [27]. Thus, the opposite effects of *Igf-1r* deficiency in HD males and females may reflect an inherent difference in IIS between males and females in the C57BL/6J background that could be exacerbated by HD pathology. In this regard, IGF-1 levels have been shown to decrease in an age-dependent manner in the R6/2 HD mouse model, associating IGF-I levels with the body weight loss that occurs in HD patients [41]. However, in the N171-82Q HD mouse model studied here, IGF-1 levels were higher in all HD females regardless of *Igf-1r* gene status and were also elevated in HD; *Igf-1r*⁺/⁻ males. These differences may be due to the fact that here IGF-1 levels were measured here at an early disease time point on C57BL/6J genetic background, which has been shown to produce low levels of circulating IGF-1 [42]. High levels of GH (growth hormone) and IGF-1 have been reported in HD patients [19,43,44], with no differences in IGF-1 levels between genders. Only in HD male patients, the high levels of IGF-1 were correlated with increased cognitive decline [44].

AKT activation is known to have anti-apoptotic effects and being neuroprotective in Huntington's disease through the direct phosphorylation of huntingtin at serine 421 [17]. In the N171-82Q mouse model, the transgene expresses the N-terminal 171 residues of human huntingtin with 82 polyglutamines, and therefore lacks serine 421. Thus, the possible neuroprotective effects through the direct phosphorylation of mutant huntingtin are not modelled in this study.

In *C. elegans*, a reduction of IIS has been shown to protect from toxic aggregation in different proteinopathies, including HD [25,45]. Nonetheless, in the R6/2 HD mouse model, IGF-1 administration has been shown to lead to some beneficial effects, including protection against diabetes and hind-limb clasping, but not on motor function [24]. Recently, administration of IGF-1 has been proven to rescue Huntington's disease phenotypes in YAC128 mice [23]. These paradoxical beneficial effects of both a reduction and an increase in IIS have also been shown in AD models. In worms and mice, IIS reduction leads to protection from toxicity associated with the aggregation of human Abeta [27,28,46]. Interestingly, in one of the studies, diminished

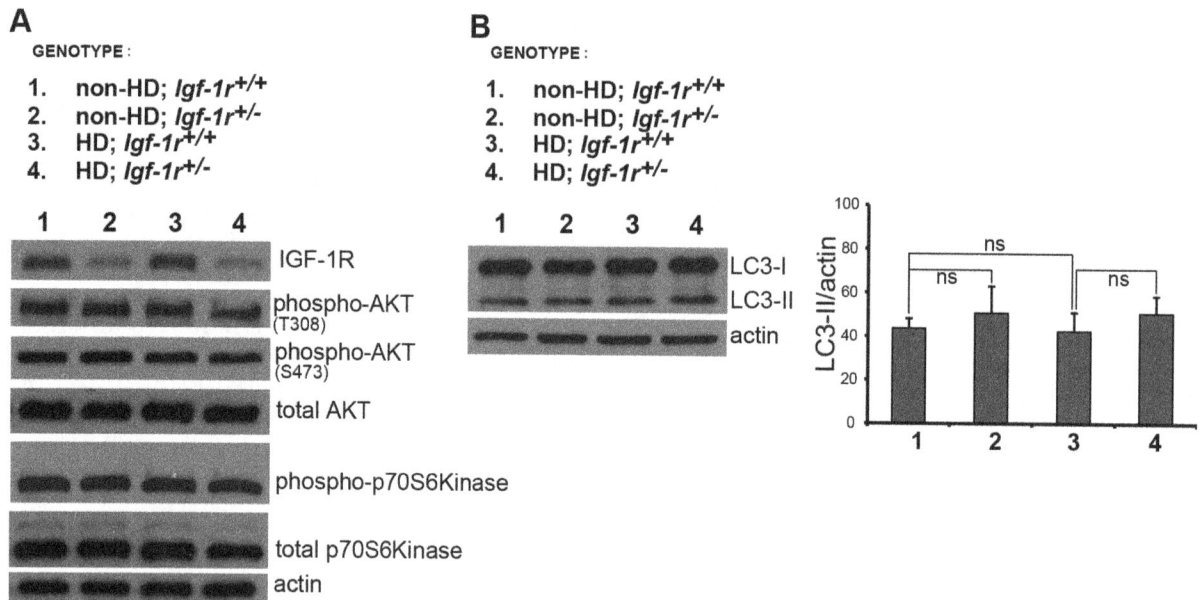

Figure 5. *Igf-1r* hemizygosity has no effect on AKT and S6K activation or autophagosome numbers in HD mice. A. *Igf-1r* deficiency leads to a significant decrease in IGF-1R protein levels (p = 0.0057) but does not significantly affect AKT phosphorylation at Ser473 or Thr308, nor the phosphorylation of S6K at Threonine 389 in half-brain homogenates of 12 weeks old female mice of the indicated genotypes. Representative images are presented. For densitometry analysis, four different samples for each genotype were used (n = 4 per group). Further analysis is presented in Figure S3. **B.** *Igf-1r* hemizygosity does not affect autophagosome numbers. Brain homogenates from 12 week-old females of the indicated genotypes were subjected to western blot analysis to assess LC3 levels. The graph reports the quantitative analysis of LC3-II levels relative to actin from four different brain samples for each genotype. The *p* values for the densitometric analyses were determined by using Student's *t*-test (n = 4). Data are expressed as mean ± s.e.m. *P<0.05; **P<0.01; ***P<0.001. ns = non-significant.

expression of *Irs2* in the AD mice protected females but not males [28] just as we observed here. IIS reduction has also been linked to a compaction of the deposited Abeta plaques [27,46], that could correlate with the changes in huntingtin cerebellar inclusion sizes in the present study. However, as in the HD case, an increase in IIS (by administration of IGF-I) has also been shown to protect from Abeta mediated toxicity [47]. Thus, as is the case for AD, both an increase and a decrease in IIS may have some potential therapeutic value in HD models, perhaps affecting different features of the disease, which could also be influenced by sex, at least in the mouse.

We have recently published that long-term *Igf-1r* depletion or chemical inhibition impaired autophagy, which was unexpected given the literature on short-term effects of IGF1 administration. Our previous *in vitro* and *in vivo* data suggested that IGF-1R inhibition decreases autophagosome formation by reducing endocytosis, a step which is tightly controlled by the mTORC2 complex activity [32]. However, here we show that the *Igf-1r* hemizygosity (which causes, as expected, a 50% reduction in the receptor levels) does not have an obvious effect on downstream mTOR signalling or autophagosome numbers *in vivo*. We have recently proposed that a complex auto-regulatory feedback loop mechanism allows the mTORC1 complex activity to be sustained when IGF-1R activity is reduced in cell-based systems [32]. It is worth noting that, in this context, even with a 80% reduction of the IGF-1R receptor levels, cells were capable of activating the mTORC1 downstream signalling modules upon IGF-1 stimulation [32]. Such a scenario may explain how the mTORC1 pathway activity is quite tightly buffered and controlled in the long term in mammalian systems. Moreover, the mTORC2 activity (as assessed by AKT phosphorylation on serine 473) was overall not affected by *Igf-1r* heterozygosis in the HD mice. It is quite possible

that a reduction of IGF-1R signalling of greater than 50% (along the lines we reported previously [32]) may be required to consistently impact on mTORC2 signalling (and autophagy). One should also note that the LC3-II only assess steady-state levels of the protein (which correlates for autophagosomes number), making difficult to infer about any possible and concomitant change in the rate of synthesis and/or flux through the pathway [48]. Hence, we cannot exclude the possibility that the decreased aggregate numbers in the cerebellum of HD; *Igf-1r* hemizygous mice compared to control littermates, may be resulting from differential acute nutrient/IGF1/insulin signalling in the mice that may be sufficient to create a short-term relative difference in autophagy sufficient to impact on huntingtin aggregate numbers, even if the "steady-state" activity of the mTOR pathway were unchanged in these mice.

Overall, altering the very refined pathway of IIS in different proteinopathies leads to differential outcomes in different disease model systems. Intriguingly, both diminishing and increasing IIS pathway seem to lead to some beneficial effects in models of HD, although in HD males, we show here that diminishing IIS could also lead to some deleterious effects.

Methods

Ethics statement

All procedures were carried out with the appropriate UK Home Office and MRC Harwell Ethical Committee approval.

Mice

Transgenic mice expressing the first 171 residues of huntingtin with 82 CAG repeats [49] were maintained in hemizygozity by backcrossing to C57BL/6J (B6) for more than 10 generations (both from Jackson Laboratories). *Igf-1r*$^{+/-}$ mice, described elsewhere and available from http://www.emma.rm.cnr.it were maintained as hemizygotes by backcrossing to C57BL/6J. Genotyping was carried out by PCR of DNA from the ear clips, using the primers recommended by the distributor (http://www.emma.rm.cnr.it) To generate double mutants and their appropriate control littermates, we crossed hemizygous N171-82Q (B6 congenic) males to *Igf-1r* deficient females. We always used mice from the first generation for all the analysis performed. Observers were blind to mouse genetic status during testing.

Behavioural phenotype

We assessed modified SHIRPA, rotarod and grip strength, as previously described [35] analysis every two weeks, from 8 weeks of age to death. A minimum of seven mice per group and gender were analysed for a specific test. Grip strength (BIOSEB, France) and rotarod tests (Accelerating model, Ugo Basile, Italy) were done in alternating weeks with the modified SHIRPA testing. Tremors onset and severity, wire manoeuvre and other tasks are monitored as part of the modified SHIRPA battery of behavioural tests. We also weighed the mice every week and checked survival, defined as time until they reach their humane end-points (in accordance with the Ethical Committee). Humane end-points were defined as the loss of more than 20% of maximum body weight or hunched appearance.

Immunoblot

Brains were frozen immediately and stored at -80°C from F1 offspring representing all four possible genotypes (doubled mutants and control littermates). We used at least n = 3 animals for each genotype and gender at 12 and 18 weeks of age, to compare an early and late stage of the disease. We added 2.5 volumes of buffer B (50 mM Tris (pH 7.5), 10% glycerol, 5 mM magnesium acetate, 0.2 mM EDTA, 0.5 mM dithiothreitol) or RIPA buffer, with protease inhibitors (complete miniEDTA-free, Roche) and phosphatase inhibitors cocktail (PhosphoStop, Roche), following homogenization in lysing matrix tubes D (MP Biomedicals, Germany) and a Fast-Prep-24 homogenizer at 4°C. Homogenates were then centrifuge at $10000 \times g$ for 15 min and the supernatant was retained. Protein concentration was determined (Bradford reagent, Sigma) and an equal amount of protein from each sample was resolved on SDS-PAGE (typically 4–12% Bis-Tris NUPAGE precast gels from Invitrogen). After transfer to PVDF membranes (GE Healthcare), membranes were blocked in 5% BSA in TBST (Tris-Buffer solution with 0.1% Tween-20) and incubated with primary antibodies overnight at 4°C. The primary antibodies assessed included rabbit anti-phospho-IGF-IR (Abcam, UK), rabbit polyclonal anti-total IGF-IRβ (Santa Cruz, USA), rabbit phospho-Akt ser427, rabbit Pan AKT, from Cell Signalling; rabbit anti-actin (Sigma), mouse anti-soluble human polyQ (MAB1537-1C2, Millipore), LC3II (Novus). Followed by secondary antibody incubation (Goat anti-rabbit IgG and anti-mouse IgG peroxidase cojungated) for 1–3 hours at room temperature, blots were developed with ECL plus detection kit (GE Healthcare). We carried out densitometry of the films using Image-J software.

Immunohistochemistry

We carried out immunohistochemistry on brain slices from mice perfused transcardially with 4% (w/v) paraformaldehyde (Sigma) in phosphate saline buffer (PBS) pH 7.4. Coronal brain cryo-sections, ±1 mm from the bregma or the whole cerebellum, at 30 μm thickness were generated to perform free-floating slices staining for inclusions at 13 weeks of age females (n = 4 per HD group). To detect mutant human huntingtin aggregates the primary antibody (MAB5374 from Millipore or the previous EM48 Chemicon) was incubated overnight, followed by secondary mouse Alexa-Fluor488 conjugated antibody (Invitrogen) and mounted on Vectashield with nuclear counterstaining DAPI (Vector labs). Confocal images were taking using Zeiss LSM 700 microscope at 60X amplification of the piriform cortex. Final image stack projections (typically the sum of 12 images per projection) were used to count the total number of inclusions per field. A total of three consecutive fields in the piriform cortex per slice, over 3 or 4 slices per mouse and 4 mice per genotype are used to account for the total number of inclusions in the piriform cortex. The counting was done by counterstaining the nuclei with DAPI, therefore excluding in the majority of the cases the somatodendritic aggregates. After manually counting the inclusions, we used the Volocity software 5.4.1 (Perkin Elmer, USA) on the Z-stack projections to verify the counting obtained and corrected by nuclei's DAPI+ per image.

To measure the size of the inclusions we used image analysis software (Cell^D, from Axioscop) over the confocal projection images taking from the granular layer of the cerebellum. We used the cerebellum because in the N171-82Q mouse model, at the selected age of 13 weeks of age, the number of inclusions/aggregates are a lot higher and clearer to detect in the cerebellum when compared to the striatum. Again coronal cryosections at 30 μm were cut and free floating staining against mutant huntingtin protein. A total of 3 confocal images (sum of 12 Z-stack at 60x magnification) adjacent to the peak of the folding granular layer per slice, over 4–5 slices per mouse and 6 mice per genotype were used to account for the analysis of inclusions in the cerebellum. The software classifies the inclusions by size and count the total of a given size range. The great majority of huntingtin inclusions present in the cerebellum of the N171-82Q model are intranuclear, as evidenced by DAPI counterstaining. The data is presented as the percentage of the total aggregates for each particular aggregate size. We classified the inclusion sizes into 4 categories, from the smallest aggregates (0–0.3 μm^2) to the biggest inclusions found (1.8–4.5 μm^2).

Seprion ligand ELISA for polyQ aggregates

We performed Seprion ELISA as previously described [38] to quantify huntingtin aggregation. Briefly, male and female HD mice were killed at 12 weeks of age. After removing the brain, the cerebellum was separated and frozen at -80 until used. Cerebellum homogenates in RIPA buffer with protease inhibitors were subjected to ELISA detection for mutant huntingtin aggregates using MW8 primary antibody and a peroxidase (HRP)-conjugated rabbit anti-goat secondary antibody (DAKO). The product of the reaction after adding the substrate TMB (SerTec) was quantified in a plate reader at 450 nm (Biorad).

Blood measurements

Blood samples were collected in a heparin-tube by orbital bleed from mice fasted for 4 hours. We used 5 mice at 12 weeks of age per genotype and gender. After spinning, the plasma was used to quantify Igf-1 by ELISA (Mediagnost, Germany) following the manufacturer recommendations. We also used the plasma to quantify glucose.

Statistics

We determined significance levels for comparisons between groups with Student's t-test, ANOVA, ANOVA with post-hoc Bonferroni correction, non-parametric Fisher's test and Log-rank test, where appropriate.

Supporting Information

Figure S1 Grip-strength tests were performed on at least 5 mice per genotype per sex and time-point: (**A**) females and (**B**) males. No differences were observed between HD; Igf-$1r^{+/+}$ and HD; Igf-$1r^{+/-}$ mice at any time point analysed. Error bars represent $1\times$s.e.m (standard error of the mean).

Figure S2 4-hour fasted glucose measured (mmol/L) in females (**A**) and males (**B**), shows a tendency towards higher glucose levels in HD; Igf-$1r^{+/-}$ males compared to HD; Igf-$1r^{+/+}$ mice, which is not significant (p = 0.24, more than 4 mice per group).

Figure S3 Brain homogenates of the indicated genotypes and time points were subjected to western blot analysis to assess AKT activation at ser473 and autophagosome numbers by means of LC3-II measurement controlled by actin levels. **A.** Western blots of half-brain homogenates from 12 weeks old male mice (n = 3 per group) show that AKT phosphorylation at Ser473, corrected by total levels of AKT, have a trend towards a statistically significant reduction in Non-HD; Igf-$1r^{+/-}$ when compared to Igf-$1r^{+/+}$ controls (p = 0.066), whereas no trend appears when comparing the HD groups: HD; Igf-$1r^{+/+}$ and HD; Igf-$1r^{+/-}$ mice (p = 0.40). No significant differences were found in LC3-II levels corrected by actin for any genotype. **B.** Western blots of brain homogenates from 18 weeks old female mice. AKT phosphorylation at Ser473

again shows a trend towards a reduced ratio in Non-HD; Igf-$1r^{+/-}$ when compared to Non-HD; Igf-$1r^{+/+}$ controls (p = 0.1). Again, non-significant differences appear when comparing the HD groups: HD; Igf-$1r^{+/+}$ and HD; Igf-$1r^{+/-}$ mice (p = 0.7). Not significant differences in LC3-II/actin between any of the genotypes were observed. The gels are representative of the analysis of four different brain samples for each genotype (n = 4 per group). Data are expressed as mean $\pm$ $2\times$s.e.m. ns = non-significant.

Table S1 Summary of phenotypic comparison between male, female and both combined for HD; Igf-1r+/+ and HD; Igf-1r+/− mice.

Acknowledgments

We thank Martin Holzenberger for the Igf-$1r$ deficient strain obtained through EMMA.

Author Contributions

Conceived and designed the experiments: AAA S. Corrochano MR DR SDMB. Performed the experiments: S. Corrochano MR GO S. Carter MS JM AAA. Analyzed the data: S. Corrochano MR AAA. Contributed reagents/materials/analysis tools: GPB. Wrote the paper: S. Corrochano AAA.

References

1. (1993) A novel gene containing a trinucleotide repeat that is expanded and unstable on Huntington's disease chromosomes. The Huntington's Disease Collaborative Research Group. Cell 72: 971–983.
2. Andrew SE, Goldberg YP, Kremer B, Telenius H, Theilmann J, et al. (1993) The relationship between trinucleotide (CAG) repeat length and clinical features of Huntington's disease. Nat Genet 4: 398–403.
3. Burgunder JM (2013) Translational research in Huntington's disease: opening up for disease modifying treatment. Transl Neurodegener 2: 2.
4. Caviston JP, Holzbaur EL (2009) Huntingtin as an essential integrator of intracellular vesicular trafficking. Trends Cell Biol 19: 147–155.
5. Kopito RR, Ron D (2000) Conformational disease. Nat Cell Biol 2: E207–209.
6. Zuccato C, Valenza M, Cattaneo E (2010) Molecular mechanisms and potential therapeutical targets in Huntington's disease. Physiol Rev 90: 905–981.
7. Arrasate M, Finkbeiner S (2012) Protein aggregates in Huntington's disease. Exp Neurol 238: 1–11.
8. Levine B, Klionsky DJ (2004) Development by self-digestion: molecular mechanisms and biological functions of autophagy. Dev Cell 6: 463–477.
9. Rubinsztein DC, Gestwicki JE, Murphy LO, Klionsky DJ (2007) Potential therapeutic applications of autophagy. Nat Rev Drug Discov 6: 304–312.
10. Mizushima N, Levine B, Cuervo AM, Klionsky DJ (2008) Autophagy fights disease through cellular self-digestion. Nature 451: 1069–1075.
11. Sarkar S, Ravikumar B, Floto RA, Rubinsztein DC (2009) Rapamycin and mTOR-independent autophagy inducers ameliorate toxicity of polyglutamine-expanded huntingtin and related proteinopathies. Cell Death Differ 16: 46–56.
12. Neef DW, Turski ML, Thiele DJ (2010) Modulation of heat shock transcription factor 1 as a therapeutic target for small molecule intervention in neurodegenerative disease. PLoS Biol 8: e1000291.
13. Labbadia J, Cunliffe H, Weiss A, Katsyuba E, Sathasivam K, et al. (2011) Altered chromatin architecture underlies progressive impairment of the heat shock response in mouse models of Huntington disease. J Clin Invest 121: 3306–3319.
14. Gatchel JR, Watase K, Thaller C, Carson JP, Jafar-Nejad P, et al. (2008) The insulin-like growth factor pathway is altered in spinocerebellar ataxia type 1 and type 7. Proc Natl Acad Sci U S A 105: 1291–1296.
15. Moloney AM, Griffin RJ, Timmons S, O'Connor R, Ravid R, et al. (2010) Defects in IGF-1 receptor, insulin receptor and IRS-1/2 in Alzheimer's disease indicate possible resistance to IGF-1 and insulin signalling. Neurobiol Aging 31: 224–243.
16. Lalic NM, Maric J, Svetel M, Jotic A, Stefanova E, et al. (2008) Glucose homeostasis in Huntington disease: abnormalities in insulin sensitivity and early-phase insulin secretion. Arch Neurol 65: 476–480.
17. Humbert S, Bryson EA, Cordelieres FP, Connors NC, Datta SR, et al. (2002) The IGF-1/Akt pathway is neuroprotective in Huntington's disease and involves Huntingtin phosphorylation by Akt. Dev Cell 2: 831–837.
18. Yamamoto A, Cremona ML, Rothman JE (2006) Autophagy-mediated clearance of huntingtin aggregates triggered by the insulin-signaling pathway. J Cell Biol 172: 719–731.
19. Colin E, Regulier E, Perrin V, Durr A, Brice A, et al. (2005) Akt is altered in an animal model of Huntington's disease and in patients. Eur J Neurosci 21: 1478–1488.
20. Zala D, Colin E, Rangone H, Liot G, Humbert S, et al. (2008) Phosphorylation of mutant huntingtin at S421 restores anterograde and retrograde transport in neurons. Hum Mol Genet 17: 3837–3846.
21. Rangone H, Pardo R, Colin E, Girault JA, Saudou F, et al. (2005) Phosphorylation of arfaptin 2 at Ser260 by Akt Inhibits PolyQ-huntingtin-induced toxicity by rescuing proteasome impairment. J Biol Chem 280: 22021–22028.
22. Rangone H, Poizat G, Troncoso J, Ross CA, MacDonald ME, et al. (2004) The serum- and glucocorticoid-induced kinase SGK inhibits mutant huntingtin-induced toxicity by phosphorylating serine 421 of huntingtin. Eur J Neurosci 19: 273–279.
23. Lopes C, Ribeiro M, Duarte AI, Humbert S, Saudou F, et al. (2014) IGF-1 intranasal administration rescues Huntington's disease phenotypes in YAC128 mice. Molecular neurobiology 49: 1126–1142.
24. Duarte AI, Petit GH, Ranganathan S, Li JY, Oliveira CR, et al. (2011) IGF-1 protects against diabetic features in an in vivo model of Huntington's disease. Exp Neurol 231: 314–319.
25. Cohen E, Bieschke J, Percivalle RM, Kelly JW, Dillin A (2006) Opposing activities protect against age-onset proteotoxicity. Science 313: 1604–1610.
26. Kaletsky R, Murphy CT (2010) The role of insulin/IGF-like signaling in C. elegans longevity and aging. Dis Model Mech 3: 415–419.
27. Cohen E, Paulsson JF, Blinder P, Burstyn-Cohen T, Du D, et al. (2009) Reduced IGF-1 signaling delays age-associated proteotoxicity in mice. Cell 139: 1157–1169.
28. Freude S, Hettich MM, Schumann C, Stohr O, Koch L, et al. (2009) Neuronal IGF-1 resistance reduces Abeta accumulation and protects against premature death in a model of Alzheimer's disease. FASEB J 23: 3315–3324.
29. Jia G, Cheng G, Gangahar DM, Agrawal DK (2006) Insulin-like growth factor-1 and TNF-alpha regulate autophagy through c-jun N-terminal kinase and Akt pathways in human atherosclerotic vascular smooth cells. Immunol Cell Biol 84: 448–454.
30. Bains M, Florez-McClure ML, Heidenreich KA (2009) Insulin-like growth factor-I prevents the accumulation of autophagic vesicles and cell death in Purkinje neurons by increasing the rate of autophagosome-to-lysosome fusion and degradation. J Biol Chem 284: 20398–20407.
31. Sobolewska A, Gajewska M, Zarzynska J, Gajkowska B, Motyl T (2009) IGF-I, EGF, and sex steroids regulate autophagy in bovine mammary epithelial cells via the mTOR pathway. Eur J Cell Biol 88: 117–130.
32. Renna M, Bento CF, Fleming A, Menzies FM, Siddiqi FH, et al. (2013) IGF-1 receptor antagonism inhibits autophagy. Hum Mol Genet.

33. Holzenberger M, Dupont J, Ducos B, Leneuve P, Geloen A, et al. (2003) IGF-1 receptor regulates lifespan and resistance to oxidative stress in mice. Nature 421: 182–187.

34. Wood NI, Carta V, Milde S, Skillings EA, McAllister CJ, et al. (2010) Responses to environmental enrichment differ with sex and genotype in a transgenic mouse model of Huntington's disease. PLoS One 5: e9077.

35. Corrochano S, Renna M, Carter S, Chrobot N, Kent R, et al. (2012) alpha-Synuclein levels modulate Huntington's disease in mice. Hum Mol Genet 21: 485–494.

36. Bokov AF, Garg N, Ikeno Y, Thakur S, Musi N, et al. (2011) Does reduced IGF-1R signaling in Igf1r+/− mice alter aging? PLoS One 6: e26891.

37. Ravikumar B, Vacher C, Berger Z, Davies JE, Luo S, et al. (2004) Inhibition of mTOR induces autophagy and reduces toxicity of polyglutamine expansions in fly and mouse models of Huntington disease. Nat Genet 36: 585–595.

38. Sathasivam K, Lane A, Legleiter J, Warley A, Woodman B, et al. (2010) Identical oligomeric and fibrillar structures captured from the brains of R6/2 and knock-in mouse models of Huntington's disease. Hum Mol Genet 19: 65–78.

39. Jacinto E, Facchinetti V, Liu D, Soto N, Wei S, et al. (2006) SIN1/MIP1 maintains rictor-mTOR complex integrity and regulates Akt phosphorylation and substrate specificity. Cell 127: 125–137.

40. Nadjar A, Berton O, Guo S, Leneuve P, Dovero S, et al. (2009) IGF-1 signaling reduces neuro-inflammatory response and sensitivity of neurons to MPTP. Neurobiol Aging 30: 2021–2030.

41. Pouladi MA, Xie Y, Skotte NH, Ehrnhoefer DE, Graham RK, et al. (2010) Full-length huntingtin levels modulate body weight by influencing insulin-like growth factor 1 expression. Hum Mol Genet 19: 1528–1538.

42. Rosen CJ, Dimai HP, Vereault D, Donahue LR, Beamer WG, et al. (1997) Circulating and skeletal insulin-like growth factor-I (IGF-I) concentrations in two inbred strains of mice with different bone mineral densities. Bone 21: 217–223.

43. Saleh N, Moutereau S, Durr A, Krystkowiak P, Azulay JP, et al. (2009) Neuroendocrine disturbances in Huntington's disease. PLoS One 4: e4962.

44. Saleh N, Moutereau S, Azulay JP, Verny C, Simonin C, et al. (2010) High insulinlike growth factor I is associated with cognitive decline in Huntington disease. Neurology 75: 57–63.

45. Hsu AL, Murphy CT, Kenyon C (2003) Regulation of aging and age-related disease by DAF-16 and heat-shock factor. Science 300: 1142–1145.

46. Killick R, Scales G, Leroy K, Causevic M, Hooper C, et al. (2009) Deletion of Irs2 reduces amyloid deposition and rescues behavioural deficits in APP transgenic mice. Biochem Biophys Res Commun 386: 257–262.

47. Carro E, Trejo JL, Gomez-Isla T, LeRoith D, Torres-Aleman I (2002) Serum insulin-like growth factor I regulates brain amyloid-beta levels. Nat Med 8: 1390–1397.

48. Klionsky DJ, Abdalla FC, Abeliovich H, Abraham RT, Acevedo-Arozena A, et al. (2012) Guidelines for the use and interpretation of assays for monitoring autophagy. Autophagy 8: 445–544.

49. Schilling G, Becher MW, Sharp AH, Jinnah HA, Duan K, et al. (1999) Intranuclear inclusions and neuritic aggregates in transgenic mice expressing a mutant N-terminal fragment of huntingtin. Hum Mol Genet 8: 397–407.

10

Specific Reactions of Different Striatal Neuron Types in Morphology Induced by Quinolinic Acid in Rats

Qiqi Feng[1,2♦], **Yuxin Ma**[1,3♦], **Shuhua Mu**[1], **Jiajia Wu**[1], **Si Chen**[1], **Lisi OuYang**[1], **Wanlong Lei**[1]*

1 Department of Anatomy, Zhongshan School of Medicine, Sun Yat-sen University, Guangzhou, China, **2** Department of Nephrology, The Third Affiliated Hospital of Sun Yat-sen University, Guangzhou, China, **3** Department of Anatomy, School of Basic Medicine, Guangdong Pharmaceutical University, Guangzhou, China

Abstract

Huntington's disease (HD) is a neurological degenerative disease and quinolinic acid (QA) has been used to establish HD model in animals through the mechanism of excitotoxicity. Yet the specific pathological changes and the underlying mechanisms are not fully elucidated. We aimed to reveal the specific morphological changes of different striatal neurons in the HD model. Sprague-Dawley (SD) rats were subjected to unilaterally intrastriatal injections of QA to mimic the HD model. Behavioral tests, histochemical and immunhistochemical stainings as well as Western blots were applied in the present study. The results showed that QA-treated rats had obvious motor and cognitive impairments when compared with the control group. Immunohistochemical detection showed a great loss of NeuN+ neurons and Darpp32+ projection neurons in the transition zone in the QA group when compared with the control group. The numbers of parvalbumin (Parv)+ and neuropeptide Y (NPY)+ interneurons were both significantly reduced while those of calretinin (Cr)+ and choline acetyltransferase (ChAT)+ were not changed notably in the transition zone in the QA group when compared to the controls. Parv+, NPY+ and ChAT+ interneurons were not significantly increased in fiber density while Cr+ neurons displayed an obvious increase in fiber density in the transition zone in QA-treated rats. The varicosity densities of Parv+, Cr+ and NPY+ interneurons were all raised in the transition zone after QA treatment. In conclusion, the present study revealed that QA induced obvious behavioral changes as well as a general loss of striatal projection neurons and specific morphological changes in different striatal interneurons, which may help further explain the underlying mechanisms and the specific functions of various striatal neurons in the pathological process of HD.

Editor: Gilles J. Guillemin, Macquarie University, Australia

Funding: This research was supported by the National Science Foundations of China (No. 31070941, No. 30770679) and the Major State Basic Research Development Program of China (973 Program, No. 2010CB530004). The funders had no role in study design, data collection and analysis, decision to publish, or preparation of the manuscript.

Competing Interests: The authors have declared that no competing interests exist.

* E-mail: leiwl@mail.sysu.edu.cn

♦ These authors contributed equally to this work.

Introduction

Huntington's disease (HD) is an inherited neurodegenerative disorder characterized by abnormal involuntary movements and cognitive impairment [1]. The pathological hallmark of HD is the selective neuron death in the striatum – loss of spiny projection neurons and relative sparing of aspiny interneurons [2]. The pathogenesis of HD critically involves the mutant gene huntingtin (htt) which encodes a large protein (350 kDa) with a polyglutamine stretch [3,4]. The extent of the polyglutamine expansion is correlated with the severity of symptoms, such as age of onset [5]. Despite the discovery of htt, the pathophysiology of HD and the mechanisms accounting for the selective neuron death still remain unclear. It has been suggested that excitotoxicity, mitochondrial abnormalities and transcriptional dysregulation are some important mechanisms in the progress of HD [6,7,8]. Therefore, the excitotoxin quinolinic acid (QA), mitochondrial toxin 3-nitropropionic acid (3NP) and transgenic models are used to study the pathophysiology of HD [9,10,11].

The "excitotoxicity hypothesis" of neurodegeneration has been proposed for several decades and it persists as a likely pathophysiological mechanism in HD [6,12,13]. The excitotoxin QA has

been used extensively to establish HD models in animals since it generally spares aspiny interneurons, relative to spiny projection neurons, which is more analogous to the neuropathology of HD than other excitotoxins such as kainic acid and ibotenic acid [9,14]. Furthermore, it has been demonstrated that QA is a brain endogenous excitotoxin produced and released by infiltrating macrophages and activated microglia, and acts as a neurotoxin, gliotoxin, proinflammatory mediator, pro-oxidant molecule and can alter the integrity and cohesion of the blood-brain barrier [15]. Nevertheless, the issue about the resistance of different striatal neuron types in HD is still controversial. Histologically, the striatum consists of projection neurons (90%–95% in rodents and about 80% in primates) and interneurons (5%–10% in rodents and possibly up to 20% in primates) which are subdivided into four types: parvalbumin (Parv)+, calretinin (Cr)+, neuropeptide Y/ somatostatin/neuronal nitric oxide synthase (NPY/SS/nNOS)+ and choline acetyltransferase (ChAT)+ interneurons [16]. A great amount of research applying different HD models concordantly revealed that the striatal projection neurons were vulnerable [11,17,18,19]. However, different studies provided different observations about the preservation of different striatal interneuron types in HD. For instance, plenty of evidence indicated that the striatal NPY+ interneurons were relatively spared in HD models [17,20,21,22] while several previous studies reported no such sparing [23,24]. In addition, most studies on striatal neurons in HD models mainly focused on the neuron abundance rather than the morphology. In fact, Mu *et al* revealed that the NPY+ and Cr+ interneurons were presented with an increase of fibers and varicosities in the 3NP-induced HD model [25]. It is reasonable to presume that clarifying the specific reactions of different striatal neurons in HD may help further understand the pathophysiology of HD.

The present study aimed to provide more comprehensive evidence for the QA-induced HD model in respect of behavior and histology, so as to help further comprehend the underlying pathophysiological mechanisms of HD. A series of behavioral tests, histological techniques and Western blots were applied to assess the motor and cognitive impairments, the striatal histopathological changes as well as expression levels of different marker proteins for different striatal neuron types.

Materials and Methods

Animals and experimental design

Thirty adult male Sprague-Dawley (SD) rats weighing 250–300 g (obtained from the Center for Experimental Animals of Sun Yat-sen University) were used for this study. All the animal experiments strictly adhered to the Regulations for the Administration of Affairs Concerning Experimental Animals, the Chinese national guideline for animal experiment, issued in 1988. All procedures involving animals and their care in this study were approved by the Animal Care and Use Committee of Sun Yat-sen University (Permit Number: SCXK GUANGDONG 2011-0029). All efforts were made to reduce the number of animals used. The animals were housed in an air-conditioned room under an even light-dark cycle, with food and water *ad libitum*.

The rats were randomly assigned to the QA group ($n = 10$), the control group ($n = 10$) and the normal group ($n = 10$). All rats in the QA group were injected unilaterally into the right striatum with 1 μl 100 mM QA (Sigma) [20] while animals in the control group received 1 μl vehicle, and rats in the normal group did not receive any surgery or treatment. Five days after surgery, all rats were given behavioral tests for five consecutive days. Following a ten-day survival period, fifteen animals (five from each group) were subjected to histological assessments and the rest of them were subjected to Western blots as described below.

Animal surgery

Rats in the QA group were anesthetized with ketamine (150 mg/kg). They were then positioned in a small animal stereotaxic frame (Kopf) and given unilateral injections of 1 μl QA which was dissolved in 10 mM phosphate-buffered saline (PBS) at pH 7.4 into the right side of the striatum at the following coordinate: AP = +1.0 mm; ML = 2.5 mm from bregma; DV = −5.5 mm from dura according to the atlas of Paxinos and Watson [26]. Injections were manually delivered by a Hamilton microsyringe over a period of 10 min, followed by a 5-min delay before the needle was withdrawn. The needle was withdrawn slowly over a period of additional 2 min to prevent diffusion along the needle track. Rats in the control group were treated with the same procedure but received only vehicle. Postoperatively, animals were individually placed in separate cages with free access to food and drink until they recovered from anesthesia. Five days after the surgery, animals were tested by a series of behavioral tasks.

Behavioral tests

Balance beam test. The balance beam test was carried out for rats in all groups three times a day for five consecutive days according to Shear's methods [17]. The rats were trained to travel across a suspended narrow beam (100 cm in length, 7 cm in width, 100 cm elevated above the horizontal surface of the ground) into a dark box (24.5×20×18 cm) at the other end. The completion time (the interval between the moment the rat was released to the moment it entered the dark box) and the number of paw slipping (the forelimb descending more than 1.5 cm below the surface of the beam) were recorded by two observers that were blinded to animal conditions. Animals were given 3 min to complete a trial. If the rat fell down or took more than 3 min, this trial was recorded as incomplete.

Grip strength test. Grip strength test [17] was measured three times a day for five consecutive days. Examiners were blinded to animal conditions. Grip strength was measured by recording the length of time the rat was able to hold on a steel wire (2 mm in diameter, 35 mm in length) suspended 50 cm above the horizontal surface of the ground.

Water maze task. All rats were trained with the learning trial four times a day for five consecutive days, followed by the probe trial on the last day in the water maze task [27,28]. In the learning trials, the target platform was located in different spatial locations across trials, but the visual pattern of the ball which served as a cue was consistent. During each trial, rats were released from four assigned starting points (N, S, E, W) and allowed to swim until they reached the platform within 2 min. The rats were allowed to stay on the platform for 30 sec once they reached the platform or if they failed within 2 min. The latency of reaching platform was recorded. The probe trial was administered immediately following the last learning trial. In the probe trial, the platform was removed from the tank. The animals were released into the tank and allowed to swim for 2 min, and the number of target site crossovers was recorded. The tracks were recorded by a camera and Ethovision software (Noldus, Holland) which recorded the latency of reaching platform and calculated the number of target site crossovers. This task could be acquired by learning an approach response to the visual cue, which was believed to be associated with the mnemonic functions of the striatum.

Histochemical and immunohistochemical methods

Nissl staining. After the five-day behavioral tests, five rats from each group were sacrificed for histochemical and immuno-histochemical examinations. Before the following procedures, animals were deeply anesthetized with 10% chloral hydrate (350 mg/kg), then perfused with 300 ml 0.9% saline followed by 400 ml 4% paraformaldehyde in 0.1 M phosphate buffer (PB, pH 7.4, 4°C). Brains were quickly removed and post-fixed overnight at 4°C, and were sliced into coronal sections (30 μm) on a vibratome (VIBRATOME, #053746). Sections were stained with Nissl staining according to previous classic methods [29].

Immunohistochemistry procedures. Brain sections were pre-treated with 0.3% H_2O_2 in 10 mM PBS (pH 7.4, 4°C) for 30 min. Separate series of sections were respectively incubated at 4°C for 48 h with one of the following primary antibodies: mouse anti-NeuN (1:500, Millipore), rabbit anti-Darpp32 (1:200, Cell Signaling, Danvers, MA), mouse anti-Parv (1:1,000, Sigma), rabbit anti-Cr (1:2,000, Millipore), rabbit anti-NPY (1:5,000, ABCAM) and rabbit anti-ChAT (1:1,000, Millipore). After rinsed in 10 mM PBS for three times (5 min/time), the sections were applied with secondary antibodies anti-mouse IgG or anti-rabbit IgG (both 1:200, Sigma) at room temperature for 4 h, followed by three rinses (5 min/time) in 10 mM PBS and incubation with homologous

Table 1. Measures of behavioral and histological tests in the normal group and the control group.

Test	Parameter	Norm	Cont	p #
Balance beam test	Number of paw slipping	0.15±0.10	0.17±0.16	0.933
	Completion time (sec)	18.67±4.67	19.45±7.21	0.869
Grip strength test	Hang time (sec)	11.66±3.51	11.47±4.43	0.904
Water maze test	Latency (sec)	37.09±6.30	41.42±10.77	0.558
	Number of target site crossovers	10.80±2.78	11.20±1.93	0.723
Nissl staining	Cell count (/mm²)	3224.00±365.04	3175.00±207.76	0.772
NeuN labeling	Cell count (/mm²)	2458.60±96.80	2471.20±119.13	0.917
Darpp32 labeling	Cell count (/mm²)	2007.20±56.85	1941.80±102.22	0.188
Interneuron number	Parv+ (/mm²)	79.48±1.79	78.86±2.72	0.783
	Cr+ (/mm²)	65.76±2.35	65.84±1.92	0.959
	NPY+ (/mm²)	49.20±1.48	48.90±1.95	0.828
	ChAT+ (/mm²)	69.34±2.59	69.60±1.55	0.899
Fiber density	Parv+ (/100 μm)	13.04±0.97	13.02±0.96	0.978
	Cr+ (/100 μm)	6.97±0.34	7.04±0.56	0.943
	NPY+ (/100 μm)	5.98±0.40	6.03±0.75	0.926
	ChAT+ (/100 μm)	3.06±0.24	3.16±0.40	0.777
Varicosity density	Parv+ (/100 μm)	4.36±0.71	4.04±0.79	0.599
	Cr+ (/100 μm)	6.98±1.05	7.18±1.63	0.875
	NPY+ (/100 μm)	6.22±0.79	5.80±1.10	0.540
Western blots	NeuN (OD)	1.29±0.08	1.31±0.04	0.493
	Darpp32 (OD)	1.28±0.07	1.28±0.05	0.822
	Parv+ (OD)	1.19±0.10	1.21±0.06	0.634
	Cr+ (OD)	0.67±0.08	0.68±0.05	0.731
	NPY+ (OD)	1.13±0.10	1.13±0.11	0.971
	ChAT+ (OD)	0.48±0.05	0.49±0.02	0.733

Note: values expressed as group means±SD; # normal (Norm) v.s. control (Cont), one-way ANOVA and Fisher's *post hoc* PLSD test.

peroxidase-antiperoxidase (PAP) complex (1:200, Sigma) at room temperature for 2 h. The peroxidase reaction was performed using 3, 3′-diaminobenzidine (DAB, 0.05% in 10 mM PBS, pH 7.4, Sigma) for 2–8 min, and then the sections were mounted onto gelatin-coated slides, routinely dehydrated, cleared and covered with neutral balsam for microscopic detection.

TUNEL assay. To assess apoptotic level of striatal neurons after experimental treatments, immunofluorescent detection of neurons combined with the terminal deoxynucleotidyl transferase dUTP nick labeling (TUNEL) was performed. For the present study, sections were incubated with the primary antibody mouse anti-NeuN (1:500, Millipore) at 4°C for 48 h, and subsequently with rhodamine-conjugated goat anti-mouse IgG (1:200, Jackson ImmunoResearch) at room temperature for 2 h. All sections were thereafter rinsed three times (5 min/time) in 10 mM PBS and performed with TUNEL assay (In Situ Cell Death Detection Kit, POD, Roche) according to the manufacturer's instructions. Sections were mounted on gelatin-coated slides, routinely dehydrated, cleared and covered with glycerol. Section detection and image capture were conducted on a fluorescence microscope.

Western blots

After the five-day behavioral tests, the other five rats from each group were sacrificed for Western blots. Animals were deeply anesthetized with 10% chloral hydrate (350 mg/kg), perfused with 0.9% saline, and then got decapitated. The right striatum was extracted from the brain, and then stored at −80°C before use. Western blots were carried out as previously described [25]. In brief, the tissue was homogenized in a freshly prepared lysis buffer with protease inhibitors, and then centrifuged at 12000 r/min for 30 min. The protein concentration of the homogenate was determined using the BioRad DC protein assay (BioRad Laboratories). 40 μg of total protein from each sample were subjected to an SDS–PAGE gel (10%) and transferred to a PVDF membrane (Millipore). The membrane was blocked with 5% skim milk at room temperature for 2–4 h and incubated at 4°C overnight with one of the following primary antibodies: mouse anti-NeuN (1:1000, Millipore), rabbit anti-Darpp32 (1:250, Cell Signaling), mouse anti-Parv (1:1000, Sigma), rabbit anti-Cr (1:5000, Millipore), rabbit anti-NPY (1:6000, Abcam), rabbit anti-ChAT (1:2000, Millipore) and mouse anti-β-actin (1:2000, Millipore). After washed with TBST for four times (5 min/time), the membrane was incubated with homologous HRP-conjugated secondary antibodies (1:3000, Amersham Biosciences, GE Health-care) at room temperature for 2 h, and washed again in TBST for four times (5 min/time). Blots were visualized in enhanced chemiluminescence (ECL) solution (Pierce) for 5 min and exposed to hyperfilms (Kodak) for 1–15 min.

Data collection and statistical analysis

Quantification of neuron number, fiber density and varicosity density. The investigators were blinded to which

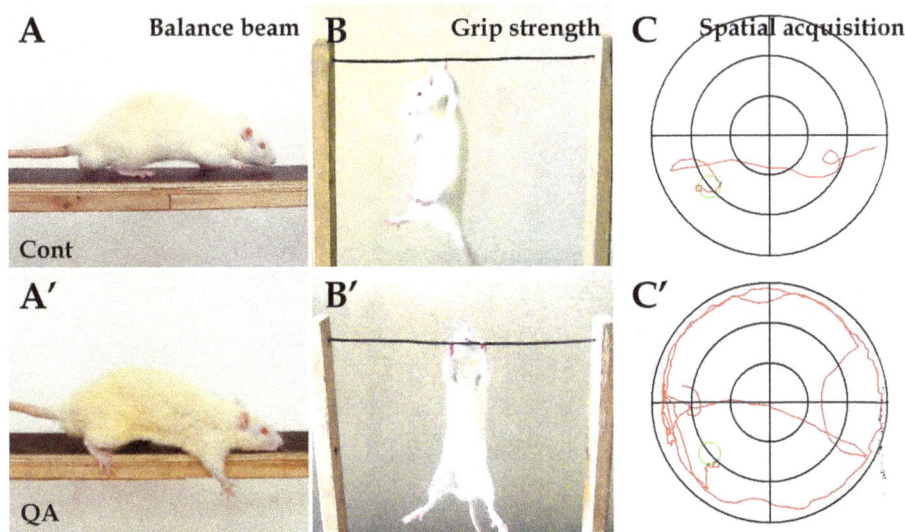

Figure 1. Experimental tests for behavioral deficits induced by QA. In the balance beam test, the control rats were able to travel across the beam easily (A) while rats in the QA group had difficulty in passing across the beam with paw slipping (A′). In the grip strength test, the control rats held the wire firmly (B) while the QA-treated rats manifested hypertonia (B′). In the water maze task, the swim track of rats in the QA group was bending and often along the maze wall (C′) in comparison of the control rats (C). Cont is short for control.

group the sections belonged to when conducting the measurement. The quantification was carried out on every eighth section of the striatum (2.0 mm anterior and 0.7 mm posterior to bregma, ten to eleven sections per animal for each staining method) and the numbers of neurons, fibers and varicosities were counted throughout the depth of the section. In the Nissl-stained sections, the approximate annular zone with 50%–90% neuronal survival around the lesion core was considered the transition zone in the present study. The section was first examined under the light microscope (Olympus BHS) equipped with a camera lucida at 100× magnification, and the center of the lesion core was located which was apparent due to its severe neuron loss. Then the lesioned striatum was divided into 0.1 mm×0.1 mm zones respectively parallel and perpendicular to the ventricular edge of the ipsilateral striatum through the center of the lesion core that was just located. For convenience, an acetate overlay with the zones drawn on it was created for each case to delineate the striatal regions to be counted for each zone. The number of Nissl-stained neurons in each zone was counted at 400× magnification and neuronal survival was expressed as the percentage of neuronal abundance found in the matching zone in control animals. Zones showing 50%–90% survival of Nissl-stained neurons (i.e., zones

superior, inferior, medial and lateral to the lesion core with 50%–90% neuronal survival) were considered to be within the transition zone. For each drawn lesioned striatum with Nissl staining, two to three zones in each direction (i.e., superior, inferior, medial and lateral to the lesion core) fell within the transition zone. All the quantification of neuron number, fiber density and varicosity density was performed in these zones. The NeuN-, Darpp32-, TUNEL/NeuN-, Parv-, Cr-, NPY- and ChAT-stained sections adjacent to the corresponding Nissl-stained section were also analyzed. The accurate number of neurons was counted in the NeuN-, Darpp32-, TUNEL/NeuN-, Parv-, Cr-, NPY- and ChAT-stained sections. The quantification of fiber density was performed in the Parv-, Cr-, NPY- and ChAT-stained sections, and the numbers of intersecting processes along a 100-µm length were counted and averaged as the fiber density. The varicosity density was measured in the Parv-, Cr- and NPY-stained sections, and the numbers of varicosities along a 100-µm length were counted and averaged as the varicosity density. The final neuron number, fiber density and varicosity density of each staining method for every rat were the average of the numbers acquired from the ten to eleven equidistantly sampled sections, respectively.

Measurement of optical density in Western blots. Western blots were performed four times for each sample. The optical density (OD) was measured by the Image J 1.42q software and the OD of each marker protein was calibrated with the OD of β-actin. The final OD of each marker protein for every animal was the average of the values acquired from the four blots of each sample.

Statistical analysis. All experimental data are presented as mean±SD (standard deviation). The statistical analyses of data were performed by one-way ANOVA followed by Fisher's *post hoc* PLSD test with SPSS 16.0 software and $p<0.05$ was considered to be significant.

Result

There was no significant difference in weight among groups (data not shown). Statistical analyses were made among the QA,

Table 2. Measures of behavioral tests.

Test		Cont	QA
Balance beam test	Number of paw slipping	0.17±0.16	0.89±0.92*
	Completion time (sec)	19.45±7.21	40.36±16.48*
Grip strength test	Hang time (sec)	11.47±4.43	16.45±2.12*
Water maze test	Latency (sec)	41.42±10.77	71.53±25.34*
	Number of target site crossovers	11.20±1.93	2.10±2.69*

Note: values expressed as group means±SD; * $p<0.01$ v.s. control (Cont), one-way ANOVA and Fisher's *post hoc* PLSD test.

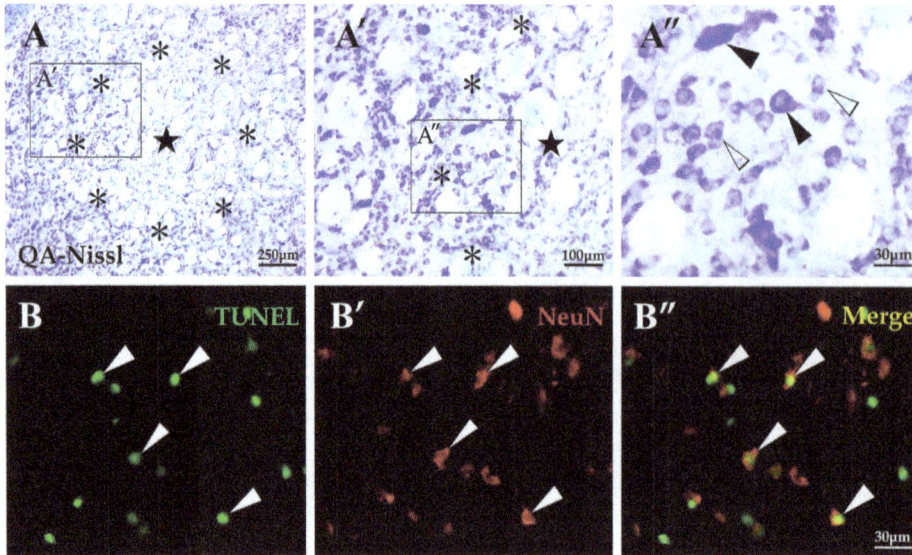

Figure 2. Histological changes and neuronal apoptosis of striatum induced by QA. In sections with Nissl staining taken from the QA-treated striatum (A-A″), the lesion core (★) was injured seriously with very few neurons survived; the annular area surrounded the lesion core, named the transition zone (*), was less injured than the lesion core with some neurons survived including several medium-sized neurons (white arrowheads in A″) and a few large-sized neurons (black arrowheads in A″); the periphery, the area outside the transition zone, appeared similar to tissues of a normal striatum. In sections with TUNEL labeling (B-B″), the apoptotic cells were mainly detected in the transition zone (white arrowheads in B) and a large proportion of them were neurons as shown in the TUNEL/NeuN double labeling section (white arrowheads in B″). Cont is short for control. Panels A′ and A″ are views of higher magnification from the boxes of Panels A and A′, respectively. Scale bars: A, 250 μm; A′, 100 μm; A″, 30 μm; B-B″, 30 μm.

the control and the normal groups, and there was no significant difference between the control group and the normal group in both behavioral tests and histological examinations. To make the following report concise and easier to understand, we provide data and statistical analyses of the normal group and the control group (Table 1) before we reveal all of our findings. In the following text, we focus on the QA group and the control group.

Motor and cognitive deficits induced by QA

To assess the motor functions of experimental rats, the balance beam test and the grip strength test were applied. In the balance beam test, one QA-treated rat failed to pass across the beam, but the other nine cases in the QA group had difficulty in initiating movement and passing across the beam in stark contrast to the control rats (Fig. 1A and A′). The number of paw slipping ($F = 7.687$, $df1 = 2$, $df2 = 26$, $p<0.01$) and the completion time ($F = 12.905$, $df1 = 2$, $df2 = 26$, $p<0.01$) in the QA group were significantly increased when compared with the control group (Table 2). In the grip strength test, rats with intrastriatal QA injections showed hypertonia with longer hang time in comparison to the control rats ($F = 6.542$, $df1 = 2$, $df2 = 27$, $p<0.01$; Fig. 1B and B′; Table 2).

The cognitive and mnemonic deficits of experimental animals were detected by the water maze task. There was no significant difference among the QA, the control and the normal groups in swim speed (QA 17.25 ± 5.89 cm/s, Cont 19.42 ± 10.03 cm/s, Norm 18.52 ± 8.01 cm/s; $F = 0.180$, $df1 = 2$, $df2 = 27$, $p>0.05$), and therefore the results reflecting cognitive functions should not have been affected by motor dysfunction in the task. QA-treated rats swam in bending routes when locating the hidden platform and often moved along the wall of the maze (Fig. 1C′). The latency of locating the platform was significantly increased in the learning trials ($F = 13.231$, $df1 = 2$, $df2 = 27$, $p<0.01$) and the number of

target site crossovers was markedly decreased in the probe trial in the QA group ($F = 42.473$, $df1 = 2$, $df2 = 27$, $p<0.01$) when compared with the control group (Table 2).

Loss of striatal projection neurons in the transition zone induced by QA

In the experimental rats treated with intrastriatal QA injections, a unilateral lesion was observed in the striatum and the exact locations were usually around the injection sites. Based on analyses of brain sections processed with Nissl staining, a severe neuron loss was observed in the lesion core and the mean lesion diameter through the center of lesion was 1.02 ± 0.13 mm (Fig. 2A and A′). The annular area surrounded the lesion core is termed transition zone (0.24 ± 0.03 mm in width) [30] in which a relatively slighter neuron loss was observed. Among the remaining cells in this zone were a few large neurons mixed with some medium-sized ones (Fig. 2A″). The transition zone has been of great interest to researchers and clinicians due to its uniqueness of cell survival and similarity to pathophysiology of HD [25,30]. Thus, we mainly focused on the transition zone and performed cell count in this area. The cell abundance of the transition zone in QA-treated rats was significantly reduced in comparison of the control animals ($F = 21.772$, $df1 = 2$, $df2 = 12$, $p<0.01$; Fig. 3A). Outside the transition zone, cells that made up a region named periphery appeared indistinguishable from those in a normal striatum in terms of quantity and appearance.

To investigate whether apoptosis participated in neuron death in the QA-induced striatal impairment, the TUNEL assay was applied in the present study. In the QA group, TUNEL-labeled cellular fragments and pyknosis were mainly found in the transition zone (371.67 ± 40.08/mm^2; Fig. 2B). Further double-labeling of TUNEL and NeuN displayed that a large proportion of cells going through apoptosis were NeuN+ neurons

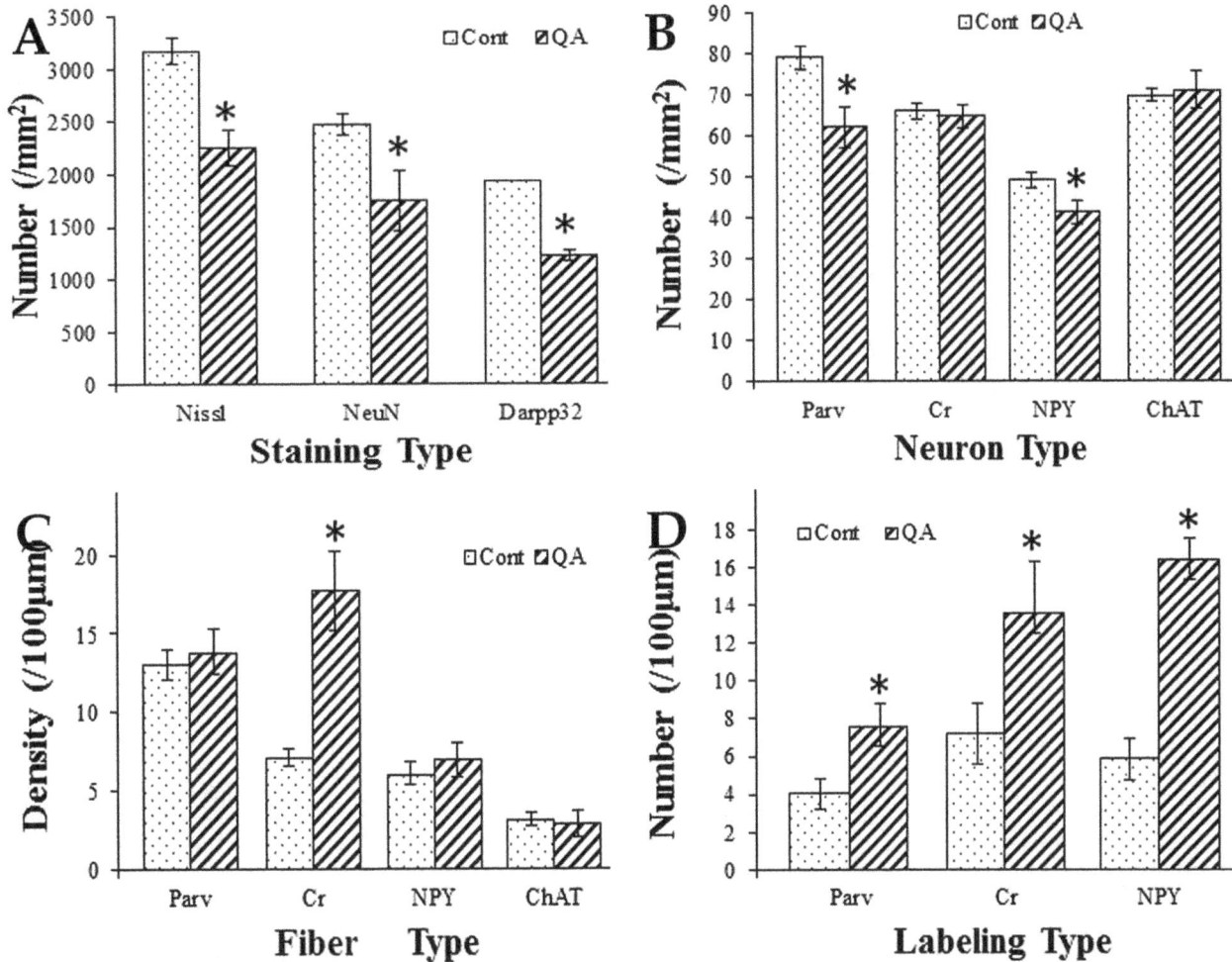

Figure 3. Histograms for comparison between the QA group and the control group. Histogram A was based on the statistical analyses of brain sections with Nissl staining as well as NeuN and Darpp32 immunolabeling. It revealed that the numbers of neurons and projection neurons in the transition zone were significantly decreased in the QA group when compared to the control group. Histograms B and C were based on the statistical analyses of brain sections with Parv, Cr, NPY and ChAT immunolabeling. The numbers of Parv+ and NPY+ interneurons were significantly decreased while those of Cr+ and ChAT+ interneurons were not notably reduced in the transition zone of the QA group when compared to the control group (B). The density of Cr+ fibers was significantly increased while those of Parv+, NPY+ and ChAT+ fibers were not notably changed in the transition zone of the QA group in comparison of the control group (C). Histogram D was based on the statistical analyses of brain sections with Parv, Cr and NPY immunolabeling. It revealed that the varicosity densities of Parv+, Cr+ and NPY+ fibers were all significantly increased in the transition zone of the QA group when compared to the control group. Values are expressed as group means±SD. * $P<0.01$ v.s. control, Student's t-test.

$(213.67\pm46.61/\text{mm}^2$; Fig. 2B″). No TUNEL labeling was observed in control and normal rats.

Histologically, the striatum consists of a vast majority of projection neurons and a small number of interneurons [16]. We applied the antibody of NeuN labeling all the neurons and the antibody of Darpp32 specific for striatal projection neurons to assess the degree of neuron loss in the QA-treated striatum. Based on the analyses of brain sections with NeuN labeling, there was a significant difference in the number of neurons in the transition zone between QA-treated rats and control rats $(F=24.005, df1=2, df2=12, p<0.01$; Fig. 3A; Fig. 4A, A′, B and B′). In sections with Darpp32 labeling, the number of projection neurons in the transition zone was significantly decreased in the QA group when compared with the control group $(F=170.562, df1=2, df2=12, p<0.01$; Fig. 3A; Fig. 4C, C′, D and D′).

Changes of striatal interneurons in the transition zone induced by QA

By means of immunohistochemistry, the four interneuron types specifically labeled by antibodies of Parv, Cr, NPY and ChAT were investigated in the transition zone. The numbers of Parv+ interneurons $(F=40.717, df1=2, df2=12, p<0.01$; Fig. 3B; Fig. 5A and B) and NPY+ interneurons $(F=22.846, df1=2, df2=12, p<0.01$; Fig. 3B; Fig. 6A and B) were significantly reduced in the QA group in comparison to the control group. In contrast to the vulnerability of Darpp32+ projection neurons as well as Parv+ and NPY+ interneurons, the Cr+ interneurons and ChAT+ interneurons were relatively resistant to excitotoxicity induced by QA. The statistical analyses showed that there was no significant difference between the QA group and the control group in the numbers of Cr+ neurons $(F=0.523, df1=2, df2=12, p>0.05$; Fig. 3B; Fig. 5C and D) and ChAT+ neurons $(F=0.347, df1=2, df2=12, p>0.05$; Fig. 3B; Fig. 6C and D).

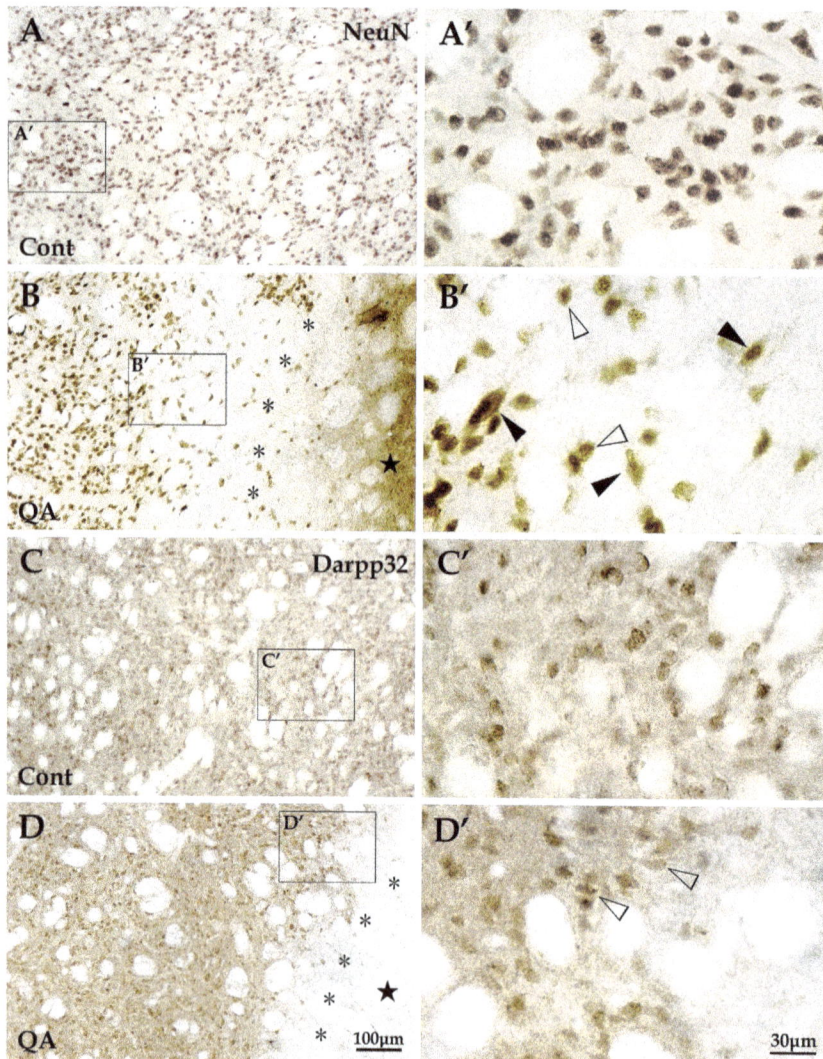

Figure 4. Changes of striatal projection neurons induced by QA. Striatal neurons, presented with NeuN labeling, were evenly distributed throughout the striatum in the control group (A and A') while the NeuN+ cells in the QA group (B and B') were extremely scarce in the lesion core (★) and notably reduced in quantity in the transition zone (*). Those neurons survived in the transition zone (B') included some medium-sized neurons (white arrowheads) and a few large-sized neurons (black arrowheads). Striatal projection neurons, labeled for Darpp32, were medium in size and evenly distributed in the striatum in control rats (C and C'). The Darpp32+ projection neurons hardly survived in the lesion core and only a small proportion did in the transition zone (D and D'). Cont is short for control. Panels A'–D' are views of higher magnification from the boxes of Panels A–D, respectively. Scale bars: A–D, 100 μm; A'–D', 30 μm.

In addition to changes of neuron abundance, the interneurons in the transition zone displayed morphological changes against QA injury. Though the neuron number was not notably reduced after QA treatment, Cr+ interneurons showed an obvious increase in fiber density when compared to the controls ($F = 83.145$, $df1 = 2$, $df2 = 12$, $p < 0.01$; Fig. 3C; Fig. 5C and D''). However, the fiber densities of Parv+, NPY+ and ChAT+ interneurons were not significantly increased in the QA group in comparison of the controls (Parv+ $F = 0.873$, $df1 = 2$, $df2 = 12$, $p > 0.05$; NPY+ $F = 2.069$, $df1 = 2$, $df2 = 12$, $p > 0.05$; ChAT+ $F = 0.450$, $df1 = 2$, $df2 = 12$, $p > 0.05$; Fig. 3C; Fig. 5A' and B'; Fig. 6A'–D').

Moreover, the striatal GABAergic interneurons in the transition zone after QA treatment showed formation of varicosities along the neuronal processes. The varicosity densities of Parv+, Cr+ and NPY+ interneurons were notably increased in the QA group when compared with the controls (Parv+ $F = 21.322$, $df1 = 2$, $df2 = 12$, $p < 0.01$; Cr+ $F = 17.959$, $df1 = 2$, $df2 = 12$, $p < 0.01$; NPY+

$F = 160.422$, $df1 = 2$, $df2 = 12$, $p < 0.01$; Fig. 3D; Fig. 5A'–D'; Fig. 6A' and B'). Unlike the three types of GABAergic interneurons, the ChAT+ interneurons remained morphologically stable without varicosity formation (Fig. 6C' and D').

Marker protein changes of different striatal neurons induced by QA

To further detect changes of different striatal neurons, Western blots were applied in the present study. In line with the results from cell counts, the expression levels of NeuN ($F = 153.906$, $df1 = 2$, $df2 = 12$, $p < 0.01$), Darpp32 ($F = 89.508$, $df1 = 2$, $df2 = 12$, $p < 0.01$), Parv ($F = 170.509$, $df1 = 2$, $df2 = 12$, $p < 0.01$) and NPY ($F = 42.763$, $df1 = 2$, $df2 = 12$, $p < 0.01$) were significantly decreased while those of Cr ($F = 0.144$, $df1 = 2$, $df2 = 12$, $p > 0.05$) and ChAT ($F = 0.675$, $df1 = 2$, $df2 = 12$, $p > 0.05$) were not notably changed in the QA group when compared to the controls (Fig. 7).

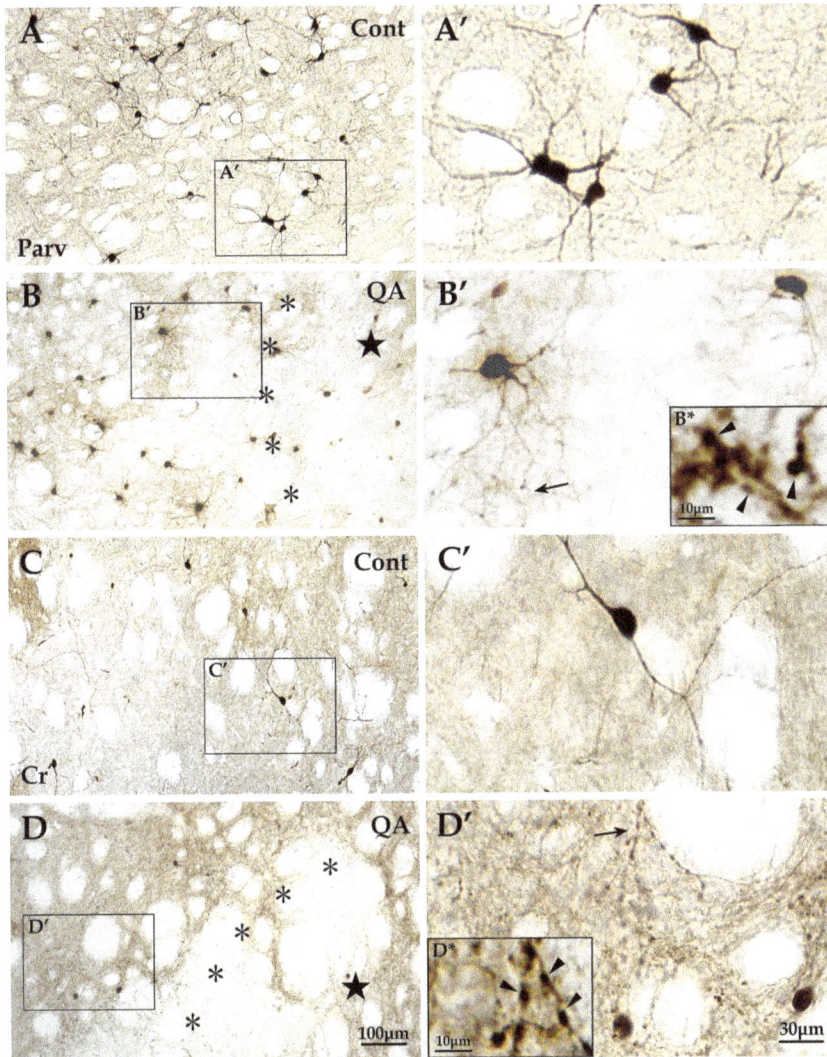

Figure 5. Reactions of Parv+ and Cr+ interneurons to QA. The Parv+ interneurons were mainly distributed in the dorsolateral striatum in the control group (A and A'). These interneurons in the QA group (B and B') were extremely scarce in the lesion core (★) and presented some changes in the transition zone (*) including decrease in neuron number and increase in the number of varicosities which formed along the neuronal processes (see the arrow in B' and the view of higher magnification in B*), but hyperplasia of fibers was not obvious. The Cr+ interneurons were mainly distributed in the medial striatum in the control rats (C and C'). In the QA group (D and D'), this interneuron type hardly survived in the lesion core but the neuron number was not notably reduced in the transition zone. However, the Cr+ interneurons reacted to QA by remarkably proliferating fibers and forming varicosities (see the arrow in D' and the view of higher magnification in D*). Panels A'–D' are views of higher magnification from the boxes of Panels A–D, respectively. Cont is short for control. Scale bars: A–D, 100 μm; A'–D', 30 μm; B* and D*, 10 μm.

Discussion

Behavioral impairments in QA-treated rats

HD is a neurodegenerative condition characterized by progressive abnormal involuntary movements (chorea, dyskinesia and dystonia) and cognitive impairment associated with perseverative behavior and impairment in strategy and planning [1,10]. Some specific neurotoxins such as QA and 3NP as well as transgenic models are used to study the pathophysiology of HD [9,10,31]. QA has long been utilized to induce HD models in rodents since it produces behavioral defects reminiscent of the human HD [9,32] and recent studies suggest that it is an endogenous metabolite of the kynurenine pathway (KP) which is critically involved in HD [12,33,34]. Previous research revealed that animals with QA treatment presented hyperactivity, significant impairment in the balance beam test and spatial learning deficits in the radial arm water maze task [17,22]. In

line with these studies, the present study detected that QA-treated rats showed motor deficits in the balance beam test and cognitive impairment in the water maze task. Furthermore, our results revealed that QA treatment induced hypertonia in the grip strength test. Several studies have reported an increase of muscular tension by the grip strength test in animals with 3NP treatment [17,25]. Shear *et al* has suggested that QA treatment produced milder behavioral effects that mimicked some of the earlier symptoms of HD, while 3NP produced more severe effects which mimicked both the later symptoms and the juvenile onset of HD [17].

Pathological pattern and existence of apoptosis in QA-treated striatum

In human and rat brains, QA is present at concentrations in the high nanomolar range (usually less than 100 nM) [35,36], but it

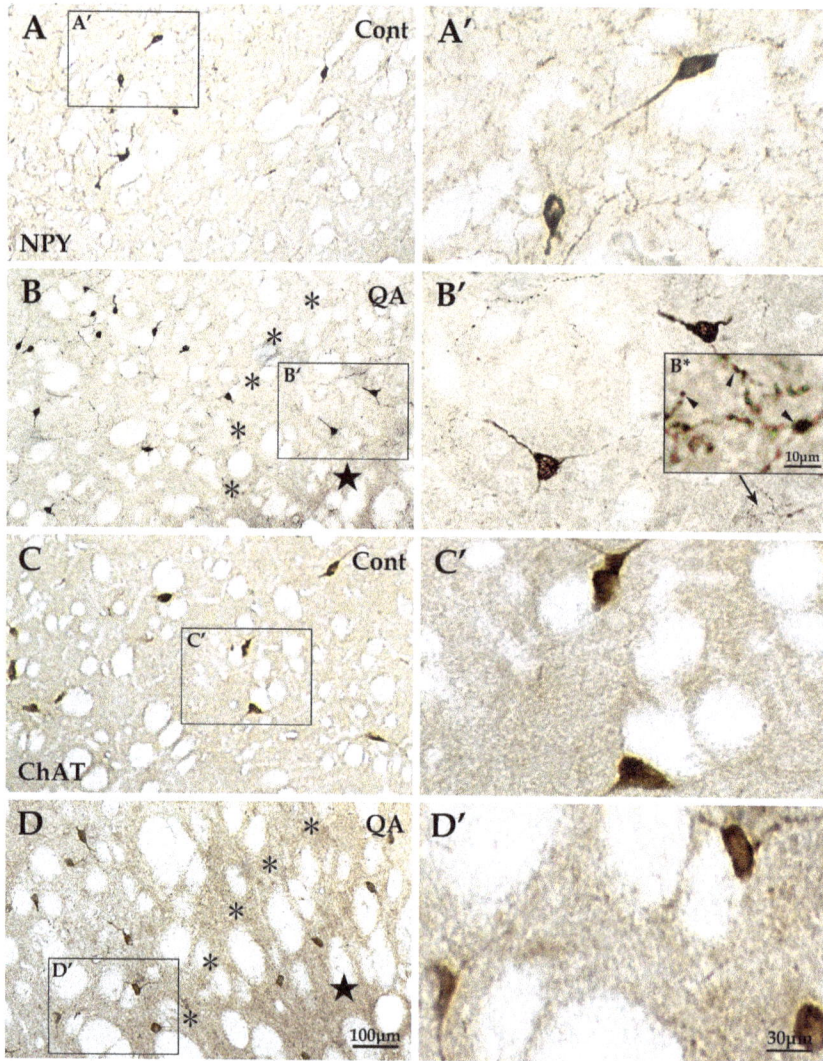

Figure 6. Reactions of NPY+ and ChAT+ interneurons to QA. The NPY+ interneurons were evenly distributed in the striatum in the control group (A and A′). This interneuron type in QA-treated rats (B and B′) hardly survived in the lesion core (★) and experienced some changes in the transition zone (*) including decrease in neuron number and increase in the number of varicosities which formed along the neuronal processes (see the arrow in B′ and the view of higher magnification in B*), but hyperplasia of fibers was not obvious. The ChAT+ interneurons were large in size and evenly distributed throughout the striatum in the control rats (C and C′) and they appeared stable in neuron abundance as well as in morphology without hyperplasia of fibers or varicosity formation in the QA-treated rats (D and D′). Panels A′–D′ are views of higher magnification from the boxes of Panels A–D, respectively. Cont is short for control. Scale bars: A–D, 100 μm; A′–D′, 30 μm; B*, 10 μm.

has been reported that the brain level of QA was increased three to four-fold in low-grade HD brain [37]. Braidy *et al* showed that QA mediated astrocytic and neuronal inflammation and damage at sub-physiological concentrations (150 nM) *in vitro* [38]. However, the *in vivo* HD animal model required intrastriatal injections of QA at much higher concentrations (50–225 mM) to produce neuronal damage [19,20,39], as it did in the present study (100 mM). The reason may be that QA acts on the brain in an acute and focal manner in the *in vivo* model while it exerts prolonged and extensive effect on the neurons during the disease progression or in the *in vitro* experiments. Thus it requires a larger amount of the excitotoxin in the animal model to produce the similar effect as it does in the pathophysiologic state.

The pathological hallmark of HD is a massive reduction of the striatal volume which results from the loss of spiny projection neurons, while the aspiny interneurons are relatively spared [40].

It has been suggested that QA can produce axon-sparing lesions closely resembling those observed in HD [14,32]. In particular, the transition zone of QA-lesioned striatum has been of great interest to researchers due to its similarity to the pathophysiology of HD [30]. The present study did detect the selective neuron death in the transition zone rather than in the lesion core where there was hardly any striatal neuron survived. The underlying mechanisms of this selective sparing of neurons are not fully elucidated. Now growing amount of evidence supports the existence of apoptosis in HD human brains [41,42,43]. Accordingly, our data found that apoptosis was a major type of neuron death in the transition zone while necrosis was the main type of neuron death in the lesion core. Research on HD animal models and postmortem tissues has also pointed that the caspase family was shown to cleave mutant htt which is closely related to the pathogenesis of HD [44,45,46]. It is well-known that the excitotoxin QA exerts its toxic effects by

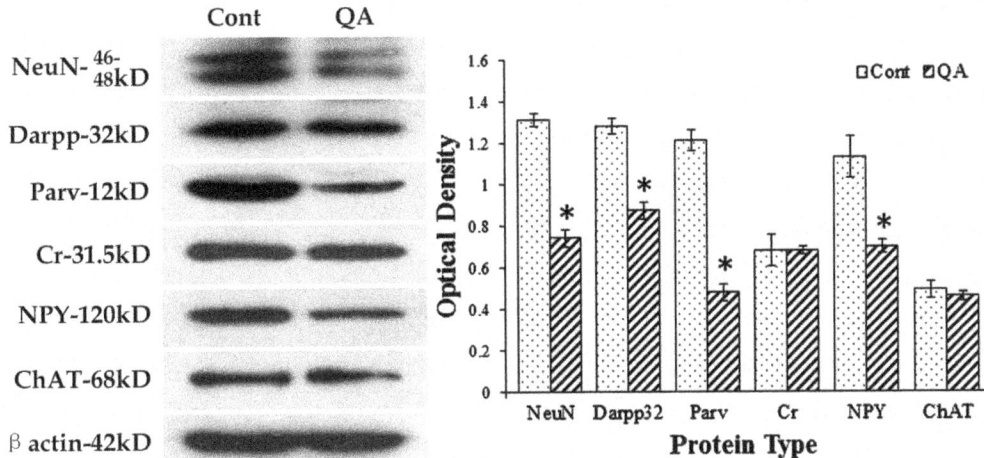

Figure 7. Western blots for marker proteins of different striatal neurons. Western blots were applied to detect the expression levels of NeuN, Darpp32, Parv, Cr, NPY and ChAT after QA treatment. β-actin was used to control for equal protein loading. In the histogram, levels indicated in the bars are expressed as optical density (OD). The ODs of NeuN, Darpp32, Parv and NPY were significantly decreased while those of Cr and ChAT were not notably changed in QA-treated striatum when compared to the controls (Cont). Values are expressed as group means±SD. * $P < 0.01$ v.s. control, Student's t-test.

overactivation of N-methyl-D-aspartate (NMDA) receptors and increased cytosolic Ca^{2+} concentrations [33]. In addition to the proven excitotoxic profile of QA, a considerable amount of evidence recently suggested that oxidative stress and energetic disturbances were major constituents of its toxic pattern [33,38,47]. Mitochondrial abnormalities, especially a deficit of energy metabolism in brains, have been reported in htt transgenic mice and it was associated with apoptotic cell death [48]. It has been proposed that prohibiting the activation process of apoptosis may be a potential neuroprotective therapy for HD [49].

Specific reactions of different striatal interneurons after QA treatment and their implications

The most intriguing findings in the present experiment were the specific reactions of different striatal interneuron types in the transition zone after QA treatment. In brief, our data showed that the Parv+ and NPY+ interneurons were relatively susceptible to QA toxicity, but to a lesser extent when compared to the projection neurons, while the Cr+ interneurons were relatively resistant and the ChAT+ interneurons seemed insensitive to QA treatment. Previous studies also revealed that the Parv+ and NPY+ striatal interneurons were relatively vulnerable to QA toxicity in rodents [17,20,50]. Figueredo-Cardenas *et al* further reported that the Parv+ neurons were relatively not impervious to QA while the NPY+ neurons were highly vulnerable in rats [51]. It is noteworthy that the Cr+ interneurons were of higher resistance to QA-mediated toxicity than the Parv+ and NPY+ neurons in the present experiment. Several chemical anatomical studies on striatal interneurons have reported that the Cr+ neurons were selectively spared in HD postmortem tissues [40,52,53]. Our assessment of neuron counts and Western blots also found that the number of Cr+ interneurons was not significantly decreased in QA-treated rats. The underlying mechanisms are still under exploration. It has been suggested that the calcium-binding protein Cr plays an important role in the maintenance of intracellular Ca^{2+} homeostasis. Its presence in some neurons

may protect them against the massive Ca^{2+} entry that may result from over-stimulation on glutamate receptors [52].

The resistance of the GABAergic interneurons against QA toxicity was also manifested with morphological changes including hyperplasia of processes and varicosities. The present experiment showed that the fiber density of Cr+ neurons was markedly increased after QA treatment. Although the absolute fiber densities of Parv+ and NPY+ neurons were not significantly increased in QA-treated rats, the numbers of these two interneurons were reduced. Thus the fibers for each individual neuron were relatively increased. Though very few experiments have been conducted in this field, our previous studies on the 3NP-induced HD model have proven that the survival of NPY+ and Cr+ interneurons in the transition zone was accompanied by an increase of fibers and varicosities [25]. It has been proposed that this may be a response to the projection neuron loss, a protective reaction, or even one of the mechanisms to exacerbate the striatal neuron loss [25,54]. The three GABAergic interneurons directly modulate precise timing of action potential firing of projection neurons [55,56]. The great loss of projection neurons can be regarded as a strong stimulus to the survived interneurons where compensatory hyperplasia of fibers and varicosities occurs.

Unlike the three GABAergic interneuron types, our data revealed that the ChAT+ interneurons remained unchanged in abundance and morphology after QA treatment. Numerous studies have consistently indicated that the cholinergic interneurons were rather resistant or insensitive in HD postmortem striatum and animal models [50,57,58]. These may result from the attribute of autonomous electrical activity, or independence to synaptic input, which suggests that the ChAT+ neurons are relatively insensitive to glutamate-receptor-dependent excitotoxicity [59].

Author Contributions

Conceived and designed the experiments: QF SM WL. Performed the experiments: YM LO. Analyzed the data: JW SC. Contributed reagents/materials/analysis tools: WL. Wrote the paper: QF YM.

References

1. Walker FO (2007) Huntington's disease. Lancet 369: 218–228.
2. Ferrante RJ, Kowall NW, Beal MF, Martin JB, Bird ED, et al. (1987) Morphologic and histochemical characteristics of a spared subset of striatal neurons in Huntington's disease. J Neuropathol Exp Neurol 46: 12–27.
3. The Huntington's Disease Collaborative Research Group (1993) A novel gene containing a trinucleotide repeat that is expanded and unstable on Huntington's disease chromosomes. Cell 72: 971–983.
4. Albin RL, Tagle DA (1995) Genetics and molecular biology of Huntington's disease. Trends Neurosci 18: 11–14.
5. Claes S, Van Zand K, Legius E, Dom R, Malfroid M, et al. (1995) Correlations between triplet repeat expansion and clinical features in Huntington's disease. Arch Neurol 52: 749–753.
6. Kim SH, Thomas CA, Andre VM, Cummings DM, Cepeda C, et al. (2011) Forebrain striatal-specific expression of mutant huntingtin protein in vivo induces cell-autonomous age-dependent alterations in sensitivity to excitotoxicity and mitochondrial function. ASN Neuro 3: e60.
7. Cowan CM, Raymond LA (2006) Selective neuronal degeneration in Huntington's disease. Curr Top Dev Biol 75: 25–71.
8. Bithell A, Johnson R, Buckley NJ (2009) Transcriptional dysregulation of coding and non-coding genes in cellular models of Huntington's disease. Biochem Soc Trans 37: 1270–1275.
9. Schwarcz R, Guidetti P, Sathyasaikumar KV, Muchowski PJ (2010) Of mice, rats and men: Revisiting the quinolinic acid hypothesis of Huntington's disease. Prog Neurobiol 90: 230–245.
10. Brouillet E, Jacquard C, Bizat N, Blum D (2005) 3-Nitropropionic acid: a mitochondrial toxin to uncover physiopathological mechanisms underlying striatal degeneration in Huntington's disease. J Neurochem 95: 1521–1540.
11. Han I, You Y, Kordower JH, Brady ST, Morfini GA (2010) Differential vulnerability of neurons in Huntington's disease: the role of cell type-specific features. J Neurochem 113: 1073–1091.
12. Bruyn RP, Stoof JC (1990) The quinolinic acid hypothesis in Huntington's chorea. J Neurol Sci 95: 29–38.
13. Doble A (1999) The role of excitotoxicity in neurodegenerative disease: implications for therapy. Pharmacol Ther 81: 163–221.
14. Roberts RC, Ahn A, Swartz KJ, Beal MF, DiFiglia M (1993) Intrastriatal injections of quinolinic acid or kainic acid: differential patterns of cell survival and the effects of data analysis on outcome. Exp Neurol 124: 274–282.
15. Guillemin GJ (2012) Quinolinic acid, the inescapable neurotoxin. FEBS J 279: 1356–1365.
16. Durieux PF, Schiffmann SN, de Kerchove DA (2011) Targeting neuronal populations of the striatum. Front Neuroanat 5: 40.
17. Shear DA, Dong J, Gundy CD, Haik-Creguer KL, Dunbar GL (1998) Comparison of intrastriatal injections of quinolinic acid and 3-nitropropionic acid for use in animal models of Huntington's disease. Prog Neuropsychopharmacol Biol Psychiatry 22: 1217–1240.
18. Guyot MC, Hantraye P, Dolan R, Palfi S, Maziere M, et al. (1997) Quantifiable bradykinesia, gait abnormalities and Huntington's disease-like striatal lesions in rats chronically treated with 3-nitropropionic acid. Neuroscience 79: 45–56.
19. Ngai LY, Herbert J (2005) Glucocorticoid enhances the neurotoxic actions of quinolinic acid in the striatum in a cell-specific manner. J Neuroendocrinol 17: 424–434.
20. Figueredo-Cardenas G, Chen Q, Reiner A (1997) Age-dependent differences in survival of striatal somatostatin-NPY-NADPH-diaphorase-containing interneurons versus striatal projection neurons after intrastriatal injection of quinolinic acid in rats. Exp Neurol 146: 444–457.
21. Meade CA, Figueredo-Cardenas G, Fusco F, Nowak TJ, Pulsinelli WA, et al. (2000) Transient global ischemia in rats yields striatal projection neuron and interneuron loss resembling that in Huntington's disease. Exp Neurol 166: 307–323.
22. Haik KL, Shear DA, Schroeder U, Sabel BA, Dunbar GL (2000) Quinolinic acid released from polymeric brain implants causes behavioral and neuroanatomical alterations in a rodent model of Huntington's disease. Exp Neurol 163: 430–439.
23. Boegman RJ, Parent A (1988) Differential sensitivity of neuropeptide Y, somatostatin and NADPH-diaphorase containing neurons in rat cortex and striatum to quinolinic acid. Brain Res 445: 358–362.
24. MacKenzie GM, Jenner P, Marsden CD (1995) The effect of nitric oxide synthase inhibition on quinolinic acid toxicity in the rat striatum. Neuroscience 67: 357–371.
25. Mu S, OuYang L, Liu B, Zhu Y, Li K, et al. (2011) Preferential interneuron survival in the transition zone of 3-NP-induced striatal injury in rats. J Neurosci Res 89: 744–754.
26. Paxinos G, Watson C (2006) The rat brain in stereotaxic coordinates. United States: ACADEMIC PRESS. 1–456 p.
27. Vorhees CV, Williams MT (2006) Morris water maze: procedures for assessing spatial and related forms of learning and memory. Nat Protoc 1: 848–858.
28. Packard MG, Knowlton BJ (2002) Learning and memory functions of the Basal Ganglia. Annu Rev Neurosci 25: 563–593.
29. Voogd J, Feirabend HKP (1981) Methods in neurobiology, vol 2. New York: Elsevier. 301–364 p.
30. Huang Q, Zhou D, Sapp E, Aizawa H, Ge P, et al. (1995) Quinolinic acid-induced increases in calbindin D28k immunoreactivity in rat striatal neurons in vivo and in vitro mimic the pattern seen in Huntington's disease. Neuroscience 65: 397–407.
31. Bates GP, Mangiarini L, Mahal A, Davies SW (1997) Transgenic models of Huntington's disease. Hum Mol Genet 6: 1633–1637.
32. Beal MF, Kowall NW, Ellison DW, Mazurek MF, Swartz KJ, et al. (1986) Replication of the neurochemical characteristics of Huntington's disease by quinolinic acid. Nature 321: 168–171.
33. Perez-De LCV, Carrillo-Mora P, Santamaria A (2012) Quinolinic Acid, an endogenous molecule combining excitotoxicity, oxidative stress and other toxic mechanisms. Int J Tryptophan Res 5: 1–8.
34. Guidetti P, Schwarcz R (2003) 3-Hydroxykynurenine and quinolinate: pathogenic synergism in early grade Huntington's disease? Adv Exp Med Biol 527: 137–145.
35. Wolfensberger M, Amsler U, Cuenod M, Foster AC, Whetsell WJ, et al. (1983) Identification of quinolinic acid in rat and human brain tissue. Neurosci Lett 41: 247–252.
36. Braidy N, Grant R, Brew BJ, Adams S, Jayasena T, et al. (2009) Effects of Kynurenine Pathway Metabolites on Intracellular NAD Synthesis and Cell Death in Human Primary Astrocytes and Neurons. Int J Tryptophan Res 2: 61–69.
37. Guidetti P, Luthi-Carter RE, Augood SJ, Schwarcz R (2004) Neostriatal and cortical quinolinate levels are increased in early grade Huntington's disease. Neurobiol Dis 17: 455–461.
38. Braidy N, Grant R, Adams S, Brew BJ, Guillemin GJ (2009) Mechanism for quinolinic acid cytotoxicity in human astrocytes and neurons. Neurotox Res 16: 77–86.
39. Kalonia H, Kumar P, Kumar A (2011) Comparative neuroprotective profile of statins in quinolinic acid induced neurotoxicity in rats. Behav Brain Res 216: 220–228.
40. Massouh M, Wallman MJ, Pourcher E, Parent A (2008) The fate of the large striatal interneurons expressing calretinin in Huntington's disease. Neurosci Res 62: 216–224.
41. Sawa A, Tomoda T, Bae BI (2003) Mechanisms of neuronal cell death in Huntington's disease. Cytogenet Genome Res 100: 287–295.
42. Dragunow M, Faull RL, Lawlor P, Beilharz EJ, Singleton K, et al. (1995) In situ evidence for DNA fragmentation in Huntington's disease striatum and Alzheimer's disease temporal lobes. Neuroreport 6: 1053–1057.
43. Thomas LB, Gates DJ, Richfield EK, O'Brien TF, Schweitzer JB, et al. (1995) DNA end labeling (TUNEL) in Huntington's disease and other neuropathological conditions. Exp Neurol 133: 265–272.
44. Portera-Cailliau C, Hedreen JC, Price DL, Koliatsos VE (1995) Evidence for apoptotic cell death in Huntington disease and excitotoxic animal models. J Neurosci 15: 3775–3787.
45. Sanchez MR, Friedlander RM (2001) Caspases in Huntington's disease. Neuroscientist 7: 480–489.
46. Hermel E, Gafni J, Propp SS, Leavitt BR, Wellington CL, et al. (2004) Specific caspase interactions and amplification are involved in selective neuronal vulnerability in Huntington's disease. Cell Death Differ 11: 424–438.
47. Tasset I, Perez-De LCV, Elinos-Calderon D, Carrillo-Mora P, Gonzalez-Herrera IG, et al. (2010) Protective effect of tert-butylhydroquinone on the quinolinic-acid-induced toxicity in rat striatal slices: role of the Nrf2-antioxidant response element pathway. Neurosignals 18: 24–31.
48. Tabrizi SJ, Workman J, Hart PE, Mangiarini L, Mahal A, et al. (2000) Mitochondrial dysfunction and free radical damage in the Huntington R6/2 transgenic mouse. Ann Neurol 47: 80–86.
49. Tarawneh R, Galvin JE (2010) Potential future neuroprotective therapies for neurodegenerative disorders and stroke. Clin Geriatr Med 26: 125–147.
50. Meade CA, Figueredo-Cardenas G, Fusco F, Nowak TJ, Pulsinelli WA, et al. (2000) Transient global ischemia in rats yields striatal projection neuron and interneuron loss resembling that in Huntington's disease. Exp Neurol 166: 307–323.
51. Figueredo-Cardenas G, Harris CL, Anderson KD, Reiner A (1998) Relative resistance of striatal neurons containing calbindin or parvalbumin to quinolinic acid-mediated excitotoxicity compared to other striatal neuron types. Exp Neurol 149: 356–372.
52. Cicchetti F, Prensa L, Wu Y, Parent A (2000) Chemical anatomy of striatal interneurons in normal individuals and in patients with Huntington's disease. Brain Res Brain Res Rev 34: 80–101.
53. Cicchetti F, Gould PV, Parent A (1996) Sparing of striatal neurons coexpressing calretinin and substance P (NK1) receptor in Huntington's disease. Brain Res 730: 232–237.
54. Kawaguchi Y (1993) Physiological, morphological, and histochemical characterization of three classes of interneurons in rat neostriatum. J Neurosci 13: 4908–4923.
55. Tepper JM, Tecuapetla F, Koos T, Ibanez-Sandoval O (2010) Heterogeneity and diversity of striatal GABAergic interneurons. Front Neuroanat 4: 150.

56. Tepper JM, Bolam JP (2004) Functional diversity and specificity of neostriatal interneurons. Curr Opin Neurobiol 14: 685–692.

57. Smith R, Chung H, Rundquist S, Maat-Schieman ML, Colgan L, et al. (2006) Cholinergic neuronal defect without cell loss in Huntington's disease. Hum Mol Genet 15: 3119–3131.

58. Davies SW, Roberts PJ (1988) Sparing of cholinergic neurons following quinolinic acid lesions of the rat striatum. Neuroscience 26: 387–393.

59. Goldberg JA, Reynolds JN (2011) Spontaneous firing and evoked pauses in the tonically active cholinergic interneurons of the striatum. Neuroscience 198: 27–43.

Genetic Deletion of Transglutaminase 2 does not Rescue the Phenotypic Deficits Observed in R6/2 and zQ175 Mouse Models of Huntington's Disease

Liliana B. Menalled[1], Andrea E. Kudwa[1], Steve Oakeshott[1], Andrew Farrar[1], Neil Paterson[1], Igor Filippov[1], Sam Miller[1], Mei Kwan[1], Michael Olsen[1], Jose Beltran[1], Justin Torello[1], Jon Fitzpatrick[1], Richard Mushlin[1], Kimberly Cox[1], Kristi McConnell[1], Matthew Mazzella[1], Dansha He[1], Georgina F. Osborne[2], Rand Al-Nackkash[2], Gill P. Bates[2], Pasi Tuunanen[3], Kimmo Lehtimaki[3], Dani Brunner[1], Afshin Ghavami[1], Sylvie Ramboz[1], Larry Park[4], Douglas Macdonald[4], Ignacio Munoz-Sanjuan[4], David Howland[4]*

1 PsychoGenics Inc., Tarrytown, New York, United States of America, 2 Department of Medical and Molecular Genetics, King's College London, London, United Kingdom, 3 Charles River Discovery Research Services, Kuopio, Finland, 4 CHDI Management/CHDI Foundation, Princeton, New Jersey, United States of America

Abstract

Huntington's disease (HD) is an autosomal dominant, progressive neurodegenerative disorder caused by expansion of CAG repeats in the huntingtin gene. Tissue transglutaminase 2 (TG2), a multi-functional enzyme, was found to be increased both in HD patients and in mouse models of the disease. Furthermore, beneficial effects have been reported from the genetic ablation of TG2 in R6/2 and R6/1 mouse lines. To further evaluate the validity of this target for the treatment of HD, we examined the effects of TG2 deletion in two genetic mouse models of HD: R6/2 CAG 240 and zQ175 knock in (KI). Contrary to previous reports, under rigorous experimental conditions we found that TG2 ablation had no effect on either motor or cognitive deficits, or on the weight loss. In addition, under optimal husbandry conditions, TG2 ablation did not extend R6/2 lifespan. Moreover, TG2 deletion did not change the huntingtin aggregate load in cortex or striatum and did not decrease the brain atrophy observed in either mouse line. Finally, no amelioration of the dysregulation of striatal and cortical gene markers was detected. We conclude that TG2 is not a valid therapeutic target for the treatment of HD.

Editor: David R. Borchelt, University of Florida, United States of America

Funding: CHDI Foundation is a privately-funded not-for-profit biomedical research organization exclusively dedicated to discovering and developing therapeutics that slow the progression of Huntington's disease. CHDI Foundation conducts research in a number of different ways; for the purposes of this manuscript, research was conducted at the contract research organizations PsychoGenics, Inc. and Charles River Discovery Research Services under a fee-for-service agreement, and at Kings College London under a sponsored research agreement. The authors listed all contributed to the conception, planning, and direction of the research; the specific roles of each author is outlined in the 'author contributions' section.

Competing Interests: The authors have declared that no competing interests exist. DH, IMS, LP and DM are employed by CHDI Management, Inc., as advisors to CHDI Foundation, Inc. LM, AK, SO, AF, NP, IF, SM, MK, MO, JB, JT, JF, RM, KC, KMC, MM, DH, DB and SR are employed by PsychoGenics, Inc. PT and KL are employed by Charles River Research Services. There are no patents, products in development or marketed products to declare. '

* Email: David.Howland@CHDIFoundation.org

Introduction

Tissue transglutaminase 2 (TG2; TGM2; human Gene ID# 7052) is a multi-functional enzyme primarily known for its calcium-dependent intra- and intermolecular cross-linking activity via isopeptide bond formation between glutamine and lysine residues [1]. TG2 has also been shown to have other enzymatic activities, such as GTPase [2], ATPase [3] and isomerase [4] activities. Genetic deletion of TG2 in mice has suggested a role for TG2 activity in mitochondrial energy function [5]. Additionally, TG2 over-activity has been associated with inflammatory diseases such as celiac disease, infectious diseases, cancer, and neurodegenerative diseases such as Huntington's disease (HD) [6–9].

HD is a genetic, autosomal dominant, progressive neurodegen-erative disorder caused by the expansion of the CAG trinucleotide repeat found in the huntingtin gene; when the repeat number exceeds 39, individuals will develop HD within an normal lifespan [10]. Clinically, the disorder is characterized by motor and cognitive deficits as well as, psychiatric problems. Histopatholog-ically, the disorder is characterized by striatal and cortical atrophy, formation of intracellular huntingtin aggregates, and gene expression changes [10].

TG2 expression and transglutaminase activity have both been demonstrated to be increased in HD patients [11–13] and in HD mouse models [14,15], which suggests a correlation with HD pathology. Additionally, genetic deletion of TG2 in two mouse models of HD, R6/1 and R6/2, resulted in improved phenotypes including reduced neuronal cell death, improved motor performance, and prolonged survival [16,17]. These reports led us to initiate a medicinal chemistry program targeting the transglutaminase activity of TG2 as a potential therapeutic strategy for the treatment of HD [18,19]. This program was recently terminated due to the lack of tractability of our TG2 inhibitors to pharmacologically modulate this enzyme in the brain. However, given the existing data derived from the genetic studies, we wanted to extend the validation of this target for the treatment of HD. We therefore repeated this study design with the R6/2 mouse model [20] as well as the zQ175 KI mouse model [21,22] to investigate the molecular, behavioral and pathophysiological association between TG2 and HD by crossing these two lines with a TG2 knockout (KO) mouse [23]. These KO mice are viable, fertile and do not present any abnormal phenotypes [23]. The behavioural effect of genetic depletion of TG2 was examined using the PhenoCube system, the procedural water T-maze test and a Go/No-go paradigm. In addition, body weight and survival were examined. We also used molecular and imaging techniques to further characterize the phenotypes of the double mutants.

In contrast to previously published findings [16,17], we report here that the genetic deletion of TG2 in either the R6/2 transgenic or zQ175 KI mice did not improve motor, cognitive, molecular, histological, or lifespan phenotypes, indicating that TG2 expression is not a determinant of disease progression in these models of HD.

Materials and Methods

1. Animals

Animals were bred in the CHDI colonies at the Jackson laboratories. Experimental mice were generated after two successive matings. The R6/2 CAG 240×TG2 KO line (CHDI-80000024-1) was generated by crossing R6/2 CAG 240 (CHDI-80000004-1, R6/2, C57Bl/6J) ovarian-transplanted females with TG2/− (CHDI-80000013-1, C57Bl/6J; [23]) male mice. Dr Graham kindly provided us with the TG2 (+/−) animals to generate the crosses. The R6/2 TG2+/− males offspring generated from that cross were then bred with TG2+/− female mice. From this second cross, we were able to generate littermates of all genotype combinations, namely: R6/2, R6/2 TG2+/−, R6/2 TG2−/−, WT (wild type), TG2+/− (heterozygous TG2 knockout) and TG2−/− (homozygous TG2 knockout). To generate the zQ175×TG2 KO line (CHDI-80000025-1), zQ175 HET (HET, CHDI-80000015-1, C57Bl/6J) females were bred with TG2−/− male mice (CHDI-80000013-1). zQ175 HET TG2+/− females and males generated from that cross were then crossed which allowed the generation of littermates of all genotype combinations, namely: HOM (zQ175 HOM), HOM TG2+/−, HOM TG2−/−, HET (zQ175 HET), HET TG2+/−, HET TG2−/−, WT, TG2+/− and TG2−/−). At 3 weeks of age, animals were weaned by sex and litter, ear tagged for identification and tail samples were collected for genotyping. At 4 weeks of age, animals were pooled into larger groups by sex and genotype. Genotypes were determined by polymerase chain reaction (PCR). CAG repeat lengths were measured by Laragen (Los Angeles, CA, USA) using standard protocols and Genemapper software as previously described [24]. The average CAG repeat length in the R6/2 mice included in the behavioral cohort from the R6/2×TG2 KO line was 247.83 (S.D. = 10.54). The average CAG repeat length of the zQ175 HOM and HET mice from the zQ175×TG2 KO line included in the behavioral cohort was 187.58 (S.D. = 6.05).

2. Ethics statement

This study was carried out in strict accordance with the recommendations in the Guide for the Care and Use of Laboratory Animals, NRC (2010). The protocols were approved by the Institutional Animal Care and Use Committee of PsychoGenics, Inc., an AAALAC International accredited institution (Unit #001213).

3. Husbandry

At Jackson laboratories, animals were housed in ventilated caging (Thoren Caging System, Inc.) with shaving bedding in 14:10 light-dark cycle.

R6/2×TG2 KO line: animals arrived at PsychoGenics Inc (Tarrytown, NY) at around 4 weeks of age. Mice were transferred from the shipping crates to opti-RAT cages (cage square inches: 144; Animal Care Systems) in the same housing groups as at the Jackson laboratories (6–8 genetically homogenous animals per cage).

zQ175×TG2 KO line: animals arrived at PsychoGenics at around 24/25 weeks of age. Mice assigned to behavioral experiments were transferred from the shipping crates to opti-RAT cages (Animal Care Systems) in the same housing groups as at the Jackson laboratories (4–6 genetically homogenous animals per cage). Animals assigned to molecular experiment were transferred from shipping crates to opti-MICE cages (cage square inches: 75; Animals Care Systems).In all cases, a scope of bedding from the crate was transfer into the opti cage upon arrival. To provide a moderate level of environmental enrichment, opti-Rat contained Enviro-dri bedding, two tunnels and 2 nylon bones while opti-Mice cages contained also Enviro-dri bedding, a tunnel and a nylon bone. Animals had free access to food (Purina 5001) and water unless otherwise specified. Animals were housed under controlled temperature (20°–24°C), humidity (30–70%) and lighting conditions (12:12 light-dark cycle). Animals from the R6/2×TG2 KO line also received supplemental wet feed from 16 weeks of age onwards.

4. Body weight

Mice from the R6/2×TG2 KO line and from the zQ175×TG2 KO line were weighed weekly from 4 weeks of age until death and from 24 to 52 weeks of age, respectively.

5. Survival

Mice were monitored upon arrival at PsychoGenics routinely, with a minimum of 2 health checks per day. Data were collected for survival analysis which included only animals either found dead or euthanized due to clear morbidity (failure to right themselves after 30 s). Once all the R6/2 mice were deceased (at 26 weeks), all of the remaining WT mice were sacrificed. Animals were euthanized either by decapitation or CO_2 exposure, following the AVMA Guidelines for Euthanasia for Animals: 2007 Edition.

6. Behavioral evaluation

Experimenters conducting behavioral experiments were blind to the genotype. A longitudinal design was used to evaluate the mice from the R6/2×TG2 KO line in the PhenoCube system at around 8, 12 and 16 weeks of age. At 14 weeks of age, mice were evaluated in the procedural water T-maze test. Survival was evaluated in this cohort during the course of the behavioral evaluation. Sample sizes are presented in Table 1.

Animals from the zQ175×TG2 KO line were examined in the PhenoCube system at around 27–28 weeks of age. After testing

Table 1. Summary of R6/2×TG2 cohorts.

Genotype	WT		TG2+/−		TG2−/−		R6/2		R6/2 TG2+/−		R6/2 TG2−/−	
Sex	M	F	M	F	M	F	M	F	M	F	M	F
Cohort 1: PhenoCube/T maze, Survival	16	16	16	15	16	14	14	13	16	16	15	16
Cohort 2: qPCR analysis - aggregation assay*	5	6 (3)	6 (4)	6 (4)	7 (4)	5 (4)	6	6	6 (5)	6 (5)	6	6
Cohort 3: MRI volumetric study	6	6	6	6	6	6	6	6	6	6	6	6

* Half of the cortex and the striatal tissues collected from each animal were used for real time qPCR analysis. The numbers in brackets indicate the sample size used for in the aggregation assay. The other half cortex was used in the aggregation assay.

Table 2. Summary of zQ175×TG2 cohorts.

Genotype	WT		TG2+/−		TG2−/−		HET		HET TG2+/−		HET TG2−/−		HOM		HOM TG2+/−		HOM TG2−/−	
Sex	M	F	M	F	M	F	M	F	M	F	M	F	M	F	M	F	M	F
Cohort 1: PhenoCube	12	12	0	0	6	12	12	12	0	0	12	18	9	12	0	0	5	7
Subset A from cohort 1:T maze and MRI volumetric study	6	6	0	0	6	6	6	6	0	0	6	6	6	6	0	0	5	6
Subset B from cohort 1: Go/no go	6	6	0	0	0	0	6	6	0	0	0	6	0	0	0	0	0	0
Cohort 2: qPCR analysis - aggregation assay*	3 (2)	4 (3)	6 (3)	6 (3)	6 (3)	6 (3)	6 (3)	6 (3)	6 (3)	6 (3)	6 (3)	6 (3)	0	0	0	0	0	0

* Half of the cortex and the striatal tissues collected from each animal were used for real time qPCR analysis. The number in brackets indicates the sample size used for in the aggregation assay. The other half striatum and cortex were used in the aggregation assay when it was different from the one used in qPCR studies. HOM: zQ175 HOM mice, HET: zQ175 HET.

was complete, animals were split in 2 cohorts, one tested on the procedural water T-maze test (28–29 weeks of age) and the other on the Go/No-go operant paradigm from 32 to 34 weeks of age (sample size presented in Table 2).

One-two weeks after animals' arrival to PGI, animals were injected with sterile transponders (T-IS 8010 FDX-B, Datamars SA) under 2% isoflurane inhalation anesthesia.

6.1 PhenoCube System. PhenoCube experiments were conducted using modified IntelliCage units (New Behavior AG), each with a camera mounted on top of the cage allowing for computer vision analysis. Each cage consisted of 4 corners with an area separated from the main arena, containing nosepokes with respective water bottles. In the central area, there were three types of climbing structures (two rods, a cubic central object and a three step staircase) providing enriched topography all within a rectangular housing unit. The corners were freely accessible through tunnels, which also serve as radio frequency identification (RFID) chip readers. Within each corner were two small recessed openings which allowed access to two water bottles situated in each corner. Access to the bottles was controlled by retractable doors controlled by a computer. Infra-red sensors detected nosepokes. While water was only available within the corners (with free or conditional access depending on the experimental protocol), food (14 mg dustless precision pellets, BioServ, NJ) was provided *ad libitum* on the cage floor. Mice were maintained on a 12:12 light/dark cycle, with red light during the dark cycle, allowing video capture (sample size provided in Table 1 and Table 2). The light intensity under red light was recorded at 7 lux using a photographic bandpass filter (LDP LLC, NJ) that eliminates long wavelength light frequencies not visible to mice [25]. Computer Vision analysis of the videos taken during the testing sessions tracked the movement and location of the mice in each cage generating data which included total distance travelled by the mice, total time immobile, locomotion, clustering, as well as rearing and climbing.

Following a period of water deprivation (16 hrs), mice were tested in the PhenoCube for 72 hrs sessions, initially under the Habituation protocol (6 hrs) and the remaining time under the Alternation protocol. Mice were removed from the experiment if the mouse did not lick and data from these mice were excluded from analysis. All R6/2 mice and corresponding control mice received supplemental HydroGel(ClearH20, ME) during the testing sessions at 16 weeks of age to ensure proper hydration.

Habituation: In this phase water was freely available in all four corners (Figure S1).

Alternation: During this phase subjects were required to alternate visits between two of the four corners (active corners) in order to gain access to water. Each mouse was assigned two adjacent active corners at random. Only one of the two nosepokes was activated in each corner, such that mice had to nosepoke on the left side in order to gain access to water in the right corner, or nosepoke to the right in the left corner (see Figure S1). After a correct alternation, a nosepoke in the correct recess resulted in the door opening and allowing access to the water bottle on that side. After 8 seconds, the door gently closed, preventing further access to water within a given visit. No penalty was imposed for initially nosepoking on the incorrect side.

6.2 Procedural water T-maze test. Mice were tested in T-mazes constructed of black Plexiglas (locally constructed at PsychoGenics, Inc, sample size presented in Table 1 and Table 2). Arms were 33 cm high and 10 cm wide, each arm was 49 cm long. Testing was performed in a dimly-lit (approximately 15 lux) room equipped with a video camera (mounted above the T-maze) and a computer and monitor. The monitor screen was covered with red transparent film to minimize light emission. The T-maze was filled with water at $25\pm1°C$, rendered opaque with Tempura non-toxic white paint. At one end of the cross-piece of the 'T', a platform was located approximately 0.5 cm below the level of the water.

In acquisition training, mice were placed in the stem of the maze and allowed to make a choice to swim into either the right or left arm to reach the escape platform, with the platform location held constant for each mouse during acquisition. A choice was defined as entry into either the left or right arm, without necessarily reaching the escape platform. Failure to leave the stem of the T-maze was defined as 'no-choice'. Any mouse that failed to reach the platform within the maximum trial duration (60 s) was placed directly onto the platform. Once an animal reached or was placed on the platform, the animal was allowed to remain there for 30 s. Animals received 8 trials per day, for a maximum of 12 days, with an inter-trial interval of approximately 15 min. The performance criterion was set at achieving 6 or more correct trials per day for 2 consecutive days. Up to 10 days of training were provided to achieve criterion. Once criterion was achieved animals progressed to reversal testing on an individual basis. In this phase the platform was placed in the opposite choice arm. Reversal performance was assessed for 6 days. Mice were monitored at all times when in the maze.

6.3 Go/No-go. Mice were tested in mouse operant chambers (Med Associates, VT) measuring 22 cm long ×18 cm wide, with 13 cm high walls (sample size presented in Table 2). Each chamber was equipped with a nosepoke recess, which could be illuminated by a small embedded light-emitting diode (LED), located centrally on the wall opposite the food magazine. Reinforcement was provided by time-limited access to a dipper containing evaporated milk (Carnation, OH). The hardware was controlled and all events were recorded by the Med-PC IV software package.

Prior to training, mice were food restricted and individually maintained at 85% of their free feeding body weights by providing them with pre-weighed rations of rodent chow on a daily basis.

Initial training. Following food restriction and two days of magazine training, all animals were trained to nosepoke via a simple free operant procedure, in which nosepoking was reinforced with 4 s access to an evaporated milk reinforcer on a response-initiated fixed-interval 20 s (FI20) schedule. The illumination of the nosepoke recess and houselight (light or dark) was counterbalanced across animals in each genotype, with the lights either on or off throughout the 40 min session. No reinforcement was delivered without a nosepoke. Animals were trained to a criterion, requiring them to obtain 40 reinforcers across two consecutive sessions, after which mice received one additional session of FI20 training.

Discrimination training. Discrimination training sessions followed completion of initial instrumental training. Discrimination sessions were also 40 min in duration, presenting the animals with both potentially reinforced and unreinforced periods, indicated by the illumination state of the nosepoke recess (the houselight was not used during this phase). The light condition presented in initial training indicated the reinforced state, such that animals were required to learn to avoid responding in the novel, unreinforced stimulus condition. No other source of illumination was utilized during discrimination training. Discrimination sessions consisted of 30 min of potentially reinforced time presented pseudorandomly in blocks of 30, 60, 90, 120 or 150 s, interspersed with 10 min of unreinforced time presented pseudorandomly in blocks of 10, 20, 30 or 60 s. Nosepoking was reinforced during the potentially reinforced periods on a response-initiated VI5 schedule with 3 s of access to the milk reinforcer, whereas nosepoking during the unreinforced period had no programmed consequence.

Discrimination performance was indexed by a discrimination ratio calculated by dividing the response rate in the reinforced condition by the sum of the response rates in the reinforced and the unreinforced conditions for each mouse for each session.

7. Tissue collection

Cortical and striatal tissues were dissected from naïve animals from the R6/2×TG2 KO line (n = 5–7 per genotype per sex, 12 weeks of age) and from the zQ175×TG2 KO line (n = 3–6 per genotype per sex, 52 weeks of age zQ175_HOM animals were not included). Tissues were kept frozen until processing. Half of the cortex and the striatal tissues were used for real time qPCR analysis. The other half cortex from the R6/2×TG2 KO line and the cortex and striatum from the zQ175×TG2 KO line were used in the aggregation assay. For *ex-vivo* MRI studies, a second cohort of naïve mice from the R6/2×TG2 line and the mice from zQ175×TG2 KO line tested in the procedural water T-maze test were perfused at 16 and 52 weeks of age respectively (Table 1 and Table 2). In brief, mice were killed by deep anesthesia with pentobarbital and transcardially perfused with 80 ml of heparinized (2.5 units/ml) saline followed by 80 ml of ice-cold 4% PFA in 0.1M PBS. Brains within skull were postfixed in the same fixative overnight and stored in solution of 0.01% sodium azide in 0.1M PBs at 4°C. Before the *ex-vivo* T2-MRI analysis of the brains, brains were rinsed with saline and embedded in perfluoropolyether (FOMBLIN).

8. Quantification of transcripts

Quantification of transcripts was performed as described previously by Menalled et al, [21]. The sample size used for each cross is presented in Table 1 and Table 2. A summary of the steps followed is described below.

Total RNA Extraction. Total mRNA was extracted using RNeasy 96 Universal Tissue Kit for RNA isolation (Cat # 74881, Qiagen, Valencia, CA). Total RNA bound to column membranes was then treated with RNase-Free DNase set (Cat # 79254, Qiagen, Valencia, CA), followed by washing steps with RW1 and RPE buffers (provided with RNeasy 96 Universal Tissue Kit). RNA was eluted with RNase-Free water.

Total RNA Quantification and Reverse Transcription. To investigate the integrity of the RNA, 2 µL of total RNA was run in 1% agarose gel. RNA was quantified using Quan-iT RiboGreen RNA Kit (Cat # R11490, Invitrogen, Carlsbad, CA) and analyzed with the SpectraMax Gemini XPS fluorescent plate reader (Molecular Devices, Sunnyvale, CA). Following the protocol previously described [21], one microgram of total RNA was reverse transcribed into cDNA.

Quantitative PCR (qPCR). Five microliters of the diluted cDNA were amplified with 12.5 µL 2× FastStart Universal Probe Master Rox (Cat # 04914058001, Roche Applied Science, Indianapolis, IN), 0.5 µL Universal Probe Library Probe (Roche Applied Science, Indianapolis, IN), 200 nM of gene specific primer- HPLC purified (Sigma-Aldrich, St. Louis, MO) in 25 µL reaction volume. The reactions were run on the ABI 7900HT Sequence Detection System (Applied Biosystems, Foster City, CA). qCPR conditions were 95°C for 10 min for activation of FastStart Taq DNA Polymerase followed by 40 cycles of 95°C for 15 seconds and 60°C for 1 minute. For primers and Universal Probe Library used for qPCR refer to Table 3).

qPCR Data Analysis. cDNAs from multiple reverse transcription reactions were pooled together and used to create qPCR standard curves and also served as a calibrator to normalize plate to plate variations. To generate the standard curve, pooled cDNA was serially diluted from 1:5 to 1:1000 in RNase-free water and assayed in triplicate in each qPCR assay. The Ct values, number of cycles required for the PCR amplicon detection to reach threshold, were plotted against the logarithm value of dilution samples and a linear trend line was obtained for each gene. Each sample cDNA (diluted 1:10) was assayed in triplicates and the Ct values averaged. Values which lie greater than 0.5 standard deviation of the average were discarded. Relative quantity of the PCR product (relative to the calibrator), the geometric means for the 3 housekeeping genes and the relative levels of the target genes were calculated as previously described [21]. *Atp5b*, *Eif4a2* and *Ubc* were used as housekeeping genes for the striatal analysis in the R6/2×TG2 KO study. *Atp5b*, *Eif4a2* and *Gadph* were used in the cortical analysis in the R6/2 CAG×TG2 KO study and in the striatal analysis of the zQ175×TG2 KO study. The relative level of the target gene was then normalized to age- and sex-matched wild type control animals.

9. Tissue preparation and quantitative western blotting

Frozen tissues were homogenized in ice cold modified RIPA buffer (50 mM Tris HCl, pH 7.5, 1% IGEPAL CA630, 0.25% SDS, 150 mM NaCl, 1 mM EDTA, 1 mM NaF, 100 mM activated Na2VO3 and Roche Applied Science's Complete Protease Inhibitor cocktail) using 500 µL per 100 mg of tissue with TissueLyser (Qiagen, Valencia, CA) and 5 mm stainless steel beads (Cat # 69989, Qiagen, Valencia, CA). Once tissues were disrupted, samples were allowed to incubate on ice for 30 min. The homogenates were then centrifuged at 10,000RPM (Eppendorf 5417R centrifuge) for 30 min at 4°C. The protein content was determined using BioRad's DC Assay Kit (Cat # 5000111, Bio-Rad, Hercules, CA).

Protein samples were denatured in Laemmli buffer (Cat # 1610737, Bio-Rad, Hercules, CA)/2-Mercapthoethanol (Cat # M3148, Sigma-Aldrich, St. Louis, MO) for 5 min at 95°C for TG2 and housekeeping proteins. Ten micrograms of denatured protein samples were separated by 4–20% SDS-PAGE Criterion Gels (Cat # 3450034, Bio-Rad, Hercules, CA). After electrophoresis, proteins were transferred from gel to Hybond-LFP PVDF membranes (Cat # RPN303LFP, GE Healthcare Bioscience, Piscataway, NJ) by electroblotting. The protein-PVDF membranes were rinsed briefly in 1× Tris-buffered saline with 0.1% Tween 20 (TBST). Non-specific binding was blocked with 5% dried milk in TBST for 1 hr. After a brief rinse in TBST, the blots were probed with primary antibody prepared with 1% dried milk in TBST for 1 h at RT. Protein-PVDF blots were washed 1×15 min followed by 3×5 min washes with TBST. Protein-PVDF blots were then incubated with secondary antibody prepared with 1% dried milk in TBST (see Table 4 for dilution) for 1 h at RT. Protein-PVDF blots were washed 1×15 min followed by 1×5 min.

Antibody binding was detected using ECL Plus Western Detection Kit (Cat # RPN2133, GE Healthcare Bioscience, Piscataway, NJ) with a Typhoon 9410 scanner (GE Healthcare Bioscience, Piscataway, NJ) using 457 nm blue laser for excitation and 520 nm emission filter at 400 V.

qWestern data analysis. Total protein from whole brain of C57BL6 mice was isolated and denatured at specific concentrations as described above. These denatured protein aliquots (of the same protein amount as target protein) served as calibrator to normalized the gel to gel variations.

The scanned images from the Typhoon were analyzed with ImageQuantTL software version 7.0 (GE Healthcare Bioscience, Piscataway, NJ), band intensities were determined using the rolling ball methods, file with band intensities was exported to EXCEL

Table 3. Quantitative Polymerase Chain Reaction (qPCR) information.

Mouse Gene ID	5′ Primer Sequence	3′ Primer Sequence	Universal Probe Library #
Bdnf II	CCGGAGAGCAGAGTCCATT	CTACCACCTCGGACAAATCC	21
Bdnf IV	GCTGCCTTGATGTTTACTTTGA	AAGGATGGTCATCACTCTTCTCA	31
Bdnf IX	GCCTTTGGAGCCTCCTCTAC	GCGGCATCCAGGTAATTTT	67
Cnr1	GGGCAAATTTCCTTGTAGCA	GGCTCAACGTGACTGAGAAA	79
Drd1a	AGGTTGAGCAGGACATACGC	TGGCTACGGGGATGTAAAAG	88
Drd2	TGAACAGGCGGAGAATGG	CTGGTGCTTGACAGCATCTC	17
Darpp32	CCACCCAAAGTCGAAGAGAC	GCTAATGGTCTGCAGGTGCT	98
Pde10A	GAAGGCTGACCGAGTGTTTC	GGGATGGAGAGAAAGATAGGC	45
Glt1	GGTCATCTTGGATGGAGGTC	ATACTGGCTGCACCAATGC	83
Htt	TCTCATCAACCACACTGACCA	GGGGGTTAAGTGCTTCGTG	77
Atp5b	GGCACAATGCAGGAAAGG	TCAGCAGGCACATAGATAGCC	77
Gadph	CAATGTGTCCGTCGTGGATCT	GTCCTCAGTGTAGCCCAAGATG	N/A
Eif4A2	GCCAGGGACTTCACAGTTTC	TTCCCTCATGATGACATCTCTTT	93
Ubc	GACCAGCAGAGGCTGATCTT	CCTCTGAGGCAGAAGGACTAA	11

for further analysis. Within each image all the raw data values of the band intensities were corrected with band intensity from calibrator, this value was referred as corrected relative quantity, calculation as follows:

Corrected Relative Quantity of Target Protein =
$(\text{Raw Data Value}^{\text{Target}})/(\text{Raw Data Value}^{\text{calibrator}})$

Corrected Relative Quantity of Housekeeping Protein 1 =
$(\text{Raw Data Value}^{\text{housekeeping1}})/(\text{Raw Data Value}^{\text{calibrator}})$

Corrected Relative Quantity of Housekeeping Protein 2 =
$(\text{Raw Data Value}^{\text{housekeeping2}})/(\text{Raw Data Value}^{\text{calibrator}})$

Corrected Relative Quantity of Housekeeping Protein 3 =
$(\text{Raw Data Value}^{\text{housekeeping3}})/(\text{Raw Data Value}^{\text{calibrator}})$

Geometric mean for the three housekeeping protein was calculated as follows:

Geometric mean = (relative quantity of housekeeping protein 1*

relative quantity of housekeeping protein 2*

relative quantity of housekeeping protein 3)$^{(1/3)}$

Relative level of target protein (TG2 and endogenous HTT) was calculated as follows:

Relative Level of Target Protein = Corrected Relative Quantity of Target Protein/Geometric mean of housekeeping Proteins

Relative level of target gene was then normalized to that of wild type (gender combined).

10. Measurement of polyQ aggregates by Seprion ligand ELISA

A 2.5% lysate was prepared with the dissected cerebral cortex from 12 week-old R6/2×TG2 KO and 52- week-old zQ175×TG2 KO (Table 1 and Table 2) in ice-cold RIPA buffer by ribolysing in lysis matrix tubes 2×30 sec at RT (Lysing matrix D; MP Biomedicals, Solon, OH) and transferring to ice for 3–

Table 4. Quantitative Western Blots Antibody information.

Mouse Gene ID	Vendor	Catalog #	Host	Antibody Dilution
TG2	Cell Signaling Technology	3557S	rabbit	1:500
ATP5B	Abcam	ab14730	mouse	1:10000
EIF4A2	Abcam	ab31218	rabbit	1:10000
GAPDH	Cell Signaling Technology	2118	rabbit	1:10000
Anti-Rabbit IgG conjugated to HRP	Cell Signaling Technology	7074	Goat	1:1000
Anti-Mouse IgG conjugated to HRP	Cell Signaling Technology	7076	Goat	1:1000

5 min to cool before the last 30 sec ribolysing. Lysates were centrifuged at 13,000 rpm for 2 min in a microfuge before they were transferred to a fresh tube on ice. Samples either used immediately or frozen on dry ice and stored at −80°C and used within 24 h.

Homogenate (15 μl) was mixed with 3 μl 10% SDS followed by 62 μl water and made up to 100 μl with 20 μl of 5× capture buffer (Microsens Biotechnologies, UK). This was transferred to the well of a Seprion ligand-coated ELISA plate (SEP1-96-01) and incubated for 1 h at 23°C. The lysate was removed and the well was washed 5× in PBS-T (PBS; 0.1% Tween) and 100 ml S830 primary antibody (diluted 1:2000 in conjugate buffer (150 mM NaCl; 4% BSA (98% electrophoretic grade); 1% dried milk; 0.1% Tween 20 in PBS) was added and incubated with shaking for 1 h at 23°C. The washing step was repeated and 100 μl horse radish peroxidase (HRP)-conjugated rabbit anti-goat secondary antibody (DAKO, Denmark) (1:2000 in conjugation buffer) was added and incubated for 45 min at 23°C. The washing step was repeated and 100 μl of TMB substrate (SerTec) (warmed to 23°C) was added and incubated in the dark at RT for 30 min. Reactions were terminated by the addition of 100 μl 0.5 M HCl and the absorption at 450 nm was measured using a plate reader (Biorad, UK).

11. *Ex vivo* T2-MRI

MRI acquisitions from the brains collected from animals from the R6/2×TG2 KO cross (Table 1) were performed using a horizontal 7 T magnet with bore size 200 mm (Bruker Biospin GmbH, Karlsruhe, Germany) equipped with Bruker BGS12-S gradient set (max. gradient strength 760 mT/m, bore 120 mm) interfaced to a Bruker PharmaScan console (Bruker Biospin GmbH, Karlsruhe, Germany) using a volume coil for transmission and surface coil for receiving (Bruker Biospin GmbH, Germany). T2-weighted MRI acquisitions from the brains collected from the animals from the zQ175×TG2 KO cross (Table 2), were performed with the use of a horizontal 7 T magnet with inner bore diameter of 160 mm (Magnex Scientific Ltd., Oxford, UK) equipped with actively shielded Magnex gradient set (max. gradient strength 400 mT/m, bore 100 mm) interfaced to a Varian DirectDrive console. Linear RF volume-coil was used for transmission and surface phased array coil for receiving (Rapid Biomedical GmbH, Rimpar, Germany).

In all cases, for ex vivo determination of total brain, striatal and cortical volumes, T2-weighted continuous multi-slice images covering the whole brain (number of slices, 21) were acquired using fast spin-echo sequence with TR = 4500 ms, echo train length ETL = 4, effective TE = 37.7 ms, matrix size of 512×256 (zeropadded to 512×512), FOV of 30*30 mm2, and a slice thickness of 0.6 mm, 4 averages. The acquired coronal images were analyzed for total brain, striatal and cortical volumes using an analysis program ran under MatLab [22].

12. Statistical analysis

Body weight, PhenoCube and Go/No go test data were evaluated using repeated measures analysis carried out with SAS (SAS Institute Inc.) using Mixed Effect Models, based on the likelihood estimation. The models were fitted using the procedure PROC MIXED [26]. Main effects of HD Genotype, TG2 Genotype, sex as well as age, day/night cycle, light/dark training condition, testing day (as appropriate) were evaluated and their interactions were considered in all the models. Significant interactions followed up with simple main effects.

In Go/No go the mean number of days to reach criterion in initial training, as well as the mean of the response rates from the final four discrimination sessions were similarly analyzed, but without the repeated measure of test day.

T-maze test. Data for acquisition were analyzed using Statview software (SAS Institute Inc.) with two-way ANOVA with the factors HD Genotype and TG2 Genotype. In addition, the proportion of mice acquiring the task each day was analyzed via Kaplan-Meier analysis. For reversal testing, data were analyzed via mixed two-way repeated-measures ANOVA with the between-subject factors HD Genotype and TG2 Genotype and Days as repeated measure.

Survival data was statistically analyzed via Kaplan-Meier analysis.

Protein expression, gene expression, and ex vivo T2-MRI data were evaluated using SAS Proc Mixed with no repeated statement and significant interactions followed up with simple main effects.

In all cases an effect was considered significant if $p < 0.05$.

All graphs, but body weight, represent data from male and female animals combined. Data are expressed as mean ± S.E.M.

Results

1. Characterization of transglutaminase 2 protein levels in R6/2×TG2 knockout line

In order to confirm that the TG2 expression levels were reduced both in the heterozygous (TG2+/−) and knockout (TG2−/−) mice, we performed western blotting on striatal lysates of 12-week-old mice from these crosses (Figure 1). No significant differences in the TG2 protein levels were detected between the WT and R6/2 mice. In the heterozygous TG2 animals, the protein level was approximately 50% of the wild type level, with a slightly lower protein level observed in the WTs compared to R6/2 mice (HD Genotype×TG2 Genotype interaction: $F_{(2,59)} = 8.51$, $p < 0.001$, simple main effects and post-hoc tests $ps < 0.05$). As expected no expression of TG2 protein was detected in the knockout animals (simple main effects and post hocs, $ps < 0.0001$).

2. TG2 depletion does not alter the body weight loss phenotype of R6/2 and zQ175 KI mice

R6/2×TG2 KO line. From the various sublines of R6/2 mice, we selected the R6/2 CAG 240 which while presenting robust deficits, offers a wider therapeutic window of intervention compared to the R6/2 CAG 110 or R6/2 CAG 160 lines [27–29] (manuscript in preparation). As expected from previous findings obtained from R6/2 animals carrying approximately 240 CAGs (manuscript in preparation, [27,28]), R6/2 mice were progressively lighter than WT controls from 6 and 7 weeks of age, for males and females respectively, although the effect was more pronounced in the males (Figure 2A–B; HD Genotype×Sex×Age interaction: $F_{(15, 2173)} = 11.02$, $p < 0.0001$; simple main effects: $ps < 0.05$). Total absence of TG2 protein resulted in a reduction in body weight, independent of R6/2 genotype or sex, which reached significance at 10, 11, 14–16 and 18–20 weeks of age, (TG2 Genotype×Age interaction: $F_{(15,2173)} = 98.52$, $p < 0.0001$; simple main effects and post hocs for ages: $ps < 0.05$).

zQ175×TG2 KO line. Consistent with the results in the R6/2 transgenic line, the zQ175 HET and, particularly, the zQ175 HOM were progressively lighter than the corresponding WT controls, with the effect being more pronounced in the males (Figure 2C–D, males and females, respectively). The effect in the males also reached significance at younger ages (29 and 26 weeks of age, for HET and HOM mice, respectively) than in the females (48 and 34 weeks of age, for zQ175 HET and HOM mice, respectively); HD Genotype×Sex×Age: $F_{(50,1475)} = 2.24$, $p < 0.0001$; simple main effects: $p < 0.05$). The TG2 KO male mice

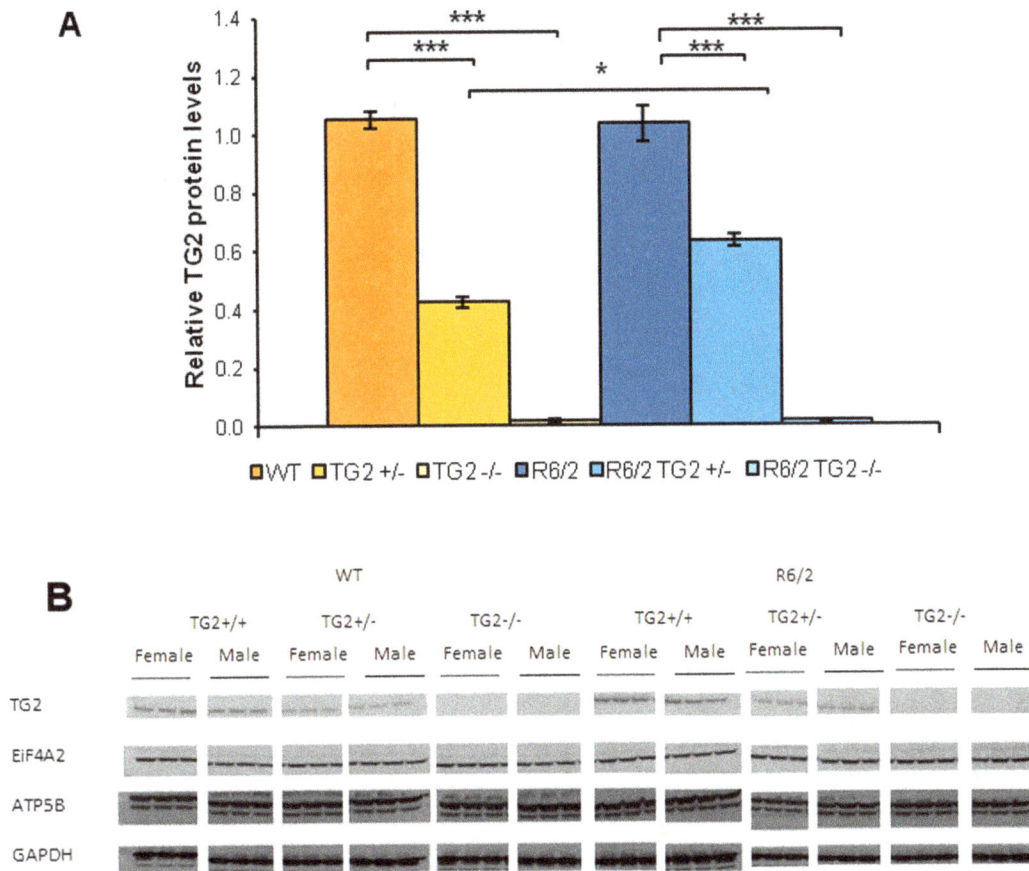

Figure 1. Transglutaminase 2 protein levels in R6/2×TG2 KO line. A. TG2 expression levels in the striatum of 12 week old animals from the R6/2×TG2 KO line (n = 11–12 per genotype). *$p < 0.05$,***$p < 0.0001$. See materials and methods' section for details regarding the calculation of TG2 protein expression levels. B. Westen blotting examples of striatal lysates of animals from the R6/2×TG2 KO line probed with antibodies that recognize TG2 and the housekeeping proteins.

presented a significantly increased body weight when compared to WT animals from 44 weeks of age (HD Genotype×TG2 Genotype×Sex×Age interaction: $F_{(50,1475)} = 3.28$, $p < 0.0001$; simple main effects and post-hocs, $ps < 0.05$).

3. TG2 depletion does not impact the survival of HD model mice

R6/2×TG2 KO line. WT mice had a normal life span during the period examined, regardless of the level of TG2 protein. The reduced lifespan characteristic of the R6/2 was not improved by the TG2 protein level (Mean survival ± S.E.M.: 18.85±0.43 weeks, 18.93±0.40 weeks and 17.42±0.45 weeks for the R6/2, R6/2 TG2+/−: and R6/2 TG2−/− respectively; Median survival: 17.71, 19.26 and 16.86 weeks for the R6/2, R6/2 TG2+/− and R6/2 TG2−/− respectively; HD Genotype log-rank test, $p < 0.0001$; TG2 Genotype log-rank test, $p > 0.8$).

zQ175×TG2 KO line. HOM and HET animals from the zQ175×TG2 cross displayed equivalent lifespan to the controls during the period examined (data not shown).

4. TG2 depletion does not improve the deficits detected in the R6/2 and zQ175 KI mice in PhenoCube System

R6/2×TG2 KO line. Overall visit frequency: R6/2 showed a progressive age-related decrease in activity when compared to

WTs in all the phases of the diurnal cycle with the exception of 8 week old mice during the light phase (Figure 3A; HD Genotype×Cycle×Age interaction: $F_{(2,319)} = 16.50$, $p < 0.0001$; simple main effects and post hocs, $ps < 0.05$). Both partial or complete reduction of the TG2 protein expression produced a decrease in overall visit frequency during the dark phase regardless of the status of the R6/2 transgene, mainly driven by male mice at 8 and 12 weeks of age (not shown, TG2 Genotype×Cycle interaction: $F_{(2, 177)} = 4.24$, $p < 0.05$, simple main effect and post hocs, $ps < 0.05$; TG2 Genotype×Age×Sex interaction: $F_{(4,301)} = 3.3$, $p < 0.05$; simple main effects and post hocs, $ps < 0.05$). As expected, mice displayed a marked increase in corner visit frequency during the dark versus light periods of the diurnal cycle irrespectively of the genotype (Cycle main effect: $F_{(1,133)} = 433.07$, $p < 0.0001$).

Mean path length: As previously observed [24], a progressive decrease in locomotion activity in the R6/2 mice was detected when compared to the WT animals (Figure 3B; HD Genotype× Age interaction: $F_{(2,36)} = 24.13$, $p < 0.0001$; simple main effect and post hocs, $ps < 0.05$). While all animals presented the expected higher levels of locomotion during the dark phase than light phase of the diurnal cycle, this was not observed in the R6/2 mice at 16 weeks of age (HD Genotype×Cycle×Age interaction: $F_{(2,36)} = 31.03$, $p < 0.0001$; simple main effect and post hocs, $ps <$

R6/2 x TG2 KO Line

zQ175 x TG2 KO Line

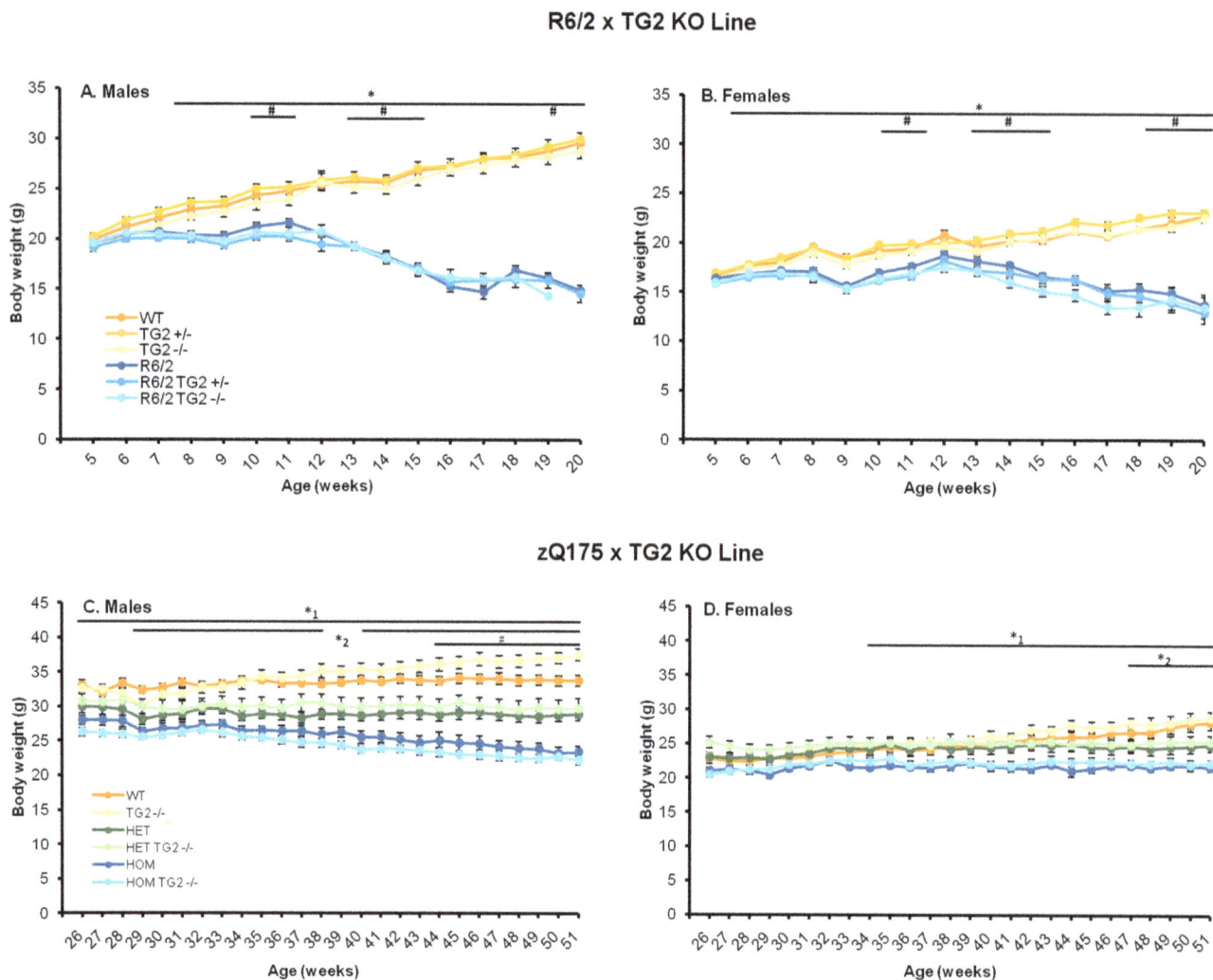

Figure 2. Body weight curves. A–B. Mean body weights of mice from the R6/2×TG2 KO line. A. Male mice (n = 14–16 per genotype). B. Female mice (n = 13–16 per genotype). C–D Mean body weights of mice from the zQ175×TG2 KO line. A. Male mice (n = 5–6 per genotype). B. Female mice (n = 6–7 per genotype). *Significant differences R6/2 vs WT,*[1] significant differences HOM vs WT, *[2] significant differences HET vs. WT, #significant TG2 genotype differences. WT: wild-type, TG2+/−: heterozygous TG2 knockout, TG2−/−: homozygous TG2 knockout, HET: zQ175 HET HOM: zQ175 HOM.

0.05). The partial or complete depletion of TG2 did not impact the animals' performance.

Percent alternations: R6/2 mice presented a decreased percent alternations between corners where water could be obtained (active corners) when compared to WT animals. This was observed both during the light and dark phases of the diurnal cycle, at 8 and 12 weeks of age, irrespectively of the TG2 expression level (Figure 3C; HD Genotype×Age×Cycle interaction: $F_{(1,141)} = 34.36$, p<0.0001; simple main effects and post hocs, ps<0.05). As expected, during the light phase WT mice presented a higher percentage of alternations than during the dark phase, regardless of the age (simple main effects and post hocs, ps<0.05). R6/2 mice, however, presented no differences in alternations during the light phase at 8 weeks of age (simple main effects and post hocs, ps<0.05). Interestingly, the percent alternations displayed by R6/2 at 12 weeks of age were below chance during the light phase. This is in alignment with an increased overall repeat visits observed in R6/2 animals in the same cycle period and age (data not shown). Surprisingly, the partial, but not the total, depletion of the TG2 protein increased alternations in R6/2

mice at 12 weeks of age, mainly in the male mice (HD Genotype×TG2 Genotype×Age interaction: $F_{(2,132)} = 3.34$, p< 0.05; TG2 Genotype×Sex interaction: $F_{(1,165)} = 3.25$, p<0.05; simple main effects and post hocs, ps<0.05). Data for this measure were not collected at 16 weeks of age since the alternation protocol was not used for R6/2 mice at this age, due to their reduced licking.

5. zQ175×TG2 KO line

Overall visit frequency: Both zQ175 HOM and HET mice showed a significantly decreased visit frequency when compared to the WT mice (Figure 4; HD Genotype main effect: $F_{(2,110)} = 6.72$, p<0.005). The absence of the TG2 protein produced a small but significant increase of activity in HOM male mice, in the dark phase of the cycle. In both female and male WT mice, the effect was, instead, a significant decrease, observed during both phases in females but only in the dark phase in males (HD Genotype×TG2 Genotype×Sex×Cycle interaction: $F_{(2,16)} = 4.11$, p<0.05; simple main effects and post hocs, ps<0.05). As expected, a marked increase in corner visit frequency during the dark versus the light

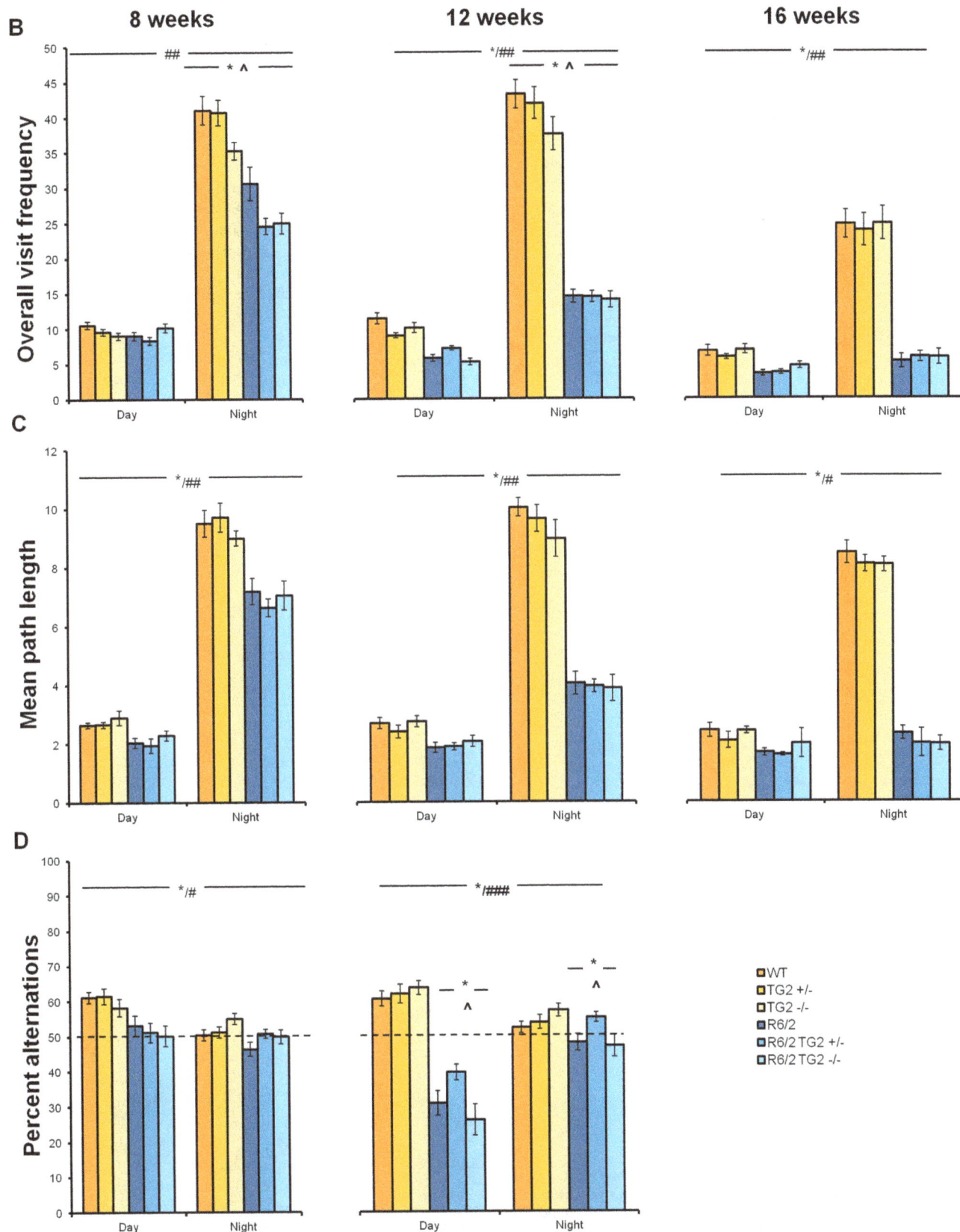

Figure 3. Behavioral data captured in the PhenoCube system as a function of genotype, age and light cycle phase in animals from the R6/2×TG2 KO line. A. Overall visit frequency. B. Mean path length. C. Percent alternations (Data for this measure were not collected at 16 weeks of age since R6/2 mice were not tested in this protocol due to reduced licking). *Significant HD genotype differences within each light phase, at each age; #: significant differences due to light phase in the diurnal cycle in the WT mice; ##significant differences due to light phase in the cycle

for each age independently of genotype; ###significant differences due to light phase in the diurnal cycle in the R6/2 mice; ^significant TG2 genotype differences. WT: wild-type, TG2+/−: heterozygous TG2 knockout, TG2−/−: homozygous TG2 knockout.

periods was observed in all mice regardless of the genotype and sex (Cycle main effect: $F_{(1,110)} = 802.22$, p<0.0001).

6. TG2 depletion does not improve the cognitive deficits of R6/2 and zQ175 KI mice

Procedural water T-maze test: R6/2×TG2 KO and zQ175×TG2 KO lines. The procedural water T-maze test allows the evaluation of cognitive abilities of animals. Mice were trained to find a submerged escape platform located in one of the arms of the T-maze without the aid of visual/light cues. Performance on this task is attributed primarily to striatal function.

R6/2×TG2 KO line: 14 weeks of age. Acquisition phase. R6/2 mice were impaired in the acquisition of the task relative to WT animals. A significantly lower proportion of R6/2 mice reached the acquisition performance criterion with successive days of training compared to WT mice (Figure 5A; Log Rank test, p< 0.05). Consequently, R6/2 required a significantly higher average number of days to reach the performance criterion relative to WT mice (Figure 5B; HD Genotype main effect: $F_{(1,123)} = 25.74$, p< 0.0001). The partial or complete depletion of TG2 protein had no impact on these features.

Reversal phase. Animals progressed to reversal testing on an individual basis once criterion was achieved in the acquisition phase. From the R6/2 TG2+/− mice, 2 mice did not reach criterion even after 10 days of training and therefore were not evaluated under the reversal conditions. Two out of 21 R6/2 TG2+/− mice and 3 out of 23 R6/2 TG2−/− mice that achieved criterion failed to complete 6 days of reversal testing due to requiring more than 6 days to meet criterion in the acquisition

phase; consequently, their data were excluded from the reversal phase. Performance in the reversal task phase improved over days of testing regardless of genotype although, as expected, R6/2 mice exhibited lower accuracy relative to WT mice as testing progressed, with R6/2 mice performing worse on each day of testing (Figure 6; HD Genotype×Session interaction: $F_{(5,590)} = 8.12$, p<0.0001). Notably, the complete absence of TG2 protein further impaired the performance of the R6/2 female mice (HD Genotype xTG2 Genotype×Sex interaction: $F_{(2,118)} = 4.90$, p<0.05: simple main effects and post hocs, p< 0.05). No effect of the partial or complete depletion of the TG2 protein was detected in the male group.

zQ175×TG2 KO line: 28–29 weeks of age. Acquisition phase. Although the zQ175 HOM required more days to reach criterion when compared to WT, this difference did not reach significance (Figure 7A–B). Consistent with the results in R6/2 mice, the complete ablation of TG2 did not impact the performance of the animals in this phase.

Reversal phase. Similar to R6/2 mice, zQ175 HOM mice exhibited impaired accuracy relative to WT, with WT mice improving in performance at a higher rate than zQ175 HOM mice (Figure 8, HD Genotype×Session interaction: $F_{(10,292)} = 3.36$, p<0.0001; simple main effects and post hocs, p<0.05). No deficits were detected in the performance of the HET mice. In agreement with our results in the R6/2×TG2 KO line, TG2 deletion significantly impaired performance on accuracy during reversal learning, in this line however, this effect was observed regardless of the zQ175 zygosity (TG2 Genotype main effect: $F_{(1,59)} = 4.29$, *p*< 0.05).

Go/No go discrimination task – zQ175×TG2 KO line. Since no cognitive deficits were detected in the zQ175 HET mice in the procedural water T-maze test, we extensively evaluated the HET mice in other assays focusing on executive function. Using a Go/No go discrimination task, we were able to uncover important cognitive deficits in discrimination learning and response inhibition in zQ175 HET mice (manuscript in preparation). For that reason we selected this assay to evaluate if TG2 ablation was able to modify the deficits observed in the zQ175 HET mice from 32 to 34 weeks of age.

Initial training. zQ175 HET mice required significantly more training sessions in order to achieve the response acquisition criterion of 40 reinforcers across two consecutive sessions (Figure 9; HD Genotype main effect: $F_{(1,31)} = 13.40$, p<0.001). The deletion of TG2 had no significant effect on this measure.

Discrimination ratio. zQ175 HET mice exhibited an impairment in discrimination performance relative to WT (Figure 10A; HD Genotype main effect: $F_{(1,31)} = 127.07$, p<0.0001). Moreover, WT, but not zQ175 HET, mice significantly improved in their discrimination performance over days of testing (HD Genotype× Session interaction: $F_{(17,515)} = 2.03$, p<0.005; simple main effect, ps<0.05). Deficits in discrimination performance in the HET mice were detected from session 4 onward (simple main effect, ps< 0.05). Interestingly, knockout TG2 mice performed better than TG2 wild type mice, regardless of zQ175 genotype (TG2 genotype main effect, $_{(1,32)} = 6.00$, p<0.05). There was also a significant interaction between light/dark condition and session, with mice trained with the stimulus light off for the reinforced condition performing better in the first session (Stimulus×Session interaction: $F_{(17,515)} = 1.95$, p<0.05; data not shown).

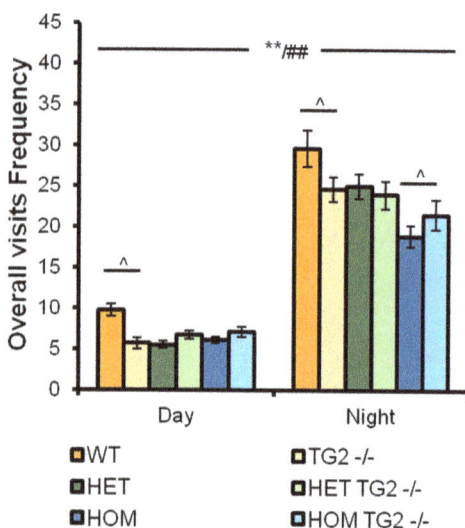

Figure 4. Overall visit frequency detected in the PhenoCube system as a function of genotype, age and light cycle phase in animals from the zQ175×TG2 KO line. *Significant HD genotype differences regardless of the light phase (in the mean path length the differences were detected between HET and WT animals); ##significant differences due to light phase in the cycle independently of genotype; ^significant TG2 genotype differences (see results method for details). WT: wild-type, TG2−/−: homozygous TG2 knockout, HET: zQ175 HET, HOM: zQ175 HOM.

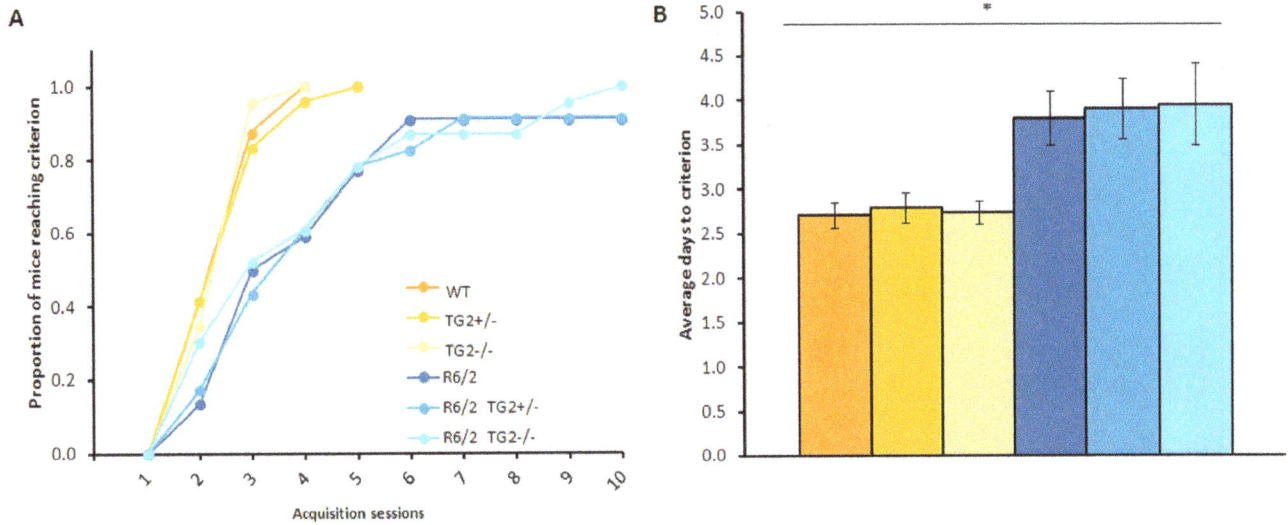

Figure 5. Acquisition of the procedural T-maze task (n = 20–24 per genotype). A. Proportion of mice acquiring the task on each test day. B. Average (±SEM) number of days to acquire the task (only animals that fulfill the acquisition criterion within 10 training days were included). *Significant HD genotype effect. WT: wild-type, TG2+/−: heterozygous TG2 knockout, TG2−/−: homozygous TG2 knockout.

Response per minute. WT mice preferentially responded at a higher rate to the reinforced stimulus, whereas zQ175 HET mice did not exhibit differential responses rates to the reinforced and unreinforced stimulus conditions (Figure 10B; HD Genotype×Reinforcement Condition interaction: $F_{(1,30)} = 47.88$, $p<0.0001$; simple main effects, $ps<0.05$). Accordingly, while zQ175 HET mice responded at a lower rate than WT mice during the reinforced condition, their response rate exceeded that of the WT mice in the unreinforced condition (simple main effects, $ps<0.05$). TG2 ablation did not affect any of these deficits observed in the HET mice.

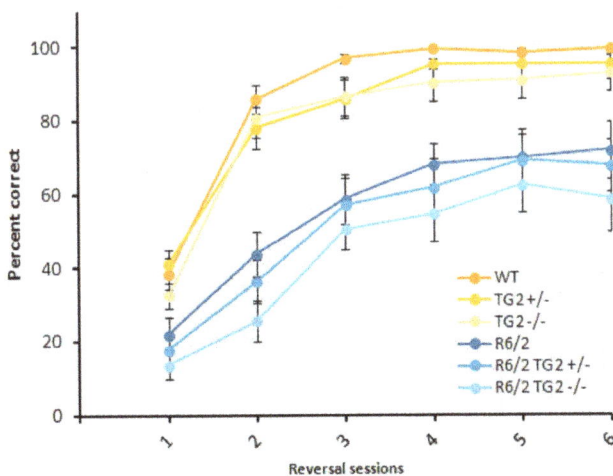

Figure 6. Reversal phase of the procedural T-maze task (platform location switched; n = 19–24 per genotype). The graph shows the mean (±SEM) percent correct for each group, on each test day. WT: wild-type, TG2+/−: heterozygous TG2 knockout, TG2−/−: homozygous TG2 knockout.

7. TG2 depletion does not modify the expression levels of dysregulated transcripts in brains of R6/2 and zQ175 KI mice

We examined whether the ablation of TG2 was able to ameliorate the dysregulation of genes that express key striatal neurotransmitter receptors and intracellular signalling molecules which have been found to be affected both in patients and in HD animal models (for a review see [30]). In addition, we examined whether the ablation of TG2 was able to ameliorate the decreased expression of brain-derived neurotrophic factor (*Bdnf*) which has also been found to be decreased in numerous HD mice and in human post-mortem tissue (for a review see [31]).

R6/2×TG2 KO line. Striatal markers. qPCR analysis revealed decreased expression of Drd2, Darpp32, Pde10a, Cnr1 and Glt1 mRNAs in the striatum of 12-week-old R6/2 mice when compared to age matched WT animals (Figure 11, left panels; HD Genotype main effects: $Fs_{(1,60)}>500.34$, $ps<0.0001$). The partial or complete absence of TG2 protein did not impact the deficits in the expression levels of those striatal markers in the R6/2 mice. However, in the WT mice, the knockout of TG2 produced a small but significant increase of Darpp32, Pde10a and Glt1 mRNA levels when compared to the heterozygous and wild type TG2 animals (HD Genotype×TG2 Genotype interaction: $Fs_{(2,60)}>3.605$, $p<0.05$; simple main effects and post hocs, $ps<0.05$).

Cortical markers. Cortical levels of the Bdnf isoforms examined, namely isoform II, IV and IX, were found to be significantly reduced in the R6/2 mice when compared to WT animals, irrespective of the TG2 protein level (Figure 11, right panels; HD Genotype main effect: $Fs_{(1,59)}>60.861$, $ps<0.0001$). Cortical mRNA levels of endogenous huntingtin (Htt) were also found to be decreased in R6/2 mice compared to WT animals (HD Genotype main effect, $Fs_{(1,59)}>6.825$, $ps<0.05$). The partial or total ablation of TG2 did not impact the deficits detected in the R6/2 animals in the cortical markers measured.

zQ175×TG2 KO line. Striatal markers. As expected [21], 52-week-old zQ175 HET mice presented a significant downregulation of Drd2, Darpp32, Pde10α, Cnr1 and Drd1a striatal mRNAs when compared to age matched WT animals (Figure 12;

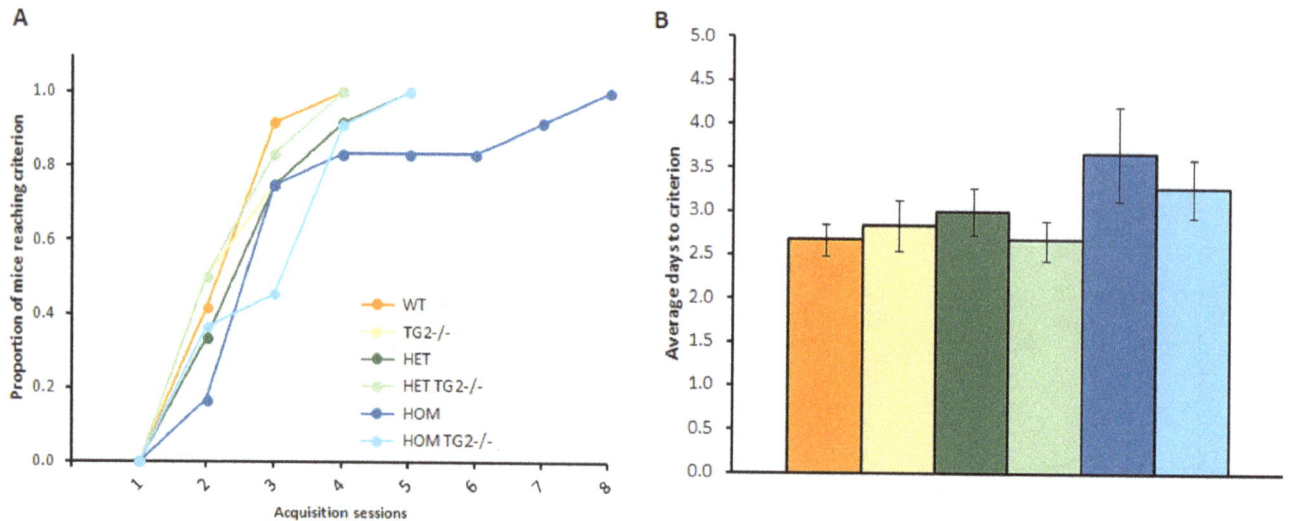

Figure 7. Acquisition of the procedural T-maze task in the zQ175×TG2 KO animals (n = 11–12, per genotype). A. Proportion of mice acquiring the task on each test day. B. Average (±SEM) number of days to acquire the task. WT: wild-type, TG2+/−: heterozygous TG2 knockout, TG2−/−: homozygous TG2 knockout, HET: zQ175 HET, HOM: zQ175 HOM.

HD Genotype main effect: $Fs_{(1,55)} > 144.62$, $ps < 0.0001$). The partial or complete depletion of TG2 protein did not impact the decreased expression of those transcripts.

8. TG2 depletion does not reduce aggregate load or attenuate brain atrophy in R6/2 and zQ175 KI mice

Using the Seprion ligand ELISA [32], we quantified the polyglutamine aggregate load in the cortex of 12-week-old animals from the R6/2×TG2 KO line and in cortex and striatum of 12-month-old heterozygous mice from the zQ175×TG2 KO line. The aggregate levels detected in the R6/2 were not impacted by the partial or total absence of TG2 protein (Figure 13A). In the zQ175 HET mice, we were unable to detect an aggregate signal in cortex at 12 months of age. The signal in striatum was comparatively low, but similar to the R6/2 results, the aggregate

levels detected in the zQ175 HET were not impacted by the partial or total depletion of TG2 protein (Figure 13B).

Using ex vivo T2-MRI analysis, we measured whole brain, striatal and cortical volumes in 16-week-old R6/2×TG2 KO animals and 52-week-old zQ175×TG2 KO animals (Figure 14).

Total brain, striatal and cortical volumes in R6/2 mice were significantly reduced when compared to the WTs, regardless of the TG2 protein level (Figure 14, top panels; HD Genotype main effect: $Fs_{(1,60)} > 90.578$, $ps < 0.0001$). Similarly, zQ175 HOM and HET mice presented significantly reduced brain volumes when compared to the WTs, regardless of the TG2 protein level (Figure 14, bottom panels; HD Genotype main effect: $Fs_{(2,60)} > 61.13$, $ps < 0.0001$; post hocs, $ps < 0.0001$). Also, in the zQ175 HOM mice those volumes were also significantly reduced when compared to the zQ175 HET mice (post hocs, $ps < 0.0001$). Whole brain and cortical volumes of females were significantly larger than those of males (not shown, Sex main effect: $F_{(1,60)} > 12.61$, $ps < 0.001$).

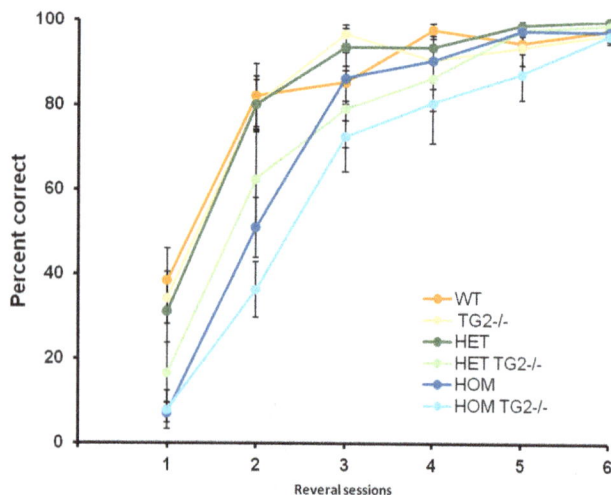

Figure 8. Reversal phase of the procedural T-maze task (platform location switched; n = 11–12 per genotype). WT: wild-type, TG2−/−: homozygous TG2 knockout, HET: zQ175 HET, HOM: zQ175 HOM.

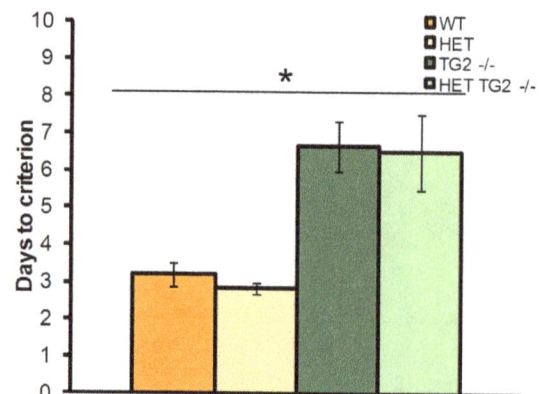

Figure 9. Mean number of days required to obtain 40 reinforcers across two consecutive sessions during the training phase (n = 6–12 per genotype). *Significant HD genotype effect. WT: wild-type, TG2−/−: homozygous TG2 knockout, HET: zQ175 HET.

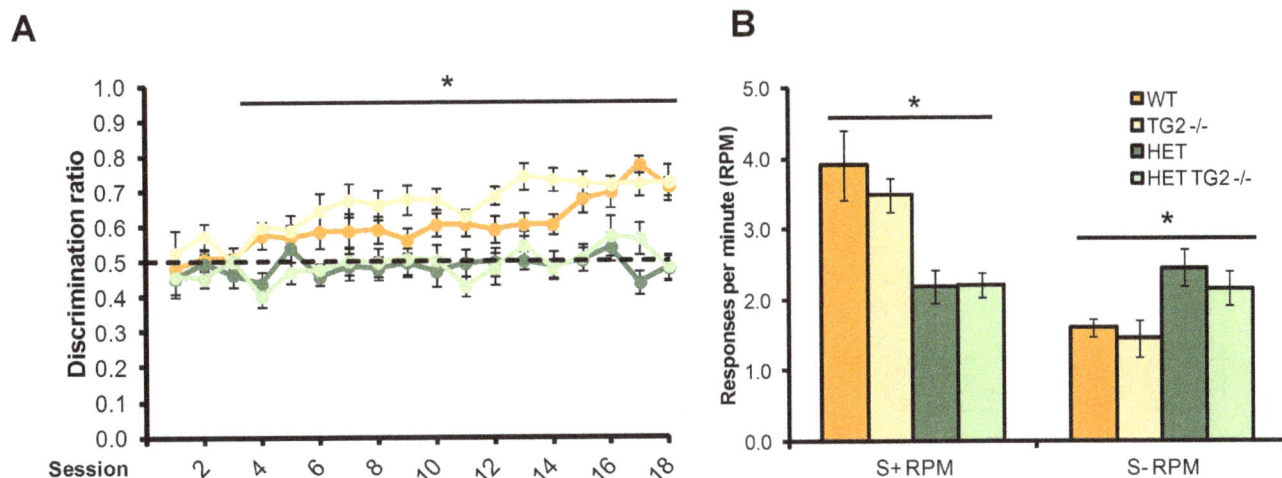

Figure 10. Discrimination performance (n = 6–12 per genotype). A. Discrimination ratio across the training period. B. Response rate for the reinforced (S+ RPM) and unreinforced (S- RPM) conditions averaged across the final four sessions for the zQ175×TG2 KO line. *Significant HD genotype effect. WT: wild-type, TG2−/−: homozygous TG2 knockout, HET: zQ175 HET.

Discussion

We employed a genetic deletion approach to further examine the possible role that TG2 plays in HD. A TG2 knockout line was crossed with both a transgenic and a knock-in mouse model of HD, the R6/2 and the zQ175 lines, respectively. We evaluated the resulting crosses using a behavioral testing battery under moderated level of environmental enrichment. In addition, we further examined the effect of the TG2 ablation using molecular and imaging techniques.

Surprisingly, we did not replicate the positive results previously reported by Bailey and Johnson using the R6/2 HD model [17]; they observed that the TG2 ablation extended the lifespan of R6/2 animals carrying 155–175 CAG repeats in a mixed background

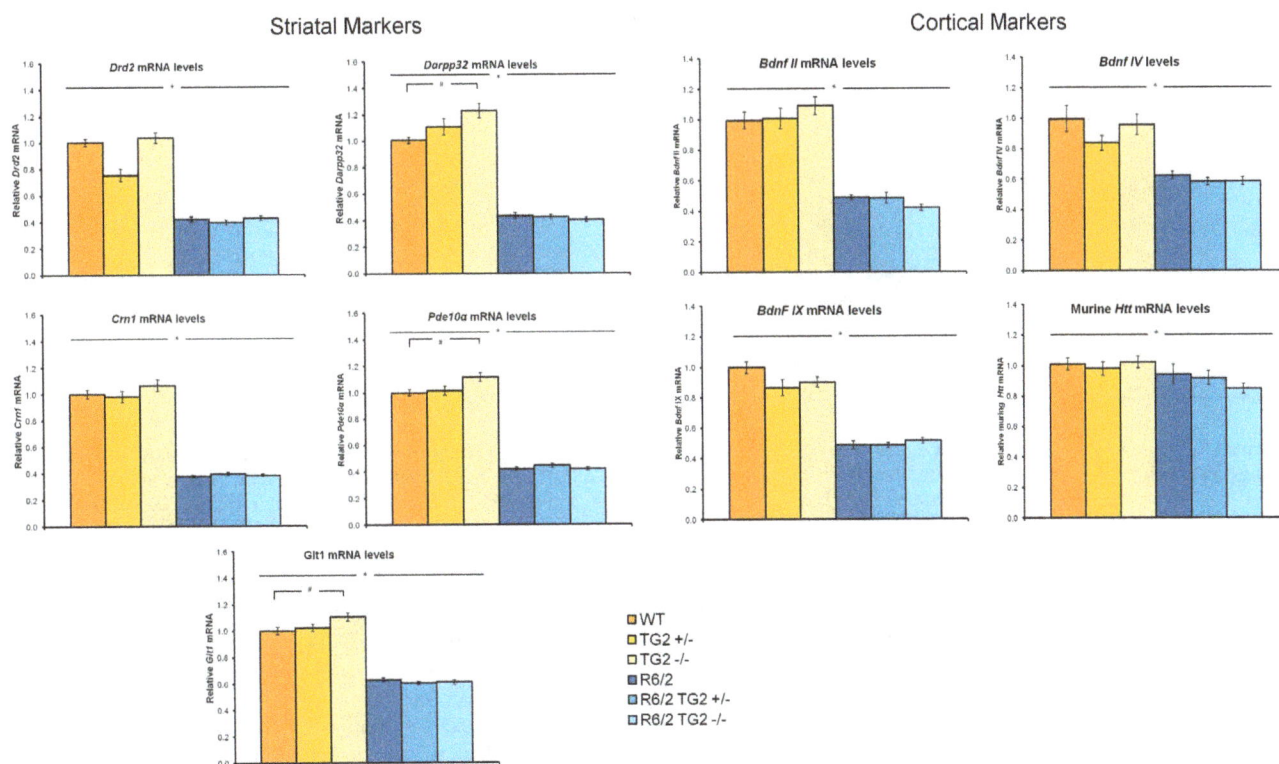

Figure 11. The relative striatal (left panels) and cortical (right panels) mRNA expression level of mice examined from the R6/2×TG2 KO line at 12 weeks of age (n = 12 per genotype). Relative mRNA levels are normalized to WT controls. For normalization, the geometric means of *Ubc*, *Eif4a2* an *Atp5b* were used. *Significant HD Genotype effect; #significant TG2 Genotype effect. WT: wild-type, TG2+/−: heterozygous TG2 knockout, TG2−/−: homozygous TG2 knockout.

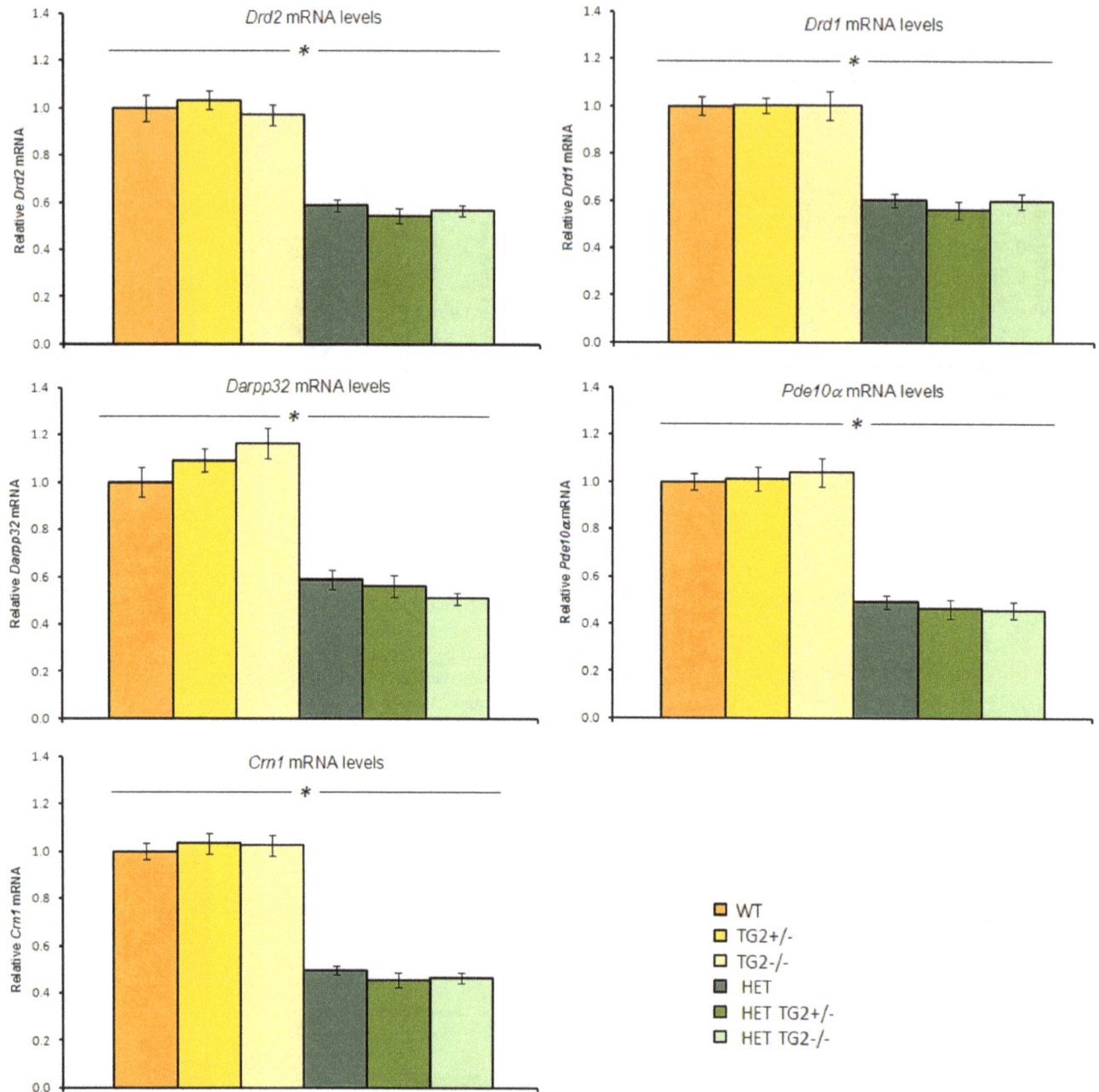

Figure 12. The relative striatal mRNA expression level of mice examined from the zQ175×TG2 KO line at 12 months of age (n = 7–12 per genotype). Relative mRNA levels are normalized to zQ175_WT TG2_WT controls. For normalization, the geometric means of *Ubc*, *Eif4a2* an *Atp5b* were used. *Significant HD Genotype effect. WT: wild-type, TG2+/−: heterozygous TG2 knockout, TG2−/−: homozygous TG2 knockout, HET: zQ175 HET.

strain [17,33], similar to results obtained with an R6/1 line [16] (see table S1 for a comparison of present results to the ones previously described). However, we were unable to replicate the increased lifespan when using R6/2 mice carrying 232–272 CAG repeats in a congenic C57BL/6J strain. It is well established that R6/2 mice carrying approximately 240 CAG repeats have a longer life span than those carrying approximately 150 CAG repeats [28,29]. It is possible that the previous report of increased survival in R6/2 mice after TG2 ablation could be modulated by the CAG repeat of the model studied. Another possible explanation as to why we did not see difference in R6/2 survival

after TG2 ablation may be because of the housing conditions utilized in our study, which have been shown previously to improve survival [34,35]. Since our goal is to uncover robust targets for HD, we provided the animals with a moderate enriched environment (namely: group housing, a range of bedding, plastic bones and tunnels) as well as easy access to food and water. These husbandry conditions produce survival data that more accurately reflects mortality due to the mutation rather than malnourishment or dehydration consequence of the motor deterioration [34]. When husbandry conditions are optimized, disease pathology is better isolated allowing more stringent evaluation of potential

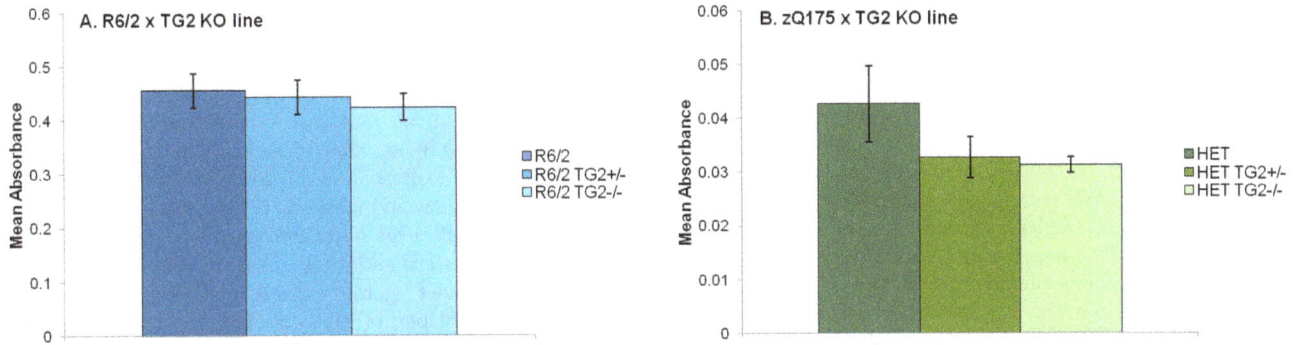

Figure 13. Seprion ligand quantification of aggregate load. A. Aggregate load in cortical tissues from 12-week-old R6/2×TG2 KO mice. The background readings obtained from the WT animals (n=3 per group) were averaged and subtracted from the readings obtained from the R6/2 animals in order to remove the baseline reading. B. Aggregate load in striatal tissues from 52-week-old zQ175×TG2 KO mice. The readings obtained from the zQ175_WT animals (n=5–7 per group) were averaged and subtracted from the readings obtained from the zQ175_HET animals in order to remove the baseline reading. WT: wild-type, TG2+/−: heterozygous TG2 knockout, TG2−/−: homozygous TG2 knockout, HET: zQ175 HET.

therapies. It is under these husbandry conditions that the ablation of TG2 failed to improve the survival of R6/2 animals. Survival analysis was not performed on the TG2×zQ175 cross since the results obtained did not warrant this long term study [21].

In our hands, TG2 ablation also did not to delay the onset of, or otherwise ameliorate, the robust locomotor deficits detected by the PhenoCube system, an automated and high throughput platform that allows unbiased evaluation of animal behavior [36]. Using a constant speed rotarod protocol, Bailey and Johnson observed a

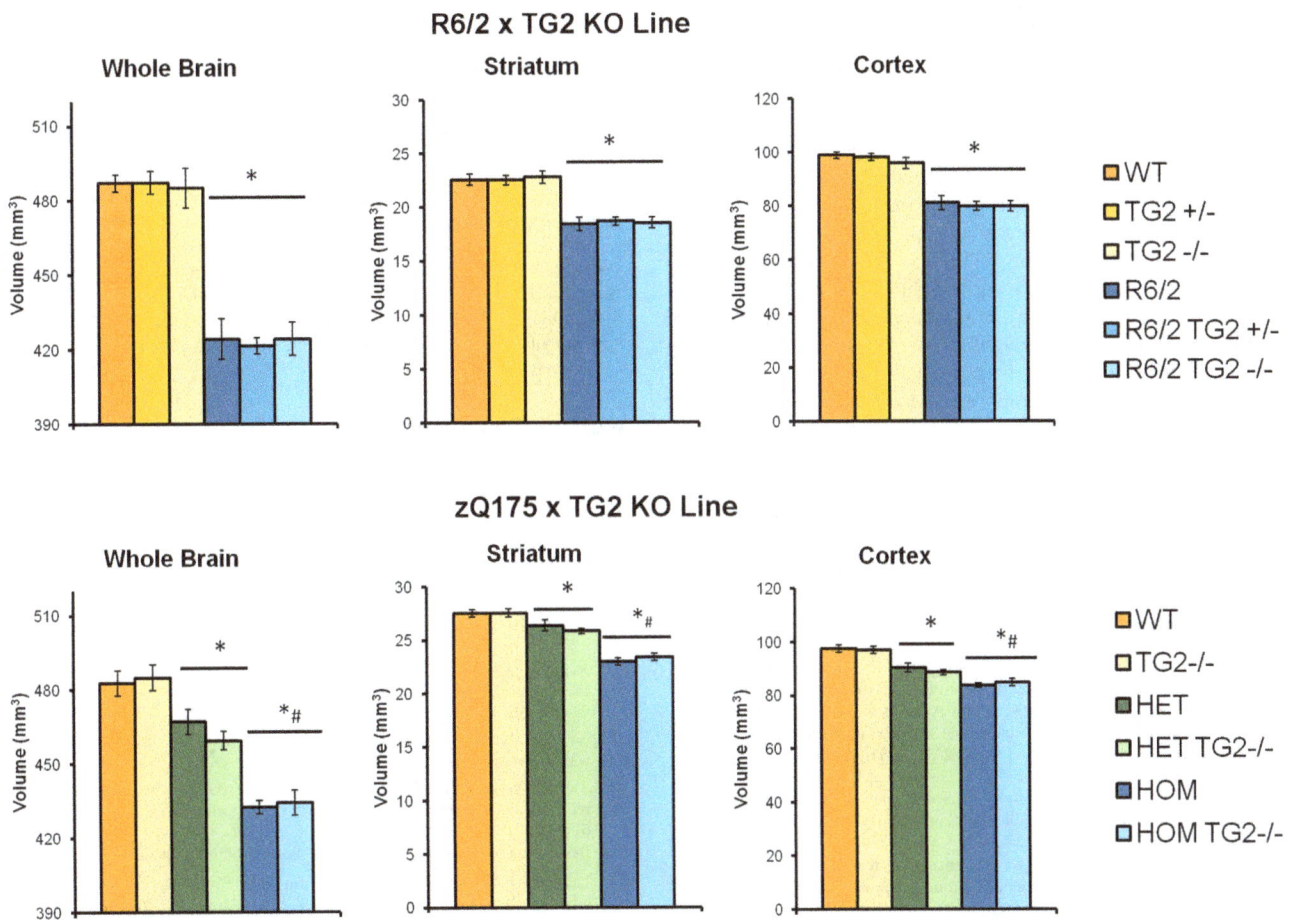

Figure 14. Whole brain, striatal and cortical volumes of 16-week-old R6/2×TG2 KO mice (top panels, n=6 per genotype per sex) and of 52-weeks-old zQ175×TG2 KO mice (bottom panels, n=6 per genotype per sex). *Significant differences compared to WT animals, #significant differences compared to HET mice. WT: wild-type, TG2+/−: heterozygous TG2 knockout, TG2−/−: homozygous TG2 knockout, HET: zQ175 HET, HOM; zQ175HOM.

delay in the onset of motor dysfunction produced after TG2 ablation, an improvement that did not translate to their ambulatory observations [17], in agreement with our results. Given the burden of cognitive decline for HD patients and their caregivers, a long term goal has been to utilize robust cognitive tests (especially those focusing on cognitive flexibility) that could be used to evaluate the effectiveness of therapies or validity of targets in mouse models. We therefore examined the ability of TG2 ablation to reverse the deficits detected in the procedural T-maze in R6/2 and zQ175 homozygous mice, as well as in the Go/No-go discrimination/response inhibition assay in zQ175 heterozygous mice, but we did not see beneficial effects. Different tests are required due to milder cognitive deficits observed in the HET mice in the T-maze at 28–29 weeks of age.

Interestingly, the TG2 ablation in R6/2 and R6/1 mice was reported to increase the number of HTT aggregates or neurons presenting aggregates, respectively [16,17]. While this was originally unexpected, *in vitro* studies have suggested that aggregates can be formed independently of TG2 through polar zippers [37,38]. Furthermore, TG2 knockout mice present impaired autophagy and an accumulation of ubiquitinated protein aggregates [39]. We did not detect an increase in aggregate load in either of the mouse models examined after TG2 ablation. TG2 has been associated with the presence of nuclear actin-cofilin stress rods in cells expressing mutant huntingtin [40]. While we did not monitor for these 'cofilin rods' in the brains of the TG2 KO crosses, the lack of amelioration of any disease phenotype in these animals suggests that TG2 activity is either not required for the formation of these rods in a physiological context, or that these rods are not relevant to disease progression in the R6/2 and zQ175 HD models. It is possible that the huntingtin aggregate burden in 12 week-old R6/2 and 52 week-old zQ175 mice prevented the detection of a minor aggregate load differences due to a ceiling effect. This seems less likely for the zQ175 mice as the Seprion signal is still relatively low at this age in the tissues examined. Alternatively, the differences with the some of the previously published studies regarding the aggregate levels may be related to the antibodies used. In the Seprion ligand-ELISA assay we used antibodies recognizing the N-terminal portion of human huntingtin protein that have been previously shown to stain HTT inclusion bodies in mouse brain tissue as well as detect oligomeric, proto-fibrillar and fibrillar aggregates using electron microscopy, atomic force microscopy (AFM) and sodium dodecyl sulphate–polyacrylamide gel electrophoresis [32,41]. Future studies will examine the role of TG2 in regulating autophagic responses in HD by investigating levels of autophagy markers such as p62 and autophagosomes as well as specifically tracking ubiquinated forms

of HTT and other proteins that are predicted to accumulate in TG2 KO mice [39].

TG2 inhibition by a novel peptide, ZDON, has been shown to normalize around 40% of the genes dysregulated in HdhQ111 immortalized striatal neurons [42]. Our data showed that TG2 ablation in the HD mouse models examined had no effect on the downregulation of expression of the group of genes examined. In agreement with Bailey and Johnson [17], we also found that TG2 ablation did not affect the histopathological endpoints examined, namely striatal, cortical and whole brain volumes.

In summary, under rigorous experimental conditions we found that the genetic ablation of TG2 does not ameliorate the disease phenotype, including physiological, molecular, neuropathological and behavioral markers in two different HD mouse models. Supporting our results, the overexpression of TG2 in R6/2 mice also did not modify the disease phenotype [43], raising additional questions about the role of TG2 activity in HD. The results of our genetic target validation work with a transglutaminase 2 null gene on the background of 2 different mouse models of HD do not support a therapeutic path aimed at TG2 inhibition for the treatment of HD.

Supporting Information

Figure S1 Graphical depiction of cage plan and water access protocol during Habituation and Alternation phases. Shaded circles signal the armed receptacles (NP: Nosepoke).

Table S1 Effect of TG2 deletion on HD mouse models: comparison of present results to previously published ones.

Acknowledgments

We wish to thank Dr Graham (Victor Chang Cardiac Research Institute, Australia) for providing the TG2 knockout animals; Brenda Lager and Simon Noble (CHDI Foundation) for the support in the generation of the experimental animals and for helpful comments on manuscript draft, respectively.

Author Contributions

Conceived and designed the experiments: DM IMS D. Howland SR LP DB AG GB AK SO LM NP. Performed the experiments: PT KL SM MK MO JB JT JF KC KM MM D. He GO RAN. Analyzed the data: RM AK LM AF GB SO IF NP PT KL. Wrote the paper: LM D. Howland DM IMS.

References

1. Greenberg CS, Birckbichler PJ, Rice RH (1991) Transglutaminases: multifunctional cross-linking enzymes that stabilize tissues. FASEB J 5: 3071–3077.
2. Im MJ, Riek RP, Graham RM (1990) A novel guanine nucleotide-binding protein coupled to the alpha 1-adrenergic receptor. II. Purification, characterization, and reconstitution. J Biol Chem 265: 18952–18960.
3. Lai TS, Slaughter TF, Peoples KA, Hettasch JM, Greenberg CS (1998) Regulation of human tissue transglutaminase function by magnesium-nucleotide complexes. Identification of distinct binding sites for Mg-GTP and Mg-ATP. J Biol Chem 273: 1776–1781.
4. Hasegawa G, Suwa M, Ichikawa Y, Ohtsuka T, Kumagai S, et al. (2003) A novel function of tissue-type transglutaminase: protein disulphide isomerase. Biochem J 373: 793–803.
5. Mastroberardino PG, Farrace MG, Viti I, Pavone F, Fimia GM, et al. (2006) "Tissue" transglutaminase contributes to the formation of disulphide bridges in proteins of mitochondrial respiratory complexes. Biochim Biophys Acta 1757: 1357–1365.
6. Molberg O, McAdam S, Sollid L (2000) Role of tissue transglutaminase in celiac disease. Journal of Pediatric Gastroenterology & Nutrition 30: 232–240.
7. Mangala L, Mehta K (2005) Tissue Transglutaminase (TG2) in Cancer Biology. In: Mehta K, Eckert R, editors. Transglutaminases: the family of enzymes with diverse functions Basel: Karger. pp. 125–138.
8. Siegel M, Khosla C (2007) Transglutaminase 2 inhibitors and their therapeutic role in disease states. Pharmacol Ther 115: 232–245.
9. Tahri-Joutei A, Pointis G (1989) Developmental changes in arginine vasopressin receptors and testosterone stimulation in Leydig cells. Endocrinology 125: 605–611.
10. Bates GP, Jones L (2002) Huntington's disease Oxford: Oxford Universtity Press.
11. Lesort M, Chun W, Johnson GV, Ferrante RJ (1999) Tissue transglutaminase is increased in Huntington's disease brain. J Neurochem 73: 2018–2027.
12. Jeitner TM, Matson WR, Folk JE, Blass JP, Cooper AJ (2008) Increased levels of gamma-glutamylamines in Huntington disease CSF. J Neurochem 106: 37–44.
13. Karpuj MV, Garren H, Slunt H, Price DL, Gusella J, et al. (1999) Transglutaminase aggregates huntingtin into nonamyloidogenic polymers, and its enzymatic activity increases in Huntington's disease brain nuclei. Proc Natl Acad Sci U S A 96: 7388–7393.

14. Dedeoglu A, Kubilus JK, Jeitner TM, Matson SA, Bogdanov M, et al. (2002) Therapeutic effects of cystamine in a murine model of Huntington's disease. J Neurosci 22: 8942–8950.

15. Karpuj MV, Becher MW, Springer JE, Chabas D, Youssef S, et al. (2002) Prolonged survival and decreased abnormal movements in transgenic model of Huntington disease, with administration of the transglutaminase inhibitor cystamine. Nat Med 8: 143–149.

16. Mastroberardino PG, Iannicola C, Nardacci R, Bernassola F, De Laurenzi V, et al. (2002) 'Tissue' transglutaminase ablation reduces neuronal death and prolongs survival in a mouse model of Huntington's disease. Cell Death Differ 9: 873–880.

17. Bailey CD, Johnson GV (2004) Tissue transglutaminase contributes to disease progression in the R6/2 Huntington's disease mouse model via aggregate-independent mechanisms. J Neurochem 92: 83–92.

18. Prime ME, Andersen OA, Barker JJ, Brooks MA, Cheng RK, et al. (2012) Discovery and structure-activity relationship of potent and selective covalent inhibitors of transglutaminase 2 for Huntington's disease. J Med Chem 55: 1021–1046.

19. Schaertl S, Prime M, Wityak J, Dominguez C, Munoz-Sanjuan I, et al. (2010) A profiling platform for the characterization of transglutaminase 2 (TG2) inhibitors. J Biomol Screen 15: 478–487.

20. Mangiarini L, Sathasivam K, Seller M, Cozens B, Harper A, et al. (1996) Exon 1 of the HD gene with an expanded CAG repeat is sufficient to cause a progressive neurological phenotype in transgenic mice. Cell 87: 493–506.

21. Menalled LB, Kudwa AE, Miller S, Fitzpatrick J, Watson-Johnson J, et al. (2012) Comprehensive behavioral and molecular characterization of a new knock-in mouse model of Huntington's disease: zQ175. PLoS One 7: e49838.

22. Heikkinen T, Lehtimaki K, Vartiainen N, Puolivali J, Hendricks SJ, et al. (2012) Characterization of neurophysiological and behavioral changes, MRI brain volumetry and 1H MRS in zQ175 knock-in mouse model of Huntington's disease. PLoS One 7: e50717.

23. Nanda N, Iismaa SE, Owens WA, Husain A, Mackay F, et al. (2001) Targeted inactivation of Gh/tissue transglutaminase II. J Biol Chem 276: 20673–20678.

24. Menalled L, El-Khodor BF, Patry M, Suarez-Farinas M, Orenstein SJ, et al. (2009) Systematic behavioral evaluation of Huntington's disease transgenic and knock-in mouse models. Neurobiol Dis 35: 319–336.

25. Jacobs GH, Fenwick JC, Calderone JB, Deeb SS (1999) Human cone pigment expressed in transgenic mice yields altered vision. J Neurosci 19: 3258–3265.

26. Singer J (1998) Using SAS PROC MIXED to fit multilevel models,hierarchical models, and individuals growth models. Journal of Educational and Behavioral Statistics 24: 323–355.

27. Cowin RM, Roscic A, Bui N, Graham D, Paganetti P, et al. (2012) Neuronal aggregates are associated with phenotypic onset in the R6/2 Huntington's disease transgenic mouse. Behav Brain Res 229: 308–319.

28. Morton AJ, Glynn D, Leavens W, Zheng Z, Faull RL, et al. (2009) Paradoxical delay in the onset of disease caused by super-long CAG repeat expansions in R6/2 mice. Neurobiol Dis 33: 331–341.

29. Dragatsis I, Goldowitz D, Del Mar N, Deng YP, Meade CA, et al. (2009) CAG repeat lengths > or = 335 attenuate the phenotype in the R6/2 Huntington's disease transgenic mouse. Neurobiol Dis 33: 315–330.

30. Cha JH (2007) Transcriptional signatures in Huntington's disease. Prog Neurobiol 83: 228–248.

31. Zuccato C, Cattaneo E (2009) Brain-derived neurotrophic factor in neurodegenerative diseases. Nat Rev Neurol 5: 311–322.

32. Sathasivam K, Lane A, Legleiter J, Warley A, Woodman B, et al. (2010) Identical oligomeric and fibrillar structures captured from the brains of R6/2 and knock-in mouse models of Huntington's disease. Hum Mol Genet 19: 65–78.

33. Bailey CD, Johnson GV (2006) The protective effects of cystamine in the R6/2 Huntington's disease mouse involve mechanisms other than the inhibition of tissue transglutaminase. Neurobiol Aging 27: 871–879.

34. Carter RJ, Hunt MJ, Morton AJ (2000) Environmental stimulation increases survival in mice transgenic for exon 1 of the Huntington's disease gene. Mov Disord 15: 925–937.

35. Wood NI, Carta V, Milde S, Skillings EA, McAllister CJ, et al. (2010) Responses to environmental enrichment differ with sex and genotype in a transgenic mouse model of Huntington's disease. PLoS One 5: e9077.

36. Balci F, Oakeshott S, Shamy JL, El-Khodor BF, Filippov I, et al. (2013) High-Throughput Automated Phenotyping of Two Genetic Mouse Models of Huntington's Disease. PLoS Curr 5.

37. Chun W, Lesort M, Tucholski J, Ross CA, Johnson GV (2001) Tissue transglutaminase does not contribute to the formation of mutant huntingtin aggregates. J Cell Biol 153: 25–34.

38. Perutz MF, Johnson T, Suzuki M, Finch JT (1994) Glutamine repeats as polar zippers: their possible role in inherited neurodegenerative diseases. Proc Natl Acad Sci U S A 91: 5355–5358.

39. D'Eletto M, Farrace MG, Rossin F, Strappazzon F, Giacomo GD, et al. (2012) Type 2 transglutaminase is involved in the autophagy-dependent clearance of ubiquitinated proteins. Cell Death Differ 19: 1228–1238.

40. Munsie L, Caron N, Atwal RS, Marsden I, Wild EJ, et al. (2011) Mutant huntingtin causes defective actin remodeling during stress: defining a new role for transglutaminase 2 in neurodegenerative disease. Hum Mol Genet 20: 1937–1951.

41. Sathasivam K, Woodman B, Mahal A, Bertaux F, Wanker EE, et al. (2001) Centrosome disorganization in fibroblast cultures derived from R6/2 Huntington's disease (HD) transgenic mice and HD patients. Hum Mol Genet 10: 2425–2435.

42. McConoughey SJ, Basso M, Niatsetskaya ZV, Sleiman SF, Smirnova NA, et al. (2010) Inhibition of transglutaminase 2 mitigates transcriptional dysregulation in models of Huntington disease. EMBO Mol Med 2: 349–370.

43. Kumar A, Kneynsberg A, Tucholski J, Perry G, van Groen T, et al. (2012) Tissue transglutaminase overexpression does not modify the disease phenotype of the R6/2 mouse model of Huntington's disease. Exp Neurol 237: 78–89.

12

Reduced Motivation in the BACHD Rat Model of Huntington Disease is Dependent on the Choice of Food Deprivation Strategy

Erik Karl Håkan Jansson[◗], Laura Emily Clemens[◗], Olaf Riess, Huu Phuc Nguyen*

Institute of Medical Genetics and Applied Genomics, University of Tuebingen, Tuebingen, Germany; and Centre for Rare Diseases, University of Tuebingen, Tuebingen, Germany

Abstract

Huntington disease (HD) is an inherited neurodegenerative disease characterized by motor, cognitive, psychiatric and metabolic symptoms. Animal models of HD show phenotypes that can be divided into similar categories, with the metabolic phenotype of certain models being characterized by obesity. Although interesting in terms of modeling metabolic symptoms of HD, the obesity phenotype can be problematic as it might confound the results of certain behavioral tests. This concerns the assessment of cognitive function in particular, as tests for such phenotypes are often based on food depriving the animals and having them perform tasks for food rewards. The BACHD rat is a recently established animal model of HD, and in order to ensure that behavioral characterization of these rats is done in a reliable way, a basic understanding of their physiology is needed. Here, we show that BACHD rats are obese and suffer from discrete developmental deficits. When assessing the motivation to lever push for a food reward, BACHD rats were found to be less motivated than wild type rats, although this phenotype was dependent on the food deprivation strategy. Specifically, the phenotype was present when rats of both genotypes were deprived to 85% of their respective free-feeding body weight, but not when deprivation levels were adjusted in order to match the rats' apparent hunger levels. The study emphasizes the importance of considering metabolic abnormalities as a confounding factor when performing behavioral characterization of HD animal models.

Editor: Xiao-Jiang Li, Emory University, United States of America

Funding: The study was funded by yearly funds allocated to the Institute of Medical Genetics and Applied Genomics by the Medical Faculty of the University of Tuebingen, to maintain animals. Erik Jansson received a stipend from the German Academic Exchange Program (DAAD: https://www.daad.de/en/) under the Procope program, project number: 54366469. The funders had no role in study design, data collection and analysis, decision to publish, or preparation of the manuscript.

Competing Interests: The authors have declared that no competing interests exist.

* Email: hoa.nguyen@med.uni-tuebingen.de

◗ These authors contributed equally to this work.

Introduction

Huntington disease (HD) is an autosomal dominantly inherited neurodegenerative disease with a prevalence of 6 per 100,000 in Europe and North America [1]. Development of HD is dependent on a single mutation that results in the extension of the CAG repeat sequence present in the gene for the Huntingtin protein [2]. HD patients display a range of symptoms that can be grouped into motor, psychiatric, cognitive and metabolic symptoms. Symptoms gradually worsen as the disease progresses, and due to the lack of disease modifying treatments HD is invariably fatal.

There are numerous transgenic animal models of HD [3], and as with any disease model, a major focus of working with these is to assess how well their phenotypes mirror symptoms found in HD patients. This is complicated due to the multitude of phenotypes that are often present, and the potential risk of some phenotypes confounding the assessment of others. The metabolic phenotypes are especially interesting in this regard. While HD patients

typically lose weight [4,5,6,7,8,9], the body weight and body composition phenotypes of transgenic animal models of HD vary [3]. Animals that express the full-length mutant huntingtin gene typically show an increased body weight, due to increased fat mass [10,11]. Although this is interesting in terms of modeling the metabolic symptoms of HD, an increase in body weight has been suggested to result in reduced performance on the rotarod [12,13], a common test of motor capacity and limb coordination.

Metabolic phenotypes are also of interest when considering tests of cognitive function, as these are often based on having food deprived animals perform certain tasks to retrieve food rewards [14]. Ideally, animals should be equally hungry and interested in food rewards when performing such tests, as studies where motivational differences are present can give misleading results [15]. Changes in body composition, such as the ones seen in HD models, are likely to either be caused by or lead to a change in *ad libitum* food consumption. Unless careful adjustments are made, such phenotypes might persist even after food deprivation. One

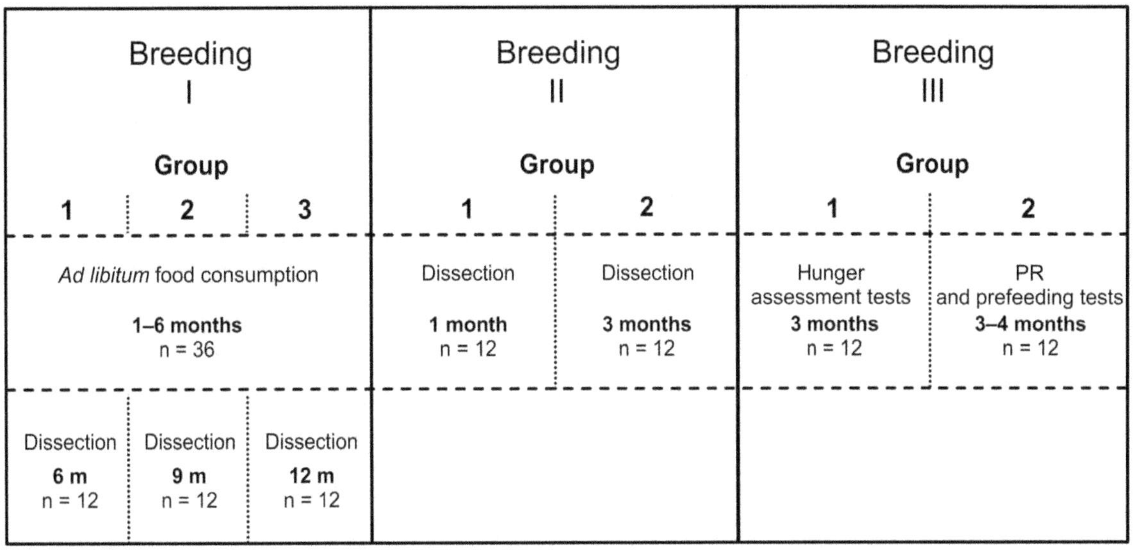

Figure 1. Overview of study groups. A total of seven groups of rats were used in the current study. These were derived from different breeding events and used in different tests, as shown in the figure. The "n" indicates the number of animals used from each genotype. Note that a total of two animals were excluded during analysis, as explained in detail under "Statistical analysis".

proposed method to avoid this when working with HD models is to adjust food deprivation levels until animals show similar consumption rates in tests where they are given brief access to food [16,17]. Similar tests are occasionally used to assess hunger and food interest, [18,19,20,21] although in HD research one should also consider that a slowed consumption rate could be caused by motor impairments. Thus, detailed knowledge about body composition and feeding behavior of an animal model, both when deprived and *ad libitum* fed, is important for planning and interpreting a variety of behavioral tests.

The BACHD rat is a recently established animal model for HD. These rats carry a large construct containing the full-length gene for human mutant Huntingtin, with its endogenous regulatory sequences [22]. Previous studies have shown that BACHD rats have motor impairments and neuropathological phenotypes reminiscent of symptoms seen among HD patients [22]. In addition, BACHD rats appear to be impaired in some cognitive tests [23]. Previous studies have indicated that BACHD rats eat less than WT rats [22], although the setup used for that particular study demanded social isolation, and its validity for assessing natural behavior has been questioned [24]. Further, although it has been pointed out that BACHD rats appear obese [22], there has not been any study on their body composition. Therefore, we performed a longitudinal study where food intake was measured in a social homecage setup, and body composition was assessed through detailed dissections. As further behavioral characterization of the BACHD rats will be dependent on tests that require food deprivation, we also sought to evaluate an optimal food deprivation strategy for BACHD rats. For this, consumption rate of reward pellets and regular food, as well as performance in a progressive ratio test with prefeedings was assessed at different levels of food deprivation.

Materials and Methods

Animals

A total of 168 male rats were used for the study. These were acquired from three separate in-house breeding events, with heterozygous BACHD males from the TG5 line [22] paired with WT females. All animals were on Sprague Dawley background. Animals were genotyped according to previously published protocols [22] and housed in type IV cages (38×55 cm), with high lids (24.5 cm from cage floor), and free access to water. Food availability and social conditions differed between the experimental groups. Rats used for *ad libitum* food intake and body composition measurements were housed in genotype-matched pairs, and had free access to food (SNIFF V1534-000 standard chow) during the entire length of their respective test. Importantly, food was provided on the cage floor and not on the cage top. Body weight was measured weekly to assess general health, and cages were changed twice per week. Rats used for hunger assessment and PR tests were housed in genotype-matched groups of three rats per cage. They had free access to food from the cage top until the age of ten weeks. At that point, the rats were food deprived as described below. Body weight was measured daily in order to assess food deprivation levels, and cages were changed weekly. The animal facility kept 21–23°C, 55–10% humidity, and was set to a partially inverted light/dark cycle with lights on/off at 02:00/14:00 during summer, and 01:00/13:00 during winter.

The seven groups of animals were used in different tests, as described below. An overview of the animal groups, and the tests, is shown in Figure 1. All experiments were approved by the local ethics committee (Regierungspraesidium Tuebingen) and carried out in accordance with the German Animal Welfare Act and the guidelines of the Federation of European Laboratory Animal Science Associations, based on European Union legislation (Directive 2010/63/EU).

Ad libitum food consumption in a social homecage environment

Ad libitum food consumption was measured using a total of 72 rats, acquired from one breeding event. At the age of five weeks, all rats were arranged into genotype-matched pairs, and housed as described above. This gave a total of 36 cages, 18 cages per genotype. Cages with WT and BACHD rats were evenly distributed over two racks, which were placed next to each other in the same housing room. Food and water intake was assessed twice weekly, when cages were changed. Cages were changed on Mondays and Thursdays during the last two hours of the light phase. At each cage-changing event, a known amount of food was placed inside each new cage, and the fresh water bottles were weighed. The weights of the old water bottles as well as the weight of the food left in each old cage were then measured to assess the amount of food and water consumed since the last cage change. The food was manually collected from the bedding of the old cages. After removing large food pieces, the bedding was sifted in a homemade sieve with a 1 mm mesh in order to collect small food pieces generated by food grinding. The animals' food and water consumption was followed in this way until the age of 26 weeks. Sifting of bedding materials started when animals were 15 weeks old.

Dissection for body composition assessment

A detailed dissection was performed in order to study the body composition of BACHD rats. Five different rat groups were sacrificed at 1, 3, 6, 9, and 12 months of age respectively, with each group being composed of 12 WT and 12 BACHD rats. The rat groups used for dissection at 6, 9, and 12 months of age were the same rats that were followed during the *ad libitum* food consumption test. The rat groups used for dissection at 1 and 3 months of age were acquired from a separate breeding. Housing conditions were identical for all animals, and according to the description above. Aside from the weekly food and water consumption assessment made during the *ad libitum* food intake test, food and water consumption were measured monthly as animals aged. When rats reached an age of interest, a dissection group was arranged based on the animals' food consumption, water intake, and body weights, so that the dissected group well represented the full group.

Rats were sacrificed in a carbon dioxide chamber two to four hours before dark-phase onset. Blood samples were collected after sacrifice, through retro-orbital bleeding. Body lengths and body weights were measured on the intact animals, with body length measured from nose tip to tail tip. Additional measurements of head, trunk, and tail lengths were measured from nose tip to back of the head, back of the head to anus, and anus to tail tip, respectively. After these external measurements, skin and subcutaneous adipose tissue deposits were removed and weighed. Then, internal organs and adipose deposits located in the abdomen and chest cavities were removed and weighed. The remaining carcass was weighed before removal of the brain. By later subtracting the brain weight, a measurement of bone and muscle weight (denoted bone/muscle) was acquired for each rat. Dissection of a given age group was carried out during four to six days, with rats of both genotypes being assessed on each day.

Hunger assessment tests

Two tests were used to assess hunger levels in WT and BACHD rats at three different food deprivation levels. A group of 24 animals with equal numbers of WT and BACHD rats was used for both tests. This group was acquired from a breeding separate from the ones used for the *ad libitum* food consumption and body composition measurements. As mentioned above, food deprivation started when the rats were ten weeks old. Body weights were compared to control data from age- and genotype-matched free-feeding animals, on a weekly basis, in order to acquire measurements of food deprivation levels (relative body weight). It should be noted that the control data was not gathered in the current study, but in previous tests. Rats were given small daily amounts of food inside their social homecages, approximately four hours after dark phase onset, to maintain food deprivation. During

the first week of food deprivation, animals were habituated to the reward pellets (Bio-Serv, Dustless Precision Pellets® F0021, purchased through Bilaney Consultants, Duesseldorf, Germany) by daily giving each cage a spoon-full of reward pellets together with the daily amount of food. Behavior assessment started one hour after dark phase onset, and was performed in the animals' housing room, using soft red light. Rats were 13 weeks old when behavioral assessment started.

Rats were assessed in both tests on each given testing occasion. The first test assessed the rats' interest in consuming 100 reward pellets. The test used a glass cage (28.5×29×29.5 cm) with mirrors, which allowed a good view of the feeding animals. At the start of each trial, a rat was placed inside the cage, and was allowed two explore it freely during two minutes. Afterwards, a glass Petri dish containing 100 reward pellets was placed inside the cage, in one of the corners that faced the experimenter. The rats were then given a total of five minutes to consume the reward pellets, while the experimenter scored their behavior. The experimenter used two timers to separately record the total time taken to consume the reward pellets, and the time each rat actually spent eating. Thus, one timer was started when the rat first discovered the pellets, and stopped either when all pellets were consumed or when five minutes had passed. The second timer was also started when the rat first discovered the pellets, but was stopped whenever the rat stopped eating, and explored the test arena. Roughly three hours were needed to assess all 24 rats. The test schedule was arranged so that entire cages of BACHD and WT rats were assessed in an alternating manner. Thus, three rats of a given genotype were assessed in sequence, followed by three rats of the other genotype. The experimenter was blinded to the animals' genotypes.

The second test assessed the rats' interest in regular food. In this test, rats were given free access to a large amount of food in their homecages. Food was made available to the rats when four hours remained of the dark phase. Identical amounts of food were placed in the cage tops, with one-minute spacing between cages, alternating between BACHD and WT cages. The remaining food was then measured each half hour, until the end of the dark phase. A final measurement was made at the end of the subsequent light phase. At each measurement, the cages were briefly inspected for larger pieces of food, as they occasionally dropped between the bars of the cage lids.

The rats were assessed in these two tests on three separate occasions. On the first, both WT and BACHD rats were deprived to 85% of their respective free-feeding body weights. In an attempt to reverse the phenotypes that were found, the food deprivation levels were then adjusted so WT and BACHD rats were at 95 and 80% of their respective free-feeding body weights. On the final trial, the previous deprivation levels were switched, so that WT and BACHD rats were at 80 and 95% of their respective free-feeding body weights. Each test occasion was separated by a week of food deprivation, to allow gradual adjustment of deprivation levels.

Progressive ratio test

A progressive ratio (PR) test was run to assess the rats' motivation to work for a food reward at two different food deprivation settings. A group of 24 animals with equal numbers of WT and BACHD rats was used for the test. This group was acquired from the same breeding as the group used for the hunger tests described above. Food deprivation was initiated and maintained as described above. Behavioral assessment started 30 minutes after dark phase onset, in a room separate from the animals' housing room, using soft red light. Rats were 11 weeks old when behavioral assessment started.

A bank of six operant conditioning chambers (Coulbourn Instruments, H10-11R-TC with H10-24 isolation boxes, purchased through Bilaney Consultants, Duesseldorf, Germany) was used to run the test. Each chamber was equipped with two retractable levers, placed 6 cm above the chamber floor, protruding 2 cm from the wall. The levers were placed on either side of a central pellet receptacle trough, which was placed 2 cm above the chamber floor. The pellet receptacle trough contained a yellow light, which was used to signal the delivery of a reward pellet in all protocols described below. The chambers also contained a red house light, on the wall opposite from the levers and pellet receptacle trough, which shined during the full duration of the training sessions. A water bottle was also available on this wall, to ensure *ad libitum* access to water during testing. All protocols were designed and run with Graphic State 4.1.04. Rats were given single daily sessions, meaning that a total of four daily runs with all six operant chambers were needed to assess the whole group. Each run assessed three WT and three BACHD rats in a determined order, so that a given rat was trained on the same time of day through the entire test. Each rat was assigned to a specific operant chamber, although this was arranged so that each operant chamber was used to assess equal numbers of WT and BACHD rats. Rats received their daily regimen of regular food four hours after the completion of the last run of the day.

During initial training, rats of both genotypes were deprived to 85% of their respective free-feeding body weights. Afterwards, all rats received two habituation sessions in the conditioning chambers. During these, both levers were retracted and a single reward pellet was delivered to the pellet trough at 10, 15, 20, 25, or 30-second intervals. The pellet delivery interval varied in a pseudo-randomized fashion so that each set of five deliveries used each given interval once. Pellet retrieval, or failure to retrieve the pellet within five seconds after delivery, lead to the start of the next pellet delivery interval. After the habituation sessions, rats were trained to lever push for a pellet reward. During these sessions, both levers were extended into the chamber, but only one was reinforced. Rats were either trained to push the right or the left lever, with the reinforced lever position being counter-balanced within the genotype groups. During training, the experimenter would reward rats for approaching, sniffing and touching the reinforced lever, until rats started to reliably push the lever on their own. During this, each lever push was rewarded with one pellet. Training continued until rats completed 100 lever pushes within a 30-minute session, without any help from the experimenter. The rats were then trained on an FR3 protocol, where they had to push the reinforced lever three times before being rewarded with a pellet. When a rat completed 100 ratios within a 30-minute session, it progressed to an FR5 protocol. Rats now had to push the reinforced lever five times before being rewarded with a pellet. Training on the FR5 protocol continued until rats completed 100 ratios within a 30-minute session, on three consecutive sessions. Afterwards, rats were trained on a PR protocol adapted from [16]. In the current protocol, the ten first ratios were of FR5 type. Afterwards, the required number of lever pushes increased after each completed ratio. During this progression, the required number of lever pushes increased in an arithmetic fashion within each block of ten ratios, but also changed between the blocks, to give an overall exponential progression. Thus, during the first, second and third block of ten ratios, the ratio requirement increased with one, three and five pushes per completed ratio, respectively. The PR sessions lasted 80 minutes. The main behavioral parameter of interest was a set of break points, defined as the first ratio where a rat made no responses on the reinforced lever during 10, 25, 50, 100, 300 or 600 seconds. Rats were trained until both genotype groups reached a stable performance, which in this case required 18 sessions. Performance during the six last sessions was defined as baseline performance.

Once stable PR performance had been reached, the rats were challenged in a set of four prefeeding tests. During these tests, the rats were fed specific amounts of reward pellets or regular food, just prior to their daily PR session. Rats were prefed by placing them in individual cages that contained the specified amount of food. Each prefeeding condition was assessed once, in the following order: 100 reward pellets, 250 reward pellets, 4.5 g of regular food, 11.25 g of regular food. Each prefeeding test was separated by two regular PR sessions to ensure that rats returned to their baseline performance.

After completion of the first round of prefeeding tests, the food deprivation level of WT rats was adjusted until they consumed food at the same rate as BACHD rats. Consumption rate was assessed daily by measuring the amount of food consumed during 15 minutes of free access to regular food, placed in the cage tops of the rats' homecages. The rats were still given daily PR sessions during food deprivation adjustments. The food consumption tests were run four hours after completion of the last PR run, i.e. at the time when the rats were usually given their daily food ration. When WT rats had reached a consumption rate equal to that of BACHD rats, six additional PR sessions were run to establish a new baseline. The prefeeding tests were then repeated in the same manner as described above. Rats were 20 weeks old at the end of the test.

Statistical analyses

All statistical analyses were conducted using GraphPad Prism v.6.01 (GraphPad Software, San Diego California USA, http://www.graphpad.com).

Food consumption in the *ad libitum* food consumption test was analyzed both in terms of the absolute amount of food consumed and the amount of food consumed relative to the animals' body weight. The main analysis of food consumption was based on the weight of large food pieces, as the food debris gathered through sifting of the bedding material also contained hair and bedding pieces. A separate analysis where food consumption was corrected for the amount of food debris was still performed. For this, the mean amount of food debris was calculated for each cage, based on their longitudinal data. This was then added to the weight of the large food pieces measured at each cage changing. For the relative food consumption, rats in a given cage were assumed to eat equal amounts of food. The approximate amount of food consumed by one of the rats was subsequently related to the mean body weight of the two rats. Two-way repeated measures ANVOAs were used to analyze body weight as well as absolute and relative food consumption. Age was used as within-subject factor, and genotype as between-subject factor.

For data gathered in the dissection study, body weight, absolute weight of adipose and bone/muscle tissues, as well as bone/muscle weight relative to body length were analyzed using regular two-way ANOVAs. The factors of interest were still age and genotype. The weights of adipose tissue, bone/muscle tissue and internal organs relative to body weight were analyzed in individual t-tests, or Mann-Whitney tests, between genotypes, within each age group. As the observed phenotypes did not vary between different adipose tissue deposits, only the combined weight of all deposits will be addressed here. One BACHD rat meant for the dissection of six months old animals died before the dissection, making that particular age group 12 WT and 11 BACHD rats.

Results from the two hunger tests were analyzed both within and between each testing occasion. For each test occasion of the reward pellet consumption test, the time needed to consume the pellets was analyzed with t-tests to compare the two genotypes. The time spent exploring the test arena was only analyzed on the first test occasion, using t-test, as rats showed essentially no interest in exploring the arena on later trials. One BACHD rat was excluded from the analysis of the last trial, as he failed to consume all reward pellets within the maximum trial time. The amount of food consumed during the food consumption test was on each test occasion analyzed with two-way repeated measures ANOVA, using time as within-subject factor, and genotype as between-subject factor. To better understand the effect of repeated testing and food deprivation levels, the time needed to consume 100 reward pellets, and the amount of food consumed during the first 30 minutes of the food consumption test were analyzed in additional detail. Thus, data from all three test-occasions were analyzed in two-way repeated measures ANOVAs, using genotype as between-subject factor, and either session number or food deprivation level as within-subject factor. Analysis of baseline performance during the PR test was also made with repeated measures two-way ANOVAs, with break point as within-subject factor, and genotype as between-subject factor. Drops in motivation during prefeeding sessions were analyzed for the 600-seconds break point, as a percentage of the ratio reached during the two preceding PR sessions. Once again, repeated two-way ANOVAs were used to analyze the results, using prefeeding condition as within-subject factor, and genotype as between-subject factor. Separate analyses were performed for prefeeding with reward pellets, and regular food. Bonferroni *post-hoc* test was used to follow up any significant effects of genotype, or interaction effects found in the two-way ANOVAs. Alpha for all analyses was set to 0.05.

Results

Ad libitum food consumption

To assess BACHD rats' growth and food consumption in a low-stress and social environment, we housed genotype-matched rats in pairs (Figure 2A), and measured their weekly body weight and food consumption. Rats of both genotypes grew steadily during the test, as indicated by the significant effect of age on body weight ($p<0.0001$, $F_{(21,1449)} =2766$) (Figure 2B). BACHD and WT rats grew at a similar rate, and showed similar body weights through the entire test, with no significant genotype effect or age x genotype interaction. The rats' food consumption also changed with age ($p<0.0001$, $F_{(20,680)} =110.5$) (Figure 2C). In general, food consumption increased gradually until the age of nine weeks, and then slowly dropped. Importantly, WT and BACHD rats consumed equal amounts of food between six and eight weeks of age, but there were a number of differences seen at older ages. At nine and ten weeks of age, BACHD rats appeared to consume more food that WT rats, although this did not reach statistical significance. Directly following this, food consumption dropped steadily among BACHD rats, while WT rats remained arguably stable until the age of 16 weeks. Due to this, BACHD rats eventually ate less than WT rats, as indicated by the significant results from the *post-hoc* analysis at 17 weeks of age and onwards ($p<0.05-0.01$). The difference in how food consumption changed with age among BACHD and WT rats was also evident in a significant age x genotype interaction ($p<0.0001$, $F_{(20,680)} =19.06$). Relating food consumption to the rats' body weight gave largely the same results, with a significant age effect ($p<0.0001$, $F_{(60,680)} =1930$) and age x genotype interaction ($p<0.0001$,

$F_{(20,680)} =12.99$) (Figure 2D). However, this analysis made the increased food intake among young BACHD rats more apparent, with the *post-hoc* test indicating significant differences between BACHD and WT at seven to ten weeks of age ($p<0.01-0.0001$). In contrast, the decreased food consumption among old BACHD rats was less apparent, with the *post-hoc* test only indicating a few significant data points at 18 to 21 weeks of age ($p<0.05-0.01$). It should be noted that BACHD rats produced less food debris compared to WT rats (Figure S1A and B). Correcting for this did not dramatically affect the food consumption phenotype, although the genotype differences became less apparent (Figure S1C). Finally, BACHD rats consumed dramatically less water compared to WT rats (Figure S1D).

Body composition of BACHD rats

In order to assess BACHD rats' body composition, we dissected BACHD and WT rats at five different ages. As expected, older rats weighed more, leading to a significant age effect on body weight ($p<0.0001$, $F_{(4,109)} =444.1$) (Figure 3A). In line with previous data, there were no differences in body weight between the genotypes in any age group, and also no significant difference in apparent growth. The body composition of BACHD rats was however different from that of WT rats. BACHD rats had significantly lower percentage of bone and muscle ($p<0.001$, all ages), and higher percentage of adipose tissue ($p<0.05-0.001$) in all age groups (Figure 3B). These differences were also apparent when analyzing the absolute weights of the respective tissues. Both WT and BACHD rats gained adipose tissue with age, as indicated by a significant age effect on the weight of total adipose tissue ($p<0.0001$, $F_{(4,109)} =142$) (Figure 3C). However, BACHD rats carried an excess amount of adipose tissue, as indicated by both a significant genotype effect ($p<0.0001$, $F_{(1,109)} =81.25$), and significant results from the *post-hoc* analysis of all groups, except the one-month old rats ($p<0.05-0.0001$). There was also a significant age x genotype interaction ($p<0.0001$, $F_{(4,109)} =7.686$) that was dependent on data from the one and three months old groups. The bone/muscle weight also increased with age for both genotypes ($p<0.0001$, $F_{(4,109)} =555.4$) (Figure 3D). However, BACHD rats were found to have significantly less bone/muscle tissue compared to WT rats in all but the one-month old age groups. This was indicated both by a significant genotype effect ($p<0.0001$, $F_{(1,109)} =70.69$), and significant results from the *post-hoc* analysis ($p<0.01-0.0001$). A significant age x genotype interaction ($p<0.001$, $F_{(4,109)} =4.18$) also indicated that there was a difference in the rats' growth. Importantly, this effect was dependent on the data of the one–month old group.

The rats' body length also increased with age for both genotypes ($p<0.0001$, $F_{(4,109)} =1517$), although a significant genotype effect ($p<0.0001$, $F_{(1,109)} =86.46$) and *post-hoc* tests ($p<0.01-0.0001$) revealed that BACHD rats were smaller than WT (Figure 3E). This was apparent in all age groups except the one-month old animals. It should, however, be noted that one-month old BACHD rats were shorter than WT rats when analyzing litter-matched groups (data not shown). The reduced body length among BACHD rats was mainly due to them having shorter tails and heads compared to WT rats (Figure S2).

BACHD rats also showed a lower amount of bone/muscle tissues in relation to their body length (Figure 3F). Rats of both genotypes gained relative amounts of bone and muscle with age ($p<0.0001$, $F_{(4,109)} =570.6$). However, BACHD rats had lower relative amounts of bone and muscle from three months of age, as evident from a significant genotype effect ($p<0.0001$, $F_{(1,109)} =47.32$) and *post-hoc* analysis ($p<0.05-0.0001$).

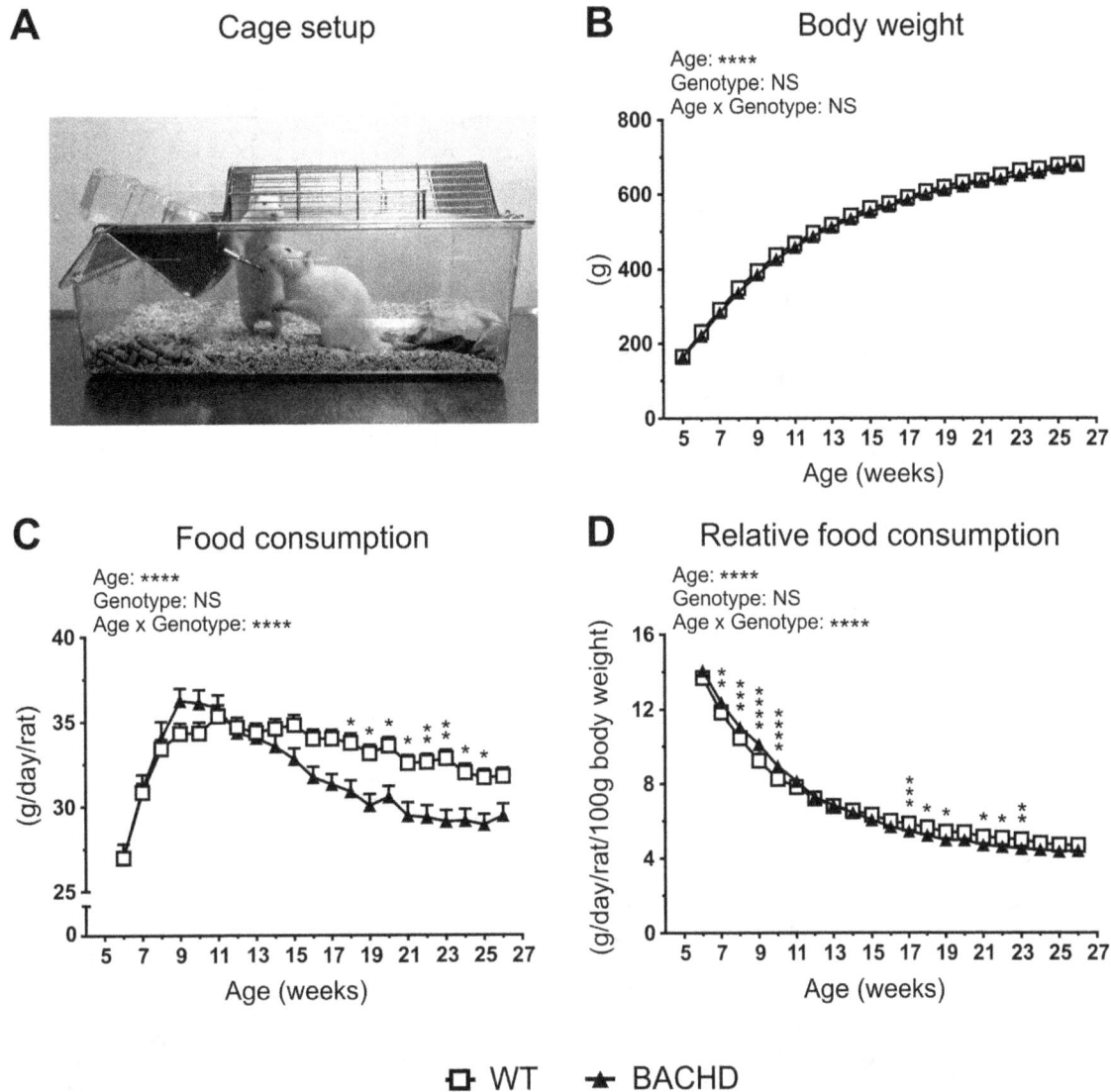

Figure 2. Body weight and food consumption. (A) Housing conditions during the *ad libitum* food consumption test. **(B)** Body weight of rats plotted against their age. **(C)** Approximate daily food consumption per rat (calculated from weekly food consumption per cage), plotted against the age of the animals. **(D)** Relative daily food consumption per rat (calculated from weekly food consumption and average body weight per cage), plotted against the age of the animals. The graphs show group mean plus standard error of the mean. Two-way ANOVA results are displayed above each graph, and significant results from *post-hoc* analysis are displayed for individual data points. Genotype differences are indicated by (p<0.05) *, (p<0.01) **, (p<0.001) *** and (p<0.0001) ****.

Assessment of hunger during food deprivation of BACHD rats

Two tests based on voluntary consumption of reward pellets and regular food, were run to assess BACHD rats' hunger level at different levels of food deprivation (Figure 4A). When both WT and BACHD rats were deprived to 85% of their respective free-feeding body weights, BACHD rats were found to consume both reward pellets and regular food at a slower rate than WT rats (Figure 4B). In the pellet consumption test, BACHD rats needed longer time to eat the reward pellets (p<0.01), but did not spend more time exploring the arena, compared to WT rats. The slower feeding speed led to a significant increase in trial time for BACHD rats (data not shown). In the food consumption test, BACHD rats were found to have eaten less than WT rats at almost all investigated intervals, as evident from the significant genotype effect (p<0.01, $F_{(1,6)} = 14.62$), and the significant results from the

post-hoc analysis (p<0.05–0.01). It should be noted that a difference in actual consumption rate was only seen during the first 30 minutes, resulting in an initial difference in the amount of food consumed, which then persisted through the remaining part of the test. This difference in behavior gave a significant time x genotype interaction (p<0.01, $F_{(9,54)} = 2.840$) in the amount of food consumed by the rats.

In an attempt to reverse the phenotypes described above, the food deprivation levels were adjusted so that BACHD and WT rats were at 80 and 95% of their respective free-feeding body weights (Figure 4C). In the pellet consumption tests, BACHD rats now needed a similar amount of time to consume the reward pellets, although there was a borderline significant trend towards BACHD rats needing more time (p = 0.0535). With the exception of one WT rat, all rats spent the entire trial eating, and showed minimal interest in exploring the test arena. In the food

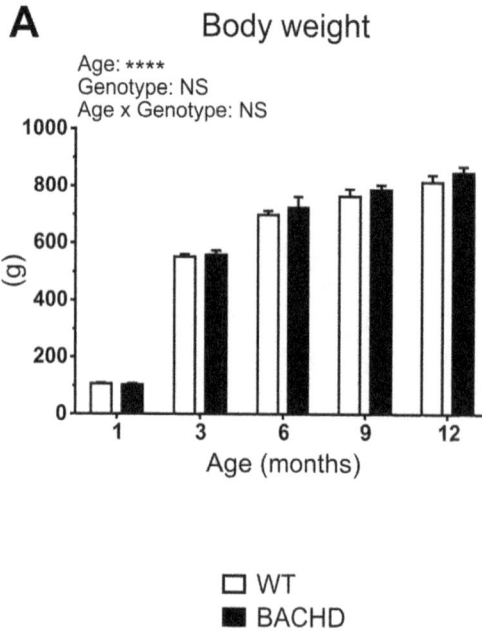

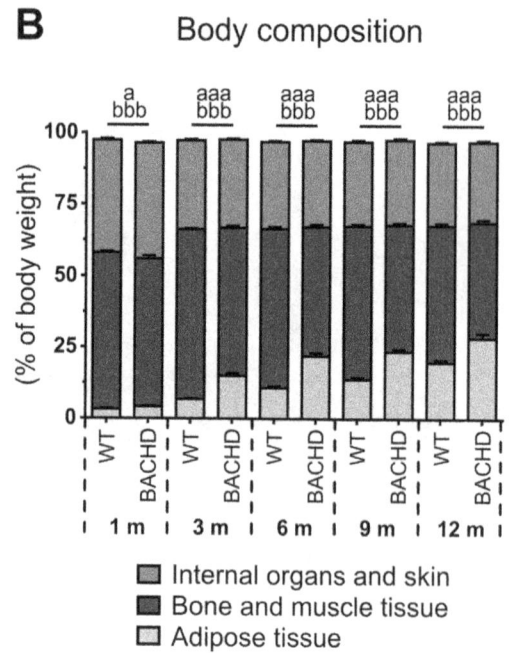

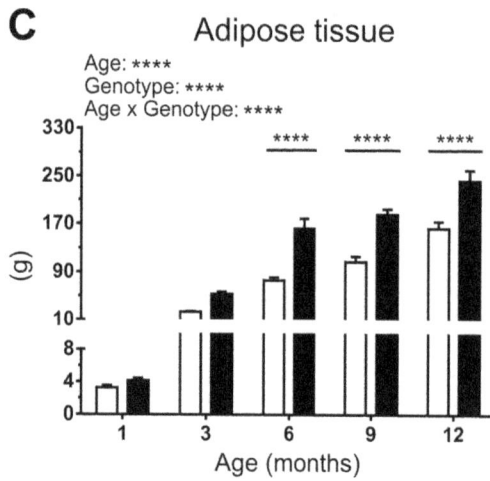

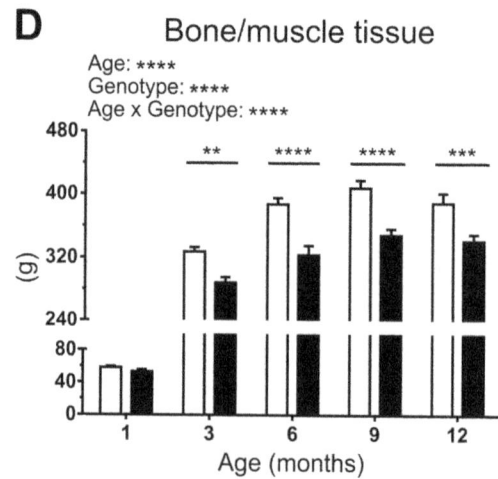

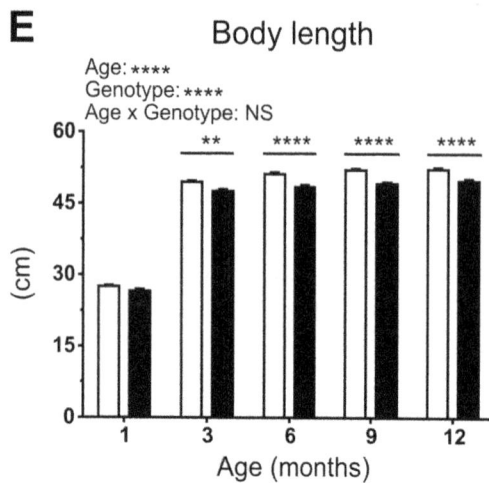

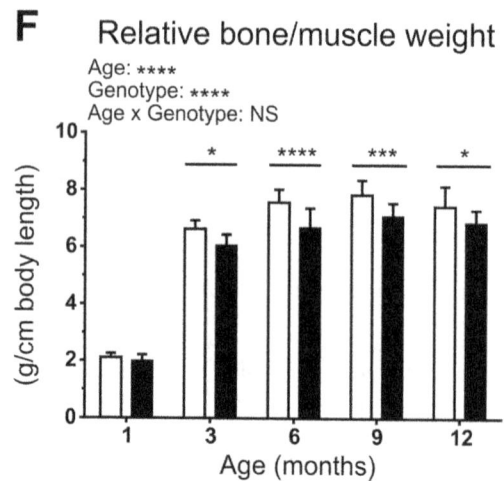

Figure 3. Body composition assessed through dissection. (A–F) Data from the dissection groups as stated in the graph titles. The graphs show group mean plus standard error of the mean. Two-way ANOVA results are displayed above each graph, and significant results from *post-hoc* analysis are displayed inside each graph. Significant genotype differences are indicated by (p<0.05) *, (p<0.01) **, (p<0.001) *** and (p<0.0001) ****. For (**B**), ANOVA was not performed, and the indicated differences concern single comparisons between WT and BACHD rats within the age groups. Significant differences are indicated with "a" and "b" for differences in the relative amount of adipose and bone/muscle tissue respectively, written according to the same grading as above.

consumption tests, BACHD and WT rats consumed food at the same rate during the first 150 minutes. During the remaining part of the test, WT rats ate more, eventually leading to a significant difference in the total amount of food consumed during the test (p<0.01). The behavioral differences led to a significant time x genotype interaction effect (p<0.0001, $F_{(9,54)}$ = 8.642).

In a final test, the food deprivation levels were adjusted so that BACHD and WT rats were at 95 and 80% of their respective free-feeding body weights (Figure 4D). At this point, BACHD rats consumed the reward pellets at the same rate as WT rats, as the aforementioned trend was no longer present. With the exception of two BACHD rats, all rats spent the entire trial eating, and showed minimal interest in exploring the test arena. One BACHD rat did not consume all reward pellets within five minutes. In the food consumption test, BACHD rats were once again found to have consumed less food than WT at all investigated intervals, resulting in a significant genotype effect (p<0.001, $F_{(1,6)}$ = 42.52), and significant results from the *post-hoc* analysis (p<0.05–0.0001). BACHD rats ate at a slower rate during the first hour. The consumption rate gradually declined among WT rats, while it gradually increased among BACHD rats, ending up at similar levels after 150 minutes. This difference in behavior gave a significant time x genotype interaction (p<0.0001, $F_{(9,54)}$ = 8.47) in the amount of food consumed by the rats.

A more detailed analysis of the results was performed with the aim of better assessing the impact of food deprivation levels on the consumption rate in the two tests. Separate two-way ANOVA analysis of the time needed to consume 100 reward pellets, using genotype as between-subject factor, and either food deprivation level or the number of test sessions as within-subject factor, revealed similar statistical results (Figure 5A). In either case, there was a significant genotype effect (p<0.05, $F_{(1,21)}$ = 5.476), and performance on the first session, where both genotypes were deprived to 85%, differed significantly between genotype groups (p<0.05). Both analyses also revealed a significant effect of their respective within-subject parameter (p<0.01, $F_{(2,42)}$ = 7.861 and 6.6333 for session and deprivation level, respectively). However, inspection of the graphed data indicated that the time needed to consume the reward pellets did not clearly decrease with increasing food deprivation levels, but did so with increased numbers of test sessions. Performing the same analyses on the amount of food consumed during the first 30 minutes of the food consumption test revealed different results (Figure 5B). Both analyses once again revealed a significant genotype effect (p< 0.01, $F_{(1,6)}$ = 15.59), and significant effects of their respective within-subject parameters (p<0.01, $F_{(2,12)}$ = 8.220 and 17.04 for session and deprivation level, respectively). *Post-hoc* analysis of data analyzed in terms of food deprivation level revealed a significant difference in consumption rate when rats of both genotypes were deprived to 85% of their free-feeding body weight. This was also found when analyzing the data in terms of the number of test sessions given to the rats, although that analysis also revealed a significant difference in consumption rate during the third session. In contrast to the results from the pellet consumption test, the consumption rate in the food consumption test appeared

to gradually increase with an increased food deprivation level, while not showing any gradual change during repeated testing.

Progressive ratio performance during different levels of food deprivation

To better assess differences in the motivational state among the rats, a progressive ratio test was run with two different food deprivation settings. All rats learned to push the lever in order to obtain a reward pellet, although there were some discrete behavioral differences between WT and BACHD rats during the initial training steps. During habituation, BACHD rats made fewer entries into the pellet receptacle (Figure S3A, B) and were initially slower at retrieving the pellets (Figure S3C). During CRF, FR3 and FR5 training, BACHD rats were generally slower at both retrieving the pellets, and returning to the reinforced lever (Figure S4 and S5).

During the fixed ratio part of the PR protocol, BACHD rats were still slower at retrieving the reward pellets, but they no longer showed an increase in lever return latencies (Figure S6). These results were largely unaffected when food deprivation levels were adjusted. WT rats tended to take longer time to complete the FR5 ratios, although this became significant only after adjustment of their deprivation level (Figure S6). Importantly, there were no overt differences between genotypes in the overall response frequency on the rewarded lever during the fixed ratios (Figure S6). The same was true for the mean number of lever pushes made on the non-reinforced lever during the entire PR session (Figure S7).

Analysis of how the rats reached a series of break points, when all were deprived to 85% of their free-feeding body weight, revealed both a significant genotype effect (p<0.01, $F_{(1,22)}$ = 10.66) and differences in the three highest break points (p< 0.01), with BACHD rats reaching lower ratios (Figure 6A). These differences were not present when the food deprivation level of WT rats had been adjusted so that their food consumption rate matched that of BACHD rats. Similarly, when all rats were deprived to 85% of their free-feeding body weight, BACHD rats responded with more pronounced drops in motivation during prefeeding of both reward pellets and regular food, as indicated by significant genotype effects (p<0.01, $F_{(1,22)}$ = 9.461 and p<0.01, $F_{(1,21)}$ = 8.343 for reward pellet and regular food prefeeding, respectively) and prefeeding x genotype interactions (p<0.001, $F_{(2,44)}$ = 11.19 and p<0.05, $F_{(1,21)}$ = 8.341 for reward pellet and regular food prefeeding, respectively) (Figure 6B). Once again, these phenotypes were not present when the food deprivation level of WT rats had been adjusted, leading to identical responses in the prefeeding tests. It should be noted that only the last break point, break point 600, was suitable for prefeeding analysis. Prefeeding induced a strong interest in water among WT rats, which dramatically affected their early break points (data not shown). It should also be noted that there was a significant difference in body weight once the food deprivation levels had been adjusted, with WT rats being significantly heavier than BACHD rats (data not shown). The WT rats weighed roughly 50 g more than BACHD rats, resulting in them being at 95% of their free-feeding body weight.

A *Reward pellet* - consumption test

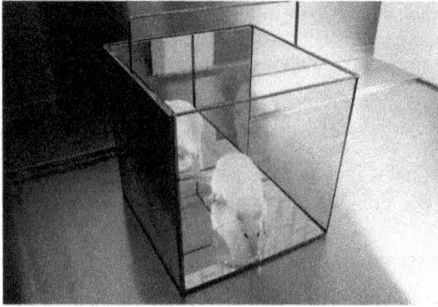

Regular food - consumption test

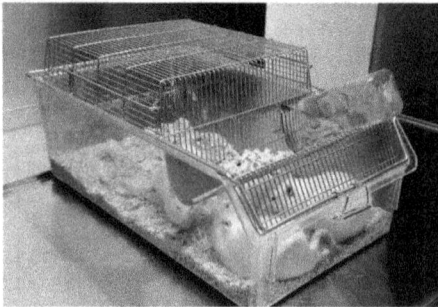

B   WT: 85%   BACHD: 85%

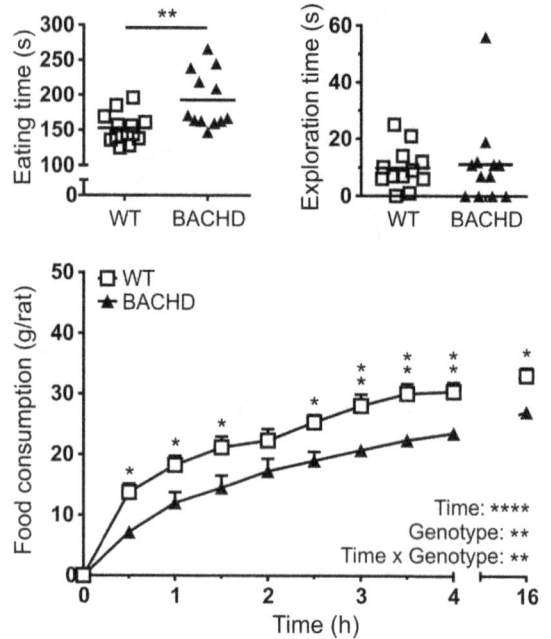

C   WT: 95%   BACHD: 80%

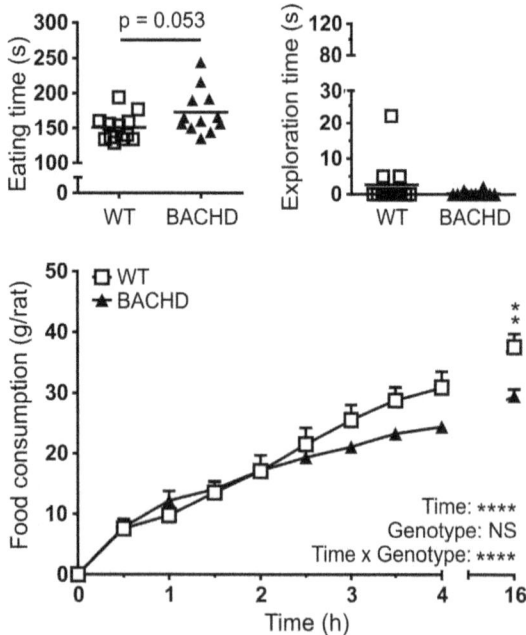

D   WT: 80%   BACHD: 95%

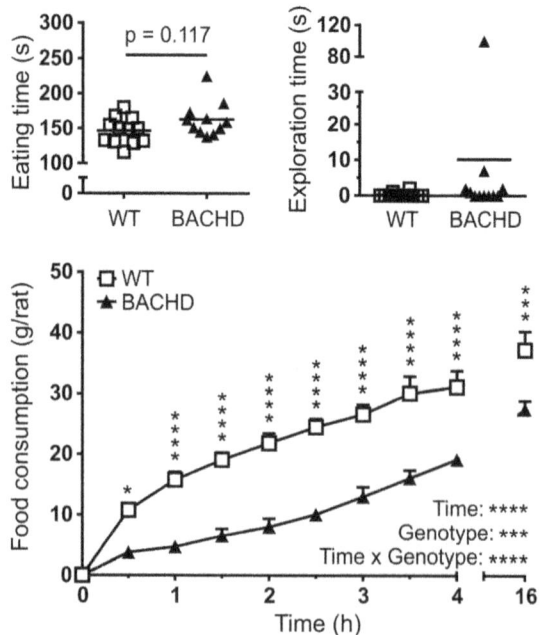

Figure 4. Hunger and food interest assessment. Setups (**A**) and performance in the two consumption tests during the first (**B**), second (**C**) and third test session (**D**), with the different food deprivation levels stated in the title of each figure panel. The time needed to eat 100 reward pellets and the time spent exploring in the reward pellet consumption setup, are displayed in the top left and right graphs of each panel, respectively. The bottom graph of each panel shows the cumulative food consumed per rat during the regular food consumption test. Scatter plots for reward pellet consumption test results indicate individual values and group mean. Line graphs for regular food consumption indicate group mean plus standard error of the mean. Statistical test results are given inside the graphs. For the regular food consumption test, two-way ANOVA results are displayed in the bottom right corner, and results from *post-hoc* analysis are shown for individual data points. Significant genotype differences are indicated by (p<0.05) *, (p<0.01) **, (p<0.001) *** and (p<0.0001) ****.

A   Reward pellet consumption

Deprivation level: **
Genotype: *
Deprivation level x Genotype: *

Session: **
Genotype: *
Session x Genotype: NS

B   Regular food consumption

Deprivation level: ***
Genotype: **
Deprivation level x Genotype: NS

Session: **
Genotype: **
Session x Genotype: **

□ WT   ▲ BACHD

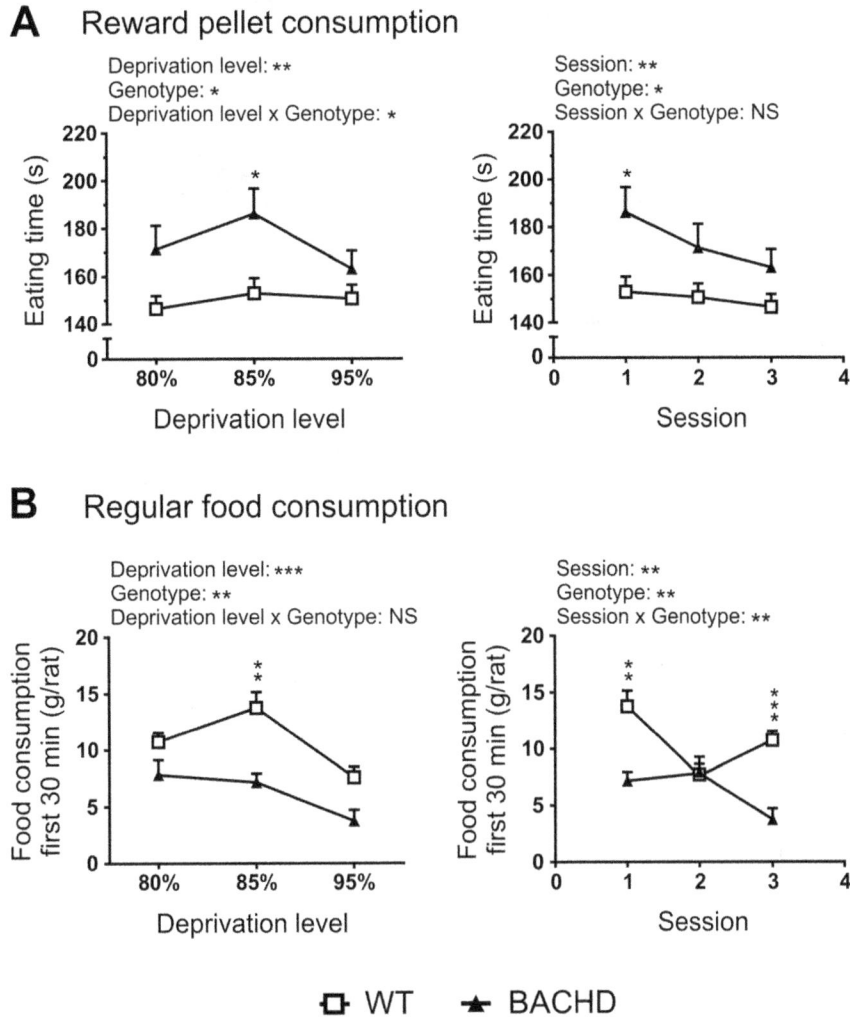

Figure 5. Impact of repeated testing and food deprivation on consumption tests. (**A**) The time needed to consume 100 reward pellets is plotted against the deprivation level (left graph) and session number (right graph). (**B**) The food consumed during the first 30 minutes of the regular food consumption test is plotted against the deprivation level (left graph) and session number (right graph). The graphs show mean plus standard error of the mean. Two-way ANOVA results are displayed above each graph, and results from *post-hoc* analysis are shown for individual data points. Significant genotype differences are indicated by (p<0.05) *, (p<0.01) **, (p<0.001) *** and (p<0.0001) ****.

Discussion

Body composition and food intake of BACHD rats

Many transgenic animal models of HD show an altered body weight compared to their WT littermates. Animals that express a fragment of the disease-causing gene typically have a reduced body weight [25,26,27], while the ones that express the full-length gene typically have an increased body weight [10,11]. We show here, that although BACHD rats did not differ from WT rats in terms of body weight, they displayed several changes in body composition. Strikingly, BACHD rats carried an excess amount of adipose tissue. This is in line with phenotypes of other full-length models of HD, as the increased body weight of BACHD and YAC128 mice has been shown to at least in part be due to an increase in adipose tissue mass [28,29]. It should be pointed out that R6/2 and N171-82Q mice, which only express a fragment of the disease-causing gene, also carry excess amounts of adipose tissue [25,30]. R6/2 mice have further been shown to maintain this increased fat mass even when they start to lose weight [25]. Thus, the increase in adipose tissue seems to be a common

phenotype of transgenic HD models, although it does not always result in obesity.

Increased amounts of adipose tissue could theoretically be the result of increased food intake, decreased home cage activity, metabolic disturbances, or a combination of the three. While BACHD mice have been shown to eat more than their WT littermates [28], R6/2 and YAC128 mice have been found to have unchanged food intake [25,29]. A previous study on BACHD rats, in which food intake was followed from three to eighteen months of age, indicated that the transgenic rats ate less than their WT littermates [22]. These results were well reproduced here, despite the different housing conditions. The current study also assessed food intake at ages younger than three months, where BACHD rats appeared to consume more food compared to WT rats. It should be noted, however, that the appearance of the food consumption phenotypes was to some degree dependent on whether or not the weight of the consumed food was normalized to the animals' body weight. The aim of this normalization was to relate the rats' food intake to a measurement of their body size, and through this investigate if the reduced food intake among

WT: 85%   BACHD: 85%   WT: 95%   BACHD: 85%

A   Baseline

B   Prefeeding

Reward pellets

Regular food

☐ WT   ▲ BACHD

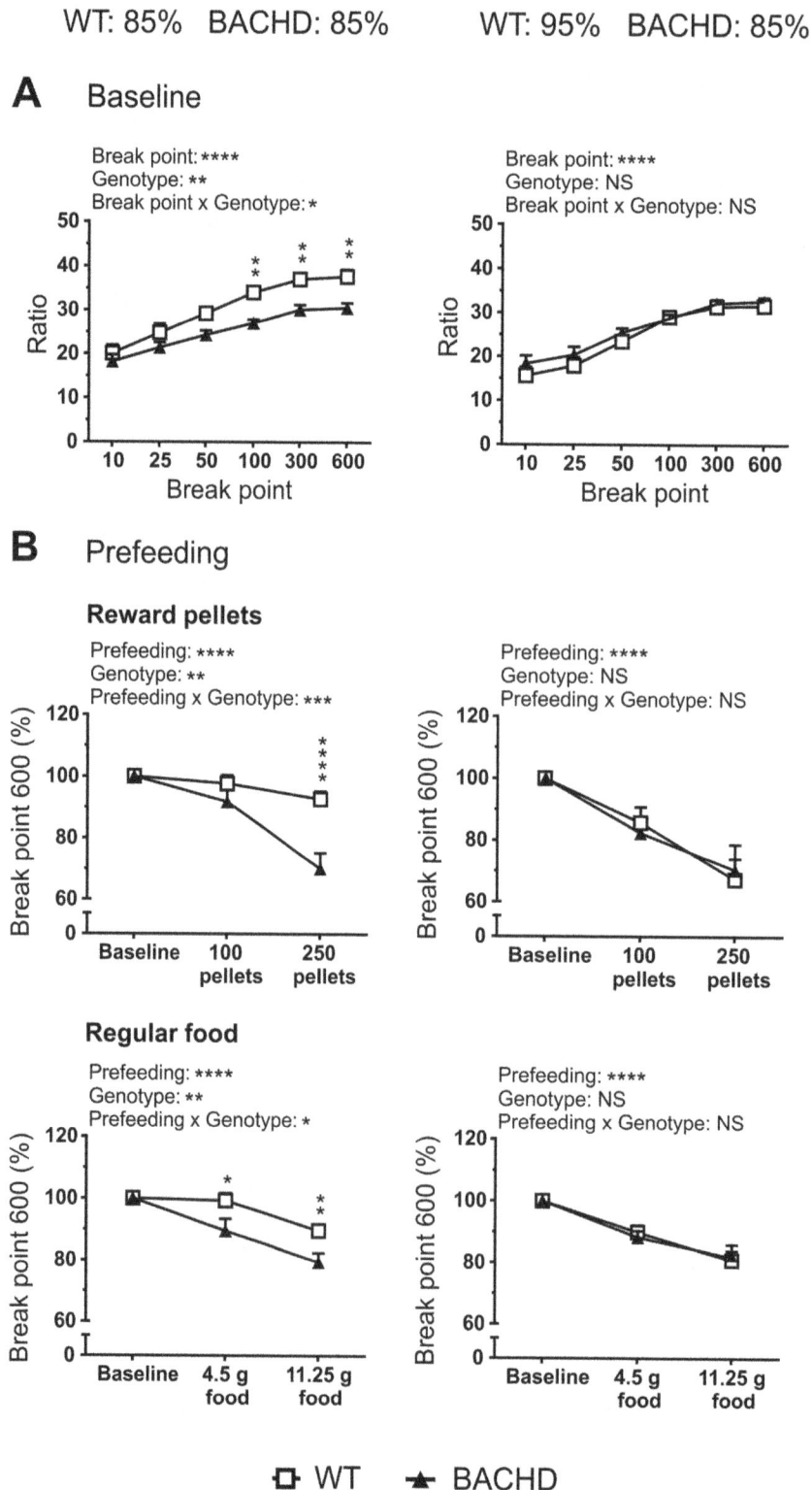

Figure 6. Progressive ratio test performance. Performance in the PR test is shown for when animals of both genotypes were deprived to 85% of their free-feeding body weight (graphs to the left in each figure panel) and when the deprivation level of WT rats had been adjusted to achieve equal food consumption rates between genotypes (graphs on the right of each figure panel). (**A**) Baseline performance during six consecutive PR sessions preceding the prefeeding tests. The ratio, where a given break point was reached, is indicated. (**B**) Performance during prefeeding with reward pellets (top panel) and regular food (bottom panel). The drop in motivation is displayed as percentage of baseline performance for break point 600. The graphs show group mean plus standard error of the mean. Two-way ANOVA results are displayed above each graph, and results from *post-hoc* analysis are shown for individual data points. Significant genotype differences are indicated by ($p<0.05$) *, ($p<0.01$) **, ($p<0.001$) *** and ($p<0.0001$) ****.

BACHD rats could be due to them being smaller than WT rats. Using body weight as an approximation of body size is, however, probably only suitable at young ages, as the body weight of older BACHD rats is distorted due to obesity. Thus, further studies are needed to reach conclusions on this matter. In addition, as food intake phenotypes are unlikely to explain the increase in adipose tissue, metabolic parameters of BACHD rats need to be further characterized. In this regard, it is important to note that the obesity phenotype of BACHD mice was abolished when the expression of mutant Huntingtin was silenced in the hypothalamus [28]. Interestingly, hypothalamic lesions can induce obesity that is not always associated with increased food intake, but can persist despite unchanged or even reduced food intake [31,32,33,34,35]. The differential effects appear to depend on which specific neuronal population is damaged [35,36], which might relate to the common phenotype of increased fat mass, but varied food intake seen across HD animal models.

In the current study, BACHD rats were shown to have a smaller body size and disproportionately lower amount of bone/muscle tissue compared to WT rats. Information about similar parameters is scarce for other HD models, although YAC128 mice have been shown to have unchanged lean body mass [29], while R6/2 mice show a progressive reduction in lean body mass as they age [25]. These are both in contrast to the bone/muscle phenotype seen in BACHD rats, as the lower amount of bone/muscle tissue seen in the current study did not seem to progress with age. Instead, the body size and bone/muscle phenotypes seen in the BACHD rats appeared to be caused by discrete developmental deficits and stunted growth. It is unlikely that these phenotypes were the result of malnutrition during testing, as food was available *ad libitum* on the cage floor. It is possible, however, that BACHD pups might have had difficulties when competing for mothers' milk, leading to malnutrition at early ages. Such factors have been shown to affect the growth of animals from large litters [37]. Alternatively, the growth of BACHD rats might be disturbed on a molecular level, as Huntingtin has been shown to be important during fetal development [38]. The fact that BACHD rats had smaller heads compared to WT rats is particularly interesting, as similar symptoms have been seen in HD gene-carriers [39]. Thus, the discrete developmental deficits found in the BACHD rats might be closely connected to developmental deficits of human patients.

Food deprivation and motivation of BACHD rats

Behavioral assessment of HD animal models through the use of operant conditioning tests is of interest, as cognitive symptoms are common in HD patients and might become valuable to clinically track disease progression and treatment effects [40,41,42]. Many conditioning protocols require food deprivation in order to both efficiently train the animals to perform a given task and to maintain high performance. However, food deprivation of HD models requires extra care as they can be expected to have changes in body composition. To better understand how to optimally food deprive BACHD rats, we assessed their interest in food in a total of three different tests.

Free intake of reward pellets and regular food is sometimes used to assess an animal's hunger level and interest in food [18,19,20,21]. In the current study, WT and BACHD rats deprived to 85% of their free-feeding body weight did not seem to differ in their interest in consuming 100 reward pellets, although BACHD rats needed more time to eat all pellets. Food deprivation levels were then adjusted in an attempt to reverse the phenotypes, however, this did not seem to affect the rats' behavior. Instead, both the time spent exploring the arena and the time needed to consume all pellets decreased with repeated testing. The training

effect on the consumption rate eventually led to BACHD rats consuming the reward pellets at an equal rate compared to WT rats. There were indications that rats deprived to 95% of their free-feeding body weight spent more time exploring the arena compared to rats deprived to 80%, but this generally concerned one or two rats of an entire group of twelve. As the current protocol did not appear to be sensitive even to large changes in food deprivation levels, it is unlikely to be a suitable test for assessing discrete differences in food interest. It is also clear that the apparent training effect could be misinterpreted as a food deprivation effect, if one assessed a given group of animals repeatedly with the aim of gradually adjusting their food deprivation level. The slowed consumption speed seen among BACHD rats in the pellet consumption test is, however, an interesting phenotype on its own. While eating, rats typically stood on all four paws and used their tongue to pick up the pellets. Thus, the slower feeding rate among BACHD rats is likely due to impairments in quite basic processes that are needed for eating. These could include impaired chewing, swallowing or tongue movements as well as reduced saliva production. It is tempting to hypothesize that the slower feeding speed among BACHD rats could be due to phenotypes similar to the tongue protrusion symptoms that are often seen among HD patients [43,44]. Interestingly, there are protocols for measuring tongue protrusion [45] in rats, although these tests must be performed carefully, as the smaller head size of BACHD rats likely means that they have shorter tongues as well.

In the regular food consumption test, BACHD rats consumed less food than WT rats when both groups were deprived to 85% of their respective free-feeding body weight. Consumption rate during the first 30 minutes of the test changed in a predictable way when deprivation levels were adjusted, with more deprived rats eating at a faster rate. This suggests that the protocol was well suited for the assessment of food interest and hunger levels. Our results further showed that when BACHD and WT rats were deprived to 80 and 95% of their respective free-feeding body weights, they consumed food at an identical rate for the initial 150 minutes, indicating that the rats were equally hungry. As the test session continued, BACHD rats once again ate less than WT rats, which likely reflected differences in the rats' satiety levels. It should be noted that the feeding behavior of either genotype did not significantly differ when comparing their 80 and 85% food deprivation test sessions. Thus, although the test seems suitable to assess food interest, it does not appear to be very sensitive. Assessing food consumption in single animals, rather than in groups, would most likely improve the test's sensitivity. It would further allow separate scoring of the time spent eating and the time spent not eating, as it was done in the reward pellet consumption test. However, despite extensive habituation, we have found it difficult to get our rats to efficiently consume regular food in any other setup than their home cages. As the test did not allow separate scoring of the time the rats spent feeding and doing other activities, it was not possible to conclude if the difference in consumption rate was strictly due to a difference in hunger and food interest. This idea is especially difficult to support when considering the results of the pellet consumption test. In an attempt to reach a conclusion on the matter, we ran a PR test with prefeedings.

When both WT and BACHD rats were deprived to 85% of their respective free-feeding body weight, BACHD rats were clearly less motivated to work for food rewards in the PR test. Similar phenotypes have been found in other HD models [16,46] and they are typically discussed in terms of apathy, which is a common symptom among HD patients [47,48]. However,

BACHD rats also responded with more pronounced drops in motivation during the prefeeding tests, which would typically be interpreted as BACHD rats being less hungry compared to WT rats [49,50,51]. This would also support the idea that the BACHD rats' lower consumption rate in the first session of the food consumption test was to some degree caused by lower hunger and food interest. When the food deprivation level of WT rats was adjusted to achieve equal food consumption rates to those of the BACHD rats, all genotype differences that were previously seen in the PR test disappeared. As WT and BACHD rats did not differ during prefeeding tests, it is reasonable to assume that they were equally hungry and that the food consumption test was suitable for establishing food deprivation levels that ensured this. As they also no longer differed in baseline performance, the motivational deficit seen in the first PR test was likely dependent on a difference in hunger levels, rather than an apathy-related phenotype. It is interesting to note that after the food deprivation levels had been adjusted, BACHD rats weighed approximately 50 g less than WT rats. This difference was similar to the one found in bone/muscle tissue, suggesting that WT and BACHD rats carried a similar amount of adipose tissue. Secretion of leptin, which affects satiety and food intake [52,53], is proportional to adipose tissue mass [54], and it is possible that the food deprivation adjustment led to equal hunger and food interest due to equal levels of leptin. Importantly, higher leptin levels have been shown to reduce motivation in PR tests [55], which gives a possible explanation for the initial motivational difference.

Most of the conclusions above are based on the idea that prefeeding responses depend exclusively on hunger levels and not on other aspects of motivation. One could argue that animals that suffer from motivational deficits not related to hunger, might also respond stronger on the prefeeding tests. Thus, seeking a situation where animals respond equally to prefeeding could in itself lead to the lack of differences in PR performance. It is therefore important to note that other studies have found motivational differences despite identical responses on prefeeding tests [51], and that motivational deficits have been found in BACHD mice after adjusting deprivation levels until animals consumed food at the same rate [16]. It should also be noted that the true nature of the motivational phenotype seen here is mainly of importance when such phenotypes are being characterized. If one simply wishes to minimize motivational differences when working with BACHD rats, regardless if these are due to hunger levels or other aspects of motivation, adjusting deprivation levels so that WT and BACHD rats consume regular food at a comparable rate should suffice. Still, the current study only considered quite young animals. It is possible that older BACHD rats suffer from motor impairments that could affect the validity of the food consumption test. Also, motivational phenotypes not related to hunger might become apparent among older BACHD rats. We aim at addressing these ideas in a longitudinal study of PR performance.

Summary

In the current study, BACHD rats were found to have metabolic disturbances, which is in line with other animal models of HD. We further found that unless these phenotypes were taken into consideration during food deprivation, BACHD rats were less motivated than WT rats in a progressive ratio test. Thus, metabolic phenotypes are important to consider as possible confounding factors when assessing apathy-related phenotypes of BACHD rats. The same is likely true for other HD animal models with metabolic abnormalities.

Our results further indicated that basing the animals' food deprivation levels on their consumption rates of regular food was a convenient way to avoid motivational differences between BACHD and WT rats. Thus, previous studies that applied this method when studying apathy in HD animal models [16] likely avoided hunger-based motivational differences, and our results support the future use of this method. It is also important to consider its use in behavioral tests where the main readout is not directly related to apathy or motivation, such as [17], as motivational differences have been shown to affect animals' behavior in such tests too [15].

Supporting Information

Figure S1   Food debris and water consumption during the *ad libitum* food consumption test. (A) The approximate daily amount of food debris produced per cage (calculated from a three- to four-day average), plotted against the age of the rats. **(B)** The approximate amount of food debris per cage relative to the average food consumption per cage, plotted against the age of the rats. **(C)** The approximate daily food consumption per rat (calculated from the weekly food consumption per cage) after accounting for food debris left in the cages, plotted against the age of the rats. **(D)** The approximate daily water consumption per rat (calculated from the weekly water consumption per cage), plotted against the age of the rats. The graphs indicate group mean plus standard error of the mean. Two-way ANOVA results are displayed above each graph, and results from *post-hoc* analysis are shown for individual data points. Significant genotype differences are indicated by ($p<0.05$) *, ($p<0.01$) **, ($p<0.001$) *** and ($p<0.0001$) ****. For **(D)**, WT and BACHD rats differed highly significant (****) for all data points between 11 and 26 weeks of age.

Figure S2   Body length measurements. (A–D) Data from length measurement as stated in the graph titles. The graphs show group mean plus standard error of the mean. Two-way ANOVA results are displayed above each graph, and significant results from *post-hoc* analysis are displayed inside each graph. Significant genotype differences are indicated by ($p<0.05$) *, ($p<0.01$) **, ($p<0.001$) *** and ($p<0.0001$) ****.

Figure S3   Habituation to the operant conditioning boxes. (A) The total number of head entries made into the pellet receptacle during habituation sessions. **(B)** The total time spent with the head inside of the pellet receptacle during habituation sessions as a measurement of the duration of receptacle visits. **(C)** The mean latency to enter the pellet receptacle after the delivery of a reward pellet. The graphs indicate group mean plus standard error of the mean. Two-way ANOVA results are displayed above each graph, and results from *post-hoc* analysis are shown for individual data points. Significant genotype differences are indicated by ($p<0.05$) *, ($p<0.01$) **, ($p<0.001$) *** and ($p<0.0001$) ****.

Figure S4   Performance on the CRF protocol. Results from the final session of CRF training are shown as indicated by graph titles. Session duration measured the time the rats needed to complete 100 ratios. Retrieval latency measured the time between the release of the reinforced lever and the entry into the pellet receptacle. Lever return latency was defined as the interval between the first receptacle entry following reward delivery and the lever push that followed. Graphs indicate the performance of individual rats and group mean. Results from t-tests or Mann-Whitney tests are indicated in the graphs. Significant genotype differences are indicated by (p<0.05) *, (p<0.01) **, (p<0.001) *** and (p<0.0001) ****.

Figure S5 Performance on fixed ratio protocols. Results for several basic parameters of FR3 and FR5 protocols are shown as indicated by the graph titles. Session duration measured the time the rats needed to complete 100 ratios. Ratio duration measured the time between the first and last lever push of each ratio. Ratio interval was defined as the time between the last lever push of one ratio and the first lever push of the ratio that followed. Retrieval latency measured the time between the release of the reinforced lever and the entry into the pellet receptacle. Lever return was defined as the interval between the first receptacle entry following reward delivery and the first lever push of the ratio that followed. Scatter plots of FR3 results indicate the performance of individual rats and group mean. Results from t-tests or Mann-Whitney tests are indicated in the graphs. Only results from the final session, where rats performed at criterion, are displayed. Line graphs of FR5 results indicate group mean plus standard error of the mean, plotted against the training session. Only the three final sessions, where rats performed at criterion, are included. Two-way ANOVA results are displayed at the top right corner of each FR5 graph, and significant results from *post-hoc* analysis are shown for individual data points. Significant genotype differences are indicated by (p<0.05) *, (p<0.01) **, (p<0.001) *** and (p<0.0001) ****.

Figure S6 Performance on the fixed ratio part of the progressive ratio protocol. Results for the basic parameters of the ten FR5 ratios run at the start of each PR session. (**A**) Data from sessions where BACHD and WT rats were both deprived to 85% of their respective free-feeding body weights. (**B**) Data from sessions where food deprivation was adjusted to match the food consumption rate of BACHD and WT rats. Details for each parameter are described in the figure legend of Figure S4 and S5.

Lever push frequency was calculated based on the pushes made on the reinforced lever during the full length of a ratio, i.e. the ratio duration plus interval to subsequent ratio. Results displayed were obtained from the sessions used for baseline curves in Figure 6A. The graphs indicate group mean plus standard error of the mean. Two-way ANOVA results are displayed at the top right corner of each graph, and results from *post-hoc* analysis are shown for individual data points. Significant genotype differences are indicated by (p<0.05) *, (p<0.01) **, (p<0.001) *** and (p<0.0001) ****.

Figure S7 Mean number of errors for the fixed ratio part of the progressive ratio protocol. Errors made by the rats during the ten FR5 ratios run at the start of each PR session. (**A**) Data from sessions where BACHD and WT rats were both deprived to 85% of their respective free-feeding body weights. (**B**) Data from sessions where food deprivation was adjusted to match the food consumption rate of BACHD and WT rats. Results were obtained from the sessions used for baseline curves in Figure 6A. Graphs indicate the performance of individual rats and group mean. Results from t-tests or Mann-Whitney tests are indicated in the graphs. Significant genotype differences are indicated by (p<0.05) *, (p<0.01) **, (p<0.001) *** and (p<0.0001) ****.

Acknowledgments

The authors wish to thank Celina Tomczak for support with breeding, genotyping, animal care and data gathering.

Author Contributions

Conceived and designed the experiments: EKHJ LEC OR HPN. Performed the experiments: EKHJ LEC. Analyzed the data: EKHJ LEC. Contributed to the writing of the manuscript: EKHJ LEC HPN.

References

1. Pringsheim T, Wiltshire K, Day L, Dykesman J, Steeves T, et al. (2012) The incidence and prevalence of huntington's disease: a systematic review and meta-analysis. Mov Disord 9: 1083–1091.
2. The Huntington's disease collaborative research group (1993) A novel gene containing a trinucleotide repeat that is expanded and unstable on huntington's disease chromosomes. Cell 72: 971–983.
3. Zuccato C, Valenza M, Cattaneo E (2010) Molecular mechanism and potential therapeutocal targets in huntington's disease. Physiol Rev 90: 905–981.
4. Djoussé L, Knowlton B, Cupples LA, Marder K, Shoulson I, et al. (2002) Weight loss in early stage of huntington's disease. Neurology 59: 1325–1330.
5. Kirkwood SC, Su JL, Conneally M, Foround T (2001) Progression of symptoms in the early and middle stages of huntington disease. Arch Neurol 58: 273–278.
6. Aziz NA, van der Burg JMM, Landwehrmeyer GB, Brundin P, Stinjen T, et al. (2008) Weight loss in huntington disease increases with higher CAG repeat number. Neurology 71: 1506–1513.
7. Robbins AO, Ho AK, Barker RA (2006) Weight changes in huntington's disease. Eur J Neurol 13: e7.
8. van der Burg JMM, Björkqvist M, Brundin P (2009) Beyond the brain: widespread pathology in huntington's disease. Lancet Neurol 8: 765–774.
9. Aziz NA, van der Marck MA, Pijl H, Olde Rikkert MGM, Bloem BR, et al. (2008) Weight loss in neurodegenerative disorders. J Neurol 255: 1872–1880.
10. Gray M, Shirasaki DI, Cepeda C, André VM, Wilburn B, et al. (2008) Full-length human mutant huntingtin with a stable polyglutamine repeat can elicit progressive and selective neuropathogenesis in BACHD mice. J Neurosci 28: 6182–6195.
11. van Raamsdonk JM, Metzler M, Slow E, Pearson J, Schwab C, et al. (2007) Pheontypic abnormalities in the YAC128 mouse model of huntington disease are penetrant on multiple genetic backgrounds and modulated by strain. Neurobiol Dis 26: 189–200.
12. Kudwa AE, Menalled LB, Oakeshott S, Murphy C, Mushlin R, et al. (2013) Increased body weight of the BAC HD transgenic mouse model of huntington's disease accounts for some but not all of the observed HD-like motor deficits.

PLoS Curr 30: 5. Available: http://currents.plos.org/hd/article/increased-body-weight-of-the-bac-hd-transgenic-mouse-model-of-huntingtons-disease-accounts-for-some-but-not-all-of-the-observed-hd-like-motor-deficits/. Accessed 12 January 2014.
13. McFadyen MP, Kusek G, Bolivar VJ, Flaherty L (2003) Differences among eight inbred strains of mice in motor ability and motor learning on a rotorod. Genes Brain Behav 2: 214–219.
14. Trueman RC, Dunnett SB, Brooks SP (2012) Operant-based instrumental learning for analysis of genetically modified models of huntington's disease. Brain Res Bull 88: 261–275.
15. Youn J, Ellenbroek BA, van Eck I, Roubos S, Verhage M, et al. (2011) Finding the right motivation: Genotype-dependent differences in effective reinforcements for spatial learning. Behav Brain Res 226: 397–403.
16. Oakeshott S, Port R, Cummins-Sutphen J, Berger J, Watson-Johnson J, et al. (2012) A mixed fixed ratio/progressive ratio procedure reveals an apathy phenotype in the BAC HD and the z_Q175 KI mouse models of Huntington's disease. PLoS Curr 25: 4. Available: http://currents.plos.org/hd/article/a-mixed-fixed-ratioprogressive-ratio-procedure-reveals-an-apathy-phenotype-in-the-bac-hd-and-the-z_q175-ki-mouse-models-of-huntingtons-disease/. Accessed 13 June 2012.
17. Oakeshott S, Farrar A, Port R, Cummins-Sutphen J, Berger J, et al. (2013) Deficits in a simple visual Go/No-go discrimination task in two mouse models of huntington's disease. PLoS Curr 7: 5. Available: http://currents.plos.org/hd/article/deficits-in-a-simple-visual-gono-go-discrimination-task-in-two-mouse-models-of-huntingtons-disease/. Accessed 12 January 2014.
18. Enkel T, Berger SM, Schönig K, Tews B, Bartsch D (2014) Reduced expression of Nogo-A leads to motivational deficits in rats. Front Behav Neurosci 8: 10. Available: http://journal.frontiersin.org/Journal/10.3389/fnbeh.2014.00010/full. Accessed 7 March 2014.
19. Bradbury MJ, Campbell U, Giracello D, Chapman D, King C, et al. (2005) Metabotropic glutamate receptor mGlu5 is a mediator of appetite and energy balance in rats and mice. J Pharmacol Exp Ther 313: 395–402.

20. Roth JD, D'Souza L, Griffin PS, Athanacio J, Trevaskis JL, et al. (2012) Interactions of amylinergic and melanocortinergic systems in the control of food intake and body weight in rodents. Diabetes Obes Metab 14: 608–615.

21. Fielding SA, Brooks SP, Klein A, Bayram-Weston Z, Jones J, et al. (2012) Profiles of motor and cognitive impairment in the transgenic rat model of huntingtin's disease. Brain Res Bull 88: 223–236.

22. Yu-Taeger L, Petrasch-Parwez E, Osmand AP, Redensek A, Metzger S, et al. (2012) A novel BACHD transgenic rat exhibits characteristic neuropathological features of huntington disease. J Neurosci 32: 15426–15438.

23. Abada YK, Nguyen HP, Ellenbroek B, Schreiber R (2013) Reversal learning and associative memory impairments in a BACHD rat model for huntington disease. PLoS One 8: 10. Available: http://www.plosone.org/article/info%3Adoi%2F10.1371%2Fjournal.pone.0071633. Accessed 24 November 2013.

24. Clemens LE, Jansson EKH, Portal E, Riess O, Nguyen HP (2014) A behavioral comparison of the common laboratory rat strains lister hooded, lewis, fischer 344 and wistar in an automated homecage system. Genes Brain Behav 13: 305–21.

25. She P, Zhang Z, Marchionini D, Diaz WC, Jetton T, et al. (2011) Molecular characterization of skeletal muscle atrophy in the R6/2 mouse model of huntington's disease. Am J Physiol Endocrinol Metab 301: E49–E61.

26. Schilling G, Becher MW, Sharp AH, Jinnah HA, Duan K, et al. (1999) Intranuclear inclusions and neuritic aggregates in transgenic mice expressing a mutant N-terminal fragment of huntingtin. Hum Mol Genet 8: 397–407.

27. von Hörsten S, Schmitt I, Nguyen HP, Holzmann C, Schmidt T, et al. (2003) Transgenic rat model of huntington's disease. Hum Mol Genet 12: 617–624.

28. Hult S, Soylu R, Björklund T, Belgardt BF, Mauer J, et al. (2011) Mutant huntingtin causes metabolic imbalance by disruption of hypothalamic neurocircuits. Cell Metab 13: 428–439.

29. van Raamsdonk JM, Gibson WT, Pearson J, Murphy Z, Lu G, et al. (2006) Body weight is modulated by levels of full-length huntingtin. Hum Mol Genet 15: 1513–1523.

30. Weydt P, Pineda W, Torrence AE, Libby RT, Satterfield TF, et al. (2006) Thermoregulatory and metabolic dfects in Huntington's disease transgenic mice implicate PGC-1alpha in Huntington's disease neurodegeneration. Cell Metab 4: 349–362.

31. Hollopeter G, Erickson JC, Palmiter RD (1998) Role of neuropeptide Y in diet-, chemical and genetic-induced obesity of mice. Int J Obes Relat Metab Disord 22: 506–512.

32. Tanaka K, Shimada M, Nakao K, Kusunoki T (1978) Hypothalamic lesion induced by injection of monosodium glutamate in suckling period and subsequent development of obesity. Exp Neurol 62: 191–199.

33. Morris MJ, Tortelli CF, Filippis A, Proietto J (1998) Reduced BAT as a mechanism for obesity in the hypophagic, neuropeptide Y deficient monosodium glutamate-treated rat. Regul Pept 25: 441–447.

34. Chen W, Chen Z, Xue N, Zheng Z, Li S, et al. (2013) Effect of CB1 receptor blockade on monosodium glutamate induced hypometabolic and hypothalamic obesity in rats. Naunyn Schmiedebergs Arch Pharmacol 8: 721–732.

35. Scallet AC and Olney JW (1986) Components of hypothalamic obesity: bipiperidyl-mustard lesions add hyperphagia to monosodium glutamate-induced hyperinsulinemia. Brain Res (2): 380–384.

36. Bergen HT, Mizuno TM, Taylor J, Mobbs CV (1998) Hyperphagia and weight gain after gold-thioglucose: relation to hypothalamic neuropeptide Y and proopiomelanocortin. Endocrinology 139: 4483–4488.

37. Remmers F, Fodor M, Delemarre-van de Waal H (2008) Neonatal food restriction permanently alters rat body dimensions and energy intake. Physiol Behav 95: 208–215.

38. Nguyen GD, Molero AE, Gokhan S, Mehler MF (2013) Functions of huntingtin in germ layer specification and organogenesis. PLoS One 8: 8. Available: http://www.plosone.org/article/info%3Adoi%2F10.1371%2Fjournal.pone.0072698. Accessed 11 March 2014.

39. Lee JK, Mathews K, Schlaggar B, Perlmutter J, Paulsen JS, et al. (2012) Measures of growth in children at risk for Huntington disease. Neurology 79: 668–674.

40. Lawrence AD, Sahakian BJ, Hodges JR, Rosser AE, Lange KW, et al. (1996) Executive and mnemotic functions in early huntington's disease. Brain 119: 1633–1645.

41. Lemiere J, Decruyenaere M, Evers-Kiebooms G, Vandenbussche E, Dom R (2004) Cognitive changes in patients with huntington's disease (HD) and asymptomatic carriers of the HD mutation a longitudinal follow-up study. J Neurol 251: 935–942.

42. Harrington DL, Smith MM, Zhang Y, Carlozzi NE, Paulsen JS (2012) Cognitive domains that predict time to diagnosis in prodromal huntington disease. J Neurosurg Psychiatry 83: 612–619.

43. Meyer C, Landwehrmeyer B, Schwenke C, Doble A, Orth M, et al. (2012) Rate of change in early huntington's disease: a clinicometric analysis. Mov Disord 27: 118–124.

44. Vaccarino AL, Anderson K, Borowsky B, Duff K, Giuliano J, et al. (2011) An item response analysis of the motor and behavioral subscales of the unified huntington's disease rating scale in huntington disease gene expansion carriers. Mov Disord 26: 877–884.

45. Whisaw IQ, Tompkins GJ (1988) An optic-fiber photocell detector for measuring tongue protrusion in the rat: evaluation of recovery from localized cortical lesions. Psychol Behav 43: 397–401.

46. Trueman RC, Brooks SP, Jones L, Dunnett SB (2009) Rule learning, visuospatial function and motor performance in the HdhQ92 knock-in mouse model of Huntington's disease. Behav Brain Res 203: 215–222.

47. Paulsen JS, Ready RE, Hamilton JM, Mega MS, Cummings JL (2001) Neuropsychiatric aspects of huntington's disease. J Neurol Neurosurg Psychiatry 71: 310–314.

48. Naarding P, Janzing JGE, Eling P, van der Werf S, Kremer B (2009) Apathy is not depression in huntington's disease. J Neuropsuchiatry Clin Neurosci 21: 266–270.

49. Skjoldager P, Pierre PJ, Mittleman G (1993) Reinforcer magnitude and progressive ratio responding in the rat: effect of increased effort, prefeeding, and extinction. Learning Motivation 24: 303–343.

50. Eagle DM, Humby T, Dunnett SB, Robbins TW (1999) Effects of regional striatal lesions on motor, motivational, and executive aspects of progressive-ratio performance in rats. Behav Neurosci 133: 718–731.

51. Schmelzeis MC, Mittleman G (1996) The hippocampus and reward: effects of hippocampal lesions on progressive-ratio responding. Behav Neurosci 110: 1049–1066.

52. Halaas JL, Gajiwala KS, Maffei M, Cohen SL, Chait BT, et al. (1995) Weight-reducing effects of the plasma protein encoded by the obese gene. Science 269: 543–546.

53. Halaas JL, Boozer C, Blair-West J, Fidahusein N, Denton DA, et al. (1997) Physiological response to long-term peripheral and central leptin infusion in lean and obese mice. Proc Natl Acad Sci 94: 8878–8883.

54. Maffei M, Halaas J, Ravussin E, Pratley RE, Lee GH, et al. (1995) Leptin levels in human and rodent: Measurement of plasma leptin and ob RNA in obese and weight-reduced subjects. Nat Med 1: 1155–1161.

55. Kanoski SE, Alhadeff AL, Fortin SM, Gilbert JR, Grill HJ (2014) Leptin signaling in the medial nucleus tractus solitarius reduced food seeking and willingness to work for food. Neuropsychopharmacology 39: 605–613.

13

Striatal Synaptic Dysfunction and Hippocampal Plasticity Deficits in the Hu97/18 Mouse Model of Huntington Disease

Karolina Kolodziejczyk[1], Matthew P. Parsons[1], Amber L. Southwell[2], Michael R. Hayden[2], Lynn A. Raymond[1]*

1 Department of Psychiatry, Brain Research Centre, University of British Columbia, Vancouver, British Columbia, Canada, **2** Centre for Molecular Medicine and Therapeutics, Child and Family Research Institute, University of British Columbia, Vancouver, British Columbia, Canada

Abstract

Huntington disease (HD) is a fatal neurodegenerative disorder caused by a CAG repeat expansion in the gene (*HTT*) encoding the huntingtin protein (HTT). This mutation leads to multiple cellular and synaptic alterations that are mimicked in many current HD animal models. However, the most commonly used, well-characterized HD models do not accurately reproduce the genetics of human disease. Recently, a new 'humanized' mouse model, termed Hu97/18, has been developed that genetically recapitulates human HD, including two human *HTT* alleles, no mouse *Hdh* alleles and heterozygosity of the HD mutation. Previously, behavioral and neuropathological testing in Hu97/18 mice revealed many features of HD, yet no electrophysiological measures were employed to investigate possible synaptic alterations. Here, we describe electrophysiological changes in the striatum and hippocampus of the Hu97/18 mice. At 9 months of age, a stage when cognitive deficits are fully developed and motor dysfunction is also evident, Hu97/18 striatal spiny projection neurons (SPNs) exhibited small changes in membrane properties and lower amplitude and frequency of spontaneous excitatory postsynaptic currents (sEPSCs); however, release probability from presynaptic terminals was unaltered. Strikingly, these mice also exhibited a profound deficiency in long-term potentiation (LTP) at CA3-to-CA1 synapses. In contrast, at 6 months of age we found only subtle alterations in SPN synaptic transmission, while 3-month old animals did not display any electrophysiologically detectable changes in the striatum and CA1 LTP was intact. Together, these data reveal robust, progressive deficits in synaptic function and plasticity in Hu97/18 mice, consistent with previously reported behavioral abnormalities, and suggest an optimal age (9 months) for future electrophysiological assessment in preclinical studies of HD.

Editor: Gilberto Fisone, Karolinska Inst, Sweden

Funding: Funding was provided by the Canadian Institutes of Health Research (MOP-12699 to L.A.R. and MOP-84438 to M.R.H.) and the Cure Huntington Disease Foundation (M.R.H.). M.P.P was supported by a Michael Smith Foundation for Health Research Fellowship Award. A.L.S. was supported by a Michael Smith Foundation for Health Research Fellowship Award, Canadian Institutes of Health Research and Huntington Society of Canada. CHDI: http://chdifoundation.org/ CIHR: http://www.cihr-irsc.gc.ca/ MSF: http://www.msfhr.org/ HSC: http://huntingtonsociety.ca/ The funders had no role in study design, data collection and analysis, decision to publish, or preparation of the manuscript.

Competing Interests: The authors have declared that no competing interests exist.

* E-mail: lynn.raymond@ubc.ca

Introduction

Huntington disease (HD) is a fatal autosomal dominant neurodegenerative disorder caused by a CAG repeat expansion in the gene (*HTT*) encoding the huntingtin protein [1]. Expansion of the CAG beyond 36 repeats produces a mutated huntingtin protein (muHTT) with an expanded polyglutamine (polyQ) tract in its N-terminal region. Expression of muHTT results in profound disruption of a wide variety of cellular processes (reviewed in: [2]), including synaptic transmission and plasticity (reviewed in: [3–5]). It is of a great interest to determine whether therapeutics designed to delay or slow progression of HD can prevent or reverse these detrimental cellular changes, and how full beneficial effects.
early in disease development they should be applied to exert their

A recent and promising approach to the treatment of HD utilizes antisense oligonucleotide (ASO) technology to knock down

expression levels of muHTT. ASO administration has been employed to effectively silence the expression of a variety of genes of interest and relies on a specific design and efficient delivery of short, synthetic, modified nucleic acids. A number of preclinical and clinical studies, targeting different neurological and non-neurological disorders, have demonstrated ASO efficiency with no severe adverse effects (reviewed in: [6,7]).

ASOs targeted to muHTT, designed by exploiting the presence of single nucleotide polymorphisms (SNPs), have proven to be potent and selective in cell culture and the BACHD mouse model [8]. However, studying the effectiveness of anti-muHTT ASO therapy requires preclinical testing in an animal model that fully recapitulates the genetics of the disease and displays behavioral, cellular and synaptic deficits typical for HD. The most commonly used, well-characterized HD models do not accurately reproduce human HD genetics. Specifically, they express either mouse HTT with expanded polyQ repeats (knock-in models) or human muHTT on a mouse wild-type HTT background (fragment and full-length transgenic models; reviewed in: [9,10]). To overcome these obstacles, a new "humanized" mouse model termed Hu97/18 has been developed, and behavioral and neuropathological tests have shown it recapitulates many aspects of HD [11]. Apart from changes in motor function and reduced motor learning at 2 months of age, Hu97/18 mice show additional cognitive deficits as early as 6 months, progressing to further deficits at 9 months; these include a decline in both spatial and object recognition memory performance. Furthermore, striatal and cortical volume is significantly decreased in these animals by 12 months of age [11]. This model is unique in that it expresses only the human HD gene, heterozygous for the HD mutation (with an expanded CAG of 97 repeats), on a mouse Huntingtin *null* $(Hdh^{-/-})$ background [11], and therefore provides a valuable tool to evaluate the efficacy of selective muHTT ASO therapies.

As mentioned, HD is associated with a host of cellular and synaptic alterations and it is important for preclinical studies to determine whether a therapeutic strategy can successfully prevent or reverse such changes. While many electrophysiological signatures have been described previously in other animal models of HD [4], none have been reported for the Hu97/18 mouse model. In the present study, we describe electrophysiological changes in the striatum and hippocampus of the Hu97/18 mice. We provide evidence for robust deficits in synaptic function and plasticity that should prove essential for future assessment of the effectiveness of ASO treatment and other candidate therapeutics in preclinical studies of HD.

Materials and Methods

Ethics statement

This study was carried out in strict accordance with the requirements of Canadian Council on Animal Care (CCAC). The study was approved by the University of British Columbia Animal Care Committee, under protocol A11-0012. All efforts were made to minimize animal suffering.

Transgenic mice and brain slice preparation

Transgenic Hu18/18 and Hu97/18 mice expressing full-length human huntingtin with 18 CAG repeats (Hu18/18) or with 18 and 97 CAG repeats (Hu97/18) carried on the yeast artificial chromosome (YAC) or bacterial artificial chromosome (BAC) transgene, respectively, on the $Hdh^{-/-}$ background (strain FVB/N), were generated and maintained at the animal care facility in the Centre for Molecular Medicine and Therapeutics [11] and then transferred to the University of British Columbia Animal Research Unit approximately 2 weeks prior to experimentation. Experiments were conducted either on mice aged 9–9.5 months (9-month old group), 6–7 months (6-month old group) or 3–3.5 months (3-month old group). All reported n values represent the number of cells or slices recorded. At least 3 (typically 5 or more) animals per genotype were used for each set of experiments. All data were obtained from male mice with the exception of a small number of female mice that were used in the 6-month group. The data obtained from females at this age did not differ from the males and was therefore pooled together.

To obtain acute corticostriatal slices, the animals were killed by decapitation following deep halothane vapour anaesthesia (in accordance with the UBC Animal Care Committee, protocol A11-0012, and the Canadian Council on Animal Care). The brain was immediately removed and immersed in ice-cold oxygenated slicing medium, composed of (in mM): NaCl 125, NaHCO$_3$ 25, NaH$_2$PO$_4$ 1.25, KCl 2.5, CaCl$_2$ 0.5, MgCl$_2$ 4, D-glucose 10 (gassed

with 95% O$_2$/5% CO$_2$), pH 7.3–7.4, 300–315mOsm. Coronal slices 300 μm thick were cut on a vibratome (Leica VT1200S) and placed in a holding chamber containing oxygenated artificial cerebrospinal fluid (ACSF) at 34–36°C. The ACSF composition was the same as the slicing medium except with 2 mM CaCl$_2$ and 1 mM MgCl$_2$. After 30–45 min, slices were transferred to room temperature (RT) and kept until 8 h post-slicing. For all hippocampal experiments, slices were obtained as above but in the transverse plane at 400 μm thickness. Sections were given 30–45 minutes at 34–36°C followed by an additional 30–45 minutes at RT to recover. Hippocampal slices were used for a maximum of 6 hours following recovery.

Electrophysiology

Much of the electrophysiology was performed as described previously [12]. Slices were continuously perfused (~2–4 ml/min; RT) with oxygenated ACSF containing picrotoxin (50–100 μM; PTX, Tocris Bioscience, Bristol, UK), glycine (10 μM; Sigma-Aldrich, MO, USA) and strychnine (2 μM; Tocris Bioscience, Bristol, UK). Glycine and strychnine were omitted for all hippocampal experiments and PTX was also omitted for LTP experiments. All signals, unless stated otherwise, were filtered at 10 kHz, digitized at 10 kHz and analysed in Clampfit10.2 (Axon Instruments, CA, USA). Whole cell patch-clamp recordings were performed in voltage-clamp or current-clamp mode. For the experiments in voltage-clamp mode (paired-pulse ratio and evoked stimulation), the internal solution consisted of (in mM): caesium methanesulphonate 130, CsCl 5, NaCl 4, MgCl$_2$ 1, EGTA 5, HEPES 10, QX-314 5, Na$_2$GTP 0.5, Na$_2$-phosphocreatine 10,spermine 0.1 and MgATP 5, pH 7.3, 280–290mOsm. For the experiments in current-clamp mode, as well as spontaneous excitatory postsynaptic currents (sEPSCs) and miniature EPSC (mEPSCs) recordings, the internal solution consisted of (in mM): K-gluconate 145, MgCl$_2$ 1, HEPES 10, EGTA 1, MgATP 2, Na$_2$GTP 0.5, pH 7.3, 280–290mOsm. Pipette resistance (Rp) was 3–5 MΩ. Series resistance (Rs) was <30 MΩ and uncompensated; the data were not included in the analysis if Rs changed by >20% by the end of the experiment. For LTP experiments, glass electrodes (1–2 MΩ) were filled with ACSF and used to stimulate the Schaffer collateral pathway and record field excitatory postsynaptic potentials (fEPSPs) in CA1 stratum radiatum. Electrical stimulation (0.1 ms pulses) was increased to generate the maximal response and then reduced to the stimulation intensity that produced 30–40% of the maximal response. Responses were elicited every 20 s for at least 10 minutes prior to LTP induction. High frequency stimulation (HFS; 100 Hz for 1 s×3, 10 s inter-train interval) was applied, and responses were again recorded at 20 s intervals for 60 minutes thereafter.

sEPSCs and mEPSCs were filtered at 1 kHz, digitized at 10 kHz and analysed with Clampfit10.2 event analysis function with a detection threshold set at -8pA (SPNs) or -6pA (CA1) while recording at a holding potential of -70 mV. Decay time was measured using single exponential fitting by Clamfit10.2 event analysis function.

Evoked EPSCs (eEPSCs) were elicited by intrastriatal electrical stimulation through a glass micropipette filled with ACSF (Rp = 2–5 MΩ) placed 150–200 μm dorsal to the recorded cell. The paired-pulse ratio (PPR) was recorded at V_h of -70 mV, and when performed with different stimulation intensities (50–500 μA), a 50 ms interval was applied. NMDA peak current was measured at +40 mV 40 ms after the initial peak response (to eliminate the possibility of contamination by the fast-decaying AMPA currents, [13]). Evoked responses (at both potentials) were averages of three responses recorded at the same stimulation intensity.

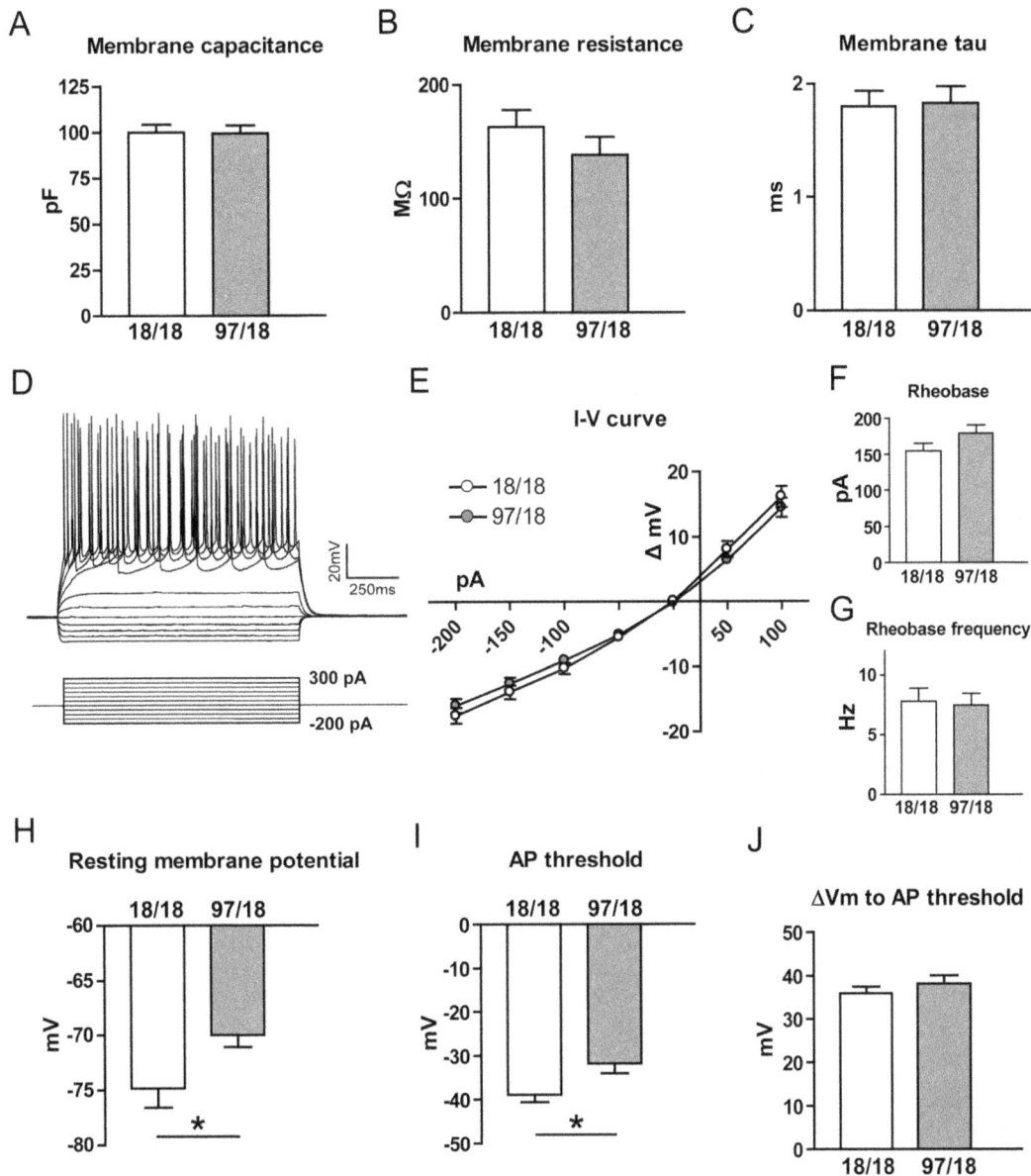

Figure 1. Alterations in basic membrane properties of Hu97/18 SPNs. (A–C): Membrane capacitance (A), membrane resistance (B), and membrane time constant (C) did not differ between Hu18/18 and Hu97/18 SPNs. Membrane capacitance measurement was pooled from the experiments with potassium-based and caesium-based internal solutions (Hu18/18 n = 46, Hu97/18 n = 44), while membrane resistance and tau were measured with potassium-based internal solution only (Hu18/18 n = 21, Hu97/18 n = 17). (D – J): Cells were patch-clamped with potassium-based solution, and membrane voltage changes in response to the injected current were recorded and analysed. (D) Representative I–V response of a Hu18/18 SPN to current injection (50pA increments from -200pA, 1 s each). (E) I–V curves showed no difference between Hu97/18 and Hu18/18 SPNs. (F) Rheobase and (G) rheobase frequency were not different between the genotypes. (H) Hu97/18 had a lower resting membrane potential than Hu18/18 SPNs (p = 0.03). (I) Action potential (AP) threshold was more depolarized in Hu97/18 SPNs (p = 0.02). (J) The change in membrane voltage from resting potential to AP threshold was not different between Hu18/18 and Hu97/18 SPNs. For the experiments in D–J, Hu18/18 n = 11 and Hu97/18 n = 12. *p<0.05 (unpaired Student's t-test).

Data analysis and statistics

Data were analysed using Clampfit10.2 (Axon Instruments, CA, USA), Microsoft Excel (Microsoft Corp., CA, USA) and Graphpad Prism5 (Graphpad Software, CA, USA). Data are presented as mean ±s.e.m. Significance was assessed with 2-tailed unpaired Student's t-tests with Welch correction or with two-way ANOVA followed by Bonferroni's *post hoc* test; P-values <0.05 were considered significant.

Results

Cellular and synaptic properties of striatal spiny projection neurons in 9 month-old Hu18/18 and Hu97/18 mice

Hu97/18 mice develop motor learning deficits as early as at 2 months of age, but memory impairments arise at 6 months of age and become fully manifest by 9 months [11]. Therefore, we began by using 9 month-old animals to assess the electrophysiological

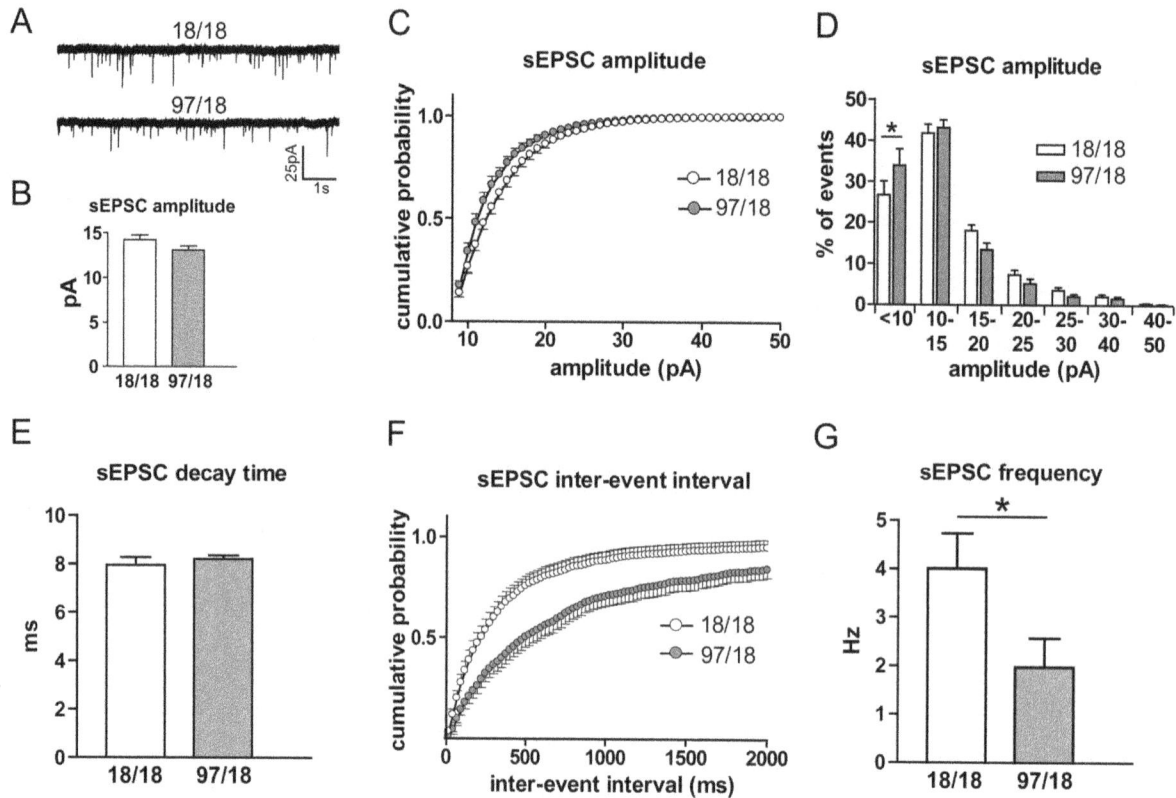

Figure 2. sEPSC amplitude and frequency change in Hu97/18 SPNs. Cells were patch-clamped with a potassium-based internal solution at $V_h = -70$ mV and sEPSCs were recorded. (A) Representative sEPSC traces for Hu18/18 (top) and Hu97/18 SPNs (bottom). (B) The average sEPSC amplitude of Hu18/18 and Hu97/18 cells (difference did not reach significance, p = 0.12). (C) Cumulative probability showed a decrease in sEPSC amplitude in Hu97/18 SPNs (significant genotype and amplitude interaction, p<0.0001). (D) Amplitude distribution analysis showed a significant increase in the percentage of small events (<10pA) and a trend towards a decrease in big events (>15pA) in Hu97/18 SPNs. (E) There was no difference in sEPSC decay time between Hu18/18 and Hu97/18 SPNs. (F) Cumulative probability showed an increase in sEPSC inter-event intervals in Hu97/18 SPNs (significant genotype and inter-event intervals interaction, p<0.0001). (G) The average sEPSC frequency was decreased in Hu97/18 SPNs (p = 0.038). For all experiments, Hu18/18 n = 20 and Hu97/18 n = 17. *P<0.05 (two-way ANOVA with Bonferroni correction, D; unpaired Student's t-test, G).

changes in the striatum and hippocampus. We identified striatal SPNs in the CPu of mouse striata as described previously [12] and first assessed passive membrane properties in voltage clamp mode ($V_h = -70$ mV). Using a potassium-based internal solution, the membrane capacitance, membrane resistance and membrane tau were not significantly different between genotypes (Fig. 1A–C). Cell firing characteristics were assessed in current clamp by recording membrane voltage changes in response to injected current steps (50pA increments starting from -200pA, 1 s each; Fig. 1D). The I–V curves were similar between the two genotypes (Fig. 1E), as was rheobase (Fig. 1F) and rheobase frequency (Fig. 1G), suggesting no changes in SPN excitability. Notably, Hu97/18 SPNs showed a significant depolarization of the resting membrane potential (p = 0.03, Fig. 1H); this change might be expected to result in an increased steady-state sodium channel inactivation. Consistent with this prediction, the action potential threshold was indeed elevated in Hu97/18 SPNs (p = 0.02, Fig. 1I) and the average change of membrane voltage from resting membrane potential to AP threshold was not different between the genotypes (Fig. 1J). Together, these results indicate that despite small changes in SPN membrane properties, the excitability of SPNs is similar for the two genotypes.

To test for alterations in synaptic transmission, we recorded spontaneous excitatory postsynaptic currents (sEPSCs) at $V_h =$

-70 mV in ACSF with the $GABA_A$ channel blocker PTX (Fig. 2A). We found a significant decrease in the amplitude of sEPSCs in Hu97/18 SPNs as shown by the cumulative probability analysis (interaction p<0.0001, Fig. 2C), although the mean difference did not reach statistical significance (p = 0.15, Fig. 2B). A more detailed analysis of amplitude distribution revealed a higher percentage of small events (<10pA, p<0.01) as well as a trend to a lower percentage of large events (15–30pA) in Hu97/18 (Fig. 2D). These data suggest the possibility of a modest decrease in postsynaptic AMPA receptor number in striatal SPNs of Hu97/18 mice. In contrast, mean sEPSC charge transfer and kinetics were not significantly different between genotypes (for the decay time, see Fig. 1E; charge transfer and rise time not shown).

Analysis of the frequency of events revealed a significant reduction in Hu97/18 compared to Hu18/18 SPNs, as shown by both the cumulative probability of inter-event intervals (interaction p<0.0001, Fig. 2F) and the mean event frequency (p = 0.038, Fig. 2G). When TTX was included in the bath solution to block action potential-driven transmitter release, we found similar genotype effects on mEPSC frequency and amplitude as we did with sEPSCs (Fig. 3A–G). In fact, the application of TTX had very little effect on the amplitude (Fig. 3D) or frequency (Fig. 3G) of spontaneous events, confirming a previous report that the majority

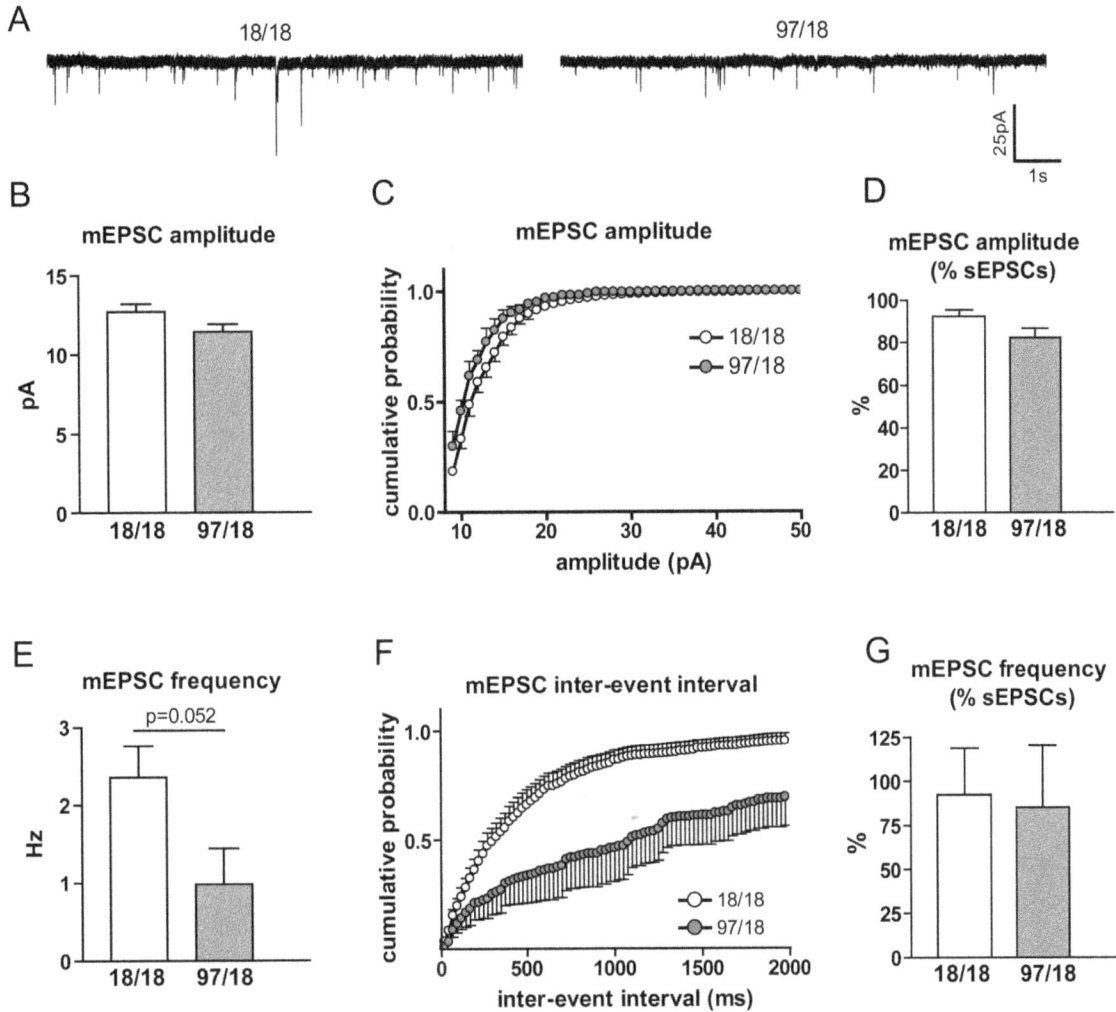

Figure 3. mEPSC amplitude and frequency change in Hu97/18 SPNs. Cells were patch-clamped with potassium-based internal solution at $V_h = -70$ mV and the initial sEPSCs were recorded. Then, TTX was added to the external solution which allowed for the extraction and analysis of mEPSCs. (A) Representative mEPSC traces for Hu18/18 (left) and Hu97/18 SPNs (right). (B) The average mEPSC amplitude of Hu18/18 and Hu97/18 cells ($p = 0.1$). (C) Cumulative probability showed a decrease in sEPSC amplitude in Hu97/18 SPNs (significant genotype and amplitude interaction, $p < 0.0001$). (D) mEPSC amplitude presented as a percentage of the initial sEPSC amplitude. There was no difference between Hu18/18 and Hu97/18 SPNs. (E) The mean mEPSC frequency trended towards a decrease in Hu97/18 SPNs but did not reach statistical significance ($p = 0.052$). (F) Cumulative probability showed an increase in mEPSC inter-event intervals in Hu97/18 SPNs (significant genotype and inter-event intervals interaction, $p < 0.0001$). (G) mEPSC frequency presented as a percentage of the initial sEPSC frequency. There was no difference between Hu18/18 and Hu97/18 SPNs. For all experiments, Hu18/18 $n = 9$ and Hu97/18 $n = 5$.

of spontaneous excitatory transmitter release in our preparation is action potential-independent [20].

The decreased sEPSC frequency is consistent with a loss of excitatory synapses on these cells, which is a signature mark of HD progression in other animal models [14,15]. On the other hand, the decreased sEPSC frequency may be linked to changes in release probability from excitatory presynaptic terminals [16]. A decrease in release probability would lead to a decrease in the frequency of postsynaptic glutamate receptor activation, which would be detected as a lower number of sEPSC events, a change that has been reported in other HD models [12,17,18]. To assess the release probability from presynaptic excitatory terminals, we patched SPNs with a caesium-based internal solution and recorded responses to paired electrical stimulation of the nearby afferents (150–200 μm from the patch-pipette; Fig. 3A). The two consecutive stimulations (50 ms apart) allowed us to calculate paired-pulse ratio (PPR), measured as the response to the second

stimulation divided by the response to the first. An increase in PPR (also known as paired-pulse facilitation) implies a lower initial probability of release, while a decrease (paired-pulse depression) indicates a higher probability. We used increasing stimulation intensities (50–500 μA) to detect any possible changes between the two genotypes that depend on the stimulus strength. At 9 months of age, no difference in PPR was observed between Hu18/18 and Hu97/18 SPNs, indicating no differences in the release probability from excitatory terminals (Fig. 4A,B). Moreover, at a stimulus intensity that generated an approximately half-maximal response, there was also no effect of genotype on PPRs with varying pulse intervals (Fig. 4C). Thus, despite a reduction in sEPSC frequency, we find no clear electrophysiological evidence of altered release probability.

The expression levels of AMPA receptors were previously shown to decrease with disease progression in a variety of HD mouse models [18,19] while NMDA receptor levels have been

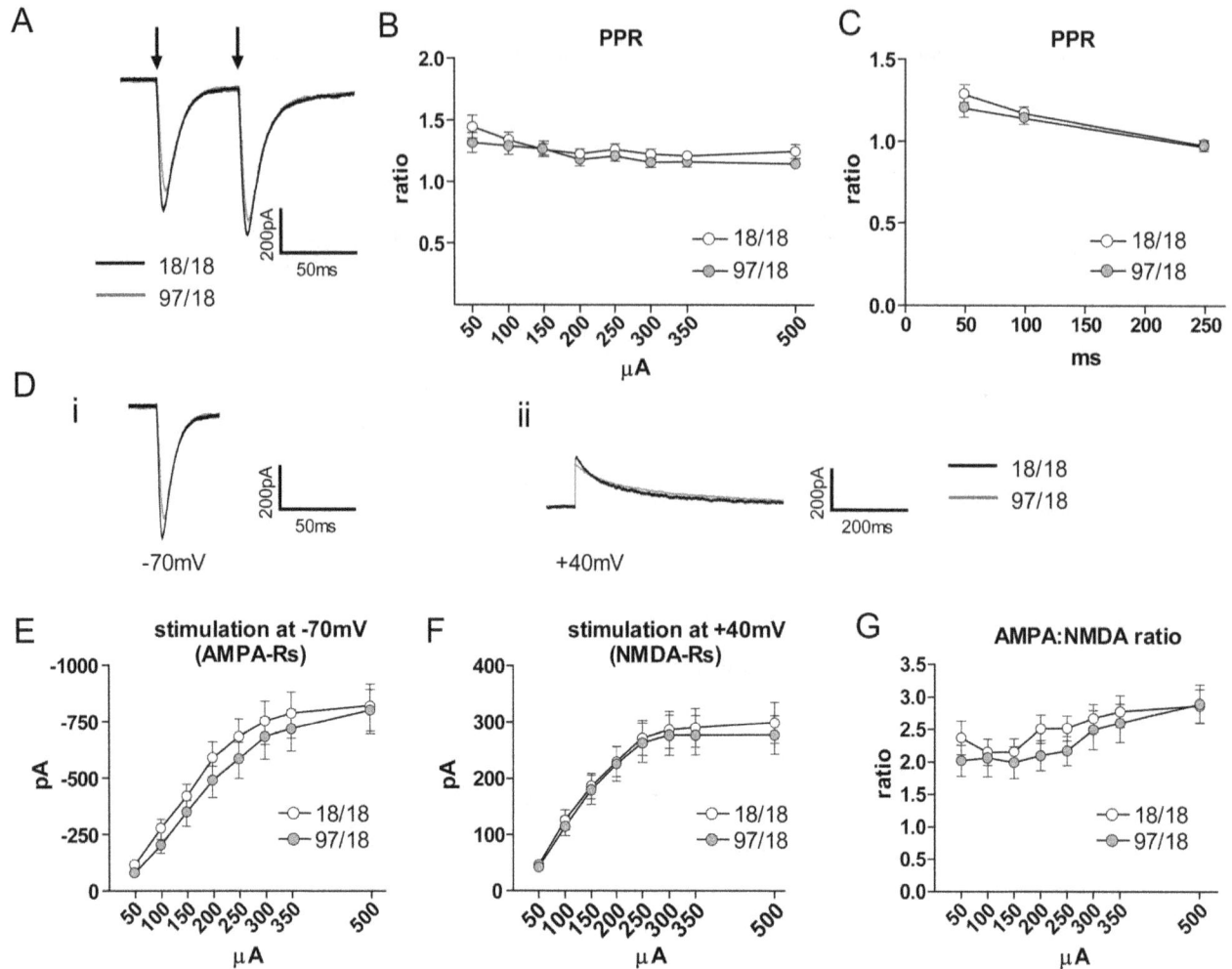

Figure. 4 Paired-pulse ratio (PPR) and AMPA:NMDA ratio are not affected in Hu97/18 SPNs. SPNs were whole-cell patch-clamped at $V_h = -$ 70 mV with caesium-based internal solution to allow for better membrane voltage control. (A) Representative traces showing responses of Hu18/18 and Hu97/18 SPNs to 200 µA paired-pulse stimulation (marked with the arrows) with 50 ms interval. Stimulus artifacts were removed. (B–C) No difference between Hu18/18 and Hu97/18 SPNs in PPR with different stimulation intensities (50–500 µA; B) and different time of inter-stimulation intervals (50, 100 and 250 ms; C) implies no change in probability of release from excitatory presynaptic terminals. For the experiments in (B), Hu18/ 18 n = 22 and Hu97/18 n = 22; for the experiments in (C), Hu18/18 n = 11 and Hu97/18 n = 14. (D) Representative responses of Hu18/18 and Hu97/18 SPN to 200 µA stimulation at $V_h = -70$ mV (i), analysed as AMPA receptor response, and at $V_h = +40$ mV (ii), analysed as NMDA receptor response at 40 ms from the initial peak. Stimulus artifacts were removed. (E) There was no statistically significant difference in the response to the stimulation at $V_h = -70$ mV between Hu18/18 (n = 22) and Hu97/18 SPNs (n = 22). The trend towards a smaller response in Hu97/18 SPNs may suggest, however, a decreased number of synaptic AMPA receptors. (F) No difference in the response to the stimulation at $V_h = +40$ mV between Hu18/18 (n = 22) and Hu97/18 SPNs (n = 21) implies no change in NMDA receptor expression levels. (G) AMPA:NMDA ratios (measured as an average from the cells where both responses to the stimulation at $V_h = -70$ mV and $V_h = +40$ mV were recorded) showed no difference between Hu18/18 (n = 19) and Hu97/18 SPNs (n = 19).

reported as increased or decreased, depending on the HD mouse model, stage of disease, and subcellular localization of the receptors [14,19,20]. Our analysis of sEPSCs has suggested that the levels of synaptic AMPA receptors may be modestly decreased in Hu97/18 SPNs (Fig. 2C–D). To evaluate levels of synaptic NMDA receptors, we measured the ratio of evoked EPSCs (eEPSCs) at negative (-70 mV) and positive (+40 mV) potentials in the same cell. Current recorded at -70 mV reflects activation of AMPA receptors only (due to cells being held at negative potential and recorded in ACSF containing a physiological concentration of Mg^{2+}, which prevents opening of NMDA receptors, and picrotoxin, which blocks $GABA_A$ receptors), while responses at +40 mV, measured 40 ms following initial peak current, reflect activation of NMDA receptors. The AMPA:NMDA ratio was then

calculated. While the mean evoked response size was slightly smaller in Hu97/18 SPNs at -70 mV (Fig. 4E), there was no significant genotype difference at this holding potential or at +40 mV (Fig. 4F). Similarly, the AMPA:NMDA ratio was unchanged (Fig. 4G).

Progressive electrophysiological differences in striatal SPNs recorded from Hu97/18 and Hu18/18 mice

After characterising electrophysiological changes in Hu97/18 SPNs at 9 months of age, we investigated whether the same alterations could be observed at an earlier time point (3 and 6 months) or rather if they represent progressive deficits. At 6 months of age, Hu97/18 mice already demonstrate many of the behavioral and cognitive deficits that become more pronounced at

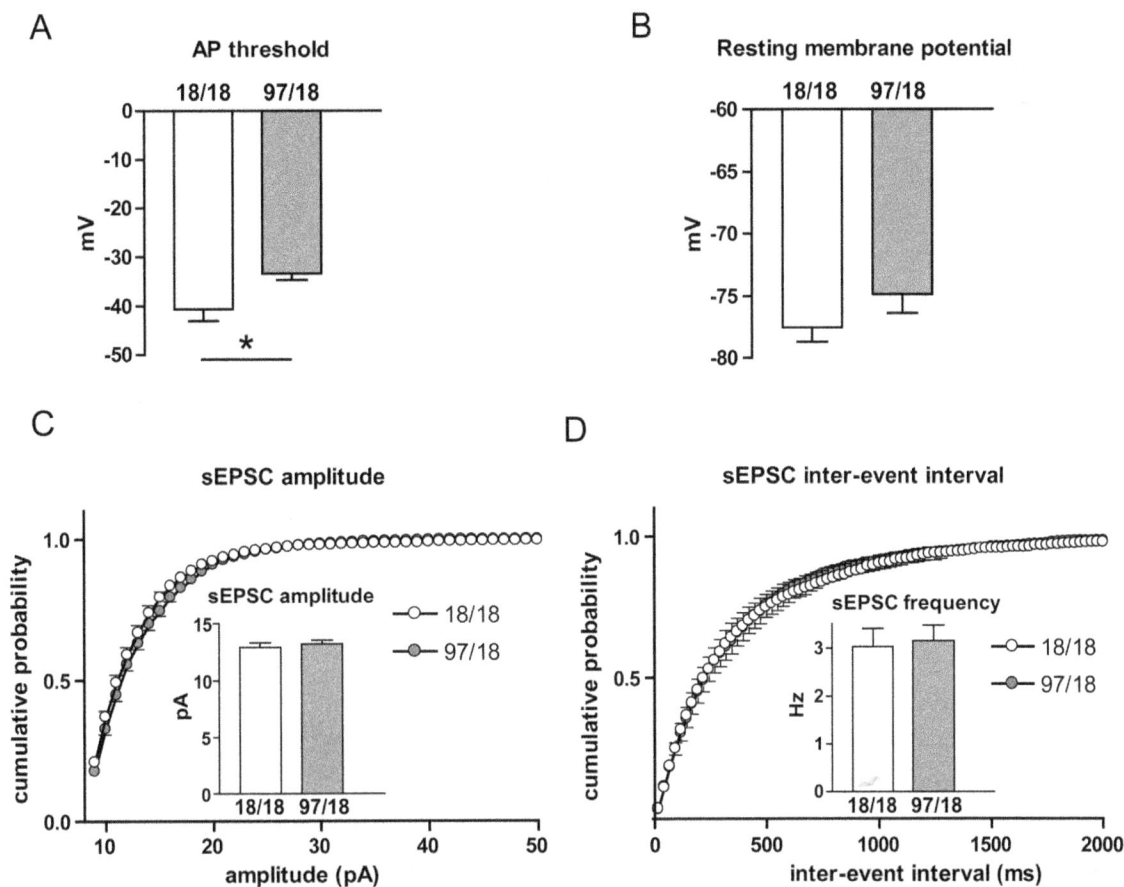

Figure 5. Subtle changes in membrane properties and unaltered sEPSC characteristics in Hu97/18 SPNs at 6 months of age. (A) At 6 months of age, action potential threshold was more depolarized in Hu97/18 SPNs. (B) No significant change in resting membrane potential was observed. sEPSC amplitude (C) and frequency (D) were unaffected in Hu97/18 SPNs at 6 months of age. For these experiments, Hu18/18 n = 13 and Hu97/18 n = 16. *p<0.05 (unpaired Student's t-test).

9 months [11], and therefore we expected to see some, if not all, of the electrophysiological changes that we recorded in older animals.

Similar to mice at 9 months of age, we observed no difference in membrane capacitance, resistance or tau. I–V curves, rheobase and rheobase frequency were also similar between Hu18/18 and Hu97/18 SPNs at 6 months of age (data not shown). However, the action potential threshold was increased (p = 0.02, Fig. 5A), similar to the results obtained from 9 month-old animals (Fig. 1I), while depolarization of the resting membrane potential appeared as a trend, but did not reach statistical significance (p = 0.18, Fig. 5B). Unlike at 9 months, there was no detectable difference in sEPSC frequency or amplitude at 6 months (Fig. 5C–D). When we examined an even earlier time point (3 months), we were unable to detect any difference in action potential threshold, resting membrane potential, sEPSC frequency or amplitude (Fig. 6 A–D). Together, these data suggest that the changes observed in Hu97/18 SPNs at 9 months of age represent progressive characteristics, and that the majority of these changes arise between 6 and 9 months of age.

Impaired hippocampal CA1 long-term potentiation in Hu97/18 mice

At 9 months, Hu97/18 mice display extensive deficits in learning and memory performance, as shown by spatial learning and novel object recognition tests [11]. To determine whether

these behavioral changes may stem from deficits in hippocampal long-term potentiation (LTP), as shown previously in other mouse models of HD [21–24], we stimulated excitatory field potentials (fEPSPs) in CA1 stratum radiatum. First, using a standard paired-pulse paradigm (at an interval of 100 ms), we found significantly reduced paired-pulse facilitation (PPF) in Hu97/18 slices (Fig. 7A–B; Hu18/18 n = 8, Hu97/18 n = 6, p = 0.021), indicating an impairment in short-term plasticity and consistent with a previous report in another HD mouse model [22]. We also observed a severe deficit in LTP in hippocampal slices from Hu97/18 mice (Fig. 7C). The presence of robust potentiation 50–60 minutes following high-frequency stimulation (HFS) in slices from Hu18/18 mice (n = 6) demonstrates that the replacement of murine HTT with human HTT does not impair LTP. On the other hand, LTP was completely absent in slices from Hu97/18 mice (n = 6, p = 0.0005 for Hu18/18 vs. Hu97/18, unpaired t-test of average fEPSP slope 50–60 minutes post-HFS). In contrast, paired pulse facilitation was normal and LTP was intact in slices from 3-month old Hu97/18 mice (Fig. 7D–F). Lastly, when we recorded CA1 pyramidal neurons under whole cell voltage-clamp at 9 months of age, we were unable to detect any genotype differences in membrane properties or mEPSC frequency or amplitude (Fig. 8A–G), demonstrating that alterations in these cellular and synaptic properties are at least somewhat specific to SPNs at this age. In all, our data support a progressive hippocampal synaptic plasticity deficit in HD and, at 9 months of age, provide an additional robust

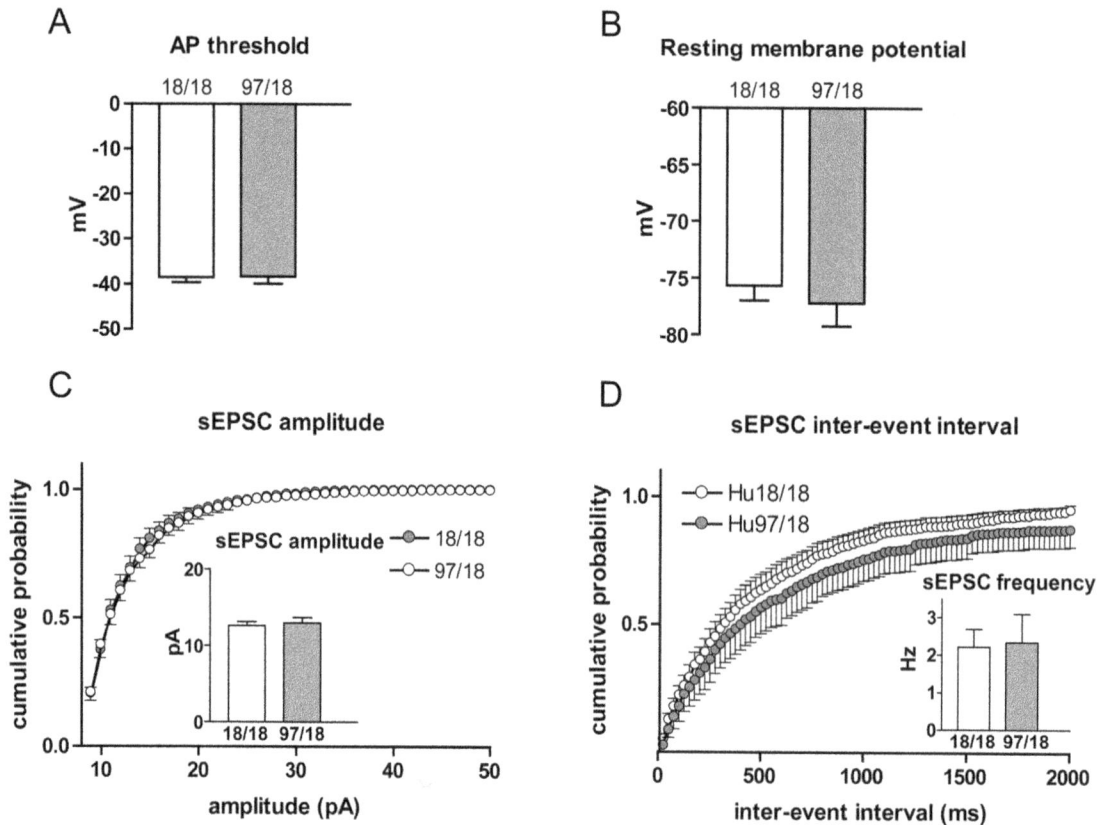

Figure 6. No changes in membrane properties and sEPSC characteristics in Hu97/18 SPNs at 3 months of age. At 3 months of age, action potential threshold (A) and resting membrane potential (B) were unaltered in Hu97/18 (n = 10), in comparison to Hu18/18 SPNs (n = 11). Likewise, sEPSC amplitude (C) and frequency (D) were unaffected in Hu97/18 (n = 8) when compared to Hu18/18 SPNs (n = 8).

electrophysiological phenotype in the humanized mouse model of HD.

Discussion

Here, we examined for the first time the electrophysiological changes that accompany behavioral and neuropathological deficits reported in the Hu97/18 mouse model [11]. Hu97/18 is a novel and unique mouse model of HD that fully recapitulates the genetics of the human disease by expressing human huntingtin heterozygous for an expanded polyglutamine tract (97 repeats) on a mouse huntingtin *null* (*Hdh*$^{-/-}$) background [11]. We describe many electrophysiological alterations in Hu97/18 SPNs, such as progressive changes in membrane properties and synaptic transmission, as well as a progressive impairment of synaptic plasticity in the hippocampus. These robust electrophysiological measures, along with the known behavioral and neuropathological changes [11], can serve as future tools to assess the efficacy of muHTT-specific ASOs [8] and other promising therapeutic options to prevent or reverse the detrimental effects of muHTT on CNS function.

Alterations in cellular and synaptic properties of striatal spiny projection neurons

Membrane capacitance, membrane resistance and tau were not altered in Hu97/18 SPNs at 6 or 9 months of age. This is not surprising, given the fact that these features are not altered in other slowly-progressing mouse models, such as YAC128 or CAG140, until 12 months of age [25]. Earlier changes in membrane

resistance were seen in the more rapidly-progressing R6/2 model, which recapitulates more accurately the phenotype of juvenile HD [17,26].

The depolarized resting membrane potential that we observed in Hu97/18 SPNs has also been noted for other HD mouse models [27,28]. It has been hypothesized that, together with large discharges from cortical afferents (detected as large, >100pA sEPSCs: [17]) and elevated input resistance, this change would directly lead to an increase in SPN excitability (as detected *in vivo*: [29]). However, Hu97/18 SPNs did not display changes in membrane resistance, nor did we observe any large-amplitude sEPSCs. Also, the current-voltage step protocol did not detect any changes in rheobase or rheobase frequency between Hu97/18 and Hu18/18 SPNs, indicating that the propagation of a signal requires similar (and not lower) stimulus intensity. This is most probably achieved by a homeostatic mechanism that involves an increase in action potential threshold. This further strengthens our conclusion that despite small changes in membrane characteristics (e.g., the depolarized resting membrane potential), Hu97/18 SPNs are not more excitable than Hu18/18 SPNs.

At 9 months of age, the sEPSC and mEPSC amplitudes were decreased in comparison to Hu18/18 SPNs, suggesting a lower number of AMPA receptors in synapses. Similar results have been previously reported in YAC128 at 1 month of age [12], but also at 7 months of age with evoked EPSCs [18] and in symptomatic R6/2 mice with AMPA bath application [19]. Therefore, this effect does not seem to be restricted to a fully symptomatic stage of HD, but more likely depends on the model of animal used and its genetic background. The Hu97/18 model is derived from

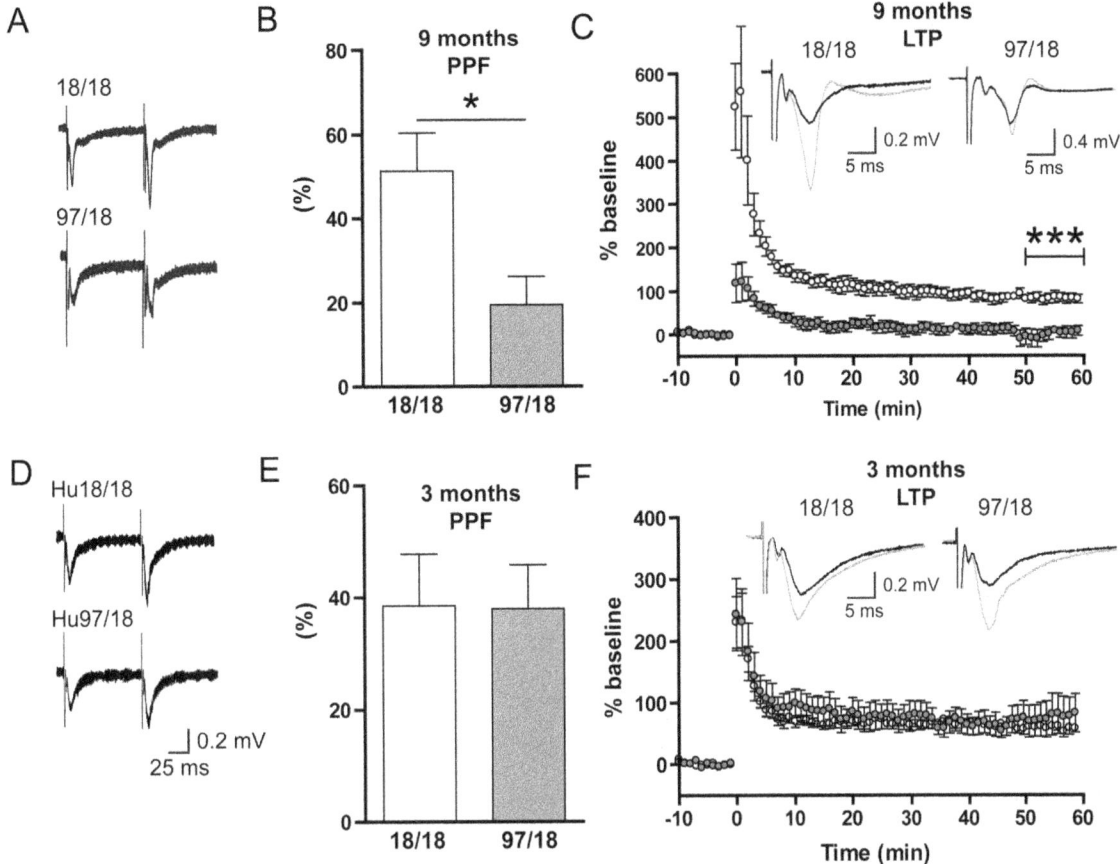

Figure 7. Long-term potentiation (LTP) is impaired in 9-month old Hu97/18 CA1. (A) Representative fEPSP traces from hippocampal slices of 9-month old Hu18/18 and Hu97/18 mice in response to two 0.1 ms pulses separated by 100 ms. fEPSPs were recorded in CA1 stratum radiatum during stimulation of the Schaffer collateral pathway. (B) Paired pulse facilitation (PPF) was measured by dividing the slope of the second response to that of the first and was expressed as percent increase. PPF was significantly lower in Hu97/18 CA1 (Hu18/18 n = 8, Hu97/18 n = 6). (C) fEPSPs were normalized to a 10-minute baseline period prior to high-frequency stimulation (HFS; 100 Hz for 1 s×3, 10 s inter-train interval). LTP was easily obtained in hippocampal slices from Hu18/18 mice (n = 6) but showed severe impairment in slices from Hu97/18 mice (n = 6). Representative traces before (black) and 50–60 minutes after (grey) HFS are shown. ***p<0.0001, t-test of average % above baseline 50–60 minutes post-HFS. (D–F) Paired pulse facilitation (D,E) and LTP (F) graphs as above but conducted in slices from 3-month old animals. n = 6 for each genotype for both (E) and (F).

BACHD mice that show changes in sEPSC amplitude at 6 months of age [30]. However, Hu97/18 mice express ~40% less muHTT than the BACHD mice [11] and so it is not surprising that the changes in sEPSCs that we observed at 9 months of age were not apparent at 6 months.

Another prominent alteration in mEPSCs and sEPSCs recorded from Hu97/18 SPNs was a decrease in frequency, which is a common change observed in HD mouse models at symptomatic stages of the disease [17,25]. This is often associated with a reduced dendritic arborization and loss of dendritic spines and excitatory synapses, both in animal models of HD [14,17,28] and in human HD patients [14]. In the present study, it was a little surprising that we did not observe a significant decrease in the size of AMPAR-mediated eEPSCs at -70 mV (see Fig. 4E), which would be expected following synaptic loss. However, the response magnitude in these experiments relies largely on electrode placement and can vary greatly from one experiment to the next. The mean eEPSC amplitude tended to be lower in Hu97/18 SPNs (see Fig. 4E); however, response size variability was too high to observe significant differences between genotypes. The alternative explanation, a decrease in release probability from presynaptic terminals, was ruled out based on no change in the paired-pulse ratio of synaptically-evoked responses.

The lack of alteration in release probability from excitatory terminals, together with the lack of large sEPSCs (suggested by others to be action-potential driven: [17]) is interesting, as it suggests no significant changes in intact corticostriatal afferents. In presymptomatic YAC72 and YAC128 mice, the release probability is significantly decreased ([12]; also observed in symptomatic YAC128: [18]), while it has been shown to be increased in pre- and symptomatic R6/2 mice [28]. Also, marked changes have been described in recordings from cortical cells from symptomatic R6/2 mice, including changes in basic membrane properties, sEPSC frequency and appearance of complex discharges [31]. Therefore, it would be interesting to examine the possibility of such changes occurring in cortical neurons from the Hu97/18 mouse model; however, these experiments are beyond the scope of this particular study.

Our finding that synaptic AMPAR current amplitude is reduced (based on sEPSC amplitude distribution), while the ratio of evoked AMPAR to NMDAR EPSC amplitude is similar between genotypes, suggests that the number of synaptic NMDA receptors may also be decreased at 9 months of age. This possibility is not entirely surprising, as although NMDA:AMPA ratio has been reported to be increased in presymptomatic YAC72 and YAC128 mice compared to controls [12,32], at symptomatic stages

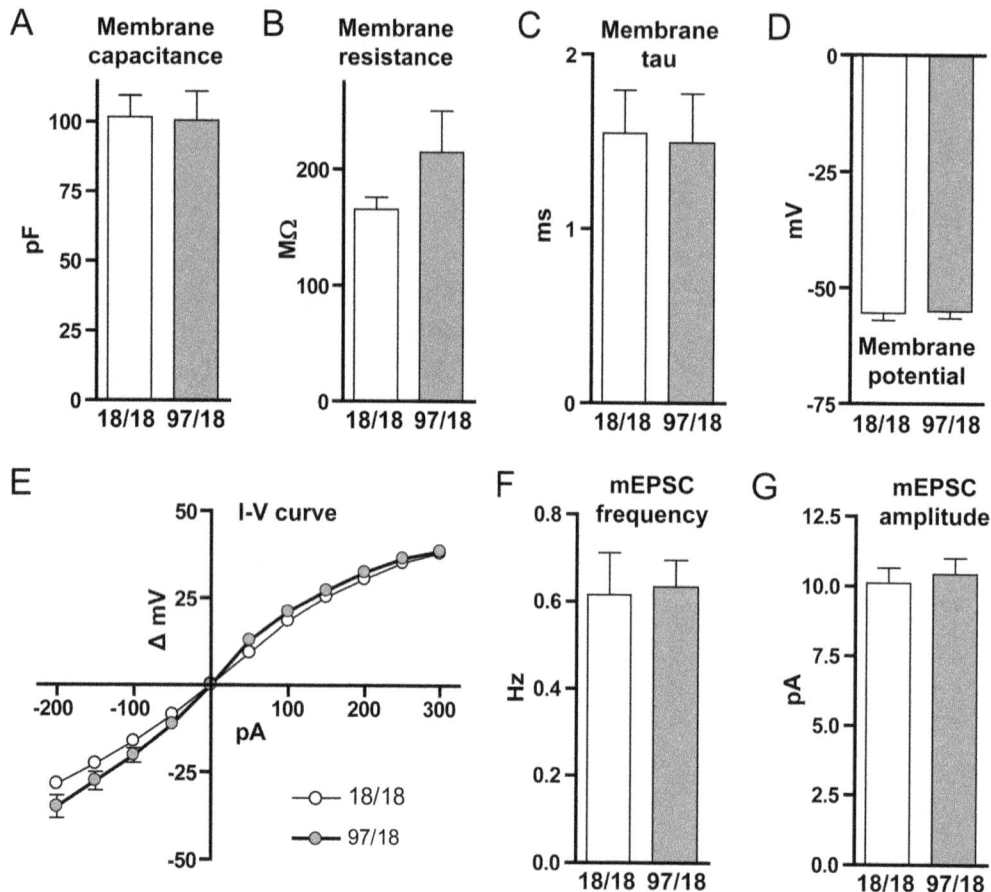

Figure 8. Whole-cell properties of CA1 pyramidal neurons from Hu18/18 and Hu97/18 mice at 9 months of age. (A–D) Whole-cell patch recordings from CA1 pyramidal neurons revealed no difference in membrane properties including membrane capacitance (Cm, Hu18/18 n = 14, Hu97/18 n = 11), membrane resistance (Rm, Hu18/18 n = 14, Hu97/18 n = 11), membrane tau (ôm, Hu18/18 n = 14, Hu97/18 n = 11) or resting membrane potential (Em, Hu18/18 n = 14, Hu97/18 n = 13). I–V plots (E, Hu18/18 n = 14, Hu97/18 n = 13), mEPSC frequency (F, Hu18/18 n = 13, Hu97/18 n = 13) and mEPSC amplitude (G, Hu18/18 n = 13, Hu97/18 n = 13) were also similar between genotypes.

YAC128 SPNs display a decrease in NMDA currents, accompanied by resistance to neurotoxicity [14]. This change could be attributed to an increase in the removal/degradation rate of NMDA receptors on the surface of SPNs [33], as well as to a mislocalization of the receptors from synaptic to extrasynaptic sites [20,34] due to an increase in calpain and STEP61 activity [33,34].

Impaired hippocampal long-term potentiation

We also recorded field potentials in CA1 stratum radiatum and found a complete absence of LTP in slices from 9-month old Hu97/18 mice 50–60 minutes following HFS. This finding is consistent with other mouse models of HD [21–24] and provides a mechanistic basis for the spatial learning deficit observed previously in Hu97/18 mice [11]. Interestingly, this learning deficit was progressive in that no impairment was seen at 3 months of age [11], a time at which we show that LTP is intact. While the molecular mechanisms underlying the observed LTP deficit at 9 months were not explored in the present study, previous work demonstrated that the LTP deficit in a knock-in mouse model of HD was restored by BDNF application directly to the slice [24] or by inducing BDNF upregulation through daily injections of an ampakine [35]. This is consistent with a role for BDNF/TrkB signalling in hippocampal plasticity [36], as well as muHTT's inhibitory effect on BDNF production [37]. The cognitive decline

associated with HD is highly debilitating and can manifest many years before the onset of cell death and overt motor symptoms. With robust and progressive deficits in both LTP and spatial memory, the Hu97/18 model is particularly suited for preclinical assessment of the effects of early treatment interventions on cognitive decline in HD.

Different genetic backgrounds of HD models and their consequences

As we have noted above, there are many similarities between the changes in Hu97/18 SPNs and those reported in other animal models. However, there are also surprising differences, such as unaltered physiology of glutamatergic input release probability and no change in SPN action potential firing properties. Furthermore, while many cellular and synaptic alterations have been reported to occur prior to measurable behavioral abnormalities, we were unable to detect any robust electrophysiological phenotype in the striatum at 6 months of age, a stage when many cognitive and motor impairments are evident. It is possible that other measures not assessed in the present study, including the extrasynaptic NMDA receptor currents [38,20], are indeed altered early in the Hu97/18 model. Nonetheless, we were surprised by the lack of electrophysiological effects at 6 months of age, and our data suggest that the bulk of synaptic deficits in the striatum occur between 6 and 9 months of age. These discrepancies may primarily stem from a different genetic background of multiple models that leads to differences in the number of CAG repeats, or muHTT expression patterns and levels (reviewed in: [9,10]; see also: [11,25,27,39,40]). BACHD mice, which the Hu97/18 model is largely based on, have not been fully described using electrophysiological methods [30]. Also, a direct comparison between BACHD and Hu97/18 could be misleading, as BACHD expresses normal levels of mouse HTT (on top of human muHTT) and its levels of muHTT are ~40% higher than those of Hu97/18 [11].

Conclusion

The Hu97/18 model is unique as it is the first animal model to fully recapitulate the genetics of human HD. It is critically important to track the changes in its phenotype, not only to expand our knowledge of HD and its progression, but also for the application and assessment of therapies in the future.

Acknowledgments

The authors would like to thank Mahsa Amirabassi for her excellent animal care.

Author Contributions

Conceived and designed the experiments: KK MPP LAR. Performed the experiments: KK MPP. Analyzed the data: KK MPP. Contributed reagents/materials/analysis tools: ALS MRH. Wrote the paper: KK MPP LAR.

References

1. The Huntington's Disease Collaborative Research Group (1993) A novel gene containing a trinucleotide repeat that is expanded and unstable on Huntington's disease chromosomes. Cell 72: 971–983.

2. Zuccato C, Valenza M, Cattaneo E (2010) Molecular mechanisms and potential therapeutical targets in Huntington's disease. Physiol Rev 90: 905–981.

3. Di Filippo M, Tozzi A, Picconi B, Ghiglieri V, Calabresi P (2007) Plastic abnormalities in experimental Huntington's disease. Curr Opin Pharmacol 7: 106–111.

4. Raymond LA, André VM, Cepeda C, Gladding CM, Milnerwood AJ, et al. (2011) Pathophysiology of Huntington's disease: time-dependent alterations in synaptic and receptor function. Neuroscience 198: 252–273.

5. Ghiglieri V, Bagetta V, Calabresi P, Picconi B (2012) Functional interactions within striatal microcircuit in animal models of Huntington's disease. Neuroscience 211: 165–184.

6. Southwell AL, Skotte NH, Bennett CF, Hayden MR (2012) Antisense oligonucleotide therapeutics for inherited neurodegenerative diseases. Trends Mol Med 18: 634–643.

7. Martinez T, Wright N, López-Fraga M, Jiménez AI, Pañeda C (2013) Silencing human genetic diseases with oligonucleotide-based therapies. Hum Genet 132: 481–493.

8. Carroll JB, Warby SC, Southwell AL, Doty CN, Greenlee S, et al. (2011) Potent and selective antisense oligonucleotides targeting single-nucleotide polymorphisms in the Huntington disease gene / allele-specific silencing of mutant huntingtin. Mol Ther 19: 2178–2185.

9. Cepeda C, Cummings DM, André VM, Holley SM, Levine MS (2010) Genetic mouse models of Huntington's disease: focus on electrophysiological mechanisms. ASN Neuro 2: e00033.

10. Pouladi MA, Morton AJ, Hayden MR (2013) Choosing an animal model for the study of Huntington's disease. Nat Rev Neurosci 14: 708–721.

11. Southwell AL, Warby SC, Carroll JB, Doty CN, Skotte NH, et al. (2013) A fully humanized transgenic mouse model of Huntington disease. Hum Mol Genet 22: 18–34.

12. Milnerwood AJ, Raymond LA (2007) Corticostriatal synaptic function in mouse models of Huntington's disease: early effects of huntingtin repeat length and protein load. J Physiol 585: 817–831.

13. Kiraly DD, Lemtiri-Chlieh F, Levine ES, Mains RE, Eipper BA (2011) Kalirin binds the NR2B subunit of the NMDA receptor, altering its synaptic localization and function. J Neurosci 31: 12554–12565.

14. Graham RK, Pouladi MA, Joshi P, Lu G, Deng Y, et al. (2009) Differential susceptibility to excitotoxic stress in YAC128 mouse models of Huntington disease between initiation and progression of disease. J Neurosci 29: 2193–2204.

15. Singaraja RR, Huang K, Sanders SS, Milnerwood AJ, Hines R, et al. (2011) Altered palmitoylation and neuropathological deficits in mice lacking HIP14. Hum Mol Genet 20: 3899–3909.

16. Thomson AM (2000) Facilitation, augmentation and potentiation at central synapses. Trends Neurosci 23: 305–312.

17. Cepeda C, Hurst RS, Calvert CR, Hernández-Echeagaray E, Nguyen OK, et al. (2003) Transient and progressive electrophysiological alterations in the corticostriatal pathway in a mouse model of Huntington's disease. J Neurosci 23: 961–969.

18. Joshi PR, Wu NP, André VM, Cummings DM, Cepeda C, et al. (2009) Age-dependent alterations of corticostriatal activity in the YAC128 mouse model of Huntington disease. J Neurosci 29: 2414–2427.

19. Cepeda C, Ariano MA, Calvert CR, Flores-Hernández J, Chandler SH, et al.

(2001) NMDA receptor function in mouse models of Huntington disease. J Neurosci Res 66: 525–539.

20. Milnerwood AJ, Gladding CM, Pouladi MA, Kaufman AM, Hines RM, et al. (2010) Early increase in extrasynaptic NMDA receptor signaling and expression contributes to phenotype onset in Huntington's disease mice. Neuron 65: 178–190.

21. Hodgson JG, Agopyan N, Gutekunst CA, Leavitt BR, LePiane F, et al. (1999) A YAC mouse model for Huntington's disease with full-length mutant huntingtin, cytoplasmic toxicity, and selective striatal neurodegeneration. Neuron 23: 181–192.

22. Usdin MT, Shelbourne PF, Myers RM, Madison DV (1999) Impaired synaptic plasticity in mice carrying the Huntington's disease mutation. Hum Mol Genet 8: 839–846.

23. Murphy KP, Carter RJ, Lione LA, Mangiarini L, Mahal A, et al. (2000) Abnormal synaptic plasticity and impaired spatial cognition in mice transgenic for exon 1 of the human Huntington's disease mutation. J Neurosci 20: 5115–5123.

24. Lynch G, Kramar EA, Rex CS, Jia Y, Chappas D, et al. (2007) Brain-derived neurotrophic factor restores synaptic plasticity in a knock-in mouse model of Huntington's disease. J Neurosci 27: 4424–4434.

25. Cummings DM, Cepeda C, Levine MS (2010) Alterations in striatal synaptic transmission are consistent across genetic mouse models of Huntington's disease. ASN Neuro 2: e00036.

26. Ariano MA, Cepeda C, Calvert CR, Flores-Hernández J, Hernández-Echeagaray E, et al. (2005) Striatal potassium channel dysfunction in Huntington's disease transgenic mice. J Neurophysiol 93: 2565–2574.

27. Levine MS, Klapstein GJ, Koppel A, Gruen E, Cepeda C, et al. (1999) Enhanced sensitivity to N-methyl-D-aspartate receptor activation in transgenic and knockin mouse models of Huntington's disease. J Neurosci Res 58: 515–532.

28. Klapstein GJ, Fisher RS, Zanjani H, Cepeda C, Jokel ES, et al. (2001) Electrophysiological and morphological changes in striatal spiny neurons in R6/2 Huntington's disease transgenic mice. J Neurophysiol 86: 2667–2677.

29. Rebec GV, Conroy SK, Barton SJ (2006) Hyperactive striatal neurons in symptomatic Huntington R6/2 mice: variations with behavioral state and repeated ascorbate treatment. Neuroscience 137: 327–336.

30. Gray M, Shirasaki DI, Cepeda C, André VM, Wilburn B, et al. (2008) Full-length human mutant huntingtin with a stable polyglutamine repeat can elicit progressive and selective neuropathogenesis in BACHD mice. J Neurosci 28: 6182–6195.

31. Cummings DM, André VM, Uzgil BO, Gee SM, Fisher YE, et al. (2009) Alterations in cortical excitation and inhibition in genetic mouse models of Huntington's disease. J Neurosci 29: 10371–10386.

32. Li L, Murphy TH, Hayden MR, Raymond LA (2004) Enhanced striatal NR2B-containing N-methyl-D-aspartate receptor-mediated synaptic currents in a mouse model of Huntington disease. J Neurophysiol 92: 2738–2746.

33. Cowan C, Fan MM, Fan J, Shehadeh J, Zhang LY, et al. (2008) Polyglutamine-modulated striatal calpain activity in YAC transgenic huntington disease mouse model: impact on NMDA receptor function and toxicity. J Neurosci 28: 12725–12735.

34. Gladding CM, Sepers MD, Xu J, Zhang LY, Milnerwood AJ, et al. (2012) Calpain and STriatal-Enriched protein tyrosine phosphatase (STEP) activation contribute to extrasynaptic NMDA receptor localization in a Huntington's disease mouse model. Hum Mol Genet 21: 3739–3752.

35. Simmons DA, Rex CS, Palmer L, Pandyarajan V, Fedulov V, et al. (2009) Up-regulating BDNF with an ampakine rescues synaptic plasticity and memory in Huntington's disease knockin mice. Proc Natl Acad Sci USA 106: 4906–4911.

36. Minichiello L (2009) TrkB signalling pathways in LTP and learning. Nat Rev Neurosci 10: 850–860.

37. Zuccato C, Ciammola A, Rigamonti D, Leavitt BR, Goffredo D, et al. (2001) Loss of huntingtin-mediated BDNF gene transcription in Huntington's disease. Science 293: 493–498.

38. Okamoto S, Pouladi MA, Talantova M, Yao D, Xia P, et al. (2009) Balance between synaptic versus extrasynaptic NMDA receptor activity influences inclusions and neurotoxicity of mutant huntingtin. Nat Med 15: 1407–1413.

39. Cummings DM, Alaghband Y, Hickey MA, Joshi PR, Hong SC, et al. (2012) A critical window of CAG repeat-length correlates with phenotype severity in the R6/2 mouse model of Huntington's disease. J Neurophysiol 107: 677–691.

40. Pouladi MA, Stanek LM, Xie Y, Franciosi S, Southwell AL, et al. (2012) Marked differences in neurochemistry and aggregates despite similar behavioural and neuropathological features of Huntington disease in the full-length BACHD and YAC128 mice. Hum Mol Genet 21: 2219–2232.

14

Nitric Oxide Dysregulation in Platelets from Patients with Advanced Huntington Disease

Albino Carrizzo[1⬠], **Alba Di Pardo**[1⬠], **Vittorio Maglione**[1], **Antonio Damato**[1], **Enrico Amico**[1], **Luigi Formisano**[2], **Carmine Vecchione**[1,3]*, **Ferdinando Squitieri**[1]*

1 IRCCS Neuromed, Pozzilli (IS), Italy, **2** Department of Science and Technology, University of Sannio, Benevento, Italy, **3** Department of Medicine and Surgery, University of Salerno, Salerno, Italy

Abstract

Nitric oxide (NO) is a biologically active inorganic molecule involved in the regulation of many physiological processes, such as control of blood flow, platelet adhesion, endocrine function, neurotransmission and neuromodulation. In the present study, for the first time, we investigated the modulation of NO signaling in platelets of HD patients. We recruited 55 patients with manifest HD and 28 gender- and age-matched healthy controls. Our data demonstrated that NO-mediated vasorelaxation, when evoked by supernatant from insulin-stimulated HD platelets, gradually worsens along disease course. The defective vasorelaxation seems to stem from a faulty release of NO from platelets of HD patients and, it is associated with impairment of eNOS phosphorylation (Ser^{1177}) and activity. This study provides important insights about NO metabolism in HD and raises the hypothesis that the decrease of NO in platelets of HD individuals could be a good tool for monitoring advanced stages of the disease.

Editor: Cristoforo Scavone, Universidade de São Paulo, Brazil

Funding: The authors have no support or funding to report.

Competing Interests: The authors have declared that no competing interests exist.

* E-mail: ferdinando.squitieri@lirh.it (FS); cvecchione@unisa.it (CV)

⬠ These authors contributed equally to this work.

Introduction

Huntington disease (HD), a dominantly transmitted neurodegenerative disorder, is characterized by the progressive striatal and cortical neurodegeneration associated with motor, cognitive and behavioral disturbances [1]. The disease-causing mutation is an expansion of a CAG trinucleotide repeat (>36 repeats) encoding a polyglutamine (polyQ) stretch in N-terminal region of huntingtin (Htt), a ubiquitous protein whose function is still unclear. Elongated polyQ stretch endows mutant Htt (mHtt) with toxic properties and results in the development of a broad array of cell dysfunctions [2]. Although the disease has traditionally been described as a disorder purely of the brain, emerging evidence indicates that abnormalities outside the central nervous system (CNS) are commonly found in HD [3]. However, whether a correlation exists between central pathology and peripheral defects is still poorly understood.

Mutant Htt has been widely described to be expressed either in central or in peripheral tissues and to exert its toxic effect in both neuronal and non-neuronal cells with similar mechanisms [4].

Previous studies highlighted the ability of mHtt to interfere with a number of molecular mechanisms in peripheral tissues, which have been suggested to virtually reflect central dysfunctions in HD and potentially useful to better understand some genetic and biochemical aspects of the disease [5,6].

Among all the several dysfunctions, the dysregulation of nitric oxide (NO)/NO synthase (NOS) pathway is suggested to potentially represent a critical contributor to HD pathology [7].

NO, known as an important signaling molecule, normally acts in many tissues and regulates a diverse range of physiological and cellular processes such as control of blood flow, platelet adhesion, neurotrasmission and neuromodulation [8]. Production of NO is mediated by different NOS isoforms in both CNS and peripheral tissues [9]. Human platelets, that normally express the endothelial form of NOS (eNOS), whose activity is regulated by phosphorylation at different Serine/Threonine residues [10], represent an important source of peripheral NO. Under pathological condition, production of NO can be either protective or toxic, depending on the stage of the disease, the isoforms of NOS involved and, the initial pathological event [7]. To date, many are the studies that described NO as a potential key mediator of neurodegeneration [11,12].

NO dysfunction in CNS has been previously demonstrated to be involved in different processes leading to progressive striatal damage and to abnormal cerebral blood flow (CBF) in both HD experimental models and patients [7,13]. However, there is no actual evidence proving NO abnormalities in peripheral blood cells.

In this study, we carried out experiments on platelets, which represent a validated peripheral model for testing potential impairment of NO regulation, obtained from patients with manifest HD. Our data highlighted defective NO metabolism in the advanced stages of HD and, for the first time, reveled a possible stage-dependent dysregulation of peripheral eNOS signaling in the disease.

Methods

Subjects

A total of 55 HD patients (11 stage I, 17 stage II, 16 stage III and 11 stage IV), and 28 gender- and age-matched healthy controls were recruited in this study. Control group was divided in two subgroups consisting of a younger control group with a mean age of 43.8±7.4 and an older control group with a mean age of 59.7±3.4 in order to match them with early (stage I and II) and late (stage III and IV) HD patients, respectively. Classification of control subjects in young and old groups has been performed in a manner similar to that described previously [14]. Subjects' demographic, clinical and genetic characteristics of both controls and HD patients are reported in Table 1. All the subjects with suspect of cardiovascular, psychiatric or neurodegenerative disorders other than HD, were excluded from this study. Most patients were taking benzodiazepines; some of the patients in stage III-IV were receiving low doses of atypical neuroleptics (olanzapine, 2.5–10 mg; risperidone, 1–3mg or tetrabenazine, 12.5–25 mg). None of the patients were taking medication for any cardiovascular diseases. Clinical examinations were conducted using the Unified Huntington's Disease Rating Scale (UHDRS) to measure motor, cognitive, behavioral and general function (Huntington Study Group, 1996) [15]. The disease stage was calculated according to the Total Functional Capacity (TFC) score [16].

Ethics Statement

All HD patients revealed a CAG repeat expansion mutation, and all of them, as well as control individuals, were requested to sign an informed consent before study recruitment. All human experiments were performed in accordance with the Declaration of Helsinki and after approval from the local Ethical Committee of Istituto Neurologico Mediterraneo IRCCS Neuromed [17].

Platelet isolation

Twenty-five millilitres of blood were collected into acid citrate dextrose (ACD: 85 mmol/L sodium citrate, 65 mmol/L citric acid, and 125 mmol/L dextrose; 2,5 ml ACD:25 ml of blood) and platelet-rich plasma was obtained by centrifugation at 130 g for 20 minutes. The resultant platelet-rich plasma (PRP) was used as source of platelets. Platelets pellet was obtained by centrifugation of PRP at 900 g for 7 minutes, and resuspended in Tyrode's solution (132 mmol/L NaCl, 4 mmol/L KCl, 1.6 mmol/L $CaCl_2$, 0.98 $MgCl_2$, 23.8 mmol/L $NaHCO_3$, 0.36 mmol/L NaH_2PO_4, 10 mmol/L glucose, 0.05 mmol/L Ca-Titriplex, and gassed with 95% O_2, 5% CO_2 and pH 7.4 at 37°C). After a further

centrifugation step (900 g, 4 minutes), washed platelets were resuspended in the same solution, allowed to equilibrate for 10 minutes at 37°C and then stimulated with insulin (10 µmol/L) for 10 minutes. Some experiments were performed in platelet pretreated with N^G-nitro-L-arginine methyl ester (L-NAME) (300 µmol/L, 30 minutes) or with 1 mmol/L 4-hydroxytempo (TEMPOL), a membrane-permeable superoxide dismutase mimetic, for 30 minutes. After stimulation, the platelet suspension was centrifuged for 2 minutes at 900 g and, increasing doses of supernatant (0.1-0.2-0.4-0.8 ml) was added to phenyleprine-precontracted arteries mounted in an organ chamber (final volume, 15 ml). Total number and purity of platelets for each preparation was assessed by flow cytometry. Total protein from each preparation was also determined. Similar number of platelets ($186\pm15\times10^6$/mL) between controls and HD patients was estimated.

Isolated vessel studies

Studies of vascular reactivity were performed on isolated vessels from C57BL6/N mice. Four ring segments (3 mm width) of thoracic aorta from each mouse were mounted between stainless steel triangles in a water-jacketed organ bath (37°C) for measurement of tension development as previously described [18,19]. Preliminary experiments demonstrated that the optimal resting tension for development of active contraction was 1 g. Vessels were gradually stretched over one-hour period to this tension. The presence of functional endothelium and smooth muscle layer were assessed in all preparations by the ability respectively of acetylcholine and nitrogliceryne (10^{-9} to 10^{-5} mol/L) to induce the relaxation of vessels precontracted with phenylephrine (10^{-9} to 10^{-6} mol/L) to obtain a similar level of precontraction in each ring (80% of initial KCl-induced contraction). Responses to vasoconstrictors were examined at this resting tension and related to maximal vasoconstriction elicited by depolarization with 80 mmol/L KCl. Responses to vasodilator supernatants obtained from stimulation of platelets were examined after achieving a preconstricted tone with increasing doses of phenylephrine (10^{-9} to 10^{-6} mol/L) to obtain a similar level of precontraction in each ring (80% of initial KCl-induced contraction).

Immunoblotting

After isolation, platelets were solubilized in lysis buffer containing: 20 mmol/L Tris-HCl, 150 mmol/L NaCl, 20 mmol/L NaF, 2 mmol/L sodium orthovanadate, 1% Nonidet, 100 µg/ml leupeptin, 100 µg/ml aprotinin, and 1 mmol/L phenylmethylsulfonyl fluoride. Then, samples were left on ice for

Table 1. Demographic and clinical data of healthy controls and HD patients.

| | | | Huntington disease stages | | | |
| | | | Early | | Late | |
	Young Controls	Old Controls	I	II	III	IV
Subjects	19	9	11	17	16	11
Male/Female	9/10	5/4	5/6	9/8	9/6	5/6
Age (years)	43.8±7.4	59.7±3.4	46.9±10.2	50.7±13.5	54.2±11.2	61.5±8.2
TFC (score)	-	-	11.5±1	7.8±0.7	4.1±1.3	1.6±0.5
CAG repeats	-	-	43.2±1.5	45.6±6.3	44.7 ± 3.4	42.3 ± 2.1

Values are given as mean ± s.d.; TFC: Total Functional Capacity, score 13-0.

30 minutes and centrifuged at 10621 g for 20 minutes, and the supernatants were used to perform immunoblot analysis. Total protein levels were determined using the Bradford method. 50 μg proteins were resolved on 8% SDS-PAGE, transferred to a nitrocellulose membrane as previously described [20] and immunoblotted with anti-phospho-eNOS S1177 (Cell Signaling, rabbit polyclonal antibody 1:800); anti-total-eNOS (Cell Signaling, mouse mAb 1:1000) and β-actin (Cell Signaling, mouse mAb 1:2000). HRP-conjugated secondary antibodies were used at 1:3000 dilution (Bio-Rad Laboratories). Protein bands were detected by ECL Prime (Amersham Biosciences) and quantitated with Quantity One software (Bio-Rad Laboratories).

Determination of platelet Nitric Oxide Synthase activity

Endothelial NOS activity was determined on platelet lysates according to the protocol published by Radomski et al. (1993) [21]. Briefly, the enzymatic activity was determined by measuring the conversion of L-[^{14}C]arginine to L-[^{14}C]citrulline. The dependence of L-arginine conversion on $Ca_2{}^+$-dependent (constitutive) NOS was confirmed in presence of ethyleneglycol bis-(2-aminoethyl ether)-N,N,N-tetraacetic acid (EGTA), and of N(G)-mono-methyl-L-arginine (L-NMMA), an inhibitor of this enzyme. The isoform specificity of this analysis is demonstrated through the use of the calcium chelator EGTA, which allows us to fractionate calcium-independent (iNOS) activity versus total NOS activity (inhibited by L-NMMA). Assay sensitivity has been shown to be just less than 1 pmol/min/mg protein for the detection of L-[^{14}C]arginine.

Measurement of NO production in platelets

Isolated platelets were centrifuged at 1500 g for 10 minutes and platelets were washed twice with a 6:1 mixture of Hank's balanced salt solution (HBSS) and ACD. Platelet suspensions (100 μL) were incubated with 1 μmol/L diaminodifluoroscein diacetate (DAF-FM DA), a photo-stable NO fluorescent indicator, in HBSS at room temperature for 30 minutes and stimulated with 10 μmol/L insulin. After incubation, fluorescence emission spectra were recorded in a 495-515 nm range in a quartz cuvette as described elsewhere [22].

Statistical analysis

One-way ANOVA followed by Turkey post-test was used to analyze protein levels, eNOS activity and DAF fluorescence measurement. Two-way ANOVA followed by Bonferroni post-test was used for the analysis of vascular reactivity studies in HD patients and controls. All data are presented as mean ± SD, except in the dose-response curve studies in which are expressed as mean ± SEM. A "p" value of less than 0.05 was considered statistically significant. F value (F) and degree of freedom (df) were also reported for each experiment. All statistical analyses were conducted with Prism statistical software.

Results

Vasorelaxation evoked by supernatant from insulin-stimulated platelets gradually alters along disease course

The supernatant from insulin-stimulated human platelets evoked a rapid dose-dependent relaxation of mice aorta rings and was abolished by NOS inhibitor, L-NAME (Figure 1A), clearly demonstrating the involvement of NO signalling in supernatant vascular action. Interestingly, our data demonstrate that the vasorelaxant effect, evoked from platelet supernatants, was markedly reduced in late stage HD patients when compared to either early HD patients or control subjects (Figure 1B). No

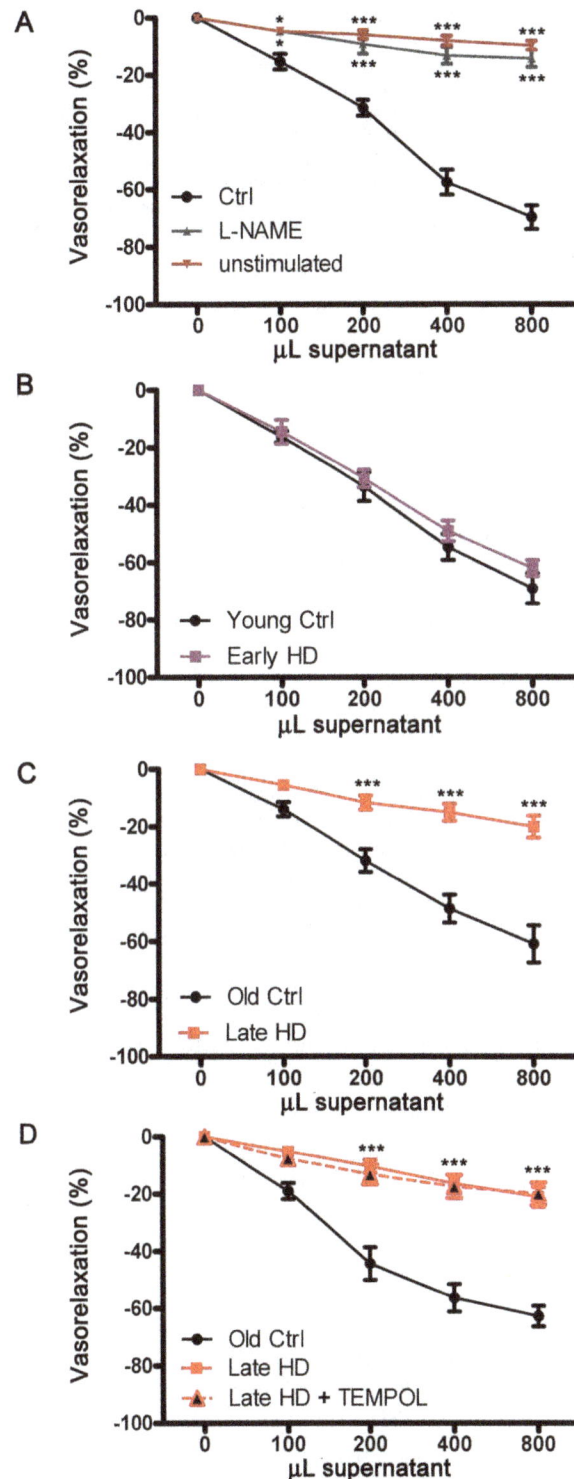

Figure 1. Vasorelaxant response to supernatants derived from insulin-stimulated platelets of HD patients. (A) Dose–response curves of phenylephrine-precontracted aorta rings to supernatants derived from insulin-stimulated and unstimulated platelets isolated from control subjects untreated and pre-treated with L-NAME. * indicates statistical significance of either Ctrls vs L-NAME-treated Ctrls or vs unstimulated samples. Ctrl n = 4; L-NAME-treated Ctrls n = 4; Unstimulated n = 4. **(B)** Dose–response curves of phenylephrine-precontracted aorta rings to supernatants derived from insulin-stimulated platelets isolated from early HD patients and young control subjects. Young Ctrl n = 13; Early HD n = 8. **(C)** Dose–response curves of

phenylephrine-precontracted aorta rings to supernatants derived from insulin-stimulated platelets isolated from late HD patients and old control subjects. * indicates statistical significance of old Ctrl vs late HD. Old Ctrl n = 6; Late HD n = 7. (**D**) Dose–response curves of phenyleph-rine-precontracted aorta rings to supernatants derived from platelets isolated from Old control subjects and late HD patients untreated and pre-treated with TEMPOL before insulin stimulation. Old Ctrl n = 3; Late HD plus Tiron n = 4. * indicates statistical significance of old Ctrl vs late HD stages treated and untreated with TEMPOL. Values are shown as mean± SEM. *, $p < 0.05$; **, $p < 0.001$; ***, $p < 0.0001$. (Two-way ANOVA followed Bonferroni post-test).

differences were observed between early HD patients and age-matched control individuals (Figure 1B). Vasorelaxation did not differ between the two control groups, excluding, therefore, any possible aging process-related effects (Figure S1 in File S1).

Next, to elucidate the putative cause of aberrant NO pathway, the potential implication of oxidative stress was explored by pre-incubating platelets from late stage HD patients with the antioxidant agent, 4-hydroxytempo. Our data indicate that the compound failed to improve the supernatant vascular effect observed in late HD patients (Figure 1C), excluding the involvement of oxidative stress in such dysfunction.

eNOS-phosphorylation is impaired in HD

To elucidate whether HD-derived platelet-mediated impaired vasorelaxation due to dysregulation of eNOS pathway, phosphor-ylation state at its serine residue 1177, was determined by biochemical studies. Levels of eNOS phosphorylation gradually decreased from stage II up stage IV HD patients in which phosphorylation signal was merely detectable (Figure 2A). eNOS phosphorylation in late stage HD patients was significantly reduced when compared with either stage I HD patients or control subjects. No significant difference was observed between early stage HD patients and healthy controls (Figure 2A). Conversely, eNOS expression did not change among all the groups (Figure 2A). In addition, no changes in the levels of β-actin were observed between HD patients and relative controls.

Furthermore, in order to clarify whether reduction of eNOS phosphorylation was associated with a defective eNOS activity along HD course, citrulline assay, the standard eNOS activity assay, was performed in platelets from different stated HD patients and healthy controls. Coherently with changes of eNOS phosphorylation, enzyme activity was found to be significantly decreased in patients with advanced HD compared to early HD patients and/or to controls subjects (Figure 2B).

NO is reduced in platelets from late stage HD patients

To test whether impaired vasorelaxant response, evoked by HD-derived platelets might be attributable to abnormal NO production, platelet-derived NO from HD patients at different stage of the disease was quantitatively determined by DAF-FM DA. Consistent with decrease of both eNOS phosphorylation and activity (Figure 2A and B), NO release was markedly reduced in patients with advanced HD compared to early stage patients as well as to control subjects (Figure 3). No differences were found between early stage patients and control individuals (Figure 3).

Discussion

Several studies highlighted peripheral abnormalities in HD and arise the hypothesis that the disease may be associated with a number of pathological changes outside the brain. A common finding across numerous studies is that peripheral cells (circulating blood lymphocytes, monocytes and platelets) represent good

candidates for biochemical studies [5,23,24], as well as for searching potential peripheral biomarkers that correlate with the onset and/or the progression of the disease [6,24].

It has been previously described an altered homeostasis of human platelets in HD [25,26] and an increased density of Adenosine A2a receptor, a protein G-coupled receptor implicated in the regulation of different biochemical processes including the release of NO, in both CNS of transgenic HD mice [13,27] and blood platelets of patients [5,6]. However, whether platelets dysfunction contributes to HD pathogenesis, or is an epiphenom-enon, remains unclear.

In this study we further examined the role of platelets in HD and postulate that the impairment of NO signaling in the peripheral district of patients might contribute to the pathology. In particular, we found that NO-mediated vasorelaxation, evoked by supernatant from HD-derived insulin-stimulated platelets was impaired in advanced HD. We also demonstrated stage-dependent changes of eNOS phosphorylation at serine residue (1177) associated with reduced eNOS activity and NO release in platelets from late stage HD patients. Importantly, as shown in Figure 1 and in Figure S1 in File S1, our results appear to be specifically related to HD pathology and not depending on aging process.

Interestingly, it has been previously shown that NO is produced in human platelets and that changes in intra-platelet NO production have important physiological and pathophysiological implications. The role of NO and its catalyzing enzyme, NOS, in neurodegenerative disease has been increasingly investigated over the past decade [27,28]. However little is known about the role of NO in HD.

NO plays an important role in the modulation of the vascular tone. It exerts vasorelaxant action and favors antiplatelet effects limiting thrombotic events [29]. Impaired NO signaling in patients might support the high incidence of cardiovascular complications, which represent one of the leading causes of death in HD [30,31].

Additionally, we observed that the progressive impairment of NO signaling along HD course seems not to depend exclusively on excessive oxidative stress. It has been previously reported that the effective half-life of NO and the vasorelaxation of aortic rings by NO is enhanced by a reduction in the concentration of superoxide radicals with superoxide dismutase (SOD) [32]. In our study, the administration of the antioxidant agent, TEMPOL, that mimics the action of SOD, did not rescue the altered vasorelaxation observed in the late stage HD patients. This result, therefore, allows us to suppose that superoxide radicals are not implicated in the impaired NO vascular action in patients with advanced HD. Interestingly, in support of this hypothesis, we found impaired activity of endothelial NOS enzyme in late stage HD patients.

Although the molecular mechanisms underlying the regulation of platelets eNOS activation and NO production are likely to be complex and will need to be further explored, we hypothesized that mHtt could affect eNOS phosphorylation through its interaction with a number of molecular targets including huntingtin-associated protein (HAP-1), CREB binding protein (CBP) and protein kinase B (AKT) [33], that have been previously described to interfere with eNOS signaling [28]. Reduction of eNOS expression and decreased NO levels in platelets from HD patients, could virtually reflect central defects and potentially clarify the molecular basis of cerebral hypoperfusion previously described in HD patients [34]. Although the clinical significance of altered eNOS/NO signal pathway is not yet elucidated, it is tempting to speculate that such impairment may be an important determinant that influences disease progression in HD.

In summary, our data indicate a gradual dysregulation of eNOS pathway in HD-derived platelets, which could represent a valuable

A

B

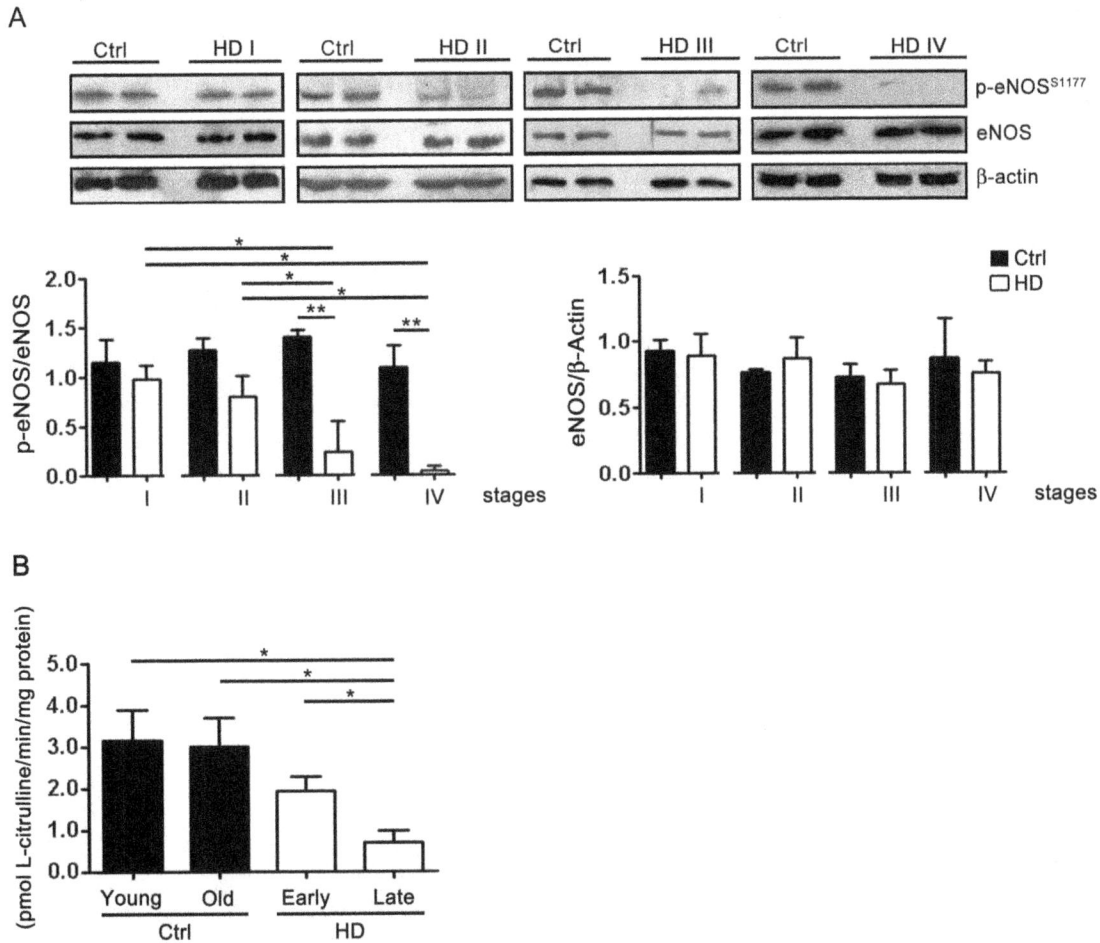

Figure 2. eNOS phosphorylation in platelets from HD patients and healthy controls. (A) Representative immunoblotting of eNOS phosphorylation at serine residue 1177 in platelets and densitometric analysis for p-eNOS[(1177)] and eNOS (left) and for eNOS and β-actin (right). **(B)** Bar graph showing endothelial NOS activity in platelets from early (I-II) and late (III-IV) stage HD patients and healthy controls. Young Ctrl n = 5; Old Ctrl n = 4; Early stage n = 9; Late stage n = 9. Data are shown as mean ± SD. *, $p < 0.05$. (One-way ANOVA followed by Tukey post test). F = 8.766; df = 26.

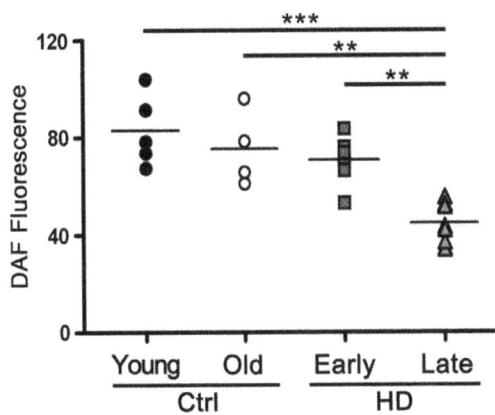

Figure 3. Production of NO in insulin-stimulated platelets from HD patients. Dot plot graph showing DAF fluorescence in platelets stimulated with insulin immediately after isolation from controls and HD patients. Lines indicate the mean values for each group. Each dot represents a single individual. Young Ctrl n = 5; Old Ctrl n = 4; Early HD n = 6; Late HD n = 6. *, $p < 0.05$; **, $p < 0.001$; ***, $p < 0.0001$. (One-way ANOVA followed by Tukey post test). F = 14.52; df = 3.

tool for determining a possible link between peripheral district and CNS. To our knowledge this is the first biological evidence of such peripheral dysregulation in HD. We believe that changes of peripheral eNOS/NO pathway during HD course could represent a potential indicator of disease severity, useful to monitor the advanced HD stages of HD. The biological characterization of late stages of HD may open new insights to therapy of advanced, untreatable patients.

Supporting Information

File S1

Aknowledgments

We are grateful to all patients for contributing to our work and to Lega Italiana Ricerca Huntington e malattie correlate (LIRH) onlus. Also, we thank Mariateresa Ambrosio and all the laboratory assistants for technical support and fruitful discussion. Vittorio Maglione is supported by a Marie Curie International Incoming Fellowship (IIF, grant ń 300197) within the 7th European Community Framework Programme.

Author Contributions

Conceived and designed the experiments: AC ADP VM CV FS. Performed the experiments: AC AD. Analyzed the data: AC ADP VM CV FS. Wrote the paper: AC ADP VM CV FS. Provided technical assistance: EA. Performed the experiments for the determination of NOS activity: LF. Read and approved the final manuscript: AC ADP VM AD EA LF CV FS.

References

1. Roos RA (2010) Huntington's disease: a clinical review. Orphanet J Rare Dis 5: 40.
2. Sugars KL, Rubinsztein DC (2003) Transcriptional abnormalities in Huntington disease. Trends Genet 19: 233–238.
3. van der Burg JM, Bjorkqvist M, Brundin P (2009) Beyond the brain: widespread pathology in Huntington's disease. Lancet Neurol 8: 765–774.
4. Sassone J, Colciago C, Cislaghi G, Silani V, Ciammola A (2009) Huntington's disease: the current state of research with peripheral tissues. Exp Neurol 219: 385–397.
5. Maglione V, Giallonardo P, Cannella M, Martino T, Frati L, et al. (2005) Adenosine A2A receptor dysfunction correlates with age at onset anticipation in blood platelets of subjects with Huntington's disease. Am J Med Genet B Neuropsychiatr Genet 139B: 101–105.
6. Maglione V, Cannella M, Martino T, De Blasi A, Frati L, et al. (2006) The platelet maximum number of A2A-receptor binding sites (Bmax) linearly correlates with age at onset and CAG repeat expansion in Huntington's disease patients with predominant chorea. Neurosci Lett 393: 27–30.
7. Deckel AW, Gordinier A, Nuttal D, Tang V, Kuwada C, et al. (2001) Reduced activity and protein expression of NOS in R6/2 HD transgenic mice: effects of L-NAME on symptom progression. Brain Res 919: 70–81.
8. Puca AA, Carrizzo A, Ferrario A, Villa F, Vecchione C (2012) Endothelial nitric oxide synthase, vascular integrity and human exceptional longevity. Immun Ageing 9: 26.
9. Forstermann U, Sessa WC (2012) Nitric oxide synthases: regulation and function. European Heart Journal 33: 829–837, 837a–837d.
10. Mount PF, Kemp BE, Power DA (2007) Regulation of endothelial and myocardial NO synthesis by multi-site eNOS phosphorylation. J Mol Cell Cardiol 42: 271–279.
11. Calabrese V, Bates TE, Stella AM (2000) NO synthase and NO-dependent signal pathways in brain aging and neurodegenerative disorders: the role of oxidant/antioxidant balance. Neurochem Res 25: 1315–1341.
12. Schulz JB, Matthews RT, Beal MF (1995) Role of nitric oxide in neurodegenerative diseases. Curr Opin Neurol 8: 480–486.
13. Perez-Severiano F, Escalante B, Vergara P, Rios C, Segovia J (2002) Age-dependent changes in nitric oxide synthase activity and protein expression in striata of mice transgenic for the Huntington's disease mutation. Brain Res 951: 36–42.
14. Dukart J, Schroeter ML, Mueller K (2011) Age correction in dementia—matching to a healthy brain. PLoS One 6: e22193.
15. (1996) Unified Huntington's Disease Rating Scale: reliability and consistency. Huntington Study Group. Mov Disord 11: 136–142.
16. Marder K, Sandler S, Lechich A, Klager J, Albert SM (2002) Relationship between CAG repeat length and late-stage outcomes in Huntington's disease. Neurology 59: 1622–1624.
17. (1991) Declaration of Helsinki. Law Med Health Care 19: 264–265.
18. Gentile MT, Vecchione C, Marino G, Aretini A, Di Pardo A, et al. (2008) Resistin impairs insulin-evoked vasodilation. Diabetes 57: 577–583.
19. Vecchione C, Brandes RP (2002) Withdrawal of 3-hydroxy-3-methylglutaryl coenzyme A reductase inhibitors elicits oxidative stress and induces endothelial dysfunction in mice. Circ Res 91: 173–179.
20. Carrizzo A, Puca A, Damato A, Marino M, Franco E, et al. (2013) Resveratrol improves vascular function in patients with hypertension and dyslipidemia by modulating NO metabolism. Hypertension 62: 359–366.
21. Radomski M, Moncada S (1983) An improved method for washing of human platelets with prostacyclin. Thromb Res 30: 383–389.
22. Ku CJ, Karunarathne W, Kenyon S, Root P, Spence D (2007) Fluorescence determination of nitric oxide production in stimulated and activated platelets. Anal Chem 79: 2421–2426.
23. Squitieri F, Maglione V, Orobello S, Fornai F (2011) Genotype-, aging-dependent abnormal caspase activity in Huntington disease blood cells. J Neural Transm 118: 1599–1607.
24. Runne H, Kuhn A, Wild EJ, Pratyaksha W, Kristiansen M, et al. (2007) Analysis of potential transcriptomic biomarkers for Huntington's disease in peripheral blood. Proc Natl Acad Sci U S A 104: 14424–14429.
25. Markianos M, Panas M, Kalfakis N, Vassilopoulos D (2004) Platelet monoamine oxidase activity in subjects tested for Huntington's disease gene mutation. J Neural Transm 111: 475–483.
26. Muramatsu Y, Kaiya H, Imai H, Nozaki M, Fujimura H, et al. (1982) Abnormal platelet aggregation response in Huntington's disease. Arch Psychiatr Nervenkr 232: 191–200.
27. Deckel AW, Tang V, Nuttal D, Gary K, Elder R (2002) Altered neuronal nitric oxide synthase expression contributes to disease progression in Huntington's disease transgenic mice. Brain Res 939: 76–86.
28. Deckel AW (2001) Nitric oxide and nitric oxide synthase in Huntington's disease. J Neurosci Res 64: 99–107.
29. Loscalzo J (2001) Nitric oxide insufficiency, platelet activation, and arterial thrombosis. Circ Res 88: 756–762.
30. Kiriazis H, Jennings NL, Davern P, Lambert G, Su YD, et al. (2012) Neurocardiac dysregulation and neurogenic arrhythmias in a transgenic mouse model of Huntington's disease. Journal of Physiology-London 590: 5845–5860.
31. Mihm MJ, Amann DM, Schanbacher BL, Altschuld RA, Bauer JA, et al. (2007) Cardiac dysfunction in the R6/2 mouse model of Huntington's disease. Neurobiol Dis 25: 297–308.
32. Barton M, Cosentino F, Brandes RP, Moreau P, Shaw S, et al. (1997) Anatomic heterogeneity of vascular aging: role of nitric oxide and endothelin. Hypertension 30: 817–824.
33. Fulton D, Gratton JP, McCabe TJ, Fontana J, Fujio Y, et al. (1999) Regulation of endothelium-derived nitric oxide production by the protein kinase Akt. Nature 399: 597–601.
34. Reynolds NC Jr, Hellman RS, Tikofsky RS, Prost RW, Mark LP, et al. (2002) Single photon emission computerized tomography (SPECT) in detecting neurodegeneration in Huntington's disease. Nucl Med Commun 23: 13–18.

15

Efficacy of Selective PDE4D Negative Allosteric Modulators in the Object Retrieval Task in Female Cynomolgus Monkeys (*Macaca fascicularis*)

Jane S. Sutcliffe[1¶], **Vahri Beaumont**[2¶], **James M. Watson**[1], **Chang Sing Chew**[1], **Maria Beconi**[2], **Daniel M. Hutcheson**[1], **Celia Dominguez**[2], **Ignacio Munoz-Sanjuan**[2*]

1 Dept. of Neuroscience and CNS Safety Pharmacology, Maccine Pte Ltd, Singapore, Singapore, 2 CHDI Foundation/CHDI Management Inc., Los Angeles, California, United States of America

Abstract

Cyclic adenosine monophosphate (cAMP) signalling plays an important role in synaptic plasticity and information processing in the hippocampal and basal ganglia systems. The augmentation of cAMP signalling through the selective inhibition of phosphodiesterases represents a viable strategy to treat disorders associated with dysfunction of these circuits. The phosphodiesterase (PDE) type 4 inhibitor rolipram has shown significant pro-cognitive effects in neurological disease models, both in rodents and primates. However, competitive non-isoform selective PDE4 inhibitors have a low therapeutic index which has stalled their clinical development. Here, we demonstrate the pro-cognitive effects of selective negative allosteric modulators (NAMs) of PDE4D, D159687 and D159797 in female Cynomolgous macaques, in the object retrieval detour task. The efficacy displayed by these NAMs in a primate cognitive task which engages the corticostriatal circuitry, together with their suitable pharmacokinetic properties and safety profiles, suggests that clinical development of these allosteric modulators should be considered for the treatment of a variety of brain disorders associated with cognitive decline.

Editor: Veronique Sgambato-Faure, INSERM/CNRS, France

Funding: CHDI Foundation is a privately-funded not-for-profit biomedical research organization exclusively dedicated to discovering and developing therapeutics that slow the progression of Huntington's disease. CHDI Foundation conducts research in a number of different ways; for the purposes of this manuscript, research was conducted at the contract research organization Maccine Pte Ltd. under a fee-for-service agreement. The authors listed all contributed to the conception, study design, data collection and analysis, decision to publish, and preparation of the manuscript. The specific roles of these authors are articulated in the 'author contributions' section.

Competing Interests: The authors would like to declare the following: VB, MB, CD and IMS are employed by CHDI Management, Inc., as advisors to CHDI Foundation, Inc. JS, JW, CC, and DH are employed by Maccine Pte Ltd. There are no patents, products in development, or marketed products to declare.

* Email: ignacio.munoz@chdifoundation.org

¶ JSS and VB are co-first authors on this work.

Introduction

Cyclic nucleotide signalling pathways play essential roles in synaptic plasticity and memory formation [1–5]. The modulation of, in particular, cAMP intracellular pools in neuronal cells are essential for the mechanism of action of many psychotropic molecules, and underlies the effects of numerous G-protein coupled receptor pathways [2,6]. Phosphodiesterases (PDEs) play an important role in terminating cyclic nucleotide signalling via the hydrolysis of cyclic nucleotides [7]. There are twenty-one PDE proteins within eleven families (termed PDE1 – PDE11) with different expression patterns as well as varying affinities for cyclic nucleotides [5,6,8–11]. PDE4 inhibitors have, to date, been the most extensively investigated PDE inhibitors in the context of brain function and cognitive processes, and several studies highlight the role of cAMP and CREB signalling in neuroprotection and the modulation of neurogenesis in the dentate gyrus [12–15]. Deregulation of cyclic nucleotide and CREB signalling have been ascribed to several neurodegenerative conditions and cognitive impairment, including age-related memory loss, Alzheimer's disease (AD), and Huntington's disease (HD), amongst others.

We have a particular interest in the evaluation of PDE4 inhibitors for the treatment of Huntington's disease (HD). HD is a neurodegenerative, progressive, fatal autosomal dominant disorder characterized by loss and dysfunction of specific neuronal populations in the basal ganglia and in various cortical areas [16–20]. As a consequence, motor, psychiatric and cognitive deficits are characteristics of HD, presumably caused by dysfunctions in the cortico-basal ganglia circuitry affected in these patients. HD is caused exclusively by mutations in the *huntingtin* (*HTT*) gene. Although the exact nature of the interaction between huntingtin (HTT) protein and cyclic nucleotide signalling components is unclear, several reports point to dysregulation of cAMP pathways as a contributor to disease pathogenesis [21–30]. Loss of function of the transcriptional modulator CREB binding protein (CBP) has been postulated to contribute to the loss of neuronal function, as well as to the overall strong transcriptional deficits associated with HD, potentially through direct binding to HTT [21,28,31,32].

PDE2, 9 and 10 enzymes have also been implicated in the control of brain functions relevant to Huntington's disease (HD) [3,8,9,33–42]. Expression of PDE10 is downregulated in rodent models of the disease and in post mortem human tissues [43]. In the basal ganglia, cAMP elevation via both PDE4 and PDE10 inhibition modulates DARPP32 phosphorylation and influences behaviour during both movement and cognitive processes [4,27,40,44]. In addition, the elevation of cAMP is required for memory processes in hippocampal synaptic plasticity and memory encoding and retrieval, which are also affected in HD rodent models [9,12,37,39–41,45]. Studies in rodents, non-human primates (NHPs), and humans with rolipram and other PDE4 active-site orthosteric inhibitors have highlighted the pro-cognitive effects in a variety of tasks involving both the hippocampal and the cortico-striatal systems [9,40,41,45].

Rolipram, perhaps the most intensively studied active site PDE4 inhibitor, demonstrates preclinical efficacy in object recognition [46], water maze, and passive avoidance tasks in rodents [47], and in an object retrieval (OR) task (also called detour task) in the NHP [41]. Clinical studies using rolipram have investigated its potential utility in the treatment of affective disorders and for cognitive impairment, although its clinical development was halted due to adverse side effects including emesis and vasculitis in human and animal model studies [1,48,49], which have been observed at doses deemed too close to those necessary for efficacy. The narrow therapeutic index (TI) of rolipram prompted many investigators to pursue other strategies to separate the emetic liabilities from the beneficial effects. Such strategies have included the development of selective subtype PDE4D and PDE4B active site inhibitors [36,38,50–52], as well as the development of allosteric negative modulators (NAMs) of PDE4D [36]. In particular, a recent manuscript described the development of PDE4D NAMs with much improved TI over rolipram [36,53,54], due to their mechanism of inhibition (novel binding mode to the UCR2 domain of PDE4D7) and lack of full antagonism profile [36]. Based on a variety of tests conducted in Suncus murinus, dogs, and NHPs, these molecules were shown to have a much lower emetic potential, making them potentially useful agents for the treatment of cognitive and affective disorders. Therefore, we sought to explore whether PDE4D NAMs could affect cognitive performance relevant to HD.

Importantly, most PDE4 inhibitors in clinical development had a TI determined from studies conducted in multiple species. Typically the effective 'dose' for functional or cognitive improvement is extrapolated based on rodent tasks, whereas the adverse side effect dose is derived from toxicology studies conducted in larger species, such as dogs or NHPs. This may be misleading since in evolutionarily-divergent brain regions—such as the frontal cortex and basal ganglia—the modulation of cognitive processes in rodents versus primates (including humans) is likely to be divergent. Furthermore, the dose of psychoactive molecules might be dependent on the type and complexity of the cognitive task employed. We therefore assessed the effect of selective PDE4D NAMs in a task relevant to HD while monitoring for any adverse behaviour, including retching and emesis at the doses used during cognitive evaluation. We also monitored plasma and CSF levels of the drugs to define the exposure/efficacy relationship for potential clinical development.

The OR is a behavioral test designed to assess the functional and anatomical integrity of the frontostriatal pathway in NHPs and is adapted from an OR test used to cognitively assess children [55,56]. This paradigm has been shown to involve executive function and its components including attention, response inhibition and planning, thought to involve the frontal lobe structures of the brain [55]. Performance in this task is impaired following lesions to the prefrontal and orbitofrontal cortices in the common marmoset [57,58] and in the striatum in the capuchin monkey [59]. It has also been used to assess striatal dysfunction and cognitive impairment following SIV infection in macaques [60].

Pharmacological manipulations that elicit deficits in this task include dopaminergic depletions of the striatum in MPTP-treated monkeys [61], prefrontal serotonin depletion [62], and disruptions of this circuitry by subchronic administration of the NMDA receptor antagonist phencyclidine (PCP) [63], confirming the critical contribution of prefrontal corticostriatal circuitry. Antagonism of the D4 dopamine receptors reverse the subchronic PCP induced OR deficit [64]. Enhanced OR performance has been reported with acute dosing of the non-selective PDE4 inhibitor rolipram and with the PDE5 inhibitor sildenafil [41] in male Cynomolgus macaques (Macaca fascicularis). Other reports indicate the OR task is sensitive to nicotine, the acetylcholinesterase inhibitor donepezil [65], α7-nicotinic receptor agonists (such as GTS-21), and a GABA α5 inverse agonist [66]. Of note, elevations in cAMP signalling have been shown to impair performance in a spatial memory working task in aged (but not young) NHPs, so age is an important factor when assessing potential pro-cognitive effects of selective PDE inhibitors [67]. Therefore, the sex and age of the NHPs seem important to uncover potential cognitive effects in this task.

We evaluated both the pharmacokinetic characteristics and cognitive effects of two PDE4D NAMs, D159687 (dosed orally at 0.05, 0.5 and 5.0 mg/kg) and D159797 (dosed orally at 0.05, 0.5 and 1.0 mg/kg), and have monitored for adverse events over this dosing range. Female Cynomolgus macaques (4–6 year old) were used in this study. The two compounds display similar biochemical and cellular potencies (20–30 nM in a human cell-based assay using whole-blood [36]. D159687 and D159797 have high selectivity over other PDE enzymes, and good selectivity over the closely related enzyme PDE4B (20-fold selectivity; see [36]), setting them apart from rolipram; the latter served as a positive control in this cognitive paradigm at doses previously shown to elicit pro-cognitive effects during OR without inducing emesis (dosed at 0.003, 0.01 and 0.03 mg/kg intramuscularly) [41].

Our pharmacokinetic data indicate that the plasma clearance in NHPs of D159797 is ~10-times lower than that of D159687 (0.17 vs. 1.65 L/h/kg, respectively). Since the compounds have similar volumes of distribution, the clearance difference results in a 10-fold difference in elimination half-lives (1.24 h for D159687 and 10.4 h for D159797, respectively). Our studies replicated the pro-cognitive effects of rolipram in the OR task in young female NHPs, and demonstrate that a more robust pro-cognitive effect can be achieved with either of the PDE4D selective NAMs in this task, possibly because the dose ranging was not limited by the emergence of adverse events, as is the case with rolipram. The shorter half-life D159687 had an improved TI over D159797, which has a much longer half-life. These findings also demonstrate that selective modulation of PDE4D isoforms is sufficient for pro-cognitive benefit in this task.

Materials and Methods

The present study adhered to the Association for Assessment and Accreditation of Laboratory Animal Care (AAALAC), the National Advisory Committee on Laboratory Animal Research (NACLAR) guidelines and was approved by the Institutional Animal Care and Use Committee of Maccine Pte Ltd (IACUC protocols #46-2007 amendment 27 and #162-2009). Animals were provided with environmental enrichment such as Kong toys, mirrors, rattles and foraging boards in addition to tactile (where possible), olfactory, auditory and visual contact with con-specifics. Prior to experimental investigations animals were habituated to study personnel via positive social interaction and to experimental techniques using positive reinforcement training to minimize stress and to mitigate any adverse effects on health, well-being and behavior. Study personnel remained consistent throughout the study and veterinary care was available around the clock. The in-house veterinarian examined each subject prior to study initiation and performed blood tests and physical examinations as required. There were at minimum twice daily observations of each subject for general health, alertness, and overall behavior; any abnormal changes were immediately reported to the attending veterinarian. Following dose administration animals were monitored every 10 minutes for a minimum of 2 hours. No animal was sacrificed during these studies; however emergency procedures and humane endpoints were outlined in the IACUC protocol.

Subjects

Sixteen female, adult (4–6 years; weights 2.39–3.6 Kg) Cyno-molgus macaques (*Macaca fascicularis*) were individually housed in an AAALAC accredited, GLP compliant facility with cage environmental enrichment (such as Kong toys, mirrors, rattles and forage material) in addition to tactile (where possible), olfactory, auditory and visual contact with con-specifics. Eight animals were assigned to the object retrieval study and eight to the pharmaco-kinetic (PK) evaluation group. Animals were trained for dose administration using positive reinforcement techniques to mini-mize stress and to mitigate any adverse effects on health, wellbeing and behavior. The air-conditioned colony room was maintained at $20\pm2°C$, $50\pm20\%$ humidity with a normal 12 h light-dark cycle (on 07:00, off 19:00). Food (Primate Lab Diet 5048, Purina Mills, USA) and water were available *ad libitum* and fresh fruit was offered twice daily. All experimental procedures were approved by the Institutional Animal Care and Use Committee of Maccine Pte Ltd (IACUC protocols #46-2007 amendment 27 and #162-2009) and were in accordance with AAALAC, NACLAR and good practice [68] guidelines.

Cisterna-magna Cannulation Surgery

The eight animals assigned to the PK study were surgically prepared with indwelling cannulae inserted into the cisterna magna and connected to a subcutaneous access port to permit cerebrospinal fluid (CSF) sampling. Animals were sedated with ketamine (0.1 ml/kg of 100 mg/ml solution) and the dorsum of the head, neck, and scapular region shaved and prepared for sterile surgery. Isoflurane was delivered by mask to achieve a depth of anesthesia suitable for endotracheal intubation. Following intubation, anesthesia was maintained using isoflurane. Intraop-erative monitoring included heart rate, oxygen saturation, end-tidal carbon dioxide, eye reflexes, jaw tone, body temperature (a water circulated heating pad was used to keep animals warm), and response to surgical stimulation.

Animals were placed in sternal recumbency with added padding under the trunk, allowing the head/neck to be manipulated into a flexed position. A final surgical scrub and site preparation was performed using iodine and a sterile drape applied around the surgical site. A longitudinal incision was made in the skin on the dorsal midline of the occipital region extending caudally. In the occipital region, the incision was extended through muscle layers and planes using sharp and blunt dissection, to the ligament/membrane overlying the cisterna magna between the occipitus and the dorsal process of the atlas. The sterile catheter and port

was prepared to the correct length and filled with sterile saline. A small incision ($\sim$1–1.5 mm) was made in the membrane and the catheter carefully inserted into the cisterna magna. The catheter was tunneled under the skin to the subcutaneous space between the occipital region and the rostral portion of the head.

Muscle and skin layers were sutured with absorbable suture. A suitable analgesic was administered during induction of anesthesia and twice daily during the 48 hours postoperatively. In addition, a suitable antibiotic was administered pre-operatively and for 5 days post-operatively. Animals were allowed two weeks to recover from surgery prior to any sampling and dosing being performed. During this time, the indwelling catheters were monitored and checked for patency and observation of clear and free flowing CSF.

Compounds and Dose Formulation

Rolipram (0.3 mg/mL; Evotec, UK) was prepared fresh daily in a 10% Solutol in 90% saline (0.9% NaCl) vehicle. Rolipram formulations of 0.1 and 0.03 mg/mL were prepared from the stock 0.3 mg/mL stock solution via serial dilution. Rolipram was administered via the intramuscular route in the OR evaluation at a dose volume of 0.1 mL/kg in order to attain final dose levels of 0.03, 0.01 and 0.003 mg/kg respectively.

D159687 and D159797 (DeCode Genetics, Iceland), were supplied as the free base. Compounds had purity in excess of 97%. Dose formulations for the PK and OR study were prepared fresh daily and administered on the day of preparation. For the PK study intravenous (IV) infusions; D159687 (0.5 mg/mL) was formulated as a solution in 13% (w/v) PEG 400, 3% (w/v) Cremphor EL and 84% of 5% (w/v) Dextrose formulation. D159797 (0.5 mg/mL) was formulated in 15% (w/v) PEG 400, 1% (w/v) EtOH and 1% (w/v) Tween 80 in 0.9% NaCl vehicle. For PO administration (PK study and OR evaluation), D159687 and D159797 were prepared as solutions in a 0.5% (w/v) Poloxamer 188: 0.5% (w/v) HPMC: 0.4% Tween 80 vehicle at 5.0 mg/mL final concentration.

Pharmacokinetics of D159687 and D15979

Animal Phase. Of the eight animals surgically prepared with indwelling cisterna-magna catheters, 6 animals were initially assigned to the PK study following catheter patency checks as described above. The animals were evenly assigned to groups 1 (D159687 pharmacokinetics) and 2 (D159797 pharmacokinetics) based on their body weight measured the day prior to dosing. These animals remained in that group for the duration of the study with the exception of one animal from group 1 which had to be replaced due to cistern-magna patency issues after IV dosing and prior to the oral phase of the study.

On Day 1 of the PK study, animals were administered 1 mg/kg D159687 (group 1, n = 3) or 1 mg/kg D159797 (group 2, n = 3) by intravenous infusion (Day 1). The animals then received a 9 day wash-out prior to the commencement of the determination of oral pharmacokinetic properties. In this instance, the animals were administered 5 mg/kg D159687 (group 1, n = 3) or 5 mg/kg D159797 (group 2, n = 3) by oral gavage daily for a period of seven days (study days 11–17). Dose volume for both D159687 and D159797 was 1.0 mL/kg. The results of this study are shown on Figure 1.

On Days 1 (IV), 11 (oral, day 1), and 17 (oral, day 7), whole blood (0.5 mL) was collected from the femoral vein of each animal. CSF (150 µL) was collected from the subcutaneous port in each animal using a sterile Posigrip 'Huber point' 22G x ¾ inch needle (Access Technologies, USA) at the same time as the blood collection. The area around the port was swabbed prior to insertion of the needle and 150 µL of CSF (dead volume) was

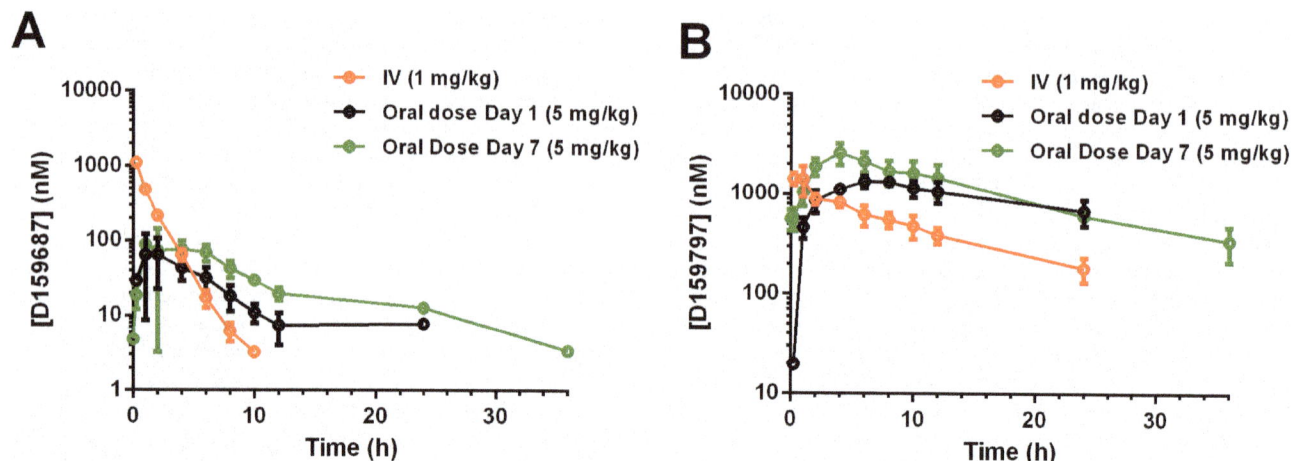

Figure 1. Pharmacokinetic analysis of PDE4D NAMs in female Cynomolgous monkeys. (A–B) Plasma exposure of D159687 (A), or D159797 (B) in female Cynomolgus monkey plasma following a single intravenous administration at 1.0 mg/kg, and on day 1 and day 7 after repeated daily oral administration at 5.0 mg/kg.

removed immediately prior to the actual CSF sample collection. Blood and CSF were collected from each animal at pre-dose and following dose administration at 0.25, 1, 2, 4, 6, 8, 10, 12, and 24 h post dose on days 1 and 11 and additional blood and CSF sample was collected at 36h post-dose on day 17. All time points were timed from the start of dose administration. Whole blood was held on wet ice until centrifugation at 4°C (3500 rpm for 10 minutes) to allow plasma separation, after which two aliquots of plasma (at least 100 μL each) were directly transferred to individually labelled tubes and stored at −70±10°C until analysis. Two CSF aliquots of 50 μL were diluted with acetonitrile (1/1, by volume) and the remaining CSF aliquots (approximately 50 μL) were snap frozen in liquid nitrogen prior to storage −70±10°C until analysis.

Bioanalysis. Concentrations of D159687 and D159797 in dose formulation, NHP plasma and CSF were determined using an HPLC-tandem mass spectrometry (LC-MS/MS) method developed at Charles Rivers Laboratory (Preclinical Services, Shrewsbury). The matrix calibration standards were prepared at concentrations of 1.00–10000 ng eq./mL in Cynomolgus control plasma for plasma, and in 1:1 by volume Cynomolgus CSF:acetonitrile for CSF. For dose formulation analysis, the calibration standards were prepared in 1:1, by volume Mobile Phase A: Mobile Phase B at concentrations of 5.00–500 ng eq./mL. Diclofenac or reserpine were used as an internal standards (IS) as indicated below. The lower limits of assay quantitation (LLOQ) for D159687 were 2.73 nM in plasma, and 2.73 nM, 5.46 nM or 13.7 nM in CSF depending on the dilution of the sample. The lower limits of assay quantitation (LLOQ) for D159797 were 2.48 nM in plasma and 2.48 nM or 12.4 nM in CSF depending on the dilution of the sample. Results of the dose formulation analysis indicated that the measured concentrations of D159687 and D159797 were within 15% of the nominal concentration for both dose routes. Therefore, all PK estimations were based on target dose levels.

CSF samples were diluted in acetonitrile (1/1, by volume), at the time of collection. Dose formulation samples were diluted in a mixture of Mobile Phase A/Mobile Phase B (1/1, by volume), to bring them to a concentration within the range of the calibration standards. Analytes were extracted by protein precipitation (test tubes were kept on ice and protected from light), as follows: An aliquot (25 μL) of samples (plasma, diluted CSF or diluted plasma),

matrix blanks, control blanks, and matrix calibration standards were placed into individual wells in 96-well plates. An aliquot (100 μL) of a solution containing diclofenac or reserpine as the internal standards (IS), (0.100 μg eq./mL in 0.1% formic acid in acetonitrile) was added to all samples except matrix blanks and solvent blanks. An aliquot (100 μL), of 0.1% formic acid in acetonitrile was added to matrix blanks. Samples were vortexed for 1-min and centrifuged for 5-min. Each supernatant was transferred to an individual well in a new 96-well plate. Immediately prior to LC-MS/MS analysis, an aliquot (50 μL) of Milli-Q water was added to each well, the plate was covered and vortexed for 1-min.

Analytes were separated by high performance liquid chromatography and quantified by mass spectrometry (LC-MS/MS). There were two mobile phases, Mobile Phase A consisted of 1.0% formic acid in water, and Mobile Phase B of 1.0% formic acid in acetonitrile. Two LC-MS/MS systems were used. The first one, used for the dosed analytes in plasma and dose formulation, consisted of an Agilent 1200 binary pump equipped with an Agilent G1367D autosampler and connected in tandem with an API5500 mass spectrometer. A Hypersil Gold (3μ, 20×2.1 mm) chromatography column at room temperature was used for analyte separation. The flow rate was maintained at 0.6 mL/min, and the gradient increased linearly from 5% to 98% Mobile Phase B in 1.2 min and held at 98% B for 0.5 min. The injection volumes were 2.5–10 μL. The second one, used for the dosed analytes in CSF and metabolites in CSF and plasma, consisted of a PE Series 200 micro pump equipped with a Leap CTC PAL autosampler and connected in tandem with an API4000 mass spectrometer. A Phenomenex Gemini (3μ, C18, 50×2.0 mm) chromatography column at room temperature was used for analyte separation. The flow rate was maintained at 0.3 mL/min, and the gradient increased linearly from 5% to 90% Mobile Phase B in 2 min and held at 90% B for 3 min. The injection volume was 30 μL.

In both instruments, the electrospray ionization source was set to scan in positive ionization mode, with a dwell time set to 100 ms. The multiple reaction monitoring (MRM) transitions were m/z 367.4 to 231.0 for D159687, m/z 403.4 to 217.0 for D159797, m/z 609.1 to 195.2 for reserpine (IS) and m/z 297.9 to 215.9 for diclofenac (IS).

A

Trial Number	Description*	Level	Pictorial Representation#
1	LOS-Line of sight	Easy	
2	LOS-Line of sight	Easy	
3	RO- Right Outside	Easy	
4	RD – Right Deep	Difficult	
5	RO – Right Outside	Easy	
6	RI - Right Inside	Easy	
7	RD- Right Deep	Difficult	
8	LO - Left Outside	Easy	
9	LD - Left Deep	Difficult	
10	LO - Left Outside	Easy	
11	LI – Left Inside	Easy	
12	LD – Left Deep	Difficult	
13	LD – Left Deep	Difficult	
14	RD – Right Deep	Difficult	
15	LD – Left Deep	Difficult	
16	RD – Right Deep	Difficult	
17**	LOS-Line of sight	Easy	

B

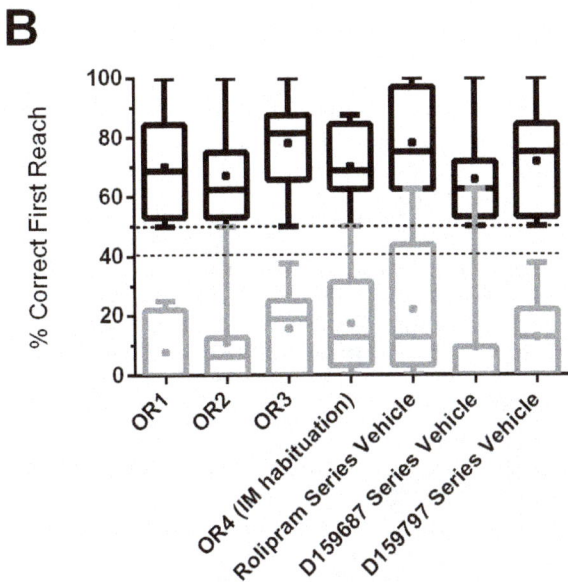

C

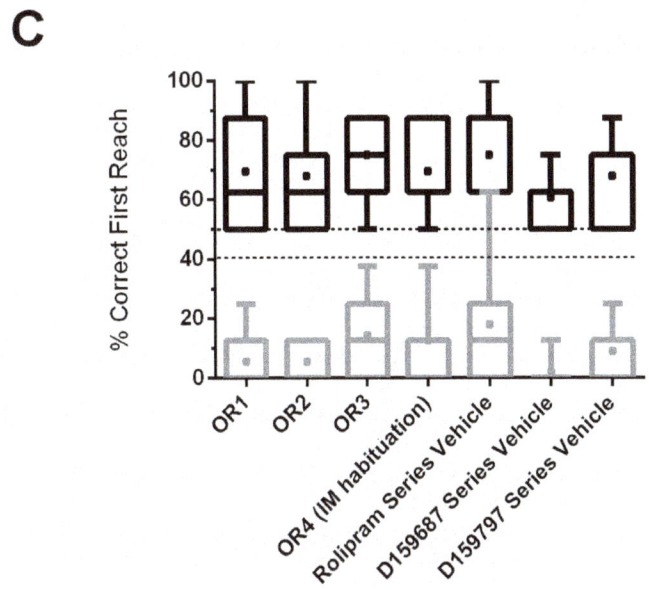

Figure 2. Object retrieval task schematic and baseline characterization. (A) Order of object retrieval task sessions for easy and difficult trials. Drawings illustrate the position of the reward in the boxes. (*) Left position will become right and right position will become left and so on in weekly

rotation throughout the study. (#) The **bold** side of the cube represents the open side of the cube. (**) Trial 17 was for reward purposes and was not included in the data analysis; (B) Box (line indicates median, * indicates mean, box represents upper and lower 25 percentiles) and whisker (maximum to minimum) plots of all animal performance during the 4 training sessions and to vehicle administration during the testing phase on both easy (grey) and difficult (black) trials. Dashed lines indicate targeted performance – performance in easy trials >50% correct first reach, and performance in difficult trials <40% correct first reach. (C) Same data as in (B) but with high performer animal 3939 excluded. Criteria are largely met by exclusion of this animal. The outlier value during the rolipram vehicle trial is due to animal 7A5D.

Pharmacokinetic Calculations. Pharmacokinetic (PK) parameters were calculated by non-compartmental analysis using WinNonlin program, version 5.2 (Scientific Consulting Inc., Palo Alto, California). A model was selected based on the vascular (IV Infusion) or extravascular (oral gavage) routes of administration. For both routes, the pre-dose concentration was used as the concentration at time zero. Plasma and CSF concentrations below the limit of quantitation were treated as absent samples for the purpose of calculating the mean plasma concentration values or for calculating pharmacokinetic parameters.

The area under the plasma concentration versus time curve (AUC) was calculated using the linear trapezoidal method (linear interpolation). When appropriate, the terminal elimination phase of the PK profile was estimated using at least the last three observed concentration values. PK parameters describing the systemic exposure of analytes of interest in plasma or CSF were estimated from observed (rather than predicted) plasma concentration values, the dosing regimen, the AUC, and the terminal elimination phase rate constant (k_{el}) for each group. The portion of the AUC from the last measurable concentration to infinity was estimated from the equation Ct/k_{el}, where Ct represents the last measurable concentration. The extrapolated portion of the AUC was used for the determination of $AUC_{(0-inf)}$. The percent bioavailability (%F) was calculated by dividing the dose normalized oral $AUC_{(0-inf)}$ by the dose normalized iv $AUC_{(0-inf)}$ times 100. The bioavailability calculations assumed concentrations were in the linear range.

Behavioural Assessments - Object Retrieval (OR)

A total of n = 8 female *Cynomolgus* monkeys aged 4–6 years were trained in the OR task and were used for these studies, following a cross-over design. Animals were trained to ensure adequate and stable performance during the dosing studies. Animals were individually housed prior to the initiation of the study. Animals were habituated to the oral gavage method using positive reinforcement techniques for a minimum of 2 weeks prior to the initiation of OR testing to mitigate any adverse impact on behaviour. To ensure accurate dosing each individual was momentarily restrained in a 'standing' type primate chair to allow easy and gentle passage of the gavage tube. The oral doses were administered in a dose volume of 1.0 mL/Kg which was followed with 5 mL of purified water to ensure no residual compound formulation remained in the gavage tube. During dose habituation and the study the same study personnel administered the compounds and thus a non-stressful, familiar routine for the animals was achieved.

The OR task [41,55] requires the subject to retrieve a food reward from a clear acrylic box (dimensions = 5×5×5 cm) with one open side which is positioned in front of the subject on a metal holder fixed to the outside of the home cage. The cube is presented to the subject with the open side facing left, right, or toward the monkey in a randomised set list of easy versus difficult trials. Food rewards (raisins or cubes of fruit pieces 1–2 cm^2) were placed on the outer edge, inner edge, line of sight (all easy), or deep within the box (difficult). Each test session consisted of 17 trials [41], with an initial Easy phase of 3 easy trials followed by a Random phase

of 9 trials (4 difficult and 5 easy, presented randomly for each session), followed by a Difficult phase of 4 difficult trials and finally one final Easy Trial (Figure 2A). The final easy trial was included for reward purposes and although the number of attempts was recorded the data were not used for analysis. For successive test sessions, the subject was presented with the trials in an order exactly the reverse of the previous session (previous left side exposure became right side exposure and vice-versa). Individual trials within one OR session were terminated if there were no reaches or successful retrieval of the reward within 2 minutes by the subject. The acrylic box was cleaned between trials to minimize cues which may influence subsequent task performance through easier identification of the cube entrance.

Training weeks and stable baseline performance evaluation. Animals were habituated to the metal frame prior to introducing the OR cube. During training, the animals were exposed to the OR trials as depicted in Figure 2A for 4 occasions (twice a week- OR trial # T1-T4 – data not shown). Importantly, during this period of training, all animals acquired the rewards even after an incorrect first reach. OR evaluations were then subsequently conducted once per week to discourage learning and thus ensure no performance shift during the pharmacology study (Figure 2B). Animals continued to be trained once per week for a period of 3 weeks immediately prior to pharmacology (OR1- 3; Figure 2B).

Baseline performance was targeted to be an average, stable performance of >50% correct responses in the easy tasks, with less than 40% correct responses in the difficult tasks (Figure 2B). All animals evaluated during this phase met these criteria by the end of the training session, with the exception of one animal, which was a baseline 'high performer' on difficult trials (Animal 3939). Figure 2C shows the stability of the baseline performance without inclusion of this particular animal. However, this animal was included in all subsequent dosing phases. For the subsequent evaluation of compounds on OR task performance, a within-subjects design was employed for this study randomised in a Latin-square design. OR behavioural scoring was completed in a blinded fashion. Testing was conducted as follows:

Testing period (Weeks 1–16)

- Week 1: Animals were habituated to intramuscular injections daily using the 'rolipram' vehicle formulation (10% solutol (w/v), 90% saline vehicle in a 0.1 mL/Kg dose volume) Monday through Friday, and a single baseline OR trial evaluation was performed on Wednesday (OR4) (Figure 2A). Animals were dosed with vehicle 30 minutes prior to this behavioural evaluation.

- Weeks 2 to 5: Evaluation of rolipram in OR task. Following the stable baseline performance establishment (OR1 – 4), all animals were administered the 3 doses of rolipram (0.003, 0.01 and 0.03 mg/Kg) or vehicle intramuscularly 30 minutes before evaluation on the OR task, every Wednesday through Weeks 2–5 (OR5-8). All animals were dosed with vehicle on the preceding Monday and Tuesday to keep them habituated to the injections and avoid any Pavlovian conditioning to any pro-emetic effects of treatment, although no OR testing was carried out on those days. Treatment was administered at approximately the same time each day and administered via the intramuscular route at a volume of 0.1 mL/kg. Dosing was randomized per subject in a latin –square design.

- Week 6: Wash-out and habituation of the animals to handling and the oral gavage dosing procedure daily (Monday through Friday) was conducted. Animals were dosed with a 0.5% Poloxamer 188+0.5% HPMC +0.4% Tween 80 vehicle at a dose volume of 1.0 mL/Kg. This dose was washed down with approximately 5 mL of purified water. No behavioural testing was conducted during this 'wash-out' week.

- Weeks 7 to 10: The animals were given test compound D159687 every Wednesday over this 4 week period. All animals received the 3 dose levels of D159687 (0.05, 0.5 and 5.0 mg/Kg at a dose volume of 1.0 mL/Kg) or its vehicle using a Latin-square design so that all animals were tested in a randomized manner at each dose level. The test compound was administered 2 hours before evaluation on the OR task on each Wednesday (OR 9- 12). All animals were administered vehicle via oral gavage on Monday and Tuesday to keep them habituated to oral administration and to avoid any Pavlovian conditioning to any pro-emetic effects of treatment, although no testing was carried out on those days. Treatment was administered at approximately the same time each day. The doses were administered orally via gavage in a volume of 1 mL/kg and washed down with approximately 5 mL of purified water.

- Week 11: Maintenance of habituation to oral gavage/wash-out period. Animals were habituated to handling and the oral gavage dosing procedure daily (Monday through to Friday). Animals were dosed with a 0.5% Poloxamer 188+0.5% HPMC +0.4% Tween 80 vehicle at a dose volume of 1.0 mL/Kg. This dose was washed down with approximately 5 mL of purified water. No behavioural testing was conducted during this 'wash-out' week.

- Weeks 12 to 16: The animals were given test compound D159797 every Wednesday over this 4 week period. As in Week 7 to 10, animals were administered vehicle via oral gavage on Monday and Tuesday of each week to keep them habituated to oral administration and to avoid any Pavlovian conditioning to any pro-emetic effects of treatment. All animals intended to receive the 3 dose levels of D159797 (0.05, 0.5 and 1 mg/Kg) or its vehicle, randomized in a Latin-square design so that all animals were tested at each dose level (Weeks 12–15). The test compound was administered 2 hours before evaluation on the OR task on each Wednesday (OR 13–17). However, while the dose levels used were 0.05, 0.5 and 5.0 mg/Kg during week 12, the top dose level was lowered during week 13 to 1.5 mg/Kg and further reduced to 1.0 mg/Kg for weeks 13–16 following signs of retching at the highest dose (see results section). Thus the additional week was included in the dosing design (Week 16) which allowed all animals (except 7A5D) to receive a top dose of 1 mg/kg for evaluation. Deviations to the Latin square dosing design are depicted in Table S3.

Clinical Observations. Animals were closely monitored for the duration of the study, and were videotaped during task performance. Body weights were monitored weekly. Clinical observations were recorded prior to dose administration and after the completion of each OR task. Furthermore, a behavioural scoring record was used to record any changes in behaviour for each animal commencing at 5 minutes prior to dose administra-

tion and once every 10 minutes for up to 2 hours after dose administration.

Statistical Analysis. The mean percent correct first reaches, total reaches and barrier reaches for easy and difficult trials were analysed using repeat measures one-way analysis of variance (ANOVA), with dose group as the primary factor. Demonstrated observations of statistical significance were analysed via post-hoc Dunnett's analysis using the vehicle treatment as the reference control. Statistics are presented as F (DFn, DFd) and results were considered significant when $p < 0.05$ and confidence intervals were set at 95%.

Results

Pharmacokinetics

Pharmacokinetic parameters for D159687 and D159797 are presented in Figure 1, Table 1 (D159687), and Table 2 (D159797).

D159687. Following IV administration of D159687, the plasma clearance was high (1.65 L/h/kg), the volume of distribution was moderate (2.1 L/kg) and the terminal half-life was 1.24 hr. (Table 1). After the first day of oral dosing, the oral bioavailability was low (6%) and increased by approximately 2-fold (13%) after the seventh single daily dose (Figure 1A and Table 1). Consistently, the oral AUC_{0-last} increased approximately 2-fold from 447 to 869 nM h. The oral elimination half-life also increased from 3.1 to 4.3 h with multiple days of dosing. The T_{max} was quite variable between animals (2.3±1.5 h and 4.3±2.9 h at Days 1 and 7, respectively), with mean C_{max} values of 80±36 nM and 121±73 nM at Days 1 and 7, respectively. Consistent with the short terminal elimination half-life (IV), the AUC_{0-24} were similar to the AUC_{0-inf} indicating that in the absence of a change in absorption and/or clearance mechanism, D159687 will not accumulate. The low oral bioavailability was attributed to significant first pass metabolism. This conclusion was supported by the expected O-dealkylation of the compound (not shown) and was consistent with the high plasma clearance. However, contributions of dissolution limited absorption to the low oral bioavailability cannot be ruled out. The higher oral bioavailability and corresponding AUC and C_{max}, together with the approximately 2-fold increase in elimination half-life observed on day 7, after multiple oral doses, could be a consequence of a change in the clearance mechanism(s), or enhanced absorption. Given the moderate volume of distribution of the compound, it is unlikely that the increase in AUC and half-life are an artifact of an inadequate bioanalysis limit of quantitation for a drug of a bi-phasic elimination profile. While these observations suggest the possibility that D159687 is either a time-dependent inhibitor of a monkey CYP activity, or an inhibitor of an active efflux mechanism, neither of these options are favored, as the exposure of the known metabolites increased with multiple days of dosing (data not shown), and inhibition of an efflux transporter would have resulted in a more prolonged half-life. Thus, we attribute the increase in D159687 AUC with days of dosing to a moderate increase in absorption.

D159797. D159797 had a much slower clearance (0.17 L/hr/kg), with a similar volume of distribution at steady state (2.35 L/kg), and a much longer elimination half-life (13.7 hr), than D159687 (Figure 2A and Table 2). The compound had an improved oral bioavailability (57% and 66% on Day 1 and Day 7). Plasma C_{max} was higher than for D159687, with mean values of 1400±155 nM on Day 1 and 2590±656 nM on Day 7 (Table 2). The oral AUC_{0-24} increased with days of dosing as driven by the time that it took to achieve steady state concentrations with the long elimination half-life (Table 2). Given the different clearance

Table 1. Summary of plasma pharmacokinetic parameters of D159687 following single intravenous administration at 1.0 mg/kg, and on day 1 and day 7 after repeated daily oral administration at 5.0 mg/kg.

PK Parameters	Units	IV (1 mg/kg)	PO day 1 (5 mg/kg)	PO day 7 (5 mg/kg)
AUC$_{(0-last)}$	nM.h	1649±68	447±162	869±198
AUC$_{(0-inf)}$	nM.h	1657±69	477±178	920±222
AUCNorm	nM.h.kg.mg	1657±69	95±36	184±44
Cl	L/h/kg	1.65±0.07		
Vdss (area)	L/kg	2.10±0.38		
MRT (area)	h	1.27±0.17		
Oral F	%		6±2.8*	12.6±1.77*
C$_{max}$	nM		80±36	121±73
Tmax (obs)	h		2.3±1.5	4.3±2.9
t$_{1/2}$	h	1.24±0.17	3.1±0.7	4.3±1.9

Data presented as mean ± SD of 3 animals.

*Calculated from n = 2, as due to patency issues in catheter of one animal following IV dosing, one animal was replaced for po dosing, thus, it was not a cross over design.

rates and oral bioavailability of these two compounds, we tested both molecules in the OR task and monitored for potential adverse effects.

Compound exposure in CSF was measured to assess if it could be used as a surrogate for assessment of unbound compound concentration in CNS, as for most drugs examined there has shown to be a reasonable correlation (within ~3-fold)[69]. However, neither D159687 nor its known metabolites (data not shown), or D159797, were detected to any significant degree in the CSF after either IV or PO dosing (Table S1 and S2). In order to assess whether the compounds could potentially suffer from active CNS efflux, which is one mechanism that could account for the low detection in primate CSF, we conducted *in vitro* MDR1-MDCK assays with D159687 as an exemplar. These experiments showed D159687 to be low-to-moderately permeable (P$_{app}$ A-B 44 nm/s) with an efflux ratio (ER) of 0.9, demonstrating that D159687 does not act as a MDR1/Pgp substrate and active efflux from the CNS is unlikely to occur via this mechanism. This finding

is consistent with the *in vivo* PK data reported by Burgin et al. [36], who showed that the total brain: plasma AUC ratio for D159687 was ≥1 across rodents and primates.

Another potential reason why either D159687 or D159797 were not detected to any significant extent in the CSF could be due to high protein binding (both to plasma and/or brain tissue) which would limit the free (unbound) brain concentration of drug. The plasma protein binding of D159687 was measured in monkey plasma *in vitro* using equilibrium dialysis to determine if this was a significant issue. Binding was independent of incubated concentration (at 1, 5 and 10 μM) and showed that D159867 was moderate-to-highly plasma protein bound (F$_u$ 0.07). Adjustment of the total plasma AUC by F$_u$ to estimate unbound plasma AUC (AUC$_{uu}$) following oral dosing gave adjusted values of between 33 - 61 nM.h at day 1 and day 7, within the effective range for target inhibition (IC$_{50}$ of 28 nM).[36] Given that it is generally accepted that *in vitro* protein binding is a notoriously poor predictor of the central efficacy of orally administered drugs, since unbound drug

Table 2. Summary of plasma pharmacokinetic parameters of D159797 following single intravenous administration at 1.0 mg/kg, and on day 1 and day 7 after repeated daily oral administration at 5.0 mg/kg.

PK Parameters	Units	IV (1 mg/kg)	PO day 1 (5 mg/kg)	PO day 7 (5 mg/kg)
AUC$_{(0-last)}$	nM.h	11918±2087	23019±4205	39720±7924
AUC$_{(0-inf)}$	nM.h	14669±2909	42885±15527	47834±4493
AUCNorm	nM.h.kg.mg	14669±2909	8577± 3105	9567±899
Cl	L/h/kg	0.173±0.032		
Vdss (area)	L/kg	2.35±0.32		
MRT (area)	h	13.7±1.5		
Oral F	%		57.2±9.4	66.6±12.8
C$_{max}$	nM		1400±155	2590±656
Tmax (obs)	h		7.3±1.2	4±0
t$_{1/2}$	h	10.4±1.2	19.3±6.1	14.4±8.6

Data presented as mean ± SD of 3 animals.

concentration at the site of action is controlled by highly dynamic simultaneous physiological actions *in vivo* (ie permeation, target binding, metabolism, transport and movement between tissue and cellular compartments) [70,71], our results using CSF sampling cannot confirm or rule out central target engagement at the doses we tested, suggesting that CSF sampling for the PDE4D NAMs lacks the sensitivity to be used as a biomarker of free brain drug concentration, at least at the limit of detection we achieved in the CSF matrix (LOQ 10-20 nM for most samples). Thus an alternative translational endpoint would be recommended to estimate target engagement in a clinical setting.

Pro-cognitive Effects of Rolipram and selective PDE4D Negative Allosteric Modulators Evaluated via the Object Retrieval (OR) Task

The OR paradigm employed here is shown in Figure 2A. In this paradigm, we employed a cross-over randomized testing design, with weekly drug wash-out periods between the different drugs tested. A total of 8 female *Cynomolgus* monkeys (4–6 years of age) were trained with the aim to reach a stable baseline in the easy tasks, while performing consistently at less than 40% correct first reach in the difficult tasks (OR 1–4; Figure 2B). This level of performance would allow us to assess whether compounds would exhibit a pro-cognitive effect, as judged by any subsequent enhancement of the monkey's performance in the difficult trials during the dosing test periods. A consistent high level of accuracy in the easy trials (>50%) would also allow for detecting any cognitive impairment produced by drug administration. All animals selected, with the exclusion of one, met these criteria. The outlier animal, "3939", was noted to be a 'high performer' in the difficult tasks at baseline. Figure 2C shows the performance of animals over the baseline period with the exclusion of this particular animal. Additionally, a post-hoc analysis of the performance of all animals after dosing with vehicle after completion of the study (Weeks 2–16; vehicle dosing during the Rolipram trial (OR trial # 5–8, IM), D159687 (OR trial # 9–12; PO) and D159797 (OR trial # 13–17; PO), also showed that the animals did not reveal any significant shift in performance on either the mean percent correct first reach for easy trials (F[3.73, 26.09] = 0.914, p = 0.47) or difficult trials (F[3.011,21.1] = 1.2, p = 0.33; see Figure 2B). In summary, our data suggest that we can accurately evaluate drug effects without confounds in the interpretation of vehicle, route of administration, study design length (repetitive trials) or individual animal performance at baseline.

Rolipram. After establishing baseline performance, we next tested the efficacy of the PDE4 inhibitor rolipram, dosed at 0.003, 0.01 and 0.03 mg/kg intramuscularly (IM). This compound was chosen as a reference compound, as it was previously reported to show efficacy in this task at 0.01 and 0.03 mg/kg tested via IM administration [41]. Higher doses of rolipram inevitably induce emesis: in a separate study, a dose of 0.05 mg/kg IM resulted in all animals retching (Maccine, personal communication); emesis at 0.06 mg/kg was noted in Burgin *et al* [36], and in Rutten *et al*, at 0.1 mg/kg, emesis was noted in 12 of 14 monkeys.[41] For these reasons, and with the TI of rolipram already firmly established by these studies, we limited our maximum dose of rolipram in the cognitive paradigm.

No significant improvement in the mean percent correct first reach for easy level trials was observed following rolipram administration (F [3,21] = 1.641; p = 0.21), (Figure 3A and B). A significant improved OR performance was observed on rolipram dosing as determined by the mean percent correct first reach on the difficult trials (F [3,21] = 3.789; p = 0.026); (Figure 3A and D).

Post-hoc Dunnett's comparison revealed a significant increase (p< 0.05) in the mean percent correct first reaches during difficult trials at the highest dose level of rolipram (0.03 mg/Kg; 42±8%) when compared to vehicle treatment (22±8%). Figure 3D shows the individual animal performance in the difficult trials. Note that the previously identified 'high performing' animal, animal 3939, and one additional animal, 7A5D, who performed better than during the training period, showed no obvious improvement on rolipram dosing. Removal of these animals from the group mean (Figure 3C) offered some improved significance on dose effect with difficult trial performance (F [3, 15 = 6.745] p = 0.004), with a significant effect in the mean percent correct first reaches during difficult trials at the highest dose level of rolipram (0.03 mg/Kg; p<0.01). No significant change in the number of barrier reaches or total reaches were observed for either easy or difficult level trials following rolipram administration (data not shown).

Animal 5B09 was the only animal that showed adverse reactions, in response to the highest dose (0.03 mg/kg) of rolipram tested. Retching and severe salivation was seen 20 minutes post dose. Salivation became moderate 30 minutes post dose and further decreased to mild salivation by 40 minutes post dose. This is in line with previous observations underscoring the narrow therapeutic index of rolipram.

D159687. Following a 1 week wash out and oral gavage dosing habituation, we subsequently tested OR performance of the same animals following D159687 administration (0.05, 0.5 and 5.0 mg/Kg by PO gavage). All animals completed the dosing as designed. However, animal 7A5D showed some 'potential' adverse effect to dosing at the highest dose level of 5 mg/kg. While no signs of retching or emesis were observed, at 100 to 120 minutes post-dose, 7A5D was observed to be hunched up in the corner of her cage with her head down and her hands interlocked behind her head. She was responsive to interaction and would eat 'free' raisins, but was not interested in doing the OR task and did not complete the task at this dose level. However, since this observation and in subsequent unrelated studies, this animal has been frequently observed to display such behaviour, and thus these effects cannot be clearly attributed to compound effects (Maccine, personal communication).

Administration of D159687 demonstrated a significant, dose-dependent increase in the mean percent correct first reach for difficult trials when dose group was considered a factor (F[3,18] = 19.25; p<0.0001; as well as a lesser but significant increase in the mean percent correct first reach for easy level trials (F[3,18] = 4.667; p = 0.014), when including all animals in the analysis that completed the task in full (n = 7; Figure 4A). Post-hoc Dunnett's comparisons revealed a significant increase in the mean percent correct first reaches during the easy trial at 5 mg/kg (p< 0.05), and in difficult trials at both the 0.5 mg/Kg (p<0.01) and 5.0 mg/Kg (p<0.0001) dose level of D159687 (39±6% and 68±7% respectively) when compared to vehicle treatment (11±9%). Figure 4D and 4E show the individual animal performance (n = 8). Note that in the difficult trials, all animals with the exception of the 'high performer' 3939 appeared responsive to drug and improved their performance on D159687 administration. Administration of D159687 also demonstrated a significant, dose dependent decrease in the observed total number of reaches during difficult trials (F[3,18] = 16.62; p = <0.0001), but not easy trials (F[3,18] = 1.04; p = 0.40; Figure 4B). The number of barrier reaches were also significantly reduced during only the difficult trials (F[3,18] = 17.11; p = <0.0001) when dose group was considered a factor (Figure 4C). Post-hoc Dunnett's comparisons revealed a significant decrease in both the total number and barrier reaches during difficult trials at each dose

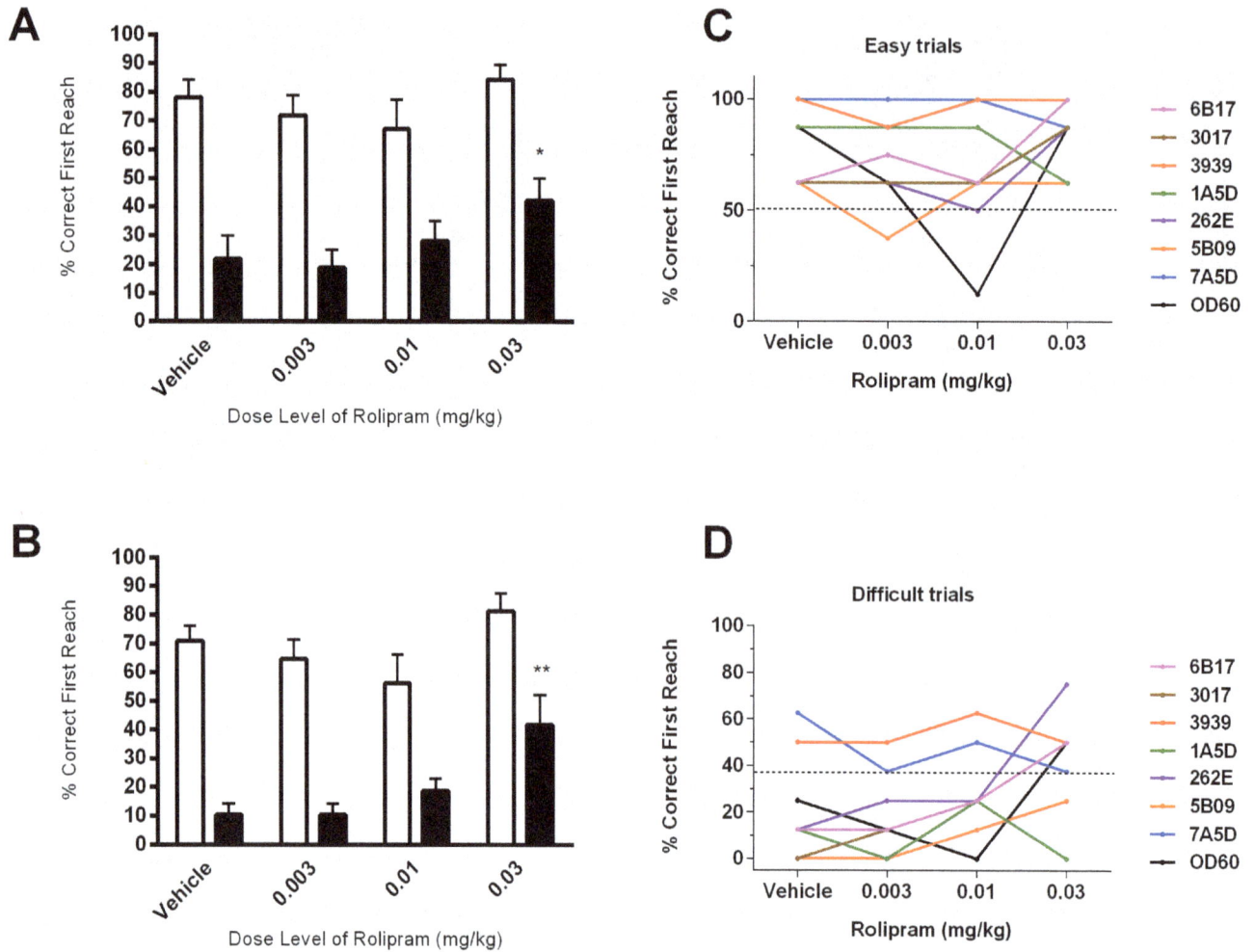

Figure 3. Influence of the PDE4 inhibitor Rolipram on the percent correct first reaches for both 'easy' and 'difficult' level OR performance. (A–B) Effects of rolipram on easy (open bars) versus difficult tasks (black bars) (A), and after exclusion of 'high baseline performing animals' 3939 and 7A5D (B). Values are shown as mean ± SEM. Asterisks denote significant differences from vehicle treatment (*p<0.05, **p<0.01) following repeat measures one-way ANOVA and Dunnett's post-hoc analysis. Individual animal performance plot in the easy trials is shown in (C) and in the difficult trials is shown in (D).

level of D159687 when compared to vehicle treatment (see Figure 4D and E for significance). The results were quantitatively much clearer than those observed with rolipram.

D159797. Following a further 1 week wash out and maintained oral gavage dosing habituation, we tested OR performance of the same animals following D159797 oral administration. The experimental dosing paradigm had been set up to originally test D159797 at equivalent doses to D159687 (0.05, 0.5 and 5.0 mg/Kg by PO gavage) using a randomized Latin-square design. We did not anticipate problems with these doses following the findings that no adverse events were seen at the highest dose during the PK evaluation, where (different) animals were dosed for seven consecutive days without any adverse events. However, on the first week of dosing (Week 12), emesis was observed in the two subjects randomised to receive the top 5 mg/Kg dose (262E and 3017). Animal 262E did not attempt the OR task, and at 2 hours post-dose was retching and salivating severely, which persisted in a milder form to 5 hours post-dose, followed by a full recovery. Animal 3017 did complete the OR task, but was observed to retch, vomit and hyper-salivate on immediate completion of the task, but then behaved normally for the rest of the observation session (5 hr.

post-dose). As a result, the top dose level was subsequently lowered to 1.5 mg/Kg on Week 13. One animal received this dose (6B17), however following the successful completion of the OR task, mild to moderate retching was also observed in this subject, which persisted intermittently for the 5 hr. post-dose observation period. Due to these clinical observations the dose levels were adjusted to a maximum dose level of 1.0 mg/Kg for D159797 for subsequent weeks. No adverse clinical observations were noted throughout the rest of the treatment. In order to make sure that all animals received the readjusted top dose of 1 mg/kg, an additional week was added to the protocol design. The dosing protocol is depicted in Table S3. However, one animal (7A5D) failed to complete the OR task at 0.5 mg/kg. In this instance, no hyper-salivation, retching or emesis was observed and the animal would take 'free' food rewards. Notably, this was the same animal that had failed to perform the task at 5 mg/kg in the previous D159687 testing period, and had, in subsequent unrelated studies, shown to exhibit the same disinterested behaviour in task performance (Maccine, personal communication). This animal was excluded from the 1 mg/kg evaluation, but we cannot ascribe the lack of performance when dosed at 0.5 mg/kg with confidence to any adverse

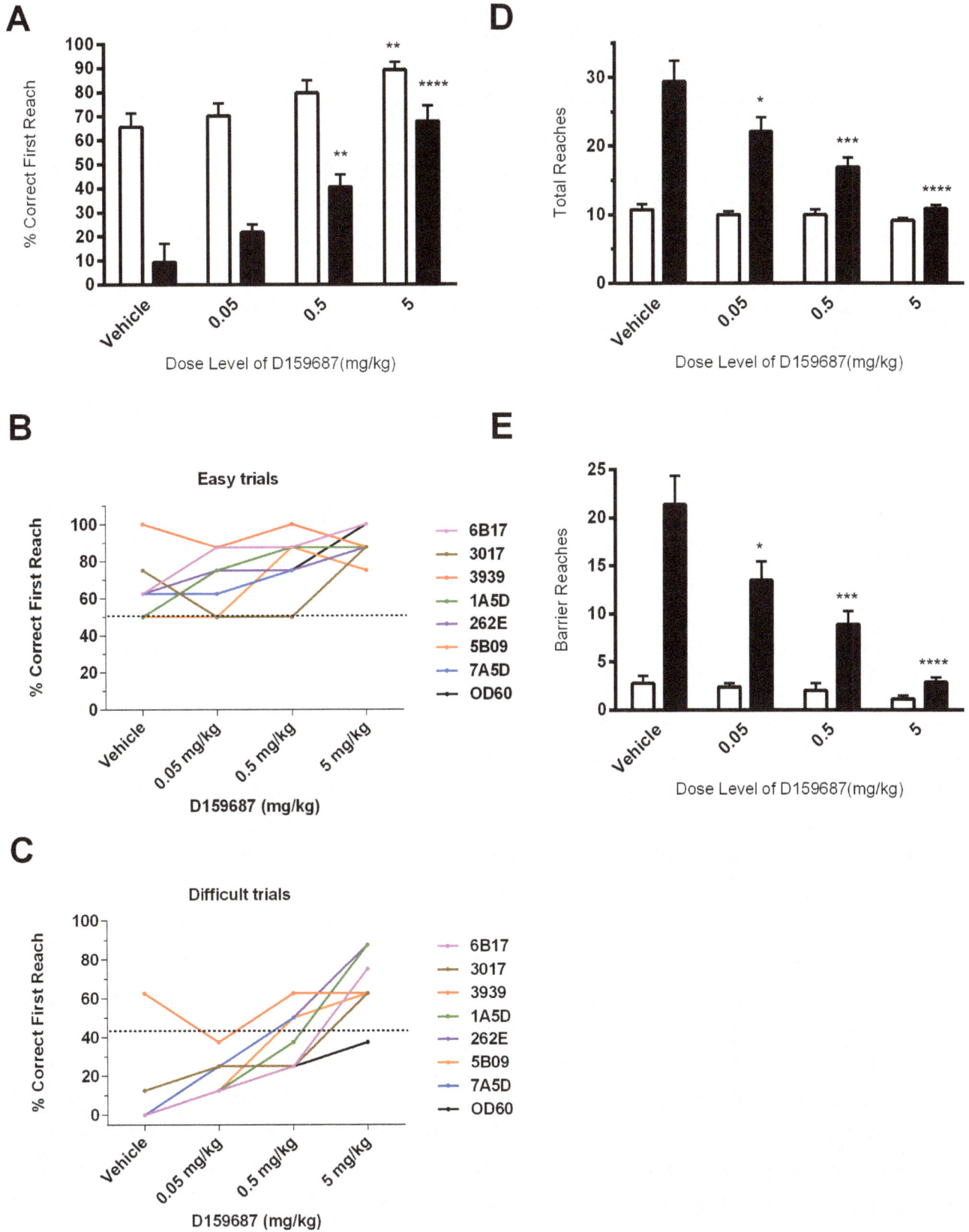

Figure 4. Influence of D159687 on OR trial performance. Effects of D159687 on easy (open bars) versus difficult task (black bars). Dose-dependent improvement in (A) mean percent correct first reach on difficult task performance, with modest improvement on easy trial performance. Individual animal performance plot in easy trials (B) and in difficult trials (C). (D–E) Dose-dependent reduction in the total number of reaches (D) and barrier reaches (E) on difficult taks. (A, D, E) Values are listed as mean ± SEM (n = 8 for vehicle, low and mid-dose groups, n = 7 for high dose group).

Asterisks denote significant differences from vehicle treatment (* p<0.05, **p<0.01 and ***p<0.001) following repeat measures one-way ANOVA and Dunnett's post-hoc analysis (n = 7, due to non-completer 7A5D).

effect of the drug at this dose level. As a result, all data presented in Figure 5 graph all data (n = 8 for vehicle, low and mid dose groups, with n = 7 for the 1 mg/kg group), but repeat measures ANOVA statistics described exclude subject 7A5D (n = 7 throughout study for all completers).

There was no significant increase in the mean percent correct first reach for easy level trials following D159797 administration (F[3,18] = 2.11; p = 0.13), but a significant increase in mean percent correct first reach for difficult level trials was observed (F[3,18] = 28.21 p<0.0001). Post-hoc Dunnett's comparisons revealed a significant increase in the mean percent correct first reaches during difficult trials at the 0.5 mg/kg (29±8%, p<0.05) and 1.0 mg/Kg (63±6%, p<0.0001) dose level of D159797 when compared to vehicle treatment (11±5%; Figure 5A). Notably and similarly to D159687 observations, in the difficult trials, all animals that completed the task showed an enhanced performance in a dose-dependent manner, and at the highest dose, every animal performed better than under vehicle conditions. Administration of D159797 also demonstrated a significant, dose dependent decrease in the observed total number of reaches during difficult trials (F[3,18] = 14.29; p = <0.0001), and in easy trials (F[3,18] = 4.543; p = 0.015; Figure 5D). The number of barrier reaches were also significantly reduced during in both easy (F[3,18] 5.04, p = 0.01) and in the difficult trials (F[3,18] = 10.62; p = 0.0003) when dose group was considered a factor (Figure 5E). Post-hoc Dunnett's comparisons revealed a significant decrease in the total number of reaches at each dose level of D159797, and a significant decrease in the number of barrier reaches at 0.5 and 1 mg/kg during difficult trials when compared to vehicle treatment (see Figure 5D and E for significance).

Discussion

We demonstrate here a robust pro-cognitive effect of two selective PDE4D NAMs in young, sexually mature female NHPs in a task that is sensitive to frontal corticostriatal function. In addition, we replicate previous findings that rolipram also exerts such pro-cognitive effects in this task; although with reduced efficacy compared to the selective PDE4D NAMs. This could, as previously suggested, be a consequence of the different binding mode for the allosteric versus orthosteric ligands [36], or possibly to the potential contribution of PDE4B to the adverse side-effect profile of rolipram [36,52–54,72], which resulted in us capping the maximum dose we used in this study, based on the well-established emetic liability noted in several studies at doses greater than 0.05 mg/kg. [36,41] It is important to note, that in our study, versus the study conducted by Rutten et al. [41], we only used female monkeys 4–6 years of age. Differences in the magnitude of the pro-cognitive effects of rolipram (our positive control) seen in the previous study, and our study, must be interpreted with this in mind. The current data obtained in female animals illustrates the same effect size at the 0.03 mg/kg dose of rolipram as that observed by Rutten et al., although significance was not observed at 0.01 mg/kg. Indeed, gender differences may be a contributing factor to the dose response profile differences between the 2 studies. Alternatively, this difference may simply reflect different group sizes (n = 12 males in the Rutten publication [41] and n = 6 in the current manuscript) or age ranges (Rutten et al studied males aged 5–12 years whilst we studied a tighter age range in females of 4–6 years of age). A direct and suitably controlled

gender/age study would be required to investigate these differences and their effect on the efficacy of these molecules.

The maximal effects of both D159687 and D159797 in the OR task were most pronounced in the difficult trials, where a potential recruitment or enhancement of synaptic function can be observed with increased task difficulty. Given that there is currently no primate genetic model of HD, task complexity in striatal-dependent behavioural tasks might serve as an alternative way to identify therapeutic compounds with cognitive-enhancing effects in disorders of the basal ganglia, such as HD, attention-deficit hyperactivity disorder (ADHD), autism or schizophrenia. Our data, in addition to the well documented pro-cognitive effects of PDE4 inhibitors in hippocampal-dependent tasks, argues for the development of PDE4 modulators with improved safety margins for a wide range of mental disorders.

For D159687, the minimum effective dose (MED) in the OR trial was 0.5 mg/kg against the primary endpoint measure of improvement in mean correct percent first reaches in difficult trials, and in which we also saw highly significant and effective reduction in total and barrier reaches during difficult trial performance. However, it should be noted that at 0.05 mg/kg PO there was a significant and effective reduction in both total reaches and barrier reaches during difficult task performance, but there was no significant improvement in mean percent correct first reaches (p = 0.14). Furthermore, we observed no evidence of adverse effects in female NHPs at doses up to 5 mg/kg in either the OR trial, where best dose effect was observed, or in the PK trial with seven day consecutive dosing, where AUC$_{(0\text{-last})}$ and C$_{max}$ were 869±198 nM.h and 121±73 nM, respectively, giving an estimated AUC$_{(0\text{-last})uu}$ and C$_{max\ uu}$ of ~61 nM.h and 8.5 nM respectively (assuming plasma F$_u$ = 0.07).

From published data [36] we know that D159687 elicits emesis at 30 mg/kg but not 10 mg/kg in NHPs, suggesting the "no adverse event limit" (NoAEL) may lie somewhere between these two doses. Taking the maximum NoAEL observed as 10 mg/kg, the therapeutic index over MED can conservatively be *estimated* as likely in excess of 20-fold (10 mg/kg/0.5 mg/kg), with the therapeutic index above best dose ~2 fold. Although we make this estimate on a dose per dose basis between our study and that of the reports of NoAEL in NHP,[36] importantly both studies use exactly the same method of administration (oral gavage), in the same formulation, suggesting that exposure would not have greatly differed between the two studies. While we believe this is a valid estimate, a dedicated within subject design to assess MED/best dose for cognitive effects versus emetic threshold dose would be needed to provide a precise TI.

For D159797, the minimum effective dose in the OR trial was also 0.5 mg/kg against all measures evaluated during difficult trial performance. Similar to D159687, beneficial activity at 0.05 mg/kg PO was apparent. There was a significant reduction in total reaches with a trend to reduction in barrier reaches during difficult task performance, but there was no significant improvement in mean percent correct first reaches (p = 0.17). At the highest dose of 1 mg/kg, the drug response was highly significant and effective in all the parameters evaluated in our hands, representing the 'best dose' level. However, conversely to D159687, emesis/retching was observed with D159797 at 1.5 mg/kg (n = 1 of 1) and 5 mg/Kg po (n = 2 of 2) during the OR trials. This was somewhat surprising to us as no signs of emesis were observed in animals tested for 7 consecutive days at 5 mg/kg during the PK evaluation for this

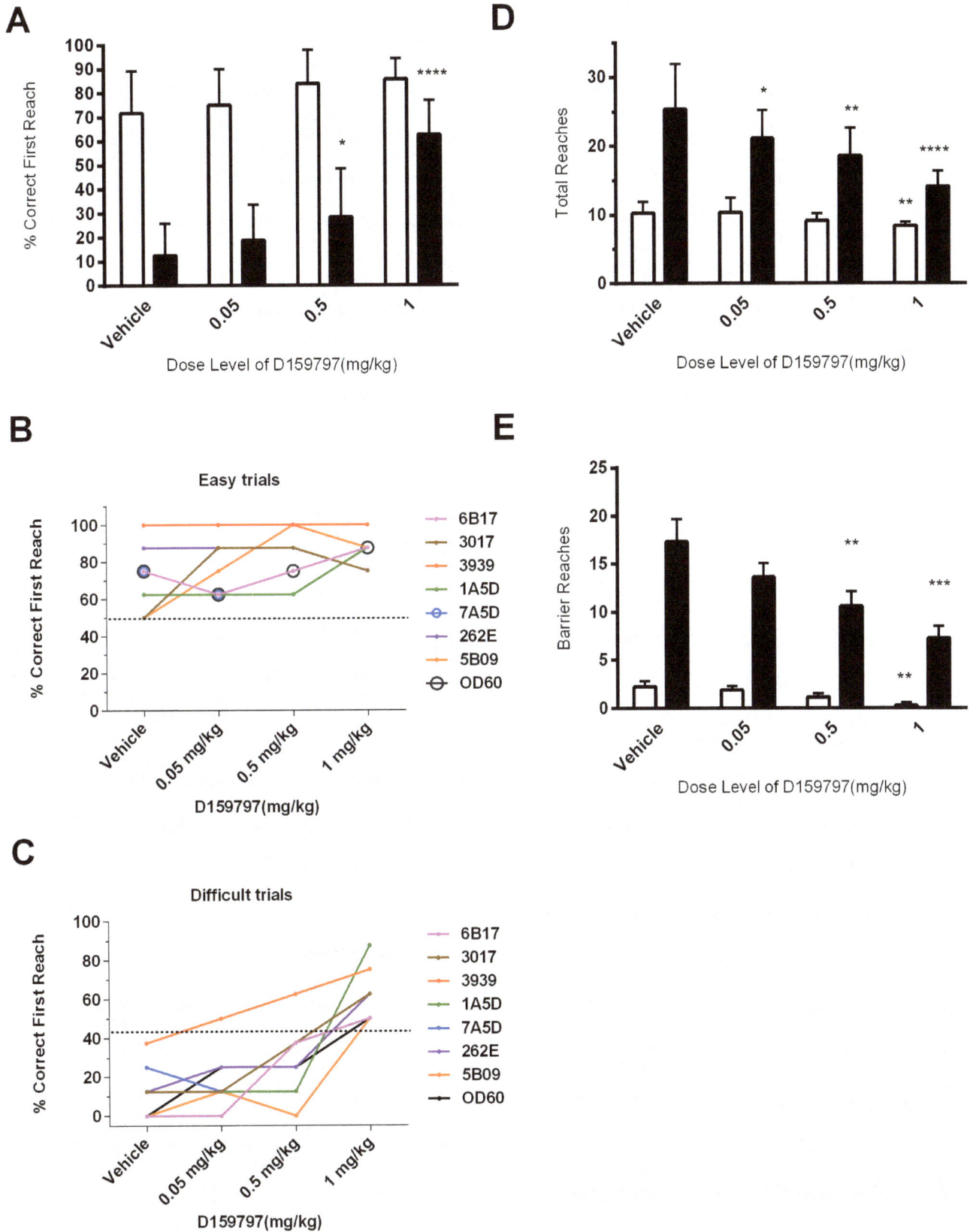

Figure 5. Influence of D159797 on OR trial performance. Effects of D159797 on easy (open bars) versus difficult tasks (black bars). Dose-dependent improvement in (A) mean percent correct first reach on difficult task performance. Individual animal performance plot in easy trials (B) and in difficult trials (C). (D–E) Dose-dependent reduction in the total number of reaches (D) and barrier reaches (E) on difficult tasks. (A, D, E) Values are listed as mean ± SEM (n = 8 for vehicle and low dose, and n = 7 for mid and high dose group). Asterisks denote significant differences from vehicle

treatment (* p<0.05, **p<0.01 and ***p<0.001) following repeat measures one-way ANOVA and Dunnett's post-hoc analysis (n = 7, due to non-completer 7A5D).

compound (n = 0 of 3). For D159797, a dose of 5 mg/kg corresponded to a plasma exposure $AUC_{(0-last)}$ and C_{max} of 39720±7924 nM.hr and 518±131.2 nM, respectively. However, the emergence of clear adverse events with D159797 at doses > 1.5 mg/kg), but not with D159687 at 5 mg/kg, suggests that there was no obvious tolerance to the effect of the PDE4D NAMs due to repeated drug administration, as D159797 was tested last in sequence. While this could have confounded the interpretation of our study if the results had been different, the choice to test D159797 last in the OR trial was deliberately chosen, based on the longer half-life of this compound, and with no *a priori* knowledge of whether long term effects would be anticipated. The extremely clear dose-dependent effects observed with the PDE4D NAMs when the dosing level was randomized in the within-subject design for each of the PDE4D NAMs tested also underscores that neither tolerance, or conversely, long-lasting effects of the compounds outliving the designated 1 week washout period, was a factor.

What pharmacokinetic parameter drives efficacy versus emesis in the PDE4 NAMs? A comparison of exposures at the reported adverse effect limit (AEL) using estimated AUCs (assuming scaling linearity) between D159687 (30 mg/kg; [36]; $AUC_{(0-last)}$ and C_{max} estimated to be ~5215 nM×hr and 726 nM) and D159797 (1.5 mg/kg; estimated $AUC_{(0-last)}$ of ~11,916 nM*h and C_{max} of 155 nM) would estimate that the AUC for D159797 is approximately 2.3-fold higher when compared to D159687. However, the C_{max} was estimated to be lower for D159797 at the AEL (726 nM for D159687 vs 155 nM) suggesting that emetic effects could be driven primarily by AUC. Additional evaluation of this class of compounds with differing exposures and clearance rates will be needed to clarify this, along with a more formal tolerability trial at higher doses to obtain a precise AEL for each compound.

In summary, our data and that obtained in rodent cognitive testing [36] suggests that this class of molecules exhibits robust cognitive effects at seemingly very low exposures. We attempted to estimate brain exposure by measuring amounts of the two compounds in primate CSF. Unfortunately, their levels were either undetectable or below the detection sensitivity using our bioanalytical methods (approximately 15 nM for each compound). Therefore, in order to further develop these molecules for clinical testing, additional measurements are required to understand target occupancy, or brain exposures needed for the beneficial (pro-cognitive) effects of these molecules versus their potential for emetic liabilities. Given both the difficulty in estimating the therapeutic index for drugs targeting this mechanism and the potential variability in responsiveness to this class of drugs, a translational non-invasive endpoint to evaluate optimal dosing and obtain evidence of a central effect is desirable. The utilization of PET imaging as a non-invasive approach to estimate occupancy at the target with existing PDE4 non-selective orthosteric ligands would be a challenging task, and currently no PDE4D selective imaging tools exist. Also, given the expected low occupancy required to elicit cognitive effects for this class of compounds in

rodents and primates, a PET imaging approach might not be feasible. Other strategies might include the use of pharmaco (ph)-MRI or quantitative (q) EEG techniques, where a relationship between dose and circuitry engagement can be garnered. Overall, based on our results and those of Burgin et al [36], we consider D159687 to be an excellent candidate molecule to conduct this additional work in to assess the potential pro-cognitive effects of PDE4D modulation in neurodegenerative and psychiatric indications.

Supporting Information

Checklist S1 ARRIVE Checklist.

Table S1 CSF concentration of D159687 following single intravenous administration at 1.0 mg/kg, and on day 1 and day 7 after repeated daily oral administration at 5.0 mg/kg.

Table S2 CSF concentration of D159797 following single intravenous administration at 1.0 mg/kg, and on day 1 and day 7 after repeated daily oral administration at 5.0 mg/kg.

Table S3 Amended dosing schedule (all doses are mg/kg) for evaluation of D159797 after retching and hypersalivation was noted in animals receiving the highest dose of 5 mg/kg during week 12 (Animals 3017 and 262E) and following 1.5 mg/kg D159797 (animal 6B17) during Week 13. Additionally, animal 7A5D was excluded from the 1 mg/kg evaluation after observations that the animal did not perform the OR task when dosed at 0.5 mg/kg D159797 (Week 12). However, subsequent evaluations with this animal (unrelated studies; Maccine communication) suggested this was a common occurrence in this animal (occasional disinterest in completing task regardless of treatment) and was deemed to be unlikely related to an adverse event caused by D159797 dosing.

Acknowledgments

DeCode graciously supplied D159687 and D159797, along with associated information on the compounds, to enable the study. The authors thank Drs Mark Gurney, Alex Kiselyov and Jakob Sigurdsson of Decode for their input and contributions to the study.

Author Contributions

Conceived and designed the experiments: JS DMH VB IMS. Performed the experiments: JS JMW CSC. Analyzed the data: JS DMH VB MB CD IMS. Wrote the paper: VB JS IMS.

References

1. Richter W, Menniti FS, Zhang HT, Conti M (2013) PDE4 as a target for cognition enhancement. Expert Opin Ther Targets 17: 1011–1027.
2. Navakkode S, Sajikumar S, Frey JU (2004) The type IV-specific phosphodiesterase inhibitor rolipram and its effect on hippocampal long-term potentiation and synaptic tagging. J Neurosci 24: 7740–7744.
3. Nishi A, Kuroiwa M, Miller DB, O'Callaghan JP, Bateup HS, et al. (2008) Distinct roles of PDE4 and PDE10A in the regulation of cAMP/PKA signaling in the striatum. J Neurosci 28: 10460–10471.
4. Nishi A, Watanabe Y, Higashi H, Tanaka M, Nairn AC, et al. (2005) Glutamate regulation of DARPP-32 phosphorylation in neostriatal neurons involves activation of multiple signaling cascades. Proc Natl Acad Sci U S A 102: 1199–1204.

5. Sanderson TM, Sher E (2013) The role of phosphodiesterases in hippocampal synaptic plasticity. Neuropharmacology 74: 86–95.
6. Oliveira RF, Terrin A, Di Benedetto G, Cannon RC, Koh W, et al. (2010) The role of type 4 phosphodiesterases in generating microdomains of cAMP: large scale stochastic simulations. PLoS One 5: e11725.
7. Frey U, Huang YY, Kandel ER (1993) Effects of cAMP simulate a late stage of LTP in hippocampal CA1 neurons. Science 260: 1661–1664.
8. Hebb AL, Robertson HA (2007) Role of phosphodiesterases in neurological and psychiatric disease. Curr Opin Pharmacol 7: 86–92.
9. Rose GM, Hopper A, De Vivo M, Tehim A (2005) Phosphodiesterase inhibitors for cognitive enhancement. Curr Pharm Des 11: 3329–3334.
10. Sharma S, Kumar K, Deshmukh R, Sharma PL (2013) Phosphodiesterases: Regulators of cyclic nucleotide signals and novel molecular target for movement disorders. Eur J Pharmacol 714: 486–497.
11. Zhang KY, Card GL, Suzuki Y, Artis DR, Fong D, et al. (2004) A glutamine switch mechanism for nucleotide selectivity by phosphodiesterases. Mol Cell 15: 279–286.
12. Li YF, Cheng YF, Huang Y, Conti M, Wilson SP, et al. (2011) Phosphodiesterase-4D knock-out and RNA interference-mediated knock-down enhance memory and increase hippocampal neurogenesis via increased cAMP signaling. J Neurosci 31: 172–183.
13. Li YF, Huang Y, Amsdell SL, Xiao L, O'Donnell JM, et al. (2009) Antidepressant- and anxiolytic-like effects of the phosphodiesterase-4 inhibitor rolipram on behavior depend on cyclic AMP response element binding protein-mediated neurogenesis in the hippocampus. Neuropsychopharmacology 34: 2404–2419.
14. Gong B, Vitolo OV, Trinchese F, Liu S, Shelanski M, et al. (2004) Persistent improvement in synaptic and cognitive functions in an Alzheimer mouse model after rolipram treatment. J Clin Invest 114: 1624–1634.
15. Sierksma AS, van den Hove DL, Pfau F, Philippens M, Bruno O, et al. (2013) Improvement of spatial memory function in APPswe/PS1dE9 mice after chronic inhibition of phosphodiesterase type 4D. Neuropharmacology.
16. Munoz-Sanjuan I, Bates GP (2011) The importance of integrating basic and clinical research toward the development of new therapies for Huntington disease. J Clin Invest 121: 476–483.
17. Rosas HD, Lee SY, Bender AC, Zaleta AK, Vangel M, et al. (2010) Altered white matter microstructure in the corpus callosum in Huntington's disease: implications for cortical "disconnection". Neuroimage 49: 2995–3004.
18. Rosas HD, Reuter M, Doros G, Lee SY, Triggs T, et al. (2011) A tale of two factors: what determines the rate of progression in Huntington's disease? A longitudinal MRI study. Mov Disord 26: 1691–1697.
19. Tabrizi SJ, Reilmann R, Roos RA, Durr A, Leavitt B, et al. (2012) Potential endpoints for clinical trials in premanifest and early Huntington's disease in the TRACK-HD study: analysis of 24 month observational data. Lancet Neurol 11: 42–53.
20. Scahill RI, Hobbs NZ, Say MJ, Bechtel N, Henley SM, et al. (2011) Clinical impairment in premanifest and early Huntington's disease is associated with regionally specific atrophy. Hum Brain Mapp.
21. Chiang MC, Lee YC, Huang CL, Chern Y (2005) cAMP-response element-binding protein contributes to suppression of the A2A adenosine receptor promoter by mutant Huntingtin with expanded polyglutamine residues. J Biol Chem 280: 14331–14340.
22. DeMarch Z, Giampa C, Patassini S, Bernardi G, Fusco FR (2008) Beneficial effects of rolipram in the R6/2 mouse model of Huntington's disease. Neurobiol Dis 30: 375–387.
23. DeMarch Z, Giampa C, Patassini S, Martorana A, Bernardi G, et al. (2007) Beneficial effects of rolipram in a quinolinic acid model of striatal excitotoxicity. Neurobiol Dis 25: 266–273.
24. Giampa C, Middei S, Patassini S, Borreca A, Marullo F, et al. (2009) Phosphodiesterase type IV inhibition prevents sequestration of CREB binding protein, protects striatal parvalbumin interneurons and rescues motor deficits in the R6/2 mouse model of Huntington's disease. Eur J Neurosci 29: 902–910.
25. Giampa C, Patassini S, Borreca A, Laurenti D, Marullo F, et al. (2009) Phosphodiesterase 10 inhibition reduces striatal excitotoxicity in the quinolinic acid model of Huntington's disease. Neurobiol Dis 34: 450–456.
26. Gines S (2003) Specific progressive cAMP reduction implicates energy deficit in presymptomatic Huntington's disease knock-in mice. Human Molecular Genetics 12: 497–508.
27. Kleiman RJ, Kimmel LH, Bove SE, Lanz TA, Harms JF, et al. (2011) Chronic suppression of phosphodiesterase 10A alters striatal expression of genes responsible for neurotransmitter synthesis, neurotransmission, and signaling pathways implicated in Huntington's disease. J Pharmacol Exp Ther 336: 64–76.
28. Obrietan K, Hoyt KR (2004) CRE-mediated transcription is increased in Huntington's disease transgenic mice. J Neurosci 24: 791–796.
29. Puerta E, Hervias I, Barros-Minones L, Jordan J, Ricobaraza A, et al. (2010) Sildenafil protects against 3-nitropropionic acid neurotoxicity through the modulation of calpain, CREB, and BDNF. Neurobiol Dis 38: 237–245.
30. Sugars KL, Brown R, Cook LJ, Swartz J, Rubinsztein DC (2004) Decreased cAMP response element-mediated transcription: an early event in exon 1 and full-length cell models of Huntington's disease that contributes to polyglutamine pathogenesis. J Biol Chem 279: 4988–4999.
31. Jung J, Bonini N (2007) CREB-binding protein modulates repeat instability in a Drosophila model for polyQ disease. Science 315: 1857–1859.
32. Mantamadiotis T, Lemberger T, Bleckmann SC, Kern H, Kretz O, et al. (2002) Disruption of CREB function in brain leads to neurodegeneration. Nat Genet 31: 47–54.
33. Reneerkens O, Rutten K, Steinbusch H, Blokland A, Prickaerts J (2009) Selective phosphodiesterase inhibitors: a promising target for cognition enhancement. Psychopharmacology 202: 419–443.
34. Asanuma M, Ogawa N, Kondo Y, Hirata H, Mori A (1993) Effects of repeated administration of rolipram, a cAMP-specific phosphodiesterase inhibitor, on acetylcholinergic indices in the aged rat brain. Arch Gerontol Geriatr 16: 191–198.
35. Bateup HS, Svenningsson P, Kuroiwa M, Gong S, Nishi A, et al. (2008) Cell type-specific regulation of DARPP-32 phosphorylation by psychostimulant and antipsychotic drugs. Nat Neurosci 11: 932–939.
36. Burgin AB, Magnusson OT, Singh J, Witte P, Staker BL, et al. (2010) Design of phosphodiesterase 4D (PDE4D) allosteric modulators for enhancing cognition with improved safety. Nat Biotechnol 28: 63–70.
37. Houslay MD, Schafer P, Zhang KYJ (2005) Keynote review: Phosphodiesterase-4 as a therapeutic target. Drug Discovery Today 10: 1503–1519.
38. Huang Z, Dias R, Jones T, Liu S, Styhler A, et al. (2007) L-454,560, a potent and selective PDE4 inhibitor with in vivo efficacy in animal models of asthma and cognition. Biochem Pharmacol 73: 1971–1981.
39. Kuroiwa M, Snyder GL, Shuto T, Fukuda A, Yanagawa Y, et al. (2011) Phosphodiesterase 4 inhibition enhances the dopamine D1 receptor/PKA/DARPP-32 signaling cascade in frontal cortex. Psychopharmacology (Berl).
40. Rodefer JS, Saland SK, Eckrich SJ (2011) Selective phosphodiesterase inhibitors improve performance on the ED/ID cognitive task in rats. Neuropharmacology.
41. Rutten K, Basile JL, Prickaerts J, Blokland A, Vivian JA (2008) Selective PDE inhibitors rolipram and sildenafil improve object retrieval performance in adult cynomolgus macaques. Psychopharmacology (Berl) 196: 643–648.
42. Marte A, Pepicelli O, Cavallero A, Raiteri M, Fedele E (2008) In vivo effects of phosphodiesterase inhibition on basal cyclic guanosine monophosphate levels in the prefrontal cortex, hippocampus and cerebellum of freely moving rats. J Neurosci Res 86: 3338–3347.
43. Kuhn A, Goldstein DR, Hodges A, Strand AD, Sengstag T, et al. (2007) Mutant huntingtin's effects on striatal gene expression in mice recapitulate changes observed in human Huntington's disease brain and do not differ with mutant huntingtin length or wild-type huntingtin dosage. Hum Mol Genet 16: 1845–1861.
44. Threlfell S, Sammut S, Menniti FS, Schmidt CJ, West AR (2009) Inhibition of Phosphodiesterase 10A Increases the Responsiveness of Striatal Projection Neurons to Cortical Stimulation. J Pharmacol Exp Ther 328: 785–795.
45. Rutten K, Lieben C, Smits L, Blokland A (2007) The PDE4 inhibitor rolipram reverses object memory impairment induced by acute tryptophan depletion in the rat. Psychopharmacology (Berl) 192: 275–282.
46. Rutten K, Prickaerts J, Blokland A (2006) Rolipram reverses scopolamine-induced and time-dependent memory deficits in object recognition by different mechanisms of action. Neurobiol Learn Mem 85: 132–138.
47. Imanishi T, Sawa A, Ichimaru Y, Miyashiro M, Kato S, et al. (1997) Ameliorating effects of rolipram on experimentally induced impairments of learning and memory in rodents. Eur J Pharmacol 321: 273–278.
48. Bertolino A, Crippa D, di Dio S, Fichte K, Musmeci G, et al. (1988) Rolipram versus imipramine in inpatients with major, "minor" or atypical depressive disorder: a double-blind double-dummy study aimed at testing a novel therapeutic approach. Int Clin Psychopharmacol 3: 245–253.
49. Hebenstreit GF, Fellerer K, Fichte K, Fischer G, Geyer N, et al. (1989) Rolipram in major depressive disorder: results of a double-blind comparative study with imipramine. Pharmacopsychiatry 22: 156–160.
50. Wang H, Peng MS, Chen Y, Geng J, Robinson H, et al. (2007) Structures of the four subfamilies of phosphodiesterase-4 provide insight into the selectivity of their inhibitors. Biochem J 408: 193–201.
51. Bruno O, Fedele E, Prickaerts J, Parker LA, Canepa E, et al. (2011) GEBR-7b, a novel PDE4D selective inhibitor that improves memory in rodents at non-emetic doses. Br J Pharmacol 164: 2054–2063.
52. Kobayashi M, Kubo S, Iwata M, Ohtsu Y, Takahashi K, et al. (2011) ASP3258, an orally active potent phosphodiesterase 4 inhibitor with low emetic activity. Int Immunopharmacol 11: 732–739.
53. Robichaud A, Savoie C, Stamatiou PB, Lachance N, Jolicoeur P, et al. (2002) Assessing the emetic potential of PDE4 inhibitors in rats. Br J Pharmacol 135: 113–118.
54. Robichaud A, Tattersall FD, Choudhury I, Rodger IW (1999) Emesis induced by inhibitors of type IV cyclic nucleotide phosphodiesterase (PDE IV) in the ferret. Neuropharmacology 38: 289–297.
55. Diamond A, Zola-Morgan S, Squire LR (1989) Successful performance by monkeys with lesions of the hippocampal formation on AB and object retrieval, two tasks that mark developmental changes in human infants. Behav Neurosci 103: 526–537.
56. Palfi S, Ferrante RJ, Brouillet E, Beal MF, Dolan R, et al. (1996) Chronic 3-nitropropionic acid treatment in baboons replicates the cognitive and motor deficits of Huntington's disease. J Neurosci 16: 3019–3025.
57. Dias R, Robbins TW, Roberts AC (1996) Primate analogue of the Wisconsin Card Sorting Test: effects of excitotoxic lesions of the prefrontal cortex in the marmoset. Behav Neurosci 110: 872–886.

58. Roberts AC, Wallis JD (2000) Inhibitory Control and Affective Processing in the Prefrontal Cortex: Neuropsychological Studies in the Common Marmoset. Cerebral Cortex 10: 252–262.

59. Roitberg BZ, Emborg ME, Sramek JG, Palfi S, Kordower JH (2002) Behavioral and Morphological Comparison of Two Nonhuman Primate Models of Huntington's Disease. Neurosurgery 50: 137–146.

60. Gray RA, Wilcox KM, Zink MC, Weed MR (2006) Impaired performance on the object retrieval-detour test of executive function in the SIV/macaque model of AIDS. AIDS Res Hum Retroviruses 22: 1031–1035.

61. Taylor JR, Elsworth JD, Roth RH, Sladek JR Jr, Redmond DE Jr (1990) Cognitive and motor deficits in the acquisition of an object retrieval/detour task in MPTP-treated monkeys. Brain 113 (Pt 3): 617–637.

62. Walker SC, Mikheenko YP, Argyle LD, Robbins TW, Roberts AC (2006) Selective prefrontal serotonin depletion impairs acquisition of a detour-reaching task. Eur J Neurosci 23: 3119–3123.

63. Jentsch JD, Redmond DE, Elsworth JD, Taylor JR, Youngren KD, et al. (1997) Enduring Cognitive Deficits and Cortical Dopamine Dysfunction in Monkeys After Long-Term Administration of Phencyclidine. Science 277: 953–955.

64. Jentsch JD, Taylor JR, Redmond DE Jr, Elsworth JD, Youngren KD, et al. (1999) Dopamine D4 receptor antagonist reversal of subchronic phencyclidine-induced object retrieval/detour deficits in monkeys. Psychopharmacology (Berl) 142: 78–84.

65. Tinsley M, Basile JL, Van-Natta K, Yeo H, Lowe DA, et al. (2007) Cognition enhancing effects of nicotinic acetylcholine alpha-7 receptor agonists in prefrontal cortex mediated tasks in adult monkeys; San Diego, USA.

66. Ballard TM, Knoflach F, Prinssen E, Borroni E, Vivian JA, et al. (2009) RO4938581, a novel cognitive enhancer acting at GABAA alpha5 subunit-containing receptors. Psychopharmacology (Berl) 202: 207–223.

67. Ramos BP, Birnbaum SG, Lindenmayer I, Newton SS, Duman RS, et al. (2003) Dysregulation of protein kinase a signaling in the aged prefrontal cortex: new strategy for treating age-related cognitive decline. Neuron 40: 835–845.

68. Diehl KH, Hull R, Morton D, Pfister R, Rabemampianina Y, et al. (2001) A good practice guide to the administration of substances and removal of blood, including routes and volumes. J Appl Toxicol 21: 15–23.

69. Friden M, Winiwarter S, Jerndal G, Bengtsson O, Wan H, et al. (2009) Structure-brain exposure relationships in rat and human using a novel data set of unbound drug concentrations in brain interstitial and cerebrospinal fluids. J Med Chem 52: 6233–6243.

70. Smith DA, Di L, Kerns EH (2010) The effect of plasma protein binding on in vivo efficacy: misconceptions in drug discovery. Nat Rev Drug Discov 9: 929–939.

71. Di L, Rong H, Feng B (2013) Demystifying brain penetration in central nervous system drug discovery. Miniperspective. J Med Chem 56: 2–12.

72. Robichaud A (2002) Deletion of phosphodiesterase 4D in mice shortens alpha2-adrenoceptor-mediated anesthesia, a behavioral correlate of emesis. Journal of Clinical Investigation 110: 1045–1052.

16

Trehalose Reverses Cell Malfunction in Fibroblasts from Normal and Huntington's Disease Patients Caused by Proteosome Inhibition

Maria Angeles Fernandez-Estevez[1,3], **Maria Jose Casarejos**[1,3], **Jose Lopez Sendon**[2,3], **Juan Garcia Caldentey**[2], **Carolina Ruiz**[2,3], **Ana Gomez**[1,3], **Juan Perucho**[1,3], **Justo García de Yebenes**[2,3], **Maria Angeles Mena**[1,3]*

1 Department of Neurobiology, Ramón y Cajal Hospital, Madrid, Spain, 2 Department of Neurology, Ramón y Cajal Hospital, Madrid, Spain, 3 CIBERNED, Instituto de Salud Carlos III, Madrid, Spain

Abstract

Huntington's disease (HD) is a neurodegenerative disorder characterized by progressive motor, cognitive and psychiatric deficits, associated with predominant loss of striatal neurons and is caused by polyglutamine expansion in the huntingtin protein. Mutant huntingtin protein and its fragments are resistant to protein degradation and produce a blockade of the ubiquitin proteasome system (UPS). In HD models, the proteasome inhibitor epoxomicin aggravates protein accumulation and the inductor of autophagy, trehalose, diminishes it. We have investigated the effects of epoxomicin and trehalose in skin fibroblasts of control and HD patients. Untreated HD fibroblasts have increased the levels of ubiquitinized proteins and higher levels of reactive oxygen species (ROS), huntingtin and the autophagy marker LAMP2A. Baseline replication rates were higher in HD than in controls fibroblasts but that was reverted after 12 passages. Epoxomicin increases the activated caspase-3, HSP70, huntingtin, ubiquitinated proteins and ROS levels in both HD and controls. Treatment with trehalose counteracts the increase in ROS, ubiquitinated proteins, huntingtin and activated caspase-3 levels induced by epoxomicin, and also increases the LC3 levels more in HD fibroblast than controls. These results suggest that trehalose could revert protein processing abnormalities in patients with Huntington's Disease.

Editor: David R. Borchelt, University of Florida, United States of America

Funding: This study has been supported in part by grants from the Spanish Ministry of Health, FIS 2010/172, CIBER 2006/05/0059, CIBERNED PI 2010/06, CIBERNED PI 2013/05, and CAM 2011/BMD-2308. The funders had no role in study design, data collection and analysis, decision to publish, or preparation of the manuscript.

Competing Interests: The authors have declared that no competing interests exist.

* E-mail: maria.a.mena@hrc.es

Introduction

Huntington's disease is an autosomal dominant neurodegenerative disorder caused by the expansion of CAG repeats in the huntingtin gene [1]. Huntingtin protein plays an important role in synaptic function, is necessary in post-embryonary period, could have antiapoptotic effects and also a protector effect against mutant huntingtin [2]. Mutant huntingtin accumulates in cells of patients with HD, translocates to the nucleous, alters gene transcription, mitochondrial function and caspase activity and leads to cell death. Mutant huntingtin inhibits 26 S proteasoma activity [3] and modulation of autophagy counteracts it [4], The toxicity induced by mutant huntingtin, can lead to defects in RNA synthesis, cell survival, ubiquitin proteasome system (UPS) and also produces cellular inclusions, impairs mitochondrial activity and activates pro-apoptotic molecules [5–8].

Macroautophagy, chaperone-mediated autophagy and ubiquitin-proteasome system, all complementary, are the mayor systems to process abnormal proteins. It has been shown that blockade of UPS results in an increase in autophagy activity that could compensate the impaired UPS function [5]. Besides UPS, another important mechanism to degrade proteins is the autophagy-lysosomal pathway [9–12]. Both systems are implicated in degradation of abnormal proteins that accumulate in neurodegenerative diseases [10,13–17].

Epoxomicin is a cell-permeable and irreversible inhibitor of proteasome activity resulting primarily in inhibition of the chymotrypsin-like activity [6]. Trehalose is a disaccharide that protects from environmental stresses by preventing protein denaturation [7,8]. Trehalose is described as a chemical chaperone that helps in protein folding interacting directly with them [8,9]. Recently, trehalose was shown to inhibit polyglutamine-mediated aggregation in vitro and in vivo models of Huntington disease [10,11].

Recent studies have shown that trehalose increases the number of autophagosomes and markers of autophagy in Human neuroblastoma cells (NB69) and prevents injuries induced by the proteasome inhibitor, epoxomicin [12]. Other studies have shown that trehalose improves dopamine cell loss and tau pathology in parkin null mice expressing knocked-in human mutant tau [18].

The purpose of our study was to investigate the epoxomicin effects on protein accumulation and cell viability in skin fibroblasts of control and HD patients. Moreover, we have studied whether the stimulation of autophagy by trehalose, as a compensatory and

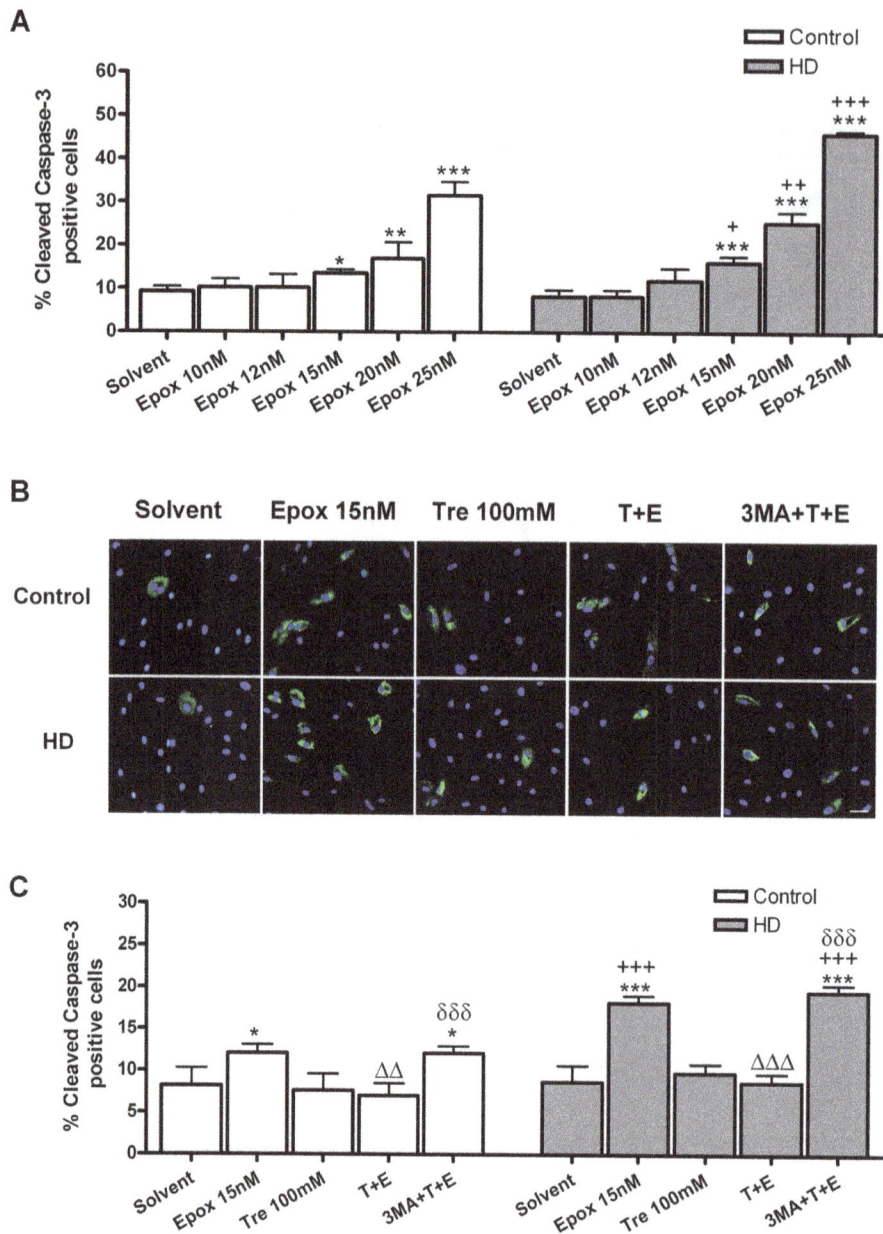

Figure 1. Epoxomicin and trehalose differential effects in cellular viability on control and HD human skin fibroblasts. (A) Dose-dependent effects of epoxomicin in caspase-3 activation, an indicator of apoptosis. (B) Photomicrographs of activated caspase-3$^+$ cells (green) and total nuclei stained with bis-benzimide (blue) after epoxomicin and trehalose treatments. (Scale bar = 20 μm). (C) Percent of activated caspase-3$^+$ cells in control and HD fibroblasts after epoxomicin and trehalose treatments. Values are expressed as the mean ± SD, $n = 4$ patients. Control cell number (mean per field) 31.87 ± 1.124, $n = 4$. HD cell number (mean per field) 44.75 ± 2.456, $n = 4$. The data of each patient was obtained using 4 replicates. Statistical analysis was performed by one-way ANOVA with repeated measures followed by Bonferroni multiple comparison test: *$p < 0.05$, **$p < 0.01$, ***$p < 0.001$ vs Solvent; +$p < 0.05$, ++$p < 0.01$, +++$p < 0.001$ HD vs controls; ΔΔ$p < 0.01$, ΔΔΔ$p < 0.001$ trehalose + epoxomicin vs epoxomicin; δδδ$p < 0.001$ 3-methyladenine + trehalose + epoxomicin vs trehalose + epoxomicin.

protective mechanism against UPS dysfunction, reverts epoxomi-cin-induced damage.

Materials and Methods

Ethics statement

This work was performed with primary human cells in culture and was approved by the Ethical Committee for the Research of the Ramón y Cajal Hospital in Madrid. Written informed consent was obtained from the subjects themselves, which

according to the Spanish Law of Biomedical Research 14/2007 and due to the nature of the study, is sufficient to perform the investigation.

Skin fibroblasts cultures

Human fibroblast were obtained from skin biopsies of healthy and Huntington's disease patients. Skin biopsies were cut up and put into a flask and grown in Amniomed medium (Genycell, EK AMG-200). After the first passage, Amniomed medium was changed to a medium containing Dulbecco's modified Eagle's

Trehalose Reverses Cell Malfunction in Fibroblasts from Normal and Huntington's Disease Patients Caused...

173

medium (DMEM) with high glucose (4.5 g/l) (Biowest, L0101–500), 4 mM L-glutamine (GIBCO, 25030–024), 1 mM sodium-pyruvate (GIBCO, 11360–039), penicillin/streptomycin/ fungizone (100 U/ml) (GIBCO, 15240–062) and 15% fetal bovine serum (USA origin) (GIBCO-Life Technologies, 16000–044). For detection of ubiquitinated proteins, the medium was replaced by a defined medium MEM/Ham's F12 1:1 (F12; PAA, E15–817, MEM; GIBCO, 041–01095), 20 nM progesterone (Sigma-Aldrich, P6149), 100 mM putrescine (Sigma-Aldrich, P5780), 30 nM sodium selenite (Sigma-Aldrich, S9133), 5 mg/ml insulin (Sigma-Aldrich, I1882) and 100 mM transferrin (Boehringuer, M1073974) supplemented with glucose 0.6% (Sigma-Aldrich G8769). Cells were maintained four days on culture before treatment with epoxomicin and trehalose.

Chemicals

Epoxomicin (Calbiochem, 324800), Trehalose (Calbiochem, 625625), Suc-Leu-Leu-Val-Tyr-AMC (Calbiochem, 539142). The BCA protein assay kit was from Pierce (Pierce, 23228, 1859078), 3-Methyladenine (Sigma-Aldrich, M9281).

Cell viability measurements and proliferation assay

Fibroblast survival was measured analysing the percentage of cells immunoreactive to cleaved caspase-3. Cultures were fixed with 4% paraformaldehyde, washed in 0.1 M phosphate-buffered saline, pH 7.4 (PBS), permeabilized with ethanol-acetic acid (19:1), and incubated at 4°C for 24 h with a rabbit polyclonal anti-cleaved caspase-3 (1/400) (Cell-Signaling, 9664P). Cells were then washed ×3 in PBS and incubated with anti-mouse Alexa

Fluor 488 (Green) (Invitrogen, A11034) for 1h at room temperature. After the final 3 washes with PBS, cover slips were mounted in anti-fading solution, 3×10^{-6} M final concentration and viewed under a fluorescent microscope. To assess antibody specificity of cleaved caspase-3, negative control was included by omission of the primary antibody.

To assay cell number and cell proliferation index, cell cultures were treated with trehalose (100 mM) for 15 min before incubating with the proteasome inhibitor epoxomicin (15 nM) for another 24 hours. Then were incubated with 50 mM BrdU (5-bromo-2'-deoxyuridine) (SIGMA-Aldrich, B-5002) for 24 h more before fixation and, for immunodetection, we used a mouse anti-BrdU antibody (1/20) (DAKO, M0744) and anti-mouse Ig-fluorescein antibody. Nuclei were stained by bis-benzimide (Hoechst33342) (SIGMA-Aldrich, B-2261) and immunostaining was visualized under fluorescent microscopy. The number of immunoreactive cells was counted in pre defined parallel strips.

Measurement of ROS production

The abundance of reactive oxygen species (ROS) was determined by using 2',7'-dichlorofluorescein diacetate (C-H2DCFH-DA; Invitrogen, C6827). Control and HD deficient fibroblasts were seeded at a density of 1×10^4 cells/cm^2 in glass cover slides pre-coated with poly-D-lysine (4.5 µg/cm^2) (SIGMA-Aldrich, P6407-5MG) at 1×10^4 cells/cm^2 three days before the experiment. After 15 min of treatment with trehalose (100 mM), the cells were incubated with the proteasome inhibitor epoxomicin (15 nM) for another 24 hours. After this time, the cells were washed twice, and incubated with 5 µM DCFH-DA in MEM free of phenol red

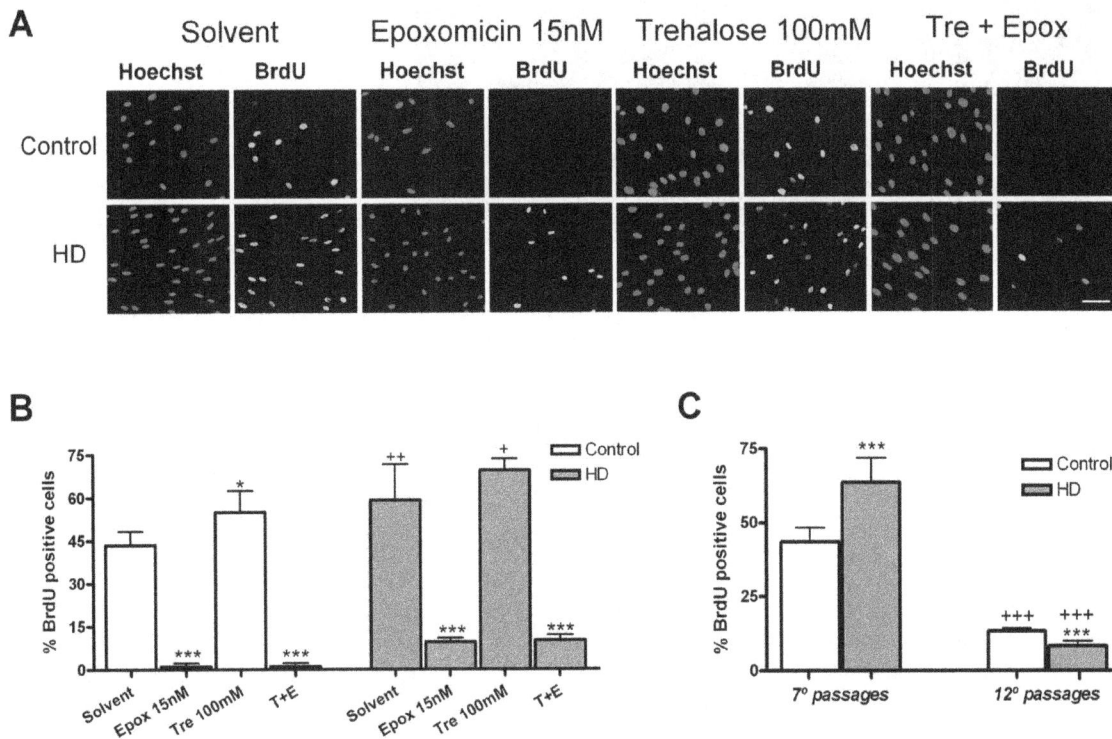

Figure 2. Effects of epoxomicin and trehalose in skin fibroblast cell cycle. (A) Photomicrographs of BrdU positive cells of dividing cells (green) and total nuclei stained with bis-benzimide (blue) from control and HD patients. (Scale bar = 20 µm). (B) Percentage of BrdU positive cells with respect to the total number. (C) Comparison of the percentage of BrdU positive cells in early and late cell passage numbers. Values are expressed as the mean ± SD, $n = 4$ patients. Control cell number (mean per field) 33.80±1.417, $n = 4$. HD cell number (mean per field) 41.56±2.025, $n = 4$. The data of each patient was obtained using 4 replicates. Statistical analysis was performed by one-way ANOVA with repeated measures followed by Bonferroni multiple comparison test: *p<0.05, ***p<0.001 vs Solvent; +p<0.05, ++p<0.01, +++p<0.001 HD vs controls.

for 30 min, at 37°C in the incubator. Then, the cells were washed twice with (PBS with 1 mM glucose), and the nuclei were stained with bis-benzimide (Hoechst 33342) added to the anti-fading solution, at a $3 \times 10M^{-6}$ final concentration. For quantitative determinations, the cover slides were observed under a fluorescent microscope using FITC (fluorescein isothiocyanate) filter and counted in 1/10 of the cover slide area; ROS positive cells were identified by fluorescence emission and total cells by bis-benzimide stained.

Immunocytochemistry

We analyzed the percentage of immunoreactive cells to LC3 (microtubule-associated protein1 *light chain* 3) and to both HSC70 (heat shock cognate 71 kDa protein) and LAMP-2A (lysosome-associated membrane protein 2-A) as markers of macro-autophagy and chaperon-mediated autophagy [15]. The fibroblast cultures were fixed with 4% paraformaldehyde, washed in 0.1 M phosphate-buffered saline, pH 7.4 (PBS), permeabilized with ethanol-acetic acid (19:1), and incubated at 4°C for 24 h with primary antibodies diluted in PBS containing 10% fetal calf serum. Rabbit polyclonal anti-LC3 antibody (MBL, PM036) was diluted at 1/200. Mouse monoclonal anti-huntingtin mAB 2166 from (Chemicon, mAB 2166) was diluted 1/500. To

measure huntingtin inside the fibroblasts we had to use the integrated Optical Density (IOD) as skin fibroblasts do not show huntingtin aggregates [14]. Mouse anti- HSC70 (heat-shock protein 70) diluted 1/100 (Abcam, Ab2788) and rabbit anti-LAMP-2A diluted 1/100 (Abcam, Ab37024). Fluorescein- and rhodamine-conjugated secondary antibodies were employed to visualize positive cells under fluorescent microscopy. Colocalization images for HSC70 and LAMP-2A were acquired using a Nikon C1 plus ECLIPSE Ti-e microscope. The number of immunoreactive cells was counted in one-seventh of the total area of the cover slides. The cells were counted in predefined parallel strips using a counting reticule inserted into the ocular.

Detection of ubiquitinated proteins

Human skin fibroblasts cultures were treated with epoxomicin (15 nM) or pre-treated with trehalose (100 mM) 15 min before the treatment with epoxomicin for 24 h. Cells were washed with PBS plus phenylmethylsulfonyl fluoride (PMSF) (SIGMA-Aldrich, P7626), scraped in 150 μL of lysis buffer [50 mM Tris HCl, 150 mM NaCl, 20 mM EDTA, 1% Triton X-100, 50 mM sodium fluoride (NaF), 20 mM N-ethyl-maleimide, 100 μM sodium ortovanadate, 1 mM PMSF and protease inhibitors

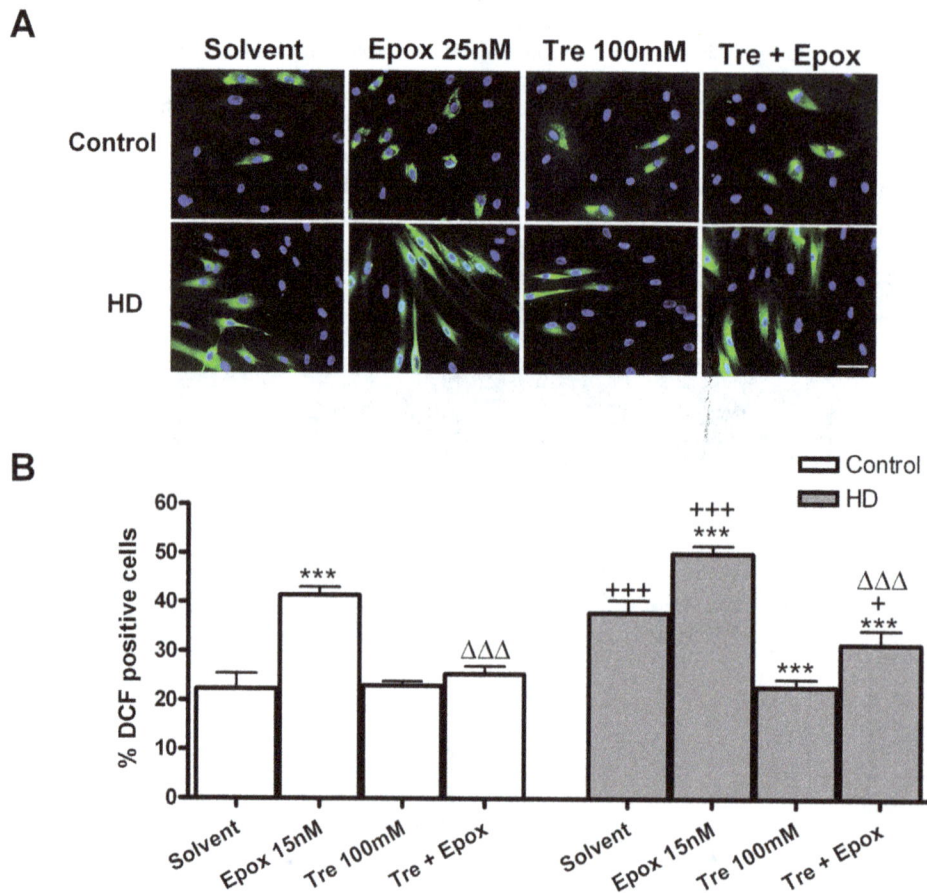

Figure 3. Epoxomicin increases ROS levels, which are reduced by trehalose in HD firboblasts. (A) 2′, 7′–dichlorofluorescin (DCF) immunocytochemistry (green) and total nuclei stained with bis-benzimide (blue) in control and HD fibroblasts and (B) percentage of DCF positive cells respect to the total number. (Scale bar = 20 μm). Values are expressed as the mean ± SD, n = 4 patients. Control cell number (mean per field) 28.83 ± 0.9280, n = 4. HD cell number (mean per field) 46.40 ± 5.247, n = 4. The data of each patient was obtained using 4 replicates. Statistical analysis was performed by one-way ANOVA with repeated measures followed by Bonferroni multiple comparison test: ***p<0.001 *vs* solvent; +p<0.05, +++ p<0.001 HD *vs* controls; ΔΔΔp<0.001 trehalose + epoxomicin *vs* epoxomicin.

cocktail (Calbiochem, 539131)] and immediately boiled for 5 min. The lysates were centrifuged at 12.000×g at 4°C for 30 min. The supernatant was used for protein determination by the BCA protein assay kit. For detection of ubiquitinated proteins by western blot, 15 μg of protein were conducted to immunoblot assay with a mouse monoclonal antibody to ubiquitin diluted 1/500 (Chemicon, MAB1510). The secondary antibodies (1/1000) followed by ECL (enhanced chemiluminescence) detection reagents (Bio-Rad, 970442/3) were used for immunodetection. Immunoblot of β-actin diluted (1/5000) (SIGMA-Aldrich, A5441) was performed to demonstrate equal protein loading. The blots were quantified by computer-assisted video.

Western blot analysis

Fibroblast cultures were homogenized with a sonicator in lysis buffer containing 20 mM Tris HCl, 10 mM potassium acetate (AcK), 1 mM dithiothreitol (DTT), 1 mM EDTA, 1 mM PMSF, 1 mM benzamidine, leupeptin, aprotinin, pepstatin 5 μg/ml each, 0.25% NP-40, pH 7.4, and then centrifuged at 12.000 g for 30 min at 4°C. For p-ERK and total ERK (microtubule-associated protein1 *light chain* 3) detection, 10 mM NaF, 2 mM sodium molibdate, 10 mM β-glicerophosphate, and 0.2 mM ortovanadate, were added to the lysis buffer. The supernatant was used for protein determination by the BCA protein assay kit and for electrophoretical separation. Samples (20–30 μg protein) were added to SDS sample loading buffer, electrophoresed in 10–15% SDS-polyacrylamide gels and then electroblotted to 0.45 μm nitrocellulose membranes, as described previously [19,20].

The antibodies used in the study were the following: the chaperone mouse anti-HSP-70 (1/750) was from Santa Cruz (Heidelberg, Germany). Mouse monoclonal anti-huntingin mAB 2166 (Chemicon, mAB 2166). Mouse monoclonal anti-ERK1/2 (SIGMA-Aldrich, M5670), Anti-P-ERK1/2 (SIGMA-Aldrich, M8159). Monoclonal anti- β-actin antibody diluted 1/5000 (SIGMA-Aldrich, A5441) diluted 1/10000 were used as a control of charge after inactivation of nitrocellulose membrane with sodium azide.

Proteasomal activity measurement

After culture treatments, cells were washed with PBS, harvested in proteasome lysis buffer and lysed by sonication (VibraCell, level 0.5 for 30 s). Lysates were centrifuged at 12.000 g at 4°C for 30 min. The protein concentration was assayed from the resulting supernatants by the BCA protein assay kit. The 20 S proteasomal chymotrypsin-like activity was quantified by monitoring the accumulation of the fluorescent cleavage product 7-amino-4-methylcoumarin (AMC) from the synthetic proteasomal substrate Suc-Leu-Leu-Val-Tyr-aminomethylcoumarin (LLVY-AMC) (Calbiochem, 539142) using the 20 S proteasome activity assay kit (Chemicon) according to the manufacturer's instruction (measurement every 30 min for 3 hours).

Statistical analysis

The results were statistically evaluated for significance with one-way ANOVA with repeated measures with two factors followed by Bonferroni multiple comparison test. The interactions between the genotype and the treatment were analyzed by two-way ANOVA followed by Bonferroni post-test. Differences were considered statistically significant when $p < 0.05$. Analysis of data was performed using the SPSS software.

Results

Epoxomicin induces the apoptotic pathway in control and HD human skin fibroblasts and trehalose protects from it

Epoxomicin activates, dose-dependently, the pro-apoptotic protein caspase-3. This effect is more pronounced in HD than in control fibroblasts (FIG. 1A). For the following experiments, we chose the 15 nM dose because was the minimum dose that discriminated both genotypes. After 24 hours of treatment, the effects of epoxomicin 15 nM in caspase-3 activation are reversed by trehalose 100 mM when added 15 min before epoxomicin and the protection is inhibited using the autophagy inhibitor 3-methyladenine (FIG. 1B–C).

Trehalose increases the number of skin proliferative cells

Trehalose 100 mM produced an increase in the number of BrdU+ fibroblasts but failed to modify the epoxomicin-induced reduction of cell division after 48 hours of treatment (FIG. 2A and 2B). The study of the cell cycle showed differences in the proliferative capacity between control and HD fibroblasts. Young HD fibroblasts had higher BrdU incorporation than aged fibroblasts that showed lower BrdU uptake in HD than in controls (FIG. 2C).

Trehalose protects from increased ROS production induced by epoxomicin

HD fibroblasts showed higher ROS levels than controls, measured as DCF positive cells with respect to total cell number (FIG. 3). Epoxomicin increased ROS levels in both control and HD fibroblasts which were reduced totally with co-treatment with trehalose 100 mM. Furthermore, trehalose could reduce the basal level of ROS in HD fibroblasts. The photomicrographs were obtained with different camera settings (FIG. 3A) to obtain a similar fluorescence intensity, because HD fibroblasts had a much higher ROS fluorescence intensity.

Trehalose protects against huntingtin and polyubiquitinated protein accumulation induced by epoxomicin in HD fibroblasts

In untreated cultures, huntingtin (HTT) and polyubiquitinated protein levels were higher in HD fibroblasts than in controls. Treatment with epoxomicin induced the accumulation of these proteins (FIG. 4A and 4B). Trehalose reduced the levels of huntingtin below baseline in control and HD fibroblasts. In addition, trehalose reduced the levels of huntingtin in epoxomicin treated HD fibroblasts (FIG. 4A). Co-treatment with trehalose partially counteracted the effect of epoxomicin in polyubiquitinated proteins. As happened with ROS levels, trehalose reduceed the basal polyubiquitinated proteins in HD fibroblasts (FIG. 4B). With respect to the proteasome activity, the chymotrypsin-like activity is reduced in HD fibroblasts. Epoxomicin further reduced this activity, at least in controls, and trehalose increased this proteasomal activity even in cultures co-treated with epoxomicin (FIG. 4C).

Effects of epoxomicin and trehalose on ERK-1/2 and HSP70 chaperone protein activation

After 24 hours of treatment, epoxomicin reduced levels of phosphorilated ERK and trehalose could not revert it in controls. In HD fibroblasts, epoxomicin increased p-ERK levels. Co-treatment with trehalose reverted the effects of the epoxomicin on p-ERK levels in HD fibroblasts (FIG. 5A). Epoxomicin greatly increased HSP70 levelsand this effect was not reverted by trehalose. (FIG. 5B).

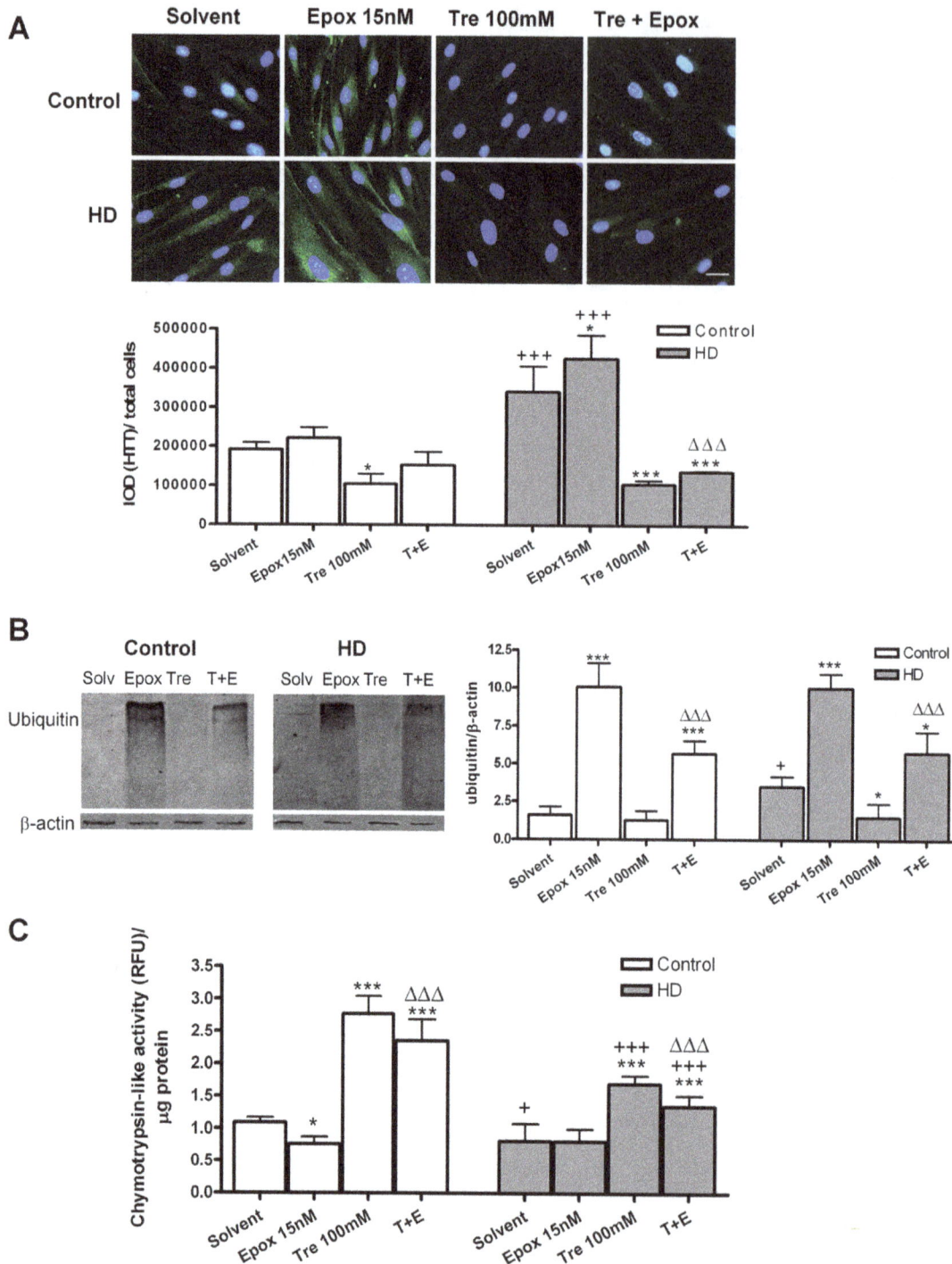

Figure 4. **Trehalose protects against accumulation of Huntingtin and poly-ubiquitinated protein induced by epoxomicin and increases UPS activity.** (A) Huntingtin immunocytochemistry (green) and total nuclei stained with bis-benzimide (blue). The histogram shows the ratio of Huntingtin (IOD) with respect to the total cell number. (Scale bar = 20 μm) (B) Ubiquitinated protein accumulation and its corresponding densitometric analysis. (C) Chymotrypsin-like proteasome activity. Values are expressed as the mean ± SD, $n = 4$ patients. Control cell number (mean per field) 32,66±1.472, $n = 4$. HD cell number (mean per field) 44,67±0.3405, $n = 4$. The data of each patient was obtained using 4 replicates. Statistical analysis was performed by one-way ANOVA with repeated measures followed by Bonferroni multiple comparison test: *$p<0.05$, ***$p<0.001$ vs solvent; +$p<0.05$, +++$p<0.001$ HD vs controls; ΔΔΔ$p<0.001$ trehalose + epoxomicin vs epoxomicin.

Effects of trehalose in macroautophagy and chaperone-mediated authophagy

The LC3 expression was upregulated in HD fibroblasts and trehalose produced a twofold increase even when epoxomicin is present in both controls and HD fibroblasts (FIG. 6A). As happened with LC3 levels, LAMP2-A levels were higher in HD fibroblasts, possibly, as a compensatory response for decreased UPS activity and ubiquitinated protein accumulation. Trehalose

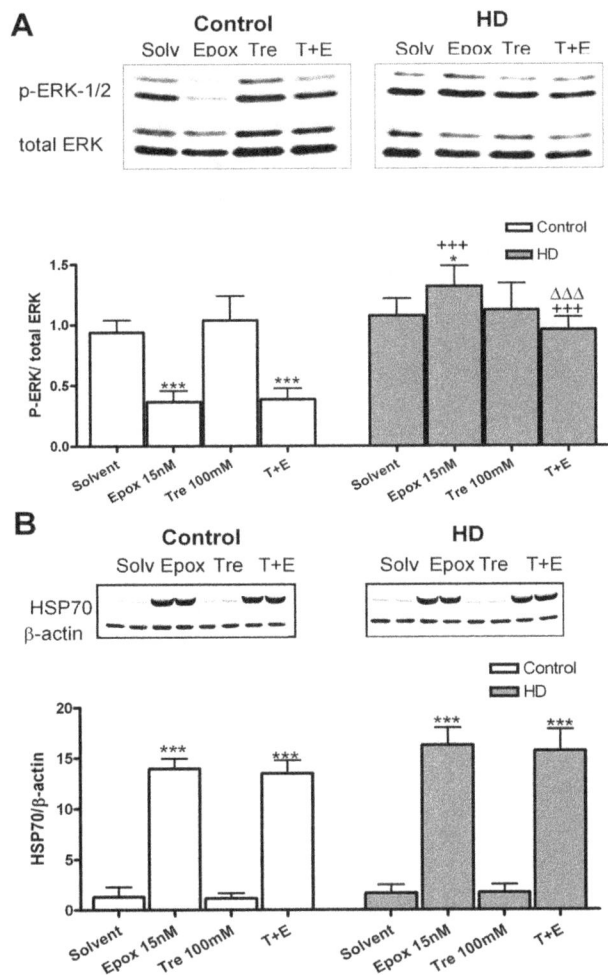

Figure 5. Effects of epoxomicin and trehalose on ERK-1/2 and HSP70 chaperone protein activation in HD fibroblasts. (A) Western blot of p-ERK-1/2 expression with regard to total ERK and its corresponding densitometric analysis in control and HD fibroblasts. (B) Western blot of HSP70 expression and its corresponding densitometric analysis. Values are expressed as the mean $\pm$ SD, $n = 4$ patients. The data of each patient was obtained using 4 replicates. Statistical analysis was performed by one-way ANOVA with repeated measures followed by Bonferroni multiple comparison test: *$p < 0.05$, ***$p < 0.001$ vs Solvent; +++$p < 0.001$ HD vs controls, $\Delta\Delta\Delta p < 0.001$ trehalose + epoxomicin vs epoxomicin. There is an interaction between epoxomicin effect and genotype in ERK activation ($F = 71.13$ with a p value $= < 0.0001$). In HD, there is an interaction between the epoxomicin and trehalose effects in ERK activation ($F = 12.67$ with a p value $= 0.0013$).

considerably increased LAMP2-A expression with or without epoxomicin treatment (FIG. 6B). HSC70 can colocalize with LAMP2-A to participate in chaperone-mediated autophagy (CMA) [15]. We showed the colocalization between these two proteins (FIG. 6C) which indicated that trehalose also increases CMA.

Discussion

We have shown, in this study, that epoxomicin produceed a differential dose-dependent increase in activation of caspase-3 in control and HD fibroblasts. Epoxomicin also increaseed ROS, ubiquitinated proteins and huntingtin accumulation in HD fibroblasts. All these changes caused by this proteasome inhibitor

are reverted by trehalose. Our experiments have revealed basal differences between HD and control fibroblasts. HD fibroblasts had higher levels of BrdU incorporation at early passage numbers. However, when we studied the proliferative rate at late passage numbers, BrdU incorporation was diminished, to a great extent in HD fibroblasts. These results suggested that HD fibroblasts suffered a faster evolution to a senescent phenotype, probably caused by their deficiency in the UPS activity [21–23]. The treatment with epoxomicin for 48 hours stopped replication 99% in control and 85% in HD fibroblasts. Furthermore, trehalose increased the replication in both HD and control fibroblasts but could not prevent the cell cycle arrest produced by epoxomicin. UPS is implicated in cell cycle [16,17] and has also shown a decreased UPS activity in senescent cells with lower replicative capacity [24], which is consistent with the cell cycle arrest caused by epoxomicin. However, we observed that HD fibroblasts had a higher replication rate than controls as described by Goetz et al [25].

Proteasomal dysfunction has been considered a mechanism of production of neurodegenerative disorders including Huntington's disease. Huntingtin protein is degraded by the ubiquitin-proteasome system and autophagy [26,27]. Abnormal UPS function has been found in HD brain and skin fibroblasts previously [28,29]. We have shown that HD fibroblasts had high levels of ubiquitinated proteins and huntingtin. We showed in this study that trehalose, as an autophagy enhancer, compensated the lack of activity in the UPS, even in fibroblasts treated with epoxomicin in both genotypes.

In HD there is abnormal mitochondrial activity and excessive production of free radicals [30–33]. Reduction of respiratory activity in HD has been found in brain but not in fibroblasts [28,34,35]. We found that HD skin fibroblasts had an increased level of ROS and a diminished chymotripsin-like activity (UPS) with respect to controls, and these effects are reverted by trehalose. In controls, trehalose also increased UPS and reversed epoxomicin-induced ROS increase. Some studies report a relation between UPS dysfunction, ROS production and mitochondrial impairment [35–37]. Increasing autophagy using trehalose improved UPS activity by mutant huntingtin elimination which could alleviate the mitochondrial impairment and reduce ROS formation.

ERK proteins belong to the MAP kinase family and are related to promoting cell survival. However, the effects of the activation of this kinase are dependent on the intensity and the maintenance of the active state. Persistent and strong activation of ERK leads to cell death [38,39], whereas a short-lived activation of ERK is associated with survival [21,40]. Furthermore, a downregulation of ERK is related to an inhibition of cell proliferation [22,23]. In our experiments we showed that ERK was downregulated in presence of epoxomicin in control fibroblasts, which is consistent with the cell cycle arrest observed in the BrdU assay. The situation was completely different in HD fibroblasts. Epoxomicin induced an ERK activation of 22% in 24 hours resulting in promotion of cell death, which is reverted with the treatment with trehalose.

HSP70 functions as a chaperone and protects neurons from protein aggregation and toxicity binding unfolded or partially folded proteins [41]. Members of the HSP40 and HSP70 chaperone families have also been found to colocalize with nuclear aggregates in several polyQ diseases, both in human and mouse brains [42,43]. In our experiments, we appreciated a huge increase in HSP70 levels when skin fibroblasts were treated with epoxomicin in both control and HD. This fact implies a protective role of HSP70 against the proteasome inhibitor effects, among which is included protein accumulation.

A

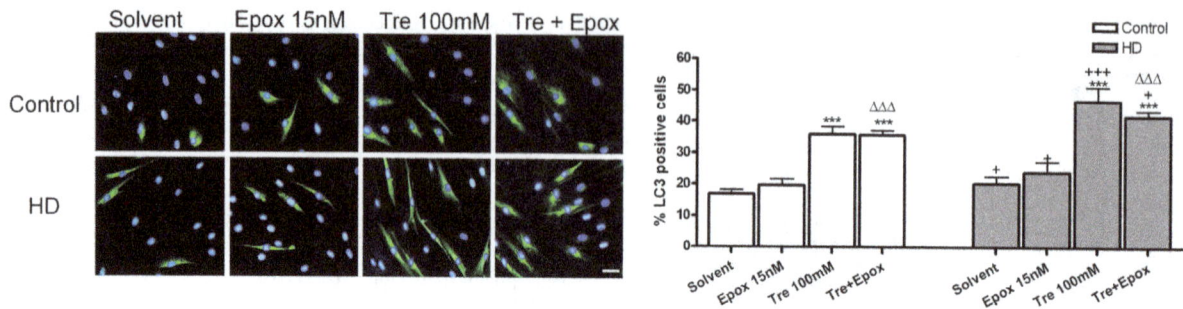

B

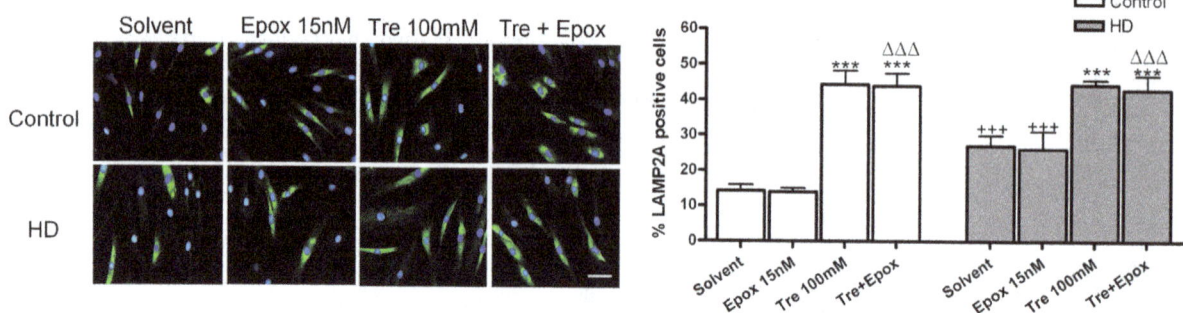

C

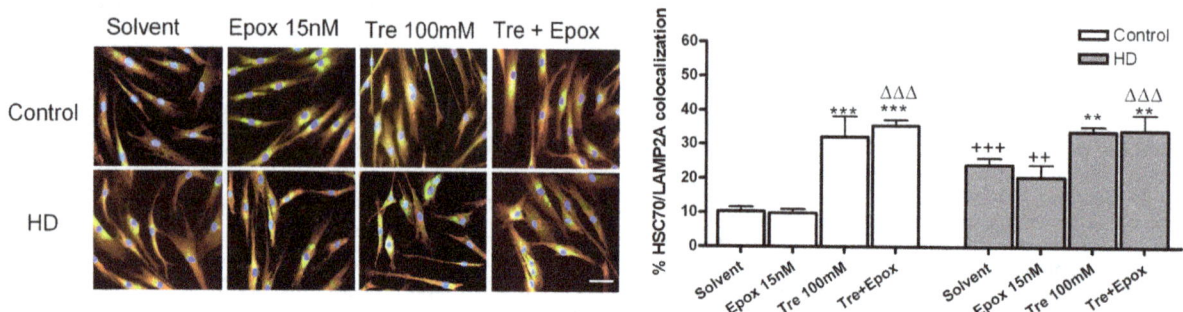

Figure 6. Macroautophagyc pathway and chaperone-mediated autophagy in control and HD human skin fibroblasts. (A) LC3 immunocytochemistry (green) and total nuclei stained with bis-benzimide (blue) and the percentage of LC3 positive cells with respect to the total cell number. (B) LAMP2A immunocytochemistry (green) and total nuclei stained with bis-benzimide (blue) and percentage of LAMP2A positive cells. (C) LAMP2A (green) and HSC70 (red) colocalization (yellow) and percentage of LAMP2A and HSC70 colocalization respect to the total cell number. (Scale bar = 20 μm). Values are expressed as the mean ± SD, $n = 4$ patients. Control cell number (mean per field) 30.94±2.012, $n = 4$. HD cell number (mean per field) 46.89±4.587, $n = 4$. The data of each patient was obtained using 4 replicates. Statistical analysis was performed by one-way ANOVA with repeated measures followed by Bonferroni multiple comparison test: **$p < 0.01$, ***$p < 0.001$ vs Solvent; +< 0.05, +$p < 0.05$, ++$p < 0.01$, +++$p < 0.001$ HD vs controls; ΔΔΔ$p < 0.001$ trehalose + epoxomicin vs epoxomicin.

UPS inhibition may induce neurodegeneration and it could be reverted by increasing autophagy [44]. LAMP-2A is a Lysosome Membrane Protein so its expression means also lysosomal activation, and LC3 is localized in the inner and outer membrane of autophagosomes [45]. We have observed an increase in autophagy, using LC3 and LAMP2-A markers, in HD and control fibroblasts treated with trehalose.

Due to the beneficial effects of trehalose in proteinopathies, as an autophagy enhancer, chemical chaperone and antioxidant, as well as its virtual absence of toxic effects even at high doses, this disaccharide is an interesting candidate for testing in clinical trials in HD patients.

Acknowledgments

The authors thank Rafael Gonzalo-Gobernado for his excellent technical microscopy assistance, Ms. Claire Marsden for editorial help and Alfonso Muriel for his assistance in statistical analysis.

Author Contributions

Conceived and designed the experiments: MFE MJC JGY MAM. Performed the experiments: MFE. Analyzed the data: MFE MJC JGY MAM. Contributed reagents/materials/analysis tools: JLS JGC CR AG JP. Wrote the paper: MFE JGY MAM.

References

1. Andrew SE, Goldberg YP, Kremer B, Telenius H, Theilmann J, et al. (1993) The relationship between trinucleotide (CAG) repeat length and clinical features of Huntington's disease. Nat Genet 4: 398–403.
2. Rubinsztein DC (2002) Lessons from animal models of Huntington's disease. Trends Genet 18: 202–209.
3. Hipp MS, Patel CN, Bersuker K, Riley BE, Kaiser SE, et al. (2012) Indirect inhibition of 26S proteasome activity in a cellular model of Huntington's disease. J Cell Biol 196: 573–587.
4. Bahr BA, Wisniewski ML, Butler D (2012) Positive lysosomal modulation as a unique strategy to treat age-related protein accumulation diseases. Rejuvenation Res 15: 189–197.
5. Pandey UB, Nie Z, Batlevi Y, McCray BA, Ritson GP, et al. (2007) HDAC6 rescues neurodegeneration and provides an essential link between autophagy and the UPS. Nature 447: 860–864.
6. Meng L, Mohan R, Kwok BH, Elofsson M, Sin N, et al. (1999) Epoxomicin, a potent and selective proteasome inhibitor, exhibits in vivo antiinflammatory activity. Proc Natl Acad Sci USA 96: 10403–10408.
7. Chen Q, Haddad GG (2004) Role of trehalose phosphate synthase and trehalose during hypoxia: from flies to mammals. J Exp Biol 207: 3125–3129.
8. Jain NK, Roy I (2009) Effect of trehalose on protein structure. Protein Sci 18: 24–36.
9. Welch WJ, Brown CR (1996) Influence of molecular and chemical chaperones on protein folding. Cell Stress Chaperones 1: 109–115.
10. Sarkar S, Davies JE, Huang Z, Tunnacliffe A, Rubinsztein DC (2007) Trehalose, a novel mTOR-independent autophagy enhancer, accelerates the clearance of mutant huntingtin and alpha-synuclein. J Biol Chem 282: 5641–5652.
11. Tanaka M, Machida Y, Niu S, Ikeda T, Jana NR, et al. (2004) Trehalose alleviates polyglutamine-mediated pathology in a mouse model of Huntington disease. Nat Med 10: 148–154.
12. Casarejos MJ, Solano R, Gómez A, Perucho J, de Yébenes JG, et al. (2011) The accumulation of neurotoxic proteins, induced by proteasome inhibition, is reverted by trehalose, an enhancer of autophagy, in human neuroblastoma cells. Neurochem Int 58: 512–520.
13. Porter AG, Jänicke RU (1999) Emerging roles of caspase-3 in apoptosis. Cell Death Differ 6: 99–104.
14. Sathasivam K, Woodman B, Mahal A, Bertaux F, Wanker EE, et al. (2001) Centrosome disorganization in fibroblast cultures derived from R6/2 Huntington's disease (HD) transgenic mice and HD patients. Hum Mol Genet 10: 2425–2435.
15. Kaushik S, Cuervo AM (2008) Chaperone-mediated autophagy. Methods Mol Biol 445: 227–244.
16. Bassermann F, Eichner R, Pagano M (2013) The ubiquitin proteasome system – Implications for cell cycle control and the targeted treatment of cancer. Biochim Biophys Acta doi: 10.1016.
17. Fasanaro P, Capogrossi MC, Martelli F (2010) Regulation of the endothelial cell cycle by the ubiquitin-proteasome system. Cardiovasc Res 85: 272–280.
18. Rodríguez-Navarro JA, Rodríguez L, Casarejos MJ, Solano RM, Gómez A, et al. (2010) Trehalose ameliorates dopaminergic and tau pathology in parkin deleted/tau overexpressing mice through autophagy activation. Neurobiol Dis 39: 423–438.
19. Solano RM, Casarejos MJ, Menendez-Cuervo J, Rodriguez-Navarro JA, Garcia de Yebenes J, et al. (2008) Glial dysfunction in parkin null mice: effects of aging. J Neurosci 28: 598–611.
20. Casarejos MJ, Solano RM, Menendez J, Rodriguez-Navarro JA, Correa C, et al. (2005) Differential effects of l-DOPA on monoamine metabolism, cell survival and glutathione production in midbrain neuronal-enriched cultures from parkin knockout and wild-type mice. J Neurochem 94: 1005–1014.
21. Xia Z, Dickens M, Raingeaud J, Davis RJ, Greenberg ME (1995) Opposing effects of ERK and JNK-p38 MAP kinases on apoptosis. Science 270: 1326–1331.
22. Fisher M, Liu B, Glennon PE, Southgate KM, Sale EM, et al. (2001) Downregulation of the ERK 1 and 2 mitogen activated protein kinases using antisense oligonucleotides inhibits proliferation of porcine vascular smooth muscle cells. Atherosclerosis 156: 289–295.
23. Jeong JC, Kim SJ, Kim YK, Kwon CH, Kim KH (2012) Lycii cortex radicis extract inhibits glioma tumor growth in vitro and in vivo through downregulation of the Akt/ERK pathway. Oncol Rep 27: 1467–1474.
24. Chondrogianni N, Stratford FL, Trougakos IP, Friguet B, Rivett AJ, et al. (2003) Central role of the proteasome in senescence and survival of human fibroblasts: induction of a senescence-like phenotype upon its inhibition and resistance to stress upon its activation. J Biol Chem 278: 28026–28037.
25. Goetz IE, Roberts E, Warren J (1981) Skin fibroblasts in Huntington disease. Am J Hum Genet 32: 187–196.
26. Qin ZH, Wang Y, Kegel KB, Kazantsev A, Apostol BL, et al. (2003) Autophagy regulates the processing of amino terminal huntingtin fragments. Hum Mol Genet 12: 3231–3244.
27. Li X, Wang CE, Huang S, Xu X, Li XJ, et al. (2010) Inhibiting the ubiquitin-proteasome system leads to preferential accumulation of toxic N-terminal mutant huntingtin fragments. Hum Mol Genet 19: 2445–2455.
28. Seo H, Sonntag KC, Isacson O (2004) Generalized brain and skin proteasome inhibition in Huntington's disease. Ann Neurol 53: 319–328.
29. Bence NF, Sampat RM, Kopito RR (2001) Impairment of the ubiquitin-proteasome system by protein aggregation. Science 292: 1552–1555.
30. Chen CM (2011) Mitochondrial dysfunction, metabolic deficits, and increased oxidative stress in Huntington's disease. Chang Gung Med J 34: 135–152.
31. Zheng Z, Diamond MI (2012) Huntington disease and the huntingtin protein. Prog Mol Biol Transl Sci 107: 189–214.
32. Arenas J, Campos Y, Ribacoba R, Martín MA, Rubio JC, et al. (1998) Complex I defect in muscle from patients with Huntington's disease. Ann Neurol 43: 397–400.
33. Browne SE (2008) Mitochondria and Huntington's disease pathogenesis: insight from genetic and chemical models. Ann N Y Acad Sci 1147: 358–382.
34. Tabrizi S, Cleeter MW, Xuereb J, Taanman JW, Cooper JM, et al. (1999) Biochemical abnormalities and excitotoxicity in Huntington's disease brain. Ann Neurol 45: 25–32.
35. del Hoyo P, García-Redondo A, de Bustos F, Molina JA, Sayed Y, et al. (2006) Oxidative stress in skin fibroblasts cultures of patients with Huntington's disease. Neurochem Res 31: 1103–1109.
36. Torres CA, Perez VI (2008) Proteasome modulates mitochondrial function during cellular senescence. Free Radic Biol Med 44: 403–414.
37. Domingues AF, Arduíno DM, Esteves AR, Swerdlow RH, Oliveira CR, et al. (2008) Mitochondria and ubiquitin-proteasomal system interplay: relevance to Parkinson's disease. Free Radic Biol Med 45: 820–825.
38. Canals S, Casarejos MJ, de Bernardo S, Solano RM, Mena MA (2003) Selective and persistent activation of extracellular signal-regulated protein kinase by nitric oxide in glial cells induces neuronal degeneration in glutathione-depleted midbrain cultures. Mol Cell Neurosci 24: 1012–1026.
39. Seo SR, Chong SA, Lee SI, Sung JY, Ahn YS, et al. (2001) Zn2+-induced ERK activation mediated by reactive oxygen species causes cell death in differentiated PC12 cells. J Neurochem 78: 600–610.
40. De Bernardo S, Canals S, Casarejos MJ, Rodriguez-Martin E, Mena MA (2003) Glia-conditioned medium induces de novo synthesis of tyrosine hydroxylase and increases dopamine cell survival by differential signaling pathways. J Neurosci Res 73: 818–830.
41. Chappell TG, Welch WJ, Schlossman DM, Palter KB, Schlesinger MJ, et al. (1986) Uncoating ATPase is a member of the 70 kilodalton family of stress proteins. cell 45: 3–13.
42. Jana NR, Tanaka M, Wang GH, Nukina N (2000) Polyglutamine length-dependent interaction of Hsp40 and Hsp70 family chaperones with truncated N-terminal huntingtin: their role in suppression of aggregation and cellular toxicity. Hum Mol Genet 9: 2009–2018.
43. Chai Y, Koppenhafer SL, Bonini NM, Paulson HL (1999) Analysis of the role of heat shock protein (Hsp) molecular chaperones in polyglutamine disease. J Neurosci 19: 10338–10347.
44. Pan T, Kondo S, Zhu W, Xie W, Jankovic J, et al. (2008) Neuroprotection of rapamycin in lactacystin-induced neurodegeneration via autophagy enhancement. Neurobiol Dis 32: 16–25.
45. Kabeya Y, Mizushima N, Ueno T, Yamamoto A, Kirisako T, et al. (2000) LC3, a mammalian homologue of yeast Apg8p, is localized in autophagosome membranes after processing. EMBO J 19: 5720–5728.

17

Allele-Specific Suppression of Mutant Huntingtin using Antisense Oligonucleotides: Providing a Therapeutic Option for all Huntington Disease Patients

Niels H. Skotte[1], Amber L. Southwell[1], Michael E. Østergaard[2], Jeffrey B. Carroll[3], Simon C. Warby[4], Crystal N. Doty[1], Eugenia Petoukhov[1], Kuljeet Vaid[1], Holly Kordasiewicz[2], Andrew T. Watt[2], Susan M. Freier[2], Gene Hung[2], Punit P. Seth[2], C. Frank Bennett[2], Eric E. Swayze[2], Michael R. Hayden[1]*

1 Centre for Molecular Medicine and Therapeutics, Child and Family Research Institute, University of British Columbia, Vancouver, British Columbia, Canada, 2 ISIS Pharmaceuticals, Carlsbad, California, United States of America, 3 Behavioral Neuroscience Program, Department of Psychology, Western Washington University, Bellingham, Washington, United States of America, 4 Center for Advanced Research in Sleep Medicine, Department of Psychiatry, University of Montréal, Montréal, Quebec, Canada

Abstract

Huntington disease (HD) is an inherited, fatal neurodegenerative disorder caused by a CAG repeat expansion in the huntingtin gene. The mutant protein causes neuronal dysfunction and degeneration resulting in motor dysfunction, cognitive decline, and psychiatric disturbances. Currently, there is no disease altering treatment, and symptomatic therapy has limited benefit. The pathogenesis of HD is complicated and multiple pathways are compromised. Addressing the problem at its genetic root by suppressing mutant huntingtin expression is a promising therapeutic strategy for HD. We have developed and evaluated antisense oligonucleotides (ASOs) targeting single nucleotide polymorphisms that are significantly enriched on HD alleles (HD-SNPs). We describe our structure-activity relationship studies for ASO design and find that adjusting the SNP position within the gap, chemical modifications of the wings, and shortening the unmodified gap are critical for potent, specific, and well tolerated silencing of mutant huntingtin. Finally, we show that using two distinct ASO drugs targeting the two allelic variants of an HD-SNP could provide a therapeutic option for all persons with HD; allele-specifically for roughly half, and non-specifically for the remainder.

Editor: Joseph C. Glorioso, University of Pittsburgh School of Medicine, United States of America

Funding: This work was supported by grants from ISIS Pharmaceuticals and the Canadian Institutes of Health Research (CIHR) (20R90174), and fellowships from the Ph.D. School for Genetic Medicine, University of Copenhagen, Denmark (NHS), Stadslæge Svend Ahrend Larsen og grosserer Jon Johannesons Fond (NHS), CIHR (ALS and NHS), Pfizer Ripples of Hope (ALS and NHS), The Huntington Society of Canada (ALS), and The Michael Smith Foundation for Health Research (ALS). MRH is a Killam University Professor and holds a Canada Research Chair. ISIS Pharmaceuticals synthesized and provided the ASOs used in this study and took part in the data generation, analysis, and manuscript preparation. None of the other funders had a role in study design, data collection and analysis, decision to publish, or preparation of the manuscript.

Competing Interests: MEØ, HK, ATW, GH, SMF, PPS, CFB, and EES are employees of, with a financial interest in, Isis Pharmaceuticals. MEØ, HK, ATW, GH, SMF, PPS, CFB, and EES have an affiliation to one of the funders, ISIS Pharmaceuticals, of this research study.

* Email: mrh@cmmt.ubc.ca

Introduction

Huntington disease (HD) is an autosomal dominant, fatal neurodegenerative disorder with a prevalence of up to 17 cases per 100,000, which makes it one of the most common inherited neurodegenerative disorders [1,2]. HD belongs to a family of polyglutamine diseases, and is caused by a mutation that expands a polyglutamine-encoding CAG repeat sequence in the huntingtin (*HTT*) gene [3]. The HTT protein is expressed ubiquitously and plays a central role in a plethora of interconnected cellular pathways [3]. The toxic effects mediated by mutant huntingtin (mHTT) are dependent on the number of CAG repeats in the gene, resulting in an inverse relationship between the age of symptom onset and the CAG repeat size [3–5]. The unaffected range is 6–35 CAG repeats, alleles with 36–39 CAGs confer

increasing risk of developing HD, and alleles with 40 CAG repeats and above are fully penetrant, causing HD within normal lifespan [3,6].

In 1983 the HD gene was mapped to the short arm of chromosome 4 and 10 years later the gene was isolated and cloned [7,8]. Even though the mutation causing HD was discovered more than two decades ago and despite tremendous progress in our understanding of the mechanisms underlying HD, there is still no efficacious therapy available to prevent the disease. Current treatment relies solely on symptomatic relief, which is most often only satisfactory in the initial phase of the disease [9,10]. Numerous drugs are being used to ameliorate the symptoms of HD including psychiatric agents, motor sedatives, and cognitive enhancers [10]. Only tetrabenazine has been approved by the FDA specifically to reduce the severity of chorea in HD [11]. Most of the potential therapeutic candidates which have been taken into clinical trials have had limited success [3]. These discouraging findings may be explained by the fact that most trials have only targeted one pathway in isolation and mHTT simultaneously disrupts multiple cellular pathways [3]. Therefore, preventing the expression of mHTT, which is the sole cause of disease, would be one of the most promising and comprehensive approaches for treating HD. Predictive testing and the identification of prodromal biomarkers in individuals positive for the HD mutation support the idea that preventative approaches are feasible [8,12]. Furthermore, the likelihood of a successful outcome is good considering that treatment can be initiated early before detrimental changes occur. This belief is furthermore supported by multiple studies. For example, it has been shown that the expression level of mHTT correlates with the onset and progression of HD features in the YAC mouse model [13], suggesting that partial reduction of mHTT would be beneficial. Furthermore, it has been demonstrated, using a conditional HD mouse model, that HD phenotypes including neuropathology and motor symptoms can be reversed by turning the HD gene off [14].

Two different gene-silencing approaches are currently under development for HD. The first and most straightforward strategy is to suppress the expression of both the wild-type (wt) and mutant protein. However, a general concern for total HTT silencing has been raised regarding the potential side effects of reducing wtHTT, whose beneficial activity for neuronal function and maintenance is well established [3]. HTT is associated with several organelles and interacts with many molecular partners playing a critical role in numerous cellular processes including transcriptional regulation, protein homeostasis, oxidative stress, axonal transport, synaptic transmission, and apoptosis suppression [3]. It is currently not completely clear how much HTT is needed to maintain these functions in adulthood, but it has been shown that HTT has a crucial role during embryogenesis, since ablation of the Huntington Disease homolog (Hdh) gene in mice results in death at embryonic day 7–9 [15–17]. Reduction of wtHTT expression to about one third causes perinatal death and abnormal development of the CNS [18]. Moreover, one study shows that loss of half of wtHTT during development causes motor dysfunction, impaired behaviour and abnormal brain morphology and pathology [15]. Lastly, a conditional deletion in the forebrain of young adult mice leads to progressive neurodegeneration [19]. These findings demonstrate that wtHTT function is essential for brain development and neuronal survival and suggest that specific silencing of mHTT expression in adulthood may be a desirable choice. There are some studies conducted in HD mouse models that support the idea that reducing both wt and mHTT is well tolerated and leads to clinical benefit [20–23]. However, alterations in molecular pathways associated with loss of normal HTT function have also been observed [24,25]. It is very difficult to predict how these findings may translate into human applications. Considering that HD patients would require life-long treatment and given the potential for side effects of long-term silencing of wtHTT, allele-specific strategies provide a valuable addition to the treatment options currently being considered.

Different approaches have been employed to achieve allele-specific silencing of mHTT by targeting disease-linked polymorphisms, including the CAG expansion [26–28], a CAG expansion-associated deletion [29], and single nucleotide polymorphisms (SNPs) enriched on HD alleles (HD-SNPs) [30–34]. Several CAG repeat-targeting silencing reagents are under pre-clinical development and have shown great promise when tested in cells from juvenile HD patients [28,35–38], whom display a more severe form of the disease with onset before the age of 20 [39]. Juvenile

HD accounts for less than 5–10% of HD patients [40] and it remains to be determined if this approach will be appropriate when the difference between the upper and lower CAG tracts is smaller, as with the majority of HD patients [41]. Some studies show that the selectivity of CAG targeted silencing reagents declines when the number of CAG repeats approaches the average size observed in the HD population [27,38,42], which suggests that this approach may not be beneficial to all HD patients [41]. Furthermore, CAG targeting strategies may be associated with the unwanted risk of reducing the expression of other CAG repeat containing transcripts, such as ataxin 3 [42,43].

As an alternative therapeutic strategy, we and others have shown that targeting HD-SNPs using RNAi or antisense-oligonucleotides (ASOs) presents a promising approach towards achieving allele-specific treatment of HD patients [32–34,44]. The heterozygosity of the SNPs in the HD population will determine the number of patients that will be amendable to this treatment strategy [41]. Since clinical trials are a considerable investment, selecting and evaluating the individual HD-SNPs becomes critical to achieve the maximal patient coverage with the lowest number of targeted SNPs. In addition to being in linkage disequilibrium with the CAG expansion, a targetable HD-SNP should ideally be found at low frequency on the wt allele to provide great specificity [44]. We have previously genotyped 234 Caucasian HD patients using a custom SNP genotyping assay and identified fifty HD-SNPs across the HTT gene that are significantly enriched on HD alleles compared to wt alleles [33,44]. Out of these, forty are heterozygous in greater than 35% of the sequenced HD population, making them potential allele-specific silencing targets. ASOs against twenty-four of these HD-SNPs have previously been screened in primary human HD fibroblasts for mRNA knock down [33]. The top candidates were counter screened for protein knock down and the best candidate displayed approximately 70% knock down of mHTT in primary neurons from BACHD mice without affecting wtHTT protein levels in primary neurons from YAC18 mice [33]. The maximal coverage, which can be achieved by targeting one of these HD-SNP is roughly half of the HD population [33]. Population genetics studies show that 75%–85% of the HD population could be treated with panel of three to five ASOs targeting these HD-SNPs [32,44]. Therefore, in addition to selecting a primary HD-SNP target, it becomes important to include supplementary HD-SNPs, which are not in linkage disequilibrium, to increase patient coverage. The majority (~90%) of the identified HTT SNPs are intronic and can only be targeted by ASOs that, unlike RNAi, do not require the endogenous microRNA processing machinery for activity [45]. ASOs promote RNase H-induced cleavage of pre-mRNA and mature mRNA preventing the generation of protein [46]. ASOs are freely taken up by neurons and can be delivered to the CNS via intrathecal injections or infusions, allowing for a rapid and controlled dosing strategy [23,47,48], making ASOs attractive candidates for therapeutic intervention.

ASO-mediated HTT knock down was demonstrated more than a decade ago using both phosphodiester and phosphorothiorated (PS) ASOs [49,50]. Since that time, the development of ASO technology has steadily progressed in both research and clinical settings. Research has focused on ASO designs that increase resistance to degradation, improve affinity and enhance specificity, thereby increasing potency and reducing undesirable off-target effects. Here, we have established a functional pipeline that allows for rapid screening and selection of potent, selective, and well tolerated ASOs in primary neurons. For our screen, we have used neurons from the humanized Hu97/18 mouse, which has human wt and mHTT transgenes, along with the corresponding SNPs associated with each human allele, and no endogenous murine Hdh [51]. Here, we evaluate both previously reported and novel ASOs in a system pertinent to the brain using a novel triage system based on protein knock down, selectivity, and toxicity to select well tolerated ASOs providing the greatest mHTT knock down while maintaining normal expression of wtHTT. This approach has resulted in identification of several promising leads and progress towards a therapeutic option for all HD patients and the screening strategy could be adapted for identification of therapeutic ASOs for other indications where allele-specific knockdown would be beneficial.

Results

ASO screening pipeline

Out of the fifty HD-SNPs previously identified [33,44], ten SNPs were selected as a starting point for efficacy studies in primary Hu97/18 neurons based on therapeutic relevance and availability of screening tools (Figure 1A). These SNPs are each heterozygous and targetable (present on the CAG expanded chromosome) in greater than 35% of the sequenced HD population as well as in available HD patient-derived fibroblast cell lines and the Hu97/18 mouse model of HD. Single ASOs were tested at ten different SNPs and the four most active ASOs

were moved forward (Figure 1B). We employed three different structure-activity relationship (SAR) studies to find the best possible ASO candidates. The first approach was to change the number and position of modifications in the wings of the ASO. Next, we conducted a microwalk of the sequence around the target SNP site and lastly, we have evaluated the effect of shortening the ASO gap from 9 to 7 nucleotides. ASOs were screened for potency and specificity. Additionally, to exclude toxic ASOs from the pipeline, we used cleavage of spectrin, a cytoskeletal protein that lines the intracellular surface of the plasma membrane and is cleaved by caspases during apoptosis [52], as a measure of neuronal tolerability.

Identification of the best targetable SNPs

The ultimate goal is to develop a panel of allele-specific ASOs that, in combination, will provide a therapeutic option to the majority of the HD patients. However, the purpose of this screen was to identify the most efficacious SNP sites and to develop the best possible ASO candidate. The selected HD-SNPs in the current study do not provide significant combinatorial advantage as they are all in high linkage disequilibrium with one another. To evaluate the activity at several SNP sites we used phosphorothioate substituted 19-mers containing five 2'-O-methoxy-ethyl (MOE; represented by "e") ribose sugars in each wing and a string of nine

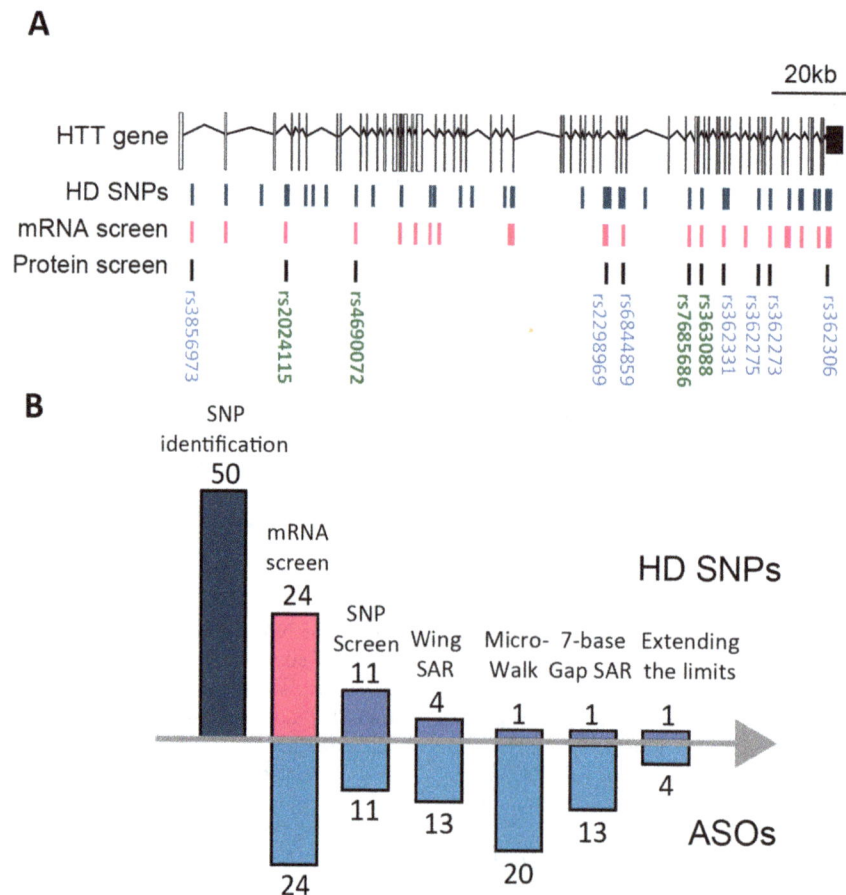

Figure 1. ASO screening pipeline. (A) HD-SNPs in the *HTT* gene: blue = HD-SNPs, pink = previous human fibroblasts screen, grey = Hu97/18 screen; green Rs numbers = SNPs identified as the most RNase-H-active sites (B) ASO development pipeline: The number of targeted SNPs and ASOs tested are shown above and below the column bars, respectively. 50 SNPs are enriched on HD alleles and ASOs targeting 24 of these were previously screened for mHTT mRNA silencing. ASOs targeting 10 SNPs were screened in primary Hu97/18 neurons for HTT protein suppression and tolerability. Then, ASOs with modifications to the wings targeting 4 of these SNPs were screened. Microwalk SAR and 7-base gap SAR was done for oligos targeting SNP Rs7685686. Lastly, higher ASO concentrations and longer treatment durations were tested.

DNA residues in the gap (5e-9-5e gapmers) [53]. Primary Hu97/18 cortical neurons were treated with bath-applied ASO on the second day in culture at 0, 16, 62.5, 250, and 1000 nM. After 6 days of treatment, the neurons were collected and the two allelic proteins were separated by electrophoresis based on differences in CAG size and assessed by Western blotting. The HTT protein was quantified and normalized to the calnexin loading control. Subsequently, membranes were re-blotted for spectrin, and the amount of cleaved spectrin (120 kDa fragment) was evaluated as an apoptosis readout with a toxicity threshold of 3-fold induction. As a positive control for spectrin cleavage, we used camptothecin, which is a topoisomerase inhibitor causing DNA damage, to induce apoptosis (Figure S1) [52,54]. Dose-response curves were generated for HTT knock down and the specificity was determined by calculating the ratio of the IC_{50} values for wtHTT and mHTT. If there was less than 50% knock down at the highest ASO concentration tested and no possibility of calculating an IC_{50} value, then the highest ASO concentration evaluated was used to calculate the ratio, which is expressed as >x fold.

ASOs A1, B1, C1, and D1 targeting rs7685686, rs4690072, rs2024115, rs363088, respectively, showed acceptable potency (34–79% mHTT remaining at 1000 nM), specificity up to 3.1 fold, and no overt toxicity (Figure 2 and Table 1). These 4 candidates were moved forward in the pipeline. The remaining ASOs showed limited HTT silencing and specificity that did not reach statistical significance with two-way ANOVA and Bonferroni post hoc test (Figure S2). None of the 10 ASOs tested displayed spectrin

cleavage above threshold (Figure S3). However, treatment with ASOs E1 and G1 for 6 days caused marked morphological changes of the neurons with increasing severity with doses starting at 250 and 500 nM, respectively (Figure S4). These findings suggest that some adverse structural changes may be occurring, and these ASOs were therefore excluded. The fact that the ASOs, having the same chemistry and design, are not equally active at all SNP sites, suggests that the location of the target SNP within the pre-mRNA sequence may play a critical role for its accessibility. It could be speculated that secondary structures in the pre-mRNA may prevent efficient ASO binding and RNase H recruitment to certain sequences.

ASO wing SAR screen

To further evaluate ASOs targeting these four SNPs and identify the ASOs with the most activity, we introduced S-constrained-ethyl (cEt; represented by "k") modifications to the wings of the 4 parent ASOs A1, B1, C1, and D1. Prior studies using these high affinity modifications in the wings found ASOs displaying improved potency without producing toxicity [55,56]. Similarly, we have found that the introduction of cEt modifications increases the potency of the ASOs significantly when used in primary neurons [33]. We have tested ASOs of three different lengths (19, 17, and 15 nucleotides) and with the incorporation of two different wing motifs, ekek-9-keke and ekk-9-kke (Figure 3A). We believed that it would be more achievable to identify ASOs with sufficient potency and then subsequently improve specificity

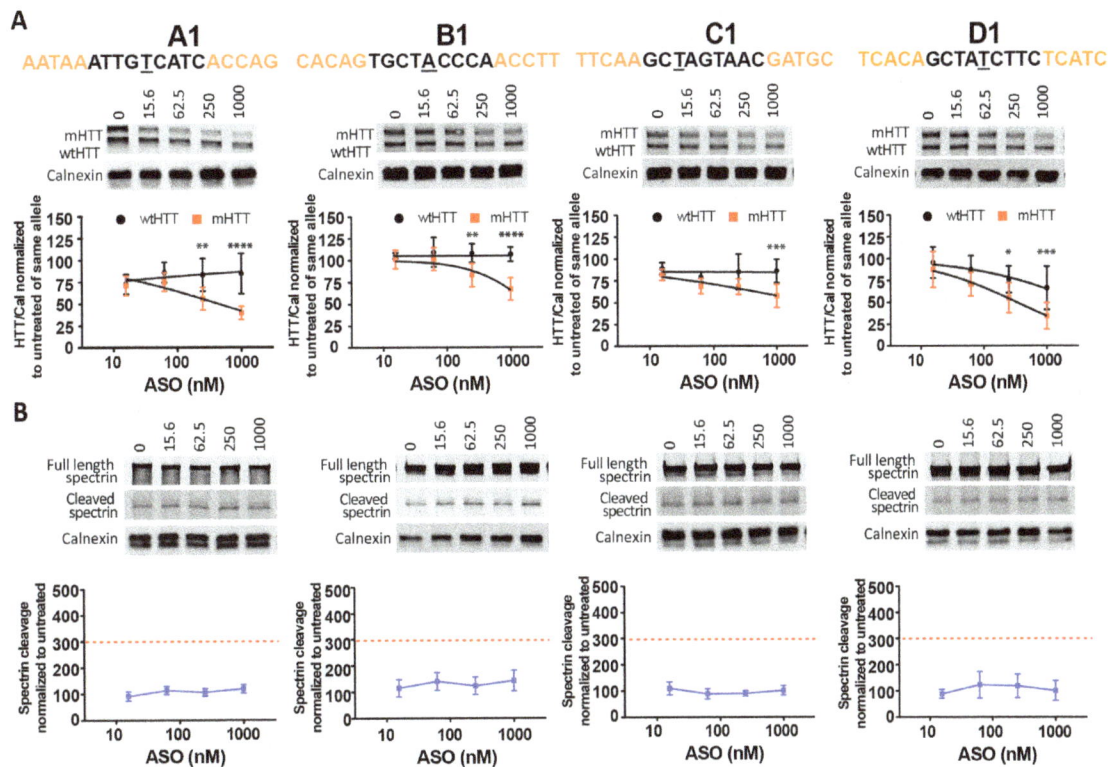

Figure 2. Selection of the best SNP targets. Primary Hu97/18 neurons were treated with 5e-9-5e ASOs targeted to 10 HD-SNPs at 6–1000 nM for 6 days. (A) HTT Western blots and quantitation for the 4 SNPs with the greatest activity. HTT levels are normalized to the internal loading control calnexin and then to the untreated sample for each allele. (B) Western blots showing full length and cleaved spectrin for the 4 ASOs. Spectrin fragment is normalized to calnexin and then to the untreated sample. Membranes were probed for HTT and reprobed for spectrin. Representative images are shown. n = 4–8 per data point. Data are presented as mean ± SD. Two way ANOVA with Bonferroni post hoc test have been performed and p values are illustrated with *, **, ***, **** for p = 0.05, 0.01, 0.001, and 0.0001. The PS backbone is black and MOE modifications are illustrated by orange. The SNP is underlined. The red dashed line represents the toxicity threshold.

Table 1. Summary of ASO protein screen in Hu97/18 primary neurons.

ASO	Notation	Rs #	Max effect		Day	IC50		Selectivity	Toxicity	Screen
			%wtHTT	%mHTT		wtHTT	mHTT			
A1	AeAeTeAeAeATTGTCATCAeCeCeAeGe	rs7685686	85	40	D6	>1000	421	>2.4	Pass	**Pass**
B1	CeAeCeAeGeTGCTACCCAAeCeCeTeTe	rs4690072	109	79	D6	>1000	>1000	ND	Pass	**Pass**
C1	TeTeCeAeAeGCTAGTAACGeAeTeGeCe	rs2024115	86	57	D6	>1000	>1000	ND	Pass	**Pass**
D1	TeCeAeCeAeGCTATCTTCTeCeAeTeCe	rs363088	66	34	D6	>1000	330	>3.1	Pass	**Pass**
E1	AeAeGeGeGeATGCTGACTTeGeGeGeCe	rs2298969	96	72	D6	>1000	>1000	ND	Pass	-
F1	CeCeTeTeCeCTCACTGAGGeAeTeGeAe	rs6844859	40	25	D6	538	234	2.3	Pass	-
G1	GeCeAeCeAeCAGTAGATGeAeGeGeGeAe	rs362331	80	70	D6	>1000	>1000	ND	Pass	-
H1	AeAeGeAeAeGCCTGATAAAeAeTeCeTe	rs362275	82	65	D6	>1000	>1000	ND	Pass	-
I1	GeAeGeCeAeGCTGCAACCTeGeGeCeAe	rs362306	52	43	D6	>1000	635	>1.6	Pass	-
J1	TeTeGeAeTeCTGTAGCAGCeAeGeCeTe	rs362273	94	84	D6	>1000	>1000	ND	Pass	-
A2	AeTkAeAkATTGTCATCAkCeCkAe	rs7685686	22	7	D6	74	9	8.2	-	-
A3	TeAkAkATTGTCATCAkCkCe	rs7685686	28	9	D6	356	40	8.9	Pass	**Pass**
B2	AeCkAeGkTGCTACCCAAkCeCkTe	rs4690072	53	35	D6	>1000	280	>3.6	-	-
B3	CeAkGkTGCTACCCAAkCkCe	rs4690072	57	34	D6	>1000	272	>3.6	-	-
C2	CeTkTeCkAAGCTAGTAAkCeGkAe	rs2024115	93	53	D6	>1000	>1000	ND	Pass	-
C3	TeTkCkAAGCTAGTAAkCkGe	rs2024115	81	44	D6	>1000	538	>1.8	Pass	-
D2	CeAkCeAkGCTATCTTCTkCeAkTe	rs363088	63	32	D6	>1000	262	>3.8	-	-
D3	AeCkAkGCTATCTTCTkCkAe	rs363088	52	33	D6	>1000	185	>5.4	-	-
A4	AeAkTeAkAeATTGTCATCAeCeCeAeGe	rs7685686	20	6	D6	57	13	4.4	Pass	-
A5	AkAeTkAeAkATTGTCATCAkCeCkAeGk	rs7685686	27	9	D6	139	14	9.9	-	-
A6	AkATkAAkATTGTCATCAkCCkAGk	rs7685686	20	7	D6	57	7	8.1	Pass	-
A7	AeTkAkAkATTGTCATCAkCkCkAe	rs7685686	14	5	D6	46	11	4.2	-	-
A8	AkTeAkAkATTGTCATCAkCkCeAk	rs7685686	14	4	D6	64	14	4.6	-	-
A11	AeAkTkTkGTCATCACCAkGe	rs7685686	27	7	D6	149	11	13.5	-	-
A20	TkTeGTCATCACCAkGkAkAe	rs7685686	24	8	D6	207	23	9.0	-	-
A21	AeTkTGTCATCACCkAkGkAe	rs7685686	52	11	D6	>1000	48	>21	-	-
A22	AeAkTTGTCATCACkCkAkGe	rs7685686	61	18	D6	>1000	78	>12.9	Pass	**Pass**
A29	AeTeAeAeAeTTGTCATCeAeCeCeAe	rs7685686	82	52	D6	>1000	>1000	ND	Pass	-
A30	AkTkAkAkAkTTGTCATCkAkCkCkAk	rs7685686	70	20	D6	>1000	38	>26.3	-	-
A31	AeTeAeAeAkTkTGTCATCAkCkCeAe	rs7685686	78	18	D6	>1000	94	>10.6	-	-
A32	AeTkAeAkAeTkTGTCATCAkCeCkAe	rs7685686	63	24	D6	>1000	77	>13.0	-	-
A33	AeTeAeAeAkTTGTCATCAkCeCeAe	rs7685686	58	25	D6	>1000	74	>13.5	Pass	-
A34	AeTeAeAeAkTkTGTCATCAkCeCkAe	rs7685686	50	13	D6	>1000	18	>55.5	-	-
A35	TeAeAeAkTkTGTCATCAkCkCeAeGe	rs7685686	76	18	D6	>1000	42	>23.8	Pass	-
A36	TeAeAeAeTkTGTCATCAkCeCeAe	rs7685686	109	32	D6	>1000	254	>3.9	Pass	-
A37	TeAeAeAkTkTGTCATCAkCkCeAe	rs7685686	70	17	D6	>1000	67	>14.9	-	-
A38	AeTeAeAeAkTkTGTCATCAkCkCe	rs7685686	86	16	D6	>1000	31.9	>31.3	Pass	**Pass**
A39	TeAeAeAkTkTGTCATCAkCkCe	rs7685686	82	14	D6	>1000	38.4	>26.0	Pass	**Pass**
A40	TeAkAkATkTGTCATCAkCkCe	rs7685686	87	25	D6	>1000	121.9	>8.2	Pass	**Pass**
A41	TeAkAkAkTkTGTCATCAkCkCe	rs7685686	72	19	D6	>1000	44.6	>22.4	Pass	**Pass**
A38	AeTeAeAeAkTkTGTCATCAkCkCe	rs7685686	82	10	D10	>1000	16.1	>62.1	Pass	**Pass**
			71	7	D15	>1000	6.8	>147.1	Pass	
			72	17	D6High	>10000	77	>130.0	Pass	
A39	TeAeAeAkTkTGTCATCAkCkCe	rs7685686	63	9	D10	>1000	17.0	>58.8	Pass	**Pass**
			60	6	D15	>1000	9.8	>102	Pass	
			81	16	D6High	>10000	68	>147.1	Pass	
A40	TeAkAkATkTGTCATCAkCkCe	rs7685686	89	20	D10	>1000	52.7	>19.0	Pass	-
			63	9	D15	>1000	17.6	>66.8	-	

Table 1. Cont.

ASO	Notation	Rs #	Max effect		Day	IC50		Selectivity	Toxicity	Screen
			%wtHTT	%mHTT		wtHTT	mHTT			
			70	23	D6High	>10000	166.	>60.0	-	
A41	TeAkAkAkTkTGTCATCAkCkCe	rs7685686	79	12	D10	>1000	8.1	>123.5	-	-
			38	6	D15	632	5.6	113	-	
			53	15	D6High	8919	67	133	-	
X1	AeTeAeAeAkTkTGCCATCAkCkCe	rs7685686	97	35	D6	ND	150	ND	Pass	**Pass**
X2	TeAeAeAkTkTGCCATCAkCkCe	rs7685686	103	34	D6	ND	134	ND	Pass	**Pass**

MOE and cEt modifications are annotated by e and k, respectively. The SNP is underlined. Maximal effect at highest dose. IC50, half maximal inhibitory concentration (nM).

than to try to enhance the potency of a highly specific ASO. Therefore, for the ASO to move forward and pass this secondary screen, we focused on identifying tolerable oligos (no visual morphological changes and less than 3-fold induction of spectrin cleavage) with good potency ($IC_{50,mHTT}$<200 nM) and moderate specificity (>5 fold). The most promising ASO series: A1, A2, and A3, is shown as an example in figure 3. We found 40 and 10 fold increase in potency for A2 and A3, respectively, compared to A1 (Figure 3B). Since the specificity for A1 (>2.4) was calculated by using the highest dose tested, it cannot be directly compared to A2 and A3 that showed allele-specific silencing of mHTT by 8.2 and 8.9 fold respectively (Table 1). A2 exhibited above threshold spectrin cleavage and was excluded, whereas the shortest molecule of the series, A3, did not show overt toxicity (Figure 3C). The remaining ASOs did not pass our selection criteria (Table 1, Figure S5 and S6), and A3 was the only ASO of the eight evaluated candidates to move forward.

In parallel, we wanted to investigate whether adding additional cEt modification to the wings of the ASO would lead to improvement in potency and specificity. To evaluate this, while maintaining the 9-base gap, three 19mer oligos, A4, A5, and A6, based on A1 were evaluated. First, we added two cEt modifications to the 5' wing (A4; ekeke-9-5e) while keeping the 3' wing only modified with MOE chemistry. Next, we mixed the modifications in both wings (A5; kekek-9-kekek), and finally replaced the MOE modifications with unmodified PS deoxynucleotides (represented by "d") and alternating cEt modifications (A6; kdkdk-9-kdkdk). All ASOs displayed excellent potency ($IC_{50,mHTT}$<14 nM) (Table 1). A4 showed reduced specificity compared to A3, whereas A5 and A6 showed comparable specificity of 9.9 and 8.1 fold, respectively. For A5 the small increase in potency and specificity unfortunately came at the cost of spectrin cleavage above threshold (Figure S7). Lastly, we evaluated two ASOs, A7 and A8, based on A2. While A2 did not meet the tolerability criteria from the previous screen, it demonstrated extremely high potency, which is an attractive property for a potential therapeutic. Greater potency translates to lower therapeutic doses, thus reducing cost and potentially reducing side effects. ASOs A7 and A8 were generated in an effort to determine if changes to the wing motif could mitigate the toxic effects of A2 while maintaining the superior potency. First, one cEt modification was added to each wing (A7; ekkk-9-kkke) and from this design the MOE and the cEt modifications were switched in each wing (A8; kekk-9-kkek). The two ASOs, A7 and A8, had a similar profile to the parent molecule, A2, displaying excellent potency ($IC_{50,mHTT}$<14 nM), but with a small reduction in specificity (4.2 and 4.6 fold). Both ASOs induced spectrin

cleavage above threshold and were therefore excluded. The strategy of changing and rearranging modifications of the wings with MOE and cEt nucleotides did not provide an ASO with a better profile than A3. Overall, our primary screen identified one tolerable candidate, A3, with good potency and moderate specificity. While it did not demonstrate the best specificity, we thought it would be easier to improve specificity with chemical modification than to improve potency. A3 was therefore used as the parent molecule for the subsequent SAR studies.

SNP Microwalk SAR

We have previously demonstrated that RNase H cleaves to the 5'-ASO/3'-RNA side of the SNP [34]. However, it is not completely clear whether the localization of the SNP position within the gap affects potency and specificity when it is moved towards either the 5' or 3' end of the molecule. This effect could presumably depend on the interaction between the ASO:RNA duplex and the RNase H enzyme. According to the crystal structure of RNase H, the enzyme makes extensive contact with the RNA:ASO heteroduplex at the 5'-RNA/3'-ASO side of the cleavage site on the RNA strand [57]. Therefore, we sought to determine if an asymmetrical wing design, providing higher affinity at either of the wings, could improve the ASO profile. First, using A3 as the parent molecule, we moved one cEt modification to the 5' wing (ekkk-9-ke) and then in turn moved the SNP site from position 4 to 14 across the gap (Figure 4A). Similarly, we moved one cEt modification to the 3' wing (ek-9-kkke) and then in turn moved the SNP site from position 2 to 12 across the gap of the ASO (Figure 4B). These 20 ASOs were first tested in a preliminary screen in primary human fibroblasts using a heterozygous cell line derived from an HD patient with the appropriate genotype at the relevant SNPs [33,44]. The fibroblast cell line was treated at a single dose of 2 µM, and HTT mRNA suppression was evaluated using a SNP-based qPCR assay. We found a clear correlation between the position of the SNP and the potency of the ASO. Moving the SNP position towards the 3' end of the gap resulted in loss of potency, whereas moving the SNP position towards the 5' end of the gap maintained potency and specificity. This was consistent between both asymmetrical wing designs (Figure 4A and B and table S1).

To investigate these preliminary findings in more detail, we selected a subset of the ASOs with favourable properties, including A11, A20, A21, and A22, to be tested for potency, specificity, and toxicity in primary neurons (Figure 4C and D). Our aim was to identify ASOs with similar or better potency and greater specificity than our parent ASO, A3. The most active ASO, A23, showed

A

5′ Wing   **ASO**   **3′ Wing**

$X_1X_2X_3X_4X_5X_6X_7X_8X_9\underline{X_{10}}X_{11}X_{12}X_{13}X_{14}X_{15}X_{16}X_{17}X_{18}X_{19}$

↓

$X_1X_2X_3X_4X_5X_6X_7X_8\underline{X_9}X_{10}X_{11}X_{12}X_{13}X_{14}X_{15}X_{16}X_{17}$

↓

$X_1X_2X_3X_4X_5X_6X_7\underline{X_8}X_9X_{10}X_{11}X_{12}X_{13}X_{14}X_{15}$

Modified wing   Unmodified Gap   Modified wing
(RNase resistant)   9 nucleotides   (RNase resistant)
                       (RNase H cleavage)

Methoxyethyl (MOE)   **Constrained Ethyl (cEt)**

Increases RNA binding and stability

B

A1   **A2**   **A3**

AATAAATTGTCATCACCAG   ATAAATTGTCATCACCA   TAAATTGTCATCACC

C

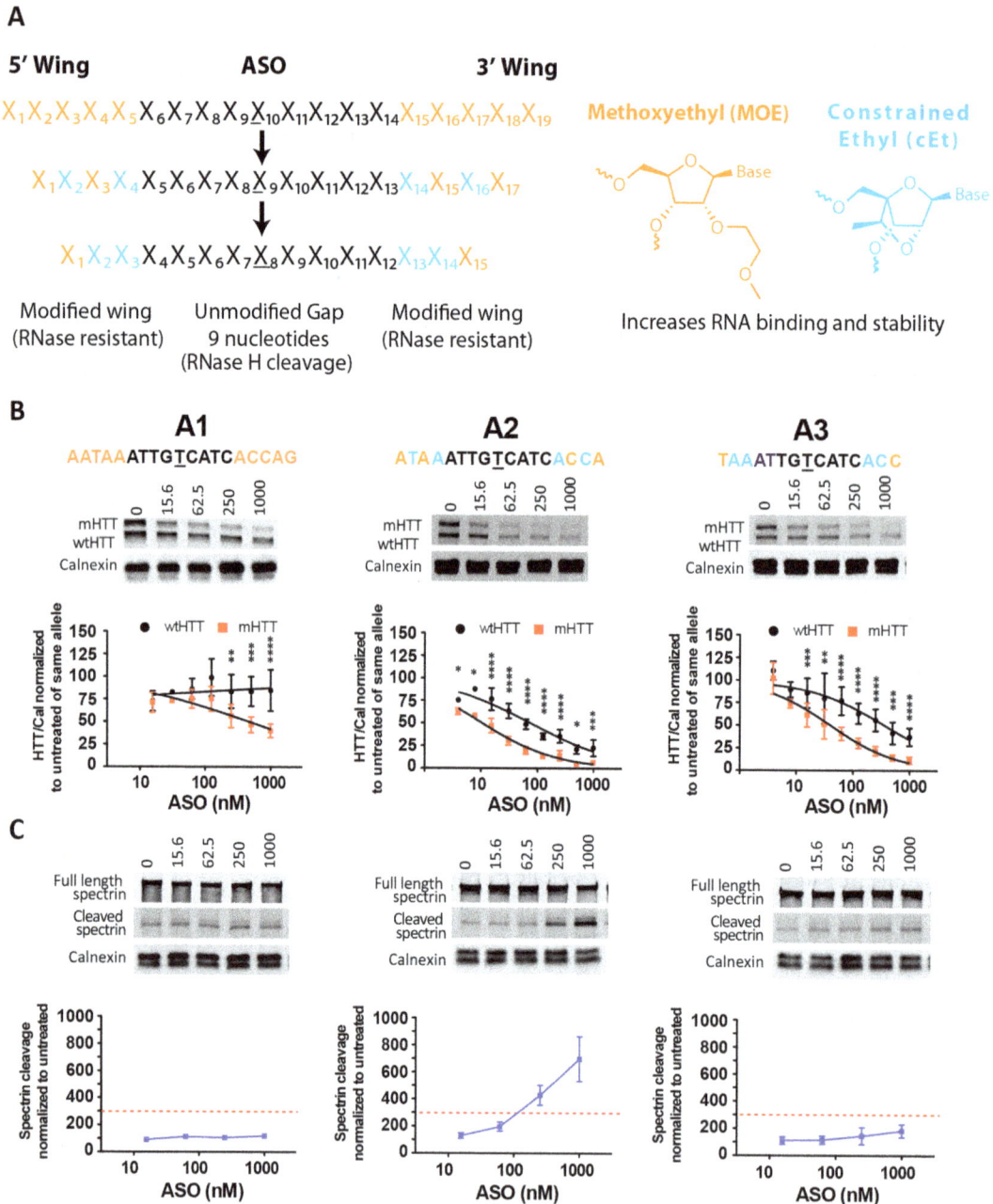

Figure 3. ASO screen at 4 SNPs using two different cEt motifs. (A) ASOs with two different cEt-modified wing motifs (ekek-9-keke and ekk-9-kke) were compared to the parent MOE oligos (5e-9-5e). Primary Hu97/18 neurons were treated with ASO at 1–1000 nM for 6 days. (B) HTT Western blot and quantitations. HTT levels are normalized to the internal loading control calnexin and then to the untreated sample for each allele. (C) Western blots showing full length and cleaved spectrin. Spectrin fragment is normalized to calnexin and then to the untreated sample. Membranes were probed for HTT and reprobed for spectrin. Representative images are shown. n = 6–8 per data point. Data are presented as mean ± SD. Two way ANOVA with Bonferroni post hoc test have been performed and p values are illustrated with *, **, ***, **** for p = 0.05, 0.01, 0.001, and 0.0001. The PS backbone is black, MOE and cEt modifications are illustrated by orange and blue, respectively. The SNP is underlined. The red dashed line represents the toxicity threshold.

better knock down of mHTT, but also greater knock down of wtHTT compared to A3, so it was not selected. A20 demonstrated the second greatest knock down of mHTT of the set and less knock down of wtHTT and was therefore chosen. The SNP positions for A21 and A22 were moved one nucleotide relative to A20. These oligos were marginally less potent, but slightly more specific and were selected for protein validation as well. A11 had an identical gap to the most promising ASO, A20, with the wing asymmetry

reversed, and was therefore included to investigate the effect of wing chemistry. The four ASOs had IC$_{50}$ values for mHTT from 11–78 nM, which is comparable to previously evaluated ASOs, suggesting that the number of modifications is more important than their distribution (Table 1). We did find an overall improvement in specificity for the four ASOs; ranging from 9 to more than 21 fold, suggesting that positioning the SNP nearer to the 5′ wing may be beneficial to specificity. However, since the

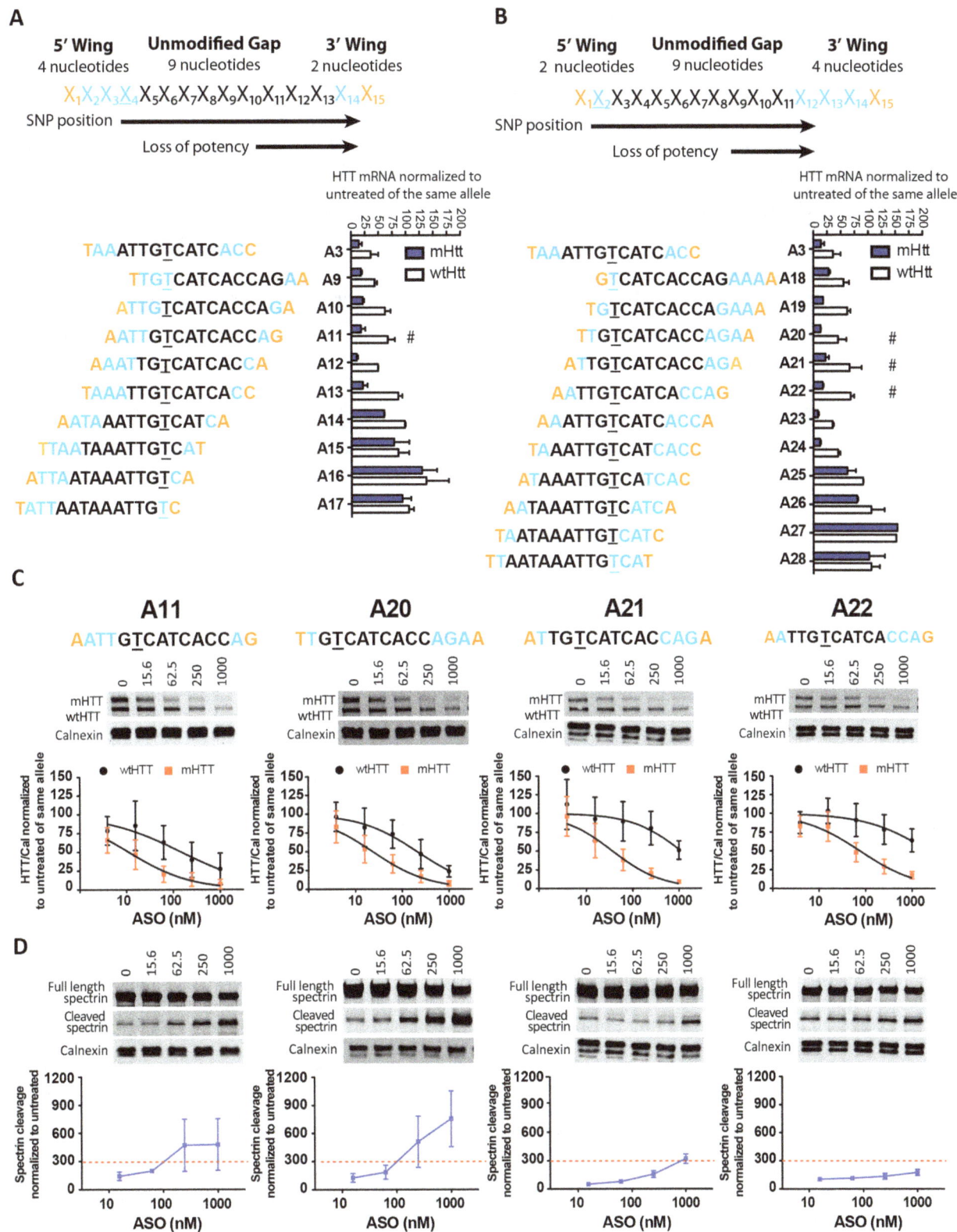

Figure 4. Microwalk of the SNP position within the gap. (A, B) Diagram of microwalk ASOs and HTT mRNA silencing in primary human HD fibroblasts. (A) Starting from A3, we moved one cEt modification to the 5′ wing (ekkk-9-ke) and moved the SNP site from position 4 to 14 (B) Similarly, we moved one cEt modification to the 3′ wing (ek-9-kkke) and moved the SNP site from position 2 to 12. mHTT and wtHTT mRNA were normalized to total RNA and then to the untreated sample. n = 2 per data point. A subset of ASOs from preliminary fibroblast screen marked by #, were evaluated in primary Hu97/18 neurons at 4–1000 nM for 6 days. (C) Western blots of HTT protein and quantitations. HTT levels are normalized to the internal loading control calnexin and then to the untreated sample for each allele. (D) Western blots showing full length and cleaved spectrin. Spectrin fragment is normalized to calnexin and then to the untreated sample. Membranes were probed for HTT and reprobed for spectrin. Representative images are shown. n = 6–10 per data point. Data are presented as mean ± SD. Two way ANOVA with Bonferroni post hoc test have been performed

and p values are illustrated with *, **, ***, **** for p = 0.05, 0.01, 0.001, and 0.0001. The PS backbone is black, MOE and cEt modifications are illustrated by orange and blue, respectively. The SNP is underlined. The red dashed line represents the toxicity threshold.

motif of the chemical modifications is different from A3, the improvement may be a combination of the two factors. ASOs A11, A20, and A21 were excluded due to increased spectrin cleavage above threshold, whereas ASO A22 was well tolerated. ASO 22 showed potency in the upper end of the range ($IC_{50,mHTT}$ = 78 nM) with robust specificity (>13 fold). However, at the highest dose of 1000 nM, A22 did cause a significant reduction in wtHTT expression of approximately 40%. Considering these data, the microwalk strategy did not provide sufficient improvement to specificity, and we therefore decided to move forward with investigation of shortening the gap of the oligo.

Shortening the gap and length of the ASO

It is well described that RNase H cleaves within the sequence of the mRNA matching the gap of the ASO [58]. Therefore, the longer the gap, the more potential secondary sites are available for cleavage. Our group has previously demonstrated that shortening the gap of the ASO can increase specificity of mHTT mRNA knock down in human fibroblasts [34]. Here, we sought to validate these findings in a system that is more relevant to the brain by both evaluating protein knock down and toxicity after ASO treatment in primary neurons. Therefore, to increase specificity by preventing secondary cleavage events, we shortened the gap from 9 to 7 bases (Figure 5A) and synthesized a panel of 15-, 16-, and 17-oligomers (A29-A41) with different chemical wing motifs (Table 1). First, we tested A29 and A30, which have either five MOE or five cEt modifications in both wings, respectively. Exclusively using MOE modifications was not sufficient to achieve adequate suppression with a shorter oligo, whereas using full cEt wings resulted in high potency ($IC_{50,mHTT}$ = 38 nM) and specificity (>26 fold). Unfortunately, A30 induced spectrin cleavage indicating that full cEt wings are not well tolerated for this specific sequence. Screening the remaining panel of ASOs, we found oligos with pronounced specificity (>56 fold) and high potency ($IC_{50,mHTT}$ values as low as 18 nM). However, the longer cEt modified ASOs (three out of five) were associated with toxicity, whereas the shorter oligos appeared more well tolerated with only one out of five inducing significant spectrin cleavage at the highest dose tested (Figure S8 and S9). Furthermore, the shorter oligos, including A38, A39, A40, and A41 showed minimal silencing of wtHTT across the doses (0–1000 nM) tested for the full panel of oligos (Figure 5B and Figure S8). Here, we confirm that by shortening the PS DNA gap, we can improve allele specificity without compromising potency or tolerability in a system pertinent to the brain.

Based on studies in non-human primates, it has become apparent that after intrathecal delivery, ASO concentration may differ significantly between areas close to or in direct contact with the cerebrospinal fluid, compared to the deeper structures of the brain [23]. Hence, it is fundamental to have a large therapeutic window, where the ASOs will be efficacious, non-toxic, and still remain specific for the mutant allele. Therefore, we wanted to determine the maximal dose of ASO that could be applied to primary neurons without overt toxicity and with minimal knock down of wtHTT. We treated primary neurons with our four lead ASO candidates at concentrations of up to 10,000 nM (Figure 5B). At the highest dose we observed spectrin cleavage just above threshold for ASO A41, whereas no spectrin cleavage above threshold was seen for ASOs A38, A39, and A40. Treatment with ASO A41 resulted in a 50% reduction of wtHTT at the highest

dose used, whereas ASOs A38, A39 and A40 showed impressive specificity of 130, 147, and 60 fold, respectively, with only minimal reduction in wtHTT at extremely high doses of ASOs (Table 1). These findings demonstrate a great therapeutic window with more than 50% knock down of mHTT and a minimal effect on wtHTT levels over more than two log scale intervals.

Since ASOs have a relatively long tissue half-life [59], it is important that specificity is maintained over time. To investigate this, we extended the treatment duration from 6 days to 10 and 15 days. As expected with longer treatment duration, increased suppression of mHTT was observed for all ASOs tested. Nonlinear regression demonstrates that IC_{50} values for lowering of mHTT decrease with longer treatment durations (A38; $IC_{50,mHTT}$ 32>16>7; A39; $IC_{50,mHTT}$ 38>17>10; A40; A41; $IC_{50,mHTT}$ 45>8>6). Despite increased activity, specificity of mHTT silencing was maintained over increased treatment durations for 3 of 4 leads. ASOs A38, A39, and A40 showed minimal silencing of wtHTT, whereas there was greater reduction in wtHTT levels after longer treatments with A41 (Figure 6 and Table 1).

To further improve the sensitivity of our triage, we wanted to explore if longer treatment durations would reveal subtle differences in tolerability. We observed increased cleavage of spectrin after 10 days of treatment with ASO A41 and after 15 days of treatment with either A40 or A41 (Figure 7), indicating that these two ASOs are not well tolerated over long treatment durations. We did not observe cleavage of spectrin above threshold for A38 and A39 after the extended treatment durations. These comprehensive analyses allowed us to characterize subtle differences between the four candidate ASOs and identify ASOs A38 and A39 as the most promising leads.

Targeting both alleles at a single HD-SNP could provide a therapy to all HD patients

The steps described here are the initial process towards the construction of a panel of ASOs to provide allele-specific silencing to the majority of HD patients. However, it will take time to achieve this goal and meanwhile all therapeutic options should be considered for the remaining HD patients until this panel is established. We have previously observed that 10.7% (7 out of 65) of HD patients are homozygous at 22 genotyped SNPs [44] and would not be treatable allele-specifically with ASOs targeted to those sites. To further investigate and substantiate these findings, we have analysed genotypes from an expanded panel of 91 SNPs [33], and similarly find that 11.5% (27 out of 234) of patients are homozygous at the SNPs tested in this assay. These data illustrate the need for an alternative approach for this group until additional allele-specific targets may be identified.

Our lead ASO candidates such as A38 or A39 that target rs7685686_A, could provide an allele-specific therapeutic option for 48.7% of the sequenced HD population [33]. Using our custom SNP genotyping assay data, we show that 44.9% of HD patients are homozygous at this SNP having an adenine on both alleles (rs7685686_A/A) (Figure 8A). Therefore, our ASOs targeting rs7685686_A could potentially provide a treatment option for a total of 93.6% of all HD patients, where approximately half would be allele-specific and the other half would be non-allele specific. Among the remaining 6.4% of the HD population, we find that 3.8% are heterozygous, with a guanine on the mutant allele and an adenine on the wt allele (rs7685686_G/A), and 2.6% are homozygous with a guanine on

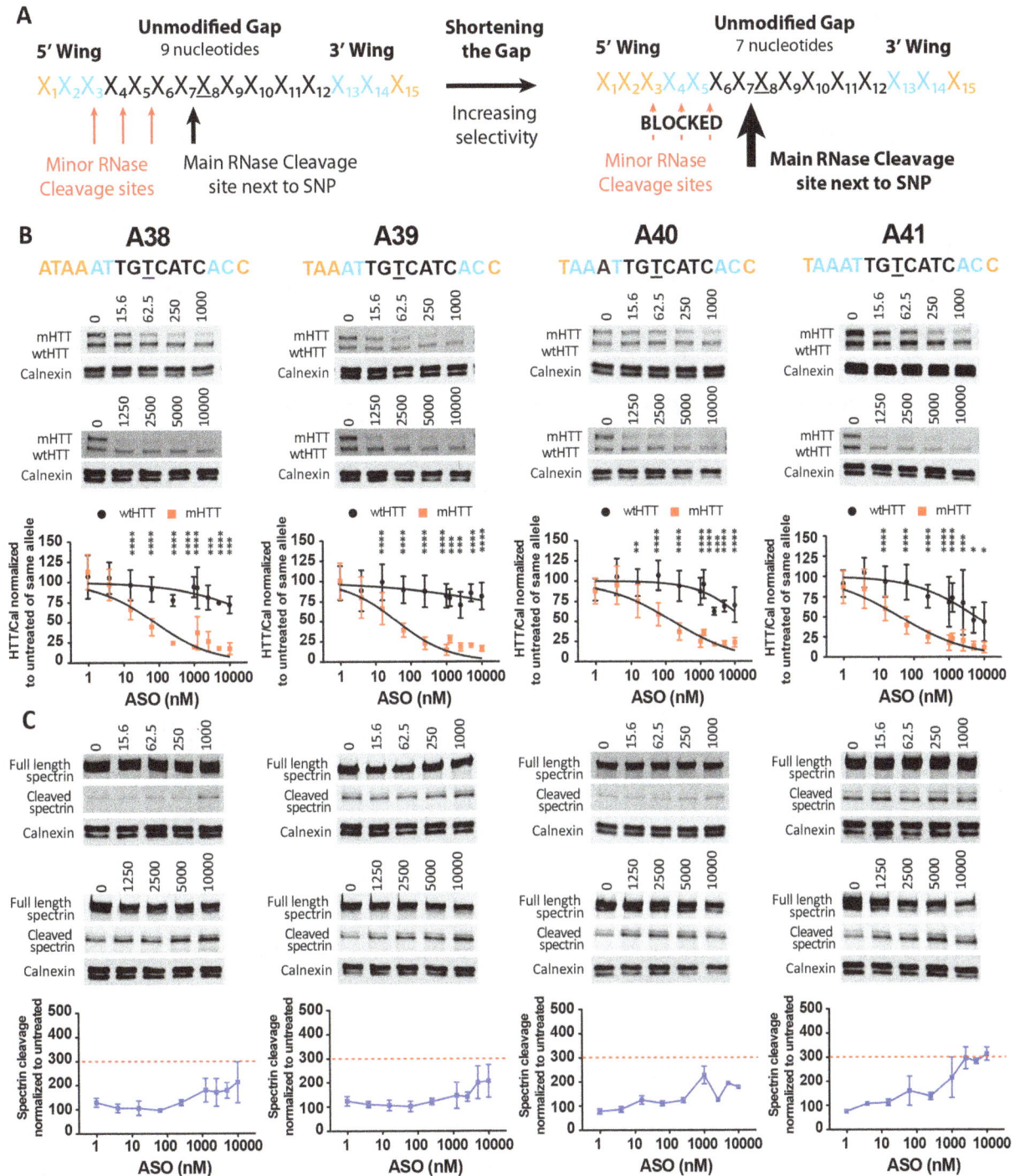

Figure 5. Shortening the gap to 7 nucleotides and evaluation at higher doses. (A) Replacing PS-nucleotides with RNase H resistant chemical modifications and shortening the gap from 9 to 7 nucleotides. The top 4 candidates are shown. Primary Hu97/18 neurons were treated with ASO at 1–10000 nM for 6 days. (B) Western blot and quantitation of HTT protein levels. HTT levels are normalized to the internal loading control calnexin and then to the untreated sample for each allele. (C) Western blots showing full length and cleaved spectrin. Spectrin fragment is normalized to calnexin and then to the untreated sample. Membranes were probed for HTT and reprobed for spectrin. Representative images are shown. n = 8–14 per data point at 0–1000 nM and n = 4–6 at 1250–10,000 nM. Data are presented as mean ± SD. Two way ANOVA with Bonferroni post hoc test have been performed and p values are illustrated with *, **, ***, **** for p = 0.05, 0.01, 0.001, and 0.0001. The PS backbone is black, MOE and cEt modifications are illustrated by orange and blue, respectively. The SNP is underlined. The red dashed line represents the toxicity threshold.

both alleles (rs7685686_G/G). Our lead ASOs targeting the adenine allele would not provide a therapeutic option for this minority of patients. Therefore, we investigated if ASOs analogous to A38 and A39 but having thymine exchanged for cytosine at the SNP position would be active against rs7685686_G (Figure 8B). To screen these oligos in an appropriate system, we used primary

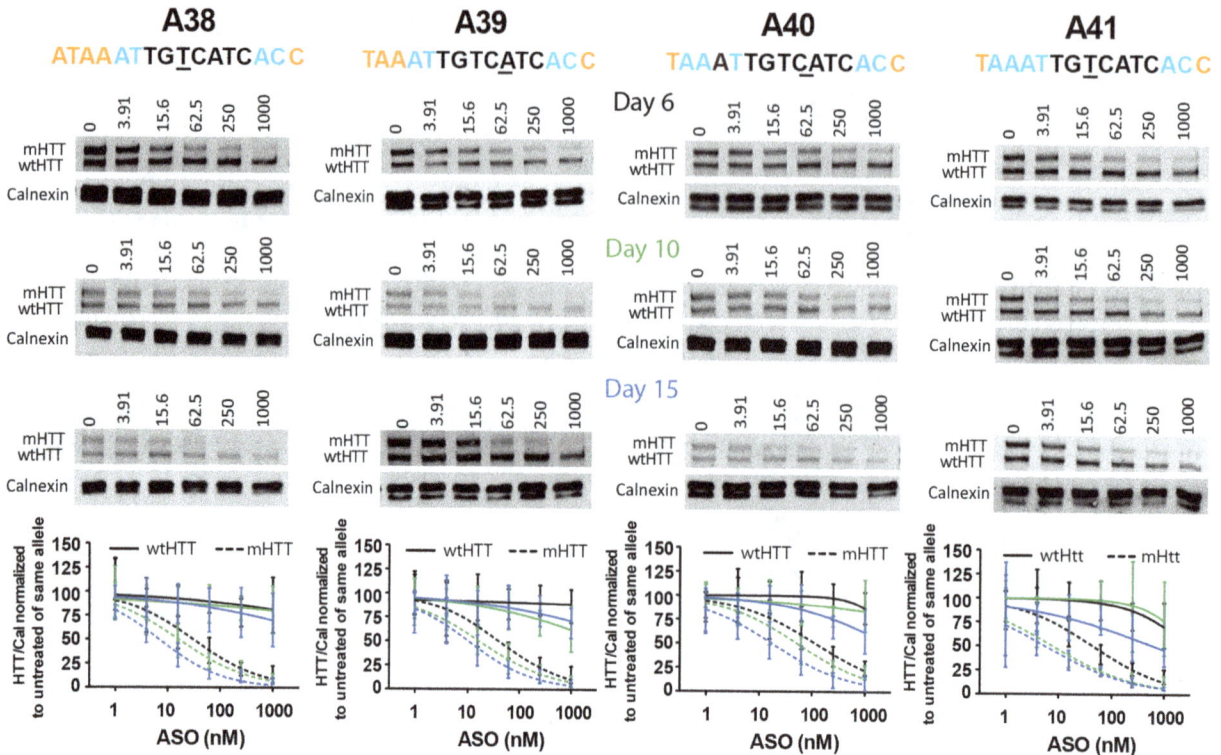

Figure 6. Increased potency with extended treatment duration. Primary Hu97/18 neurons were treated with ASO at 1–1000 nM for 6, 10, or 15 days. Western blot and quantitation of HTT protein levels. HTT levels are normalized to the internal loading control calnexin and then to the untreated sample for each allele. Representative images are shown. HTT protein levels (wtHTT = solid line, mHTT = dotted line) at day 6 (black), 10 (green), and 15 (blue). Data are presented as mean $\pm$ SD. n = 6–12 per data point. The IC_{50} values were compared using the extra-sum-of-squares F test and the F distribution and degrees of freedom F (DFn, DFd) and the associated p-values have been calculated. A38: day 6 vs. 10 $F_{(1,106)} = 7.254$, $P < 0.0082$; day 6 vs. 15 $F_{(1,109)} = 51.51$, $P < 0.0001$; day 10 vs. 15 $F_{(1,99)} = 18.88$, $P < 0.0001$; A39: $IC_{50,mHTT}$ 38 > 17 > 10; day 6 vs. 10 $F_{(1,115)} = 13.94$, $P < 0.0003$; day 6 vs. 15 $F_{(1,98)} = 25.06$, $P < 0.0001$; day 10 vs. 15 $F_{(1,21)} = 5.625$, $P < 0.0193$); A40: $IC_{50,mHTT}$ 122 > 53 > 18, day 6 vs. 10 $F_{(1,67)} = 6.030$, $P < 0.0167$; day 6 vs. 15 $F_{(1,58)} = 30.25$, $P < 0.0001$; day 10 vs. 15 $F_{(1,61)} = 12.68$, $P < 0.0007$); A41: $IC_{50,mHTT}$ 45 > 8 > 6; day 6 vs. 10 $F_{(1,85)} = 66.19$, $P < 0.0001$; day 6 vs. 15 $F_{(1,76)} = 47.82$, $P < 0.0001$; day 10 vs. 15 $F_{(1,79)} = 1.258$, $P < 0.2655$). The PS backbone is black, MOE and cEt modifications are illustrated by orange and blue, respectively. The SNP is underlined.

neurons from YAC128 mice, which carry a mutant human transgene with the guanine genotype at rs7685686 and endogenous murine Hdh gene. Because the endogenous murine Hdh genes do not share any sequence similarity to human HTT around this SNP site, we were unable to evaluate specificity and instead focused on potency and tolerability. As previously, neurons were treated with ASOs for 6 days and protein was collected for analysis. We found increased knock down of mHTT with increasing dose of ASO and, as expected, no change in the levels of endogenous murine Htt (Figure 8B). Similar to their analogs, ASOs X1 and X2 did not induce spectrin cleavage above threshold (Figure 8C). However, ASO X1 and X2 had slightly higher IC_{50} values for mHTT (150 and 134 nM, respectively) than was observed for A38 and A39, which demonstrates the impact of changing one of the 15 or 16 nucleotides in the oligo (Table 1). These ASOs provide an excellent starting point for additional SAR studies to identify ASOs targeting rs7685686_G with properties similar to ASOs A38 and A39.

Discussion

We have established a pipeline that enables us to assess the ASO activity at multiple SNP targets and further discriminate between safe and toxic oligos in a system relevant to the brain. We have identified lead ASO candidates for in vivo validation and

demonstrated that targeting two allelic variants of a single HD-SNP can be used as a therapeutic option, either allele-specific or non-specific, for all carriers of the HD mutation, using two distinct ASO drugs till additional allele-specific SNPs and supplementary ASOs are identified and developed.

Screening pipeline

Primary neurons with the appropriate genetic background including human transgenic wt and mutant HTT and without the presence of endogenous murine Htt are an ideal system for rapid *in vitro* screening of gene silencing drugs for the brain. The use of primary neurons allow us to screen for the potency and allele-specificity of a large number of ASO modifications against a great number of SNP targets, and test a wide range of ASO concentrations (0–10,000 nM), which is one to two orders of magnitude higher than other current screening systems [27,36,60,61]. Furthermore, this system provides a sensitive way to exclude toxic ASOs before they go into pre-clinical animal studies resulting in increased efficiency and reduced research costs. Providing availability of genetically appropriate mouse models, this screening approach would be amendable to other dominant monogenetic neurological disorders and can be adapted for screening ASOs, RNAi or other SNP based therapies.

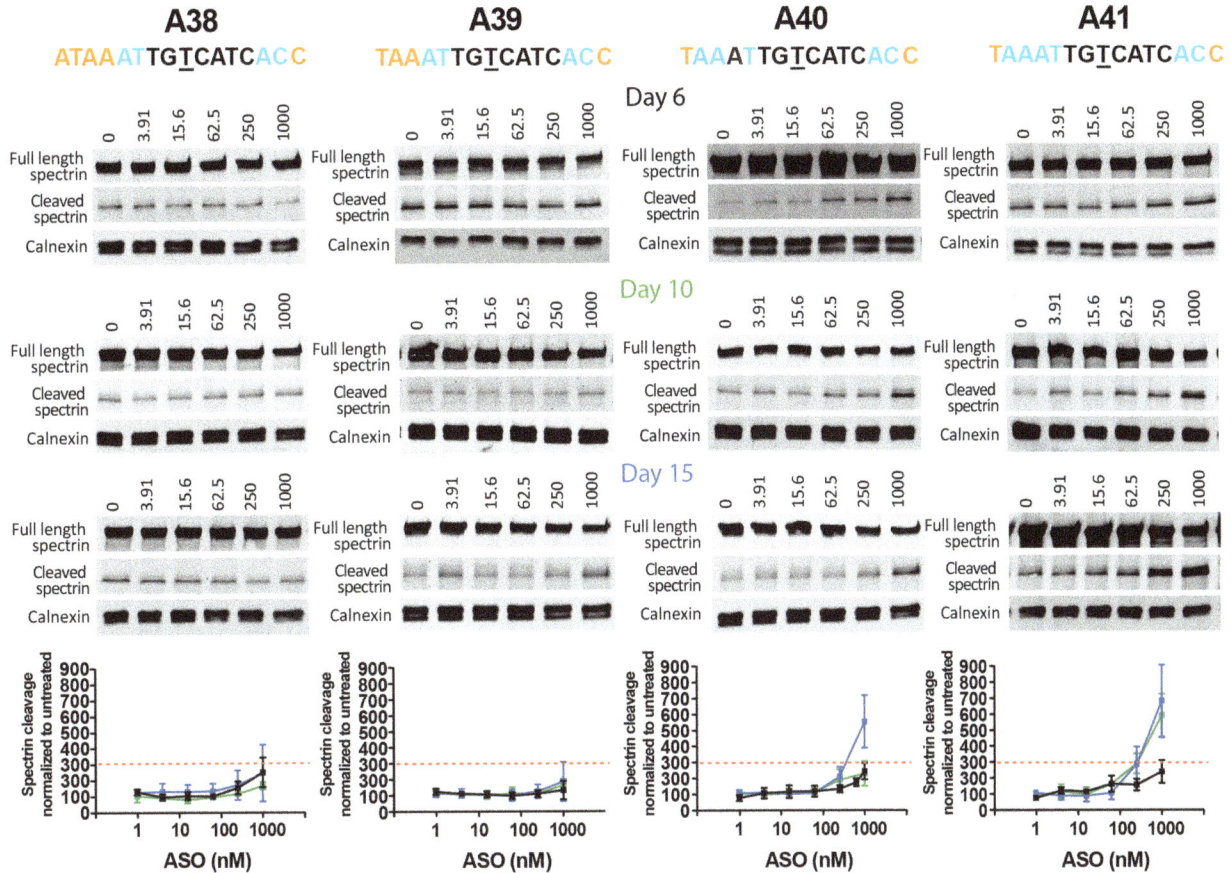

Figure 7. Spectrin cleavage after extended treatment duration. Primary Hu97/18 neurons were treated with ASO at 1–1000 nM for 6, 10, or 15 days. Western blots showing full length spectrin and cleaved spectrin (120 kDa) after 6 (black), 10 (green), and 15 (blue) days of treatment. Spectrin fragment is normalized to calnexin and then to the untreated sample. HTT membranes were reprobed for spectrin. Representative images are shown. Data are presented as mean ± SD with n=6–12 per data point. The PS backbone is black, MOE and cEt modifications are illustrated by orange and blue, respectively. The SNP is underlined. The red dashed line represents the toxicity threshold.

ASO design

Our data demonstrate that initially selecting multiple sites for evaluation is critical, since ASOs at all SNP sites are not equally active. This is most likely caused by secondary and tertiary RNA structures that can either prevent binding of the oligo to the target RNA or sterically hinder the recruitment of the RNase-H enzyme to the ASO:RNA duplex [62,63]. After identifying the SNP sites (rs7685686, rs4690072, rs2024115, rs363088) where the ASOs show the most activity, we have evaluated several ASO design strategies to facilitate potent and specific silencing of mHTT. We find that the incorporation of cEt-modified nucleotides dramatically improves potency (e.g. A29 vs. A30). However, we have not been able to clearly establish a consensus motif for wing modification that is superior to others tested. Similarly, we have not clearly isolated the individual factors that affect the safety profile of the ASO, which are comprised of multiple elements including the target, the length and sequence, and the modification motif of the wings. However, we have established that shorter oligos are generally better tolerated. We have corroborated that shortening the gap region increases specificity dramatically by decreasing the number of potential secondary RNase cleavage sites. Furthermore, our investigations have shown that there is some flexibility for the SNP position within the gap of the ASO. The SNP can be moved from the center towards the 5′ wing while maintaining potency and specificity, which allows for microwalk-

ing and identification of ASOs with a potentially better tolerability profile.

After improving the ASO design and incorporating cEt modifications in combination with MOE chemistry, we find the potency of our ASOs to be in the lower nanomolar range comparable to what has been observed in other *in vitro* systems using SiRNA, LNA oligos, single-stranded RNA, unmodified or modified RNA duplexes [27,28,36,37,61]. However, a direct comparison is not completely possible, since the actual intracellular concentration of drug will depend on delivery method e.g. free uptake versus transfection or electroporation. Furthermore, the potency will be contingent on the treatment duration and whether protein or RNA are used as a readout. Similarly, these variables in addition to the maximal concentration of drug being used may also affect the calculated specificity. Several research groups have shown promising results targeting the CAG expansion in a cell line from a juvenile HD patient (CAG 69/17) with specificity ranging from 30–71 fold. However, when using these drugs in cell lines with CAG expansions that are more representative of the general HD population (CAG 44/15, 44/21, and 47/18), specificity decreases, and there is loss of close to 50% of wtHTT expression [27,38,42]. Østergaard et al. have previously shown great specificity of >133 fold at the RNA level when targeting HD-SNPs in fibroblasts. In this study, we have found specificity of >147 fold at the protein level in primary

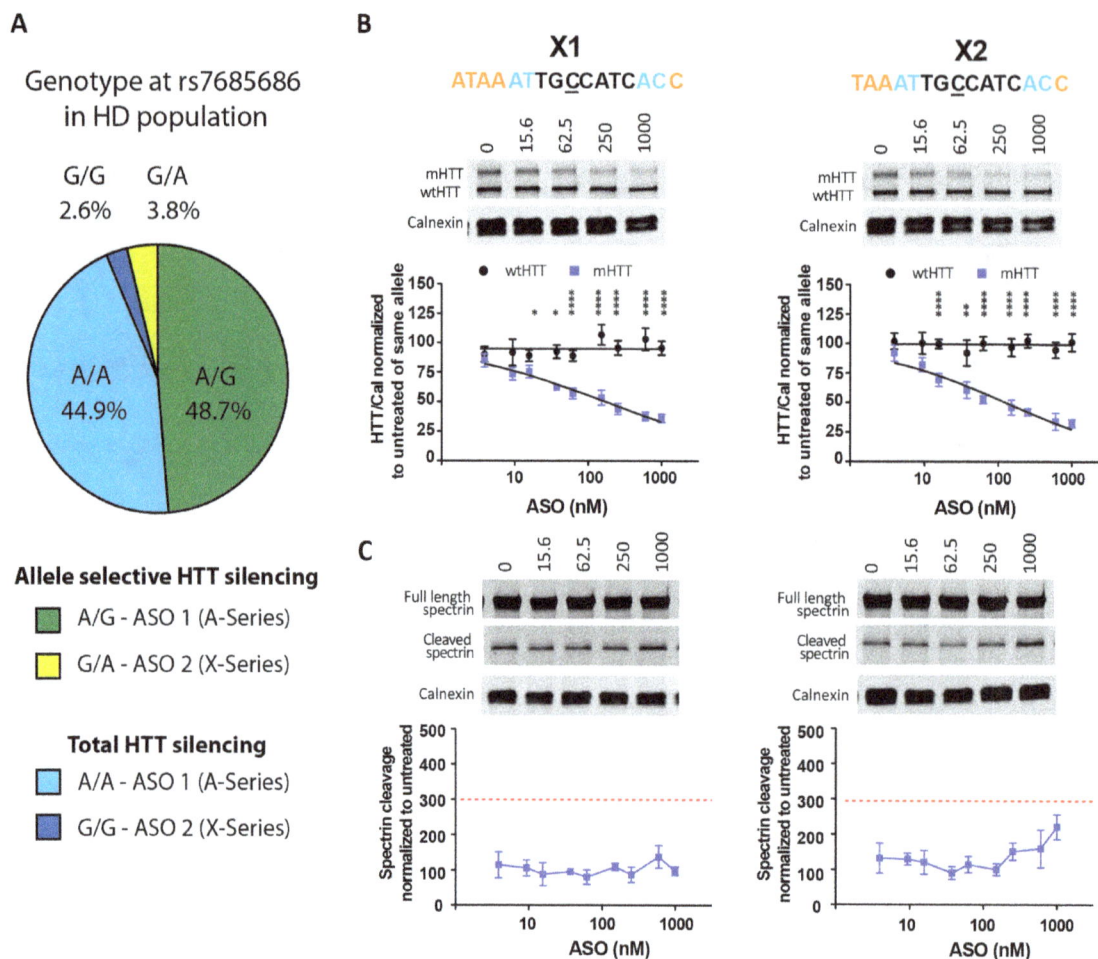

Figure 8. Targeting two variants of a single HD-SNP to provide a therapeutic option to all HD patients. (A) The genotypes for the sequenced HD population at rs7685686. Green = heterozygous HD population (rs7685686_A/G, 48.7%, targetable by A-series ASOs and rs7685686_G/A, 3.8%, targetable by X-series ASOs). Blue = homozygous HD population (rs7685686_A/A, 44.9%, targetable by A-series ASOs and rs7685686_G/G, 2.6%, targetable by X-series ASOs). Primary YAC128 neurons were treated with ASO at 16–1000 nM for 6 days. (B) Western blot and quantitation of HTT protein levels. HTT levels are normalized to the internal loading control calnexin and then to the untreated sample for each allele. (C) Western blots showing full length and cleaved spectrin. Spectrin fragment is normalized to calnexin and then to the untreated sample. Membranes were probed for HTT and reprobed for spectrin. Representative images are shown. n = 8–12 per data point. Data are presented as mean ± SD. Two way ANOVA with Bonferroni post hoc test have been performed and p values are illustrated with *, **, ***, **** for p = 0.05, 0.01, 0.001, and 0.0001. The PS backbone is represented by black. MOE and cEt modifications are illustrated by orange and blue, respectively. The SNP is underlined. The red dashed line represents the toxicity threshold.

neurons with negligible effect on wtHTT levels, which is a substantial improvement compared to most previously published studies for both SNP-targeted as well as CAG-targeted approaches suppressing mHTT protein expression [30–32,34]. Importantly, these findings are achieved without any carrier or delivery vehicle, since the ASOs are freely taken up by the neurons. We have developed two very strong lead ASOs, with low nanomolar IC_{50} values by free uptake into primary neuronal cells and impressive specificity, against rs7685686_A suitable for *in vivo* validation. Furthermore, our findings provide some insight into advantageous oligo design that can be used as a starting point for sequential screening of secondary and tertiary ASO candidates.

A therapeutic option to all HD patients

The steps described here are the initial process towards the long term goal of constructing a panel of ASOs to provide allele-specific silencing to all HD patients. We are currently in the process of re-populating our ASO pipeline using relevant HD-SNP targets that

will add additional patient coverage. We believe that screening at these complementary sites will be faster and more efficient using information garnered from this screen. Despite this increased efficiency, building a full panel of allele-specific ASOs will take significant time. Another concern that has been raised is that some people with HD may not currently be targetable with this approach. Previous genetic population studies indicate that a minority of HD patients are homozygous at all investigated HD-SNPs. Warby et al. explored a panel of 22 SNPs and found that 7 out of 67 HD patients were homozygous at these SNPs [44]. Similarly, Pfister et al. assessed 22 SNPs (18 differed from the Warby panel) in 109 patients and found that the maximal percentage of patients with at least one heterozygous SNP reached a plateau at approximately 80% [32]. This study does not provide the actual number of homozygous patients, but it can be inferred that about a fifth of patients in this study are homozygous at the 22 genotyped SNPs. To substantiate these findings, we analysed an expanded panel of 91 SNPs in 234 patients and found that 11.5%

are homozygous at the 91 SNPs in this panel [33]. These findings taken together demonstrate that we need to identify novel HD-SNPs to provide an allele-specific therapeutic option to the group of patients that are homozygous at all assayed SNPs. During the time it takes to define and validate new targets and develop new ASOs, alternative strategies have to be employed to provide the best outcome for all patients and to make sure that some therapeutic options is available to all patients. As previously mentioned, there are concerns with non-specific HTT knock down, as we cannot fully comprehend the consequences of loss of wtHTT function in the adult human brain over longer terms. However, if intermittent or short term non-specific ASO treatment could provide benefit for HD patients during the development of complementary allele-specific ASOs, it would be worth considering.

As a start, our lead ASOs targeting rs7685686_A, could provide an allele-specific therapeutic option for 48.7% of HD patients. In addition, they could provide a non-specific HTT silencing option for 44.9% of HD patients that are homozygous (rs7685686_A/A). This means that one of our lead ASOs could potentially provide a therapeutic option to 93.6% of people with HD. Since, we have found that rs7685686 is an accessible SNP site, we have explored the possibility of targeting the opposite allele at the same SNP site (e.g. 'G' vs. 'A') to provide a therapeutic option for the remaining 6.4% of patients. Targeting rs7685686_G would provide an allele-specific therapeutic option to 3.8% and a non-allele-specific option to 2.6% of HD patients.

With this strategy in mind, we designed two ASOs, X1 and X2, that are analogous to our leads, A38 and A39, and evaluated them in primary neurons from YAC128 mice. ASOs X1 and X2 showed good activity ($IC_{50, mHTT}$ of 150 and 134 nM) and were well tolerated in our screens. Overall, these findings show that two ASOs targeted to the two allelic variants of a single SNP could provide a therapeutic option for all HD patients, where roughly half would receive an allele-specific therapy and the remaining patients would receive a non-specific therapy. This strategy could potentially provide benefit during the time it takes to develop a complete allele-specific ASO panel. While there are safety concerns for long-term reduction of wtHTT, in short term, a non-specific HTT silencing therapy would likely be preferable to untreated HD.

Translation of in vitro ASO screen

We have previously demonstrated that our in vitro findings translate well to the brains of transgenic mice [33,34]. Here we show that our lead oligos, A38 and A39, induce robust suppression of mHTT while maintaining great specificity over more than two log scale intervals (100–10,000 nM). This large therapeutic window will be essential for successful in vivo efficacy and tolerability studies, since it has become apparent that therapeutic doses of ASOs delivered via the cerebrospinal fluid to the brain result in a concentration gradient of ASO across the non-human primate brain [23,64]. Ideally, the lower concentration of ASO in the deeper areas of the brains would be sufficient for mHTT suppression, whereas higher amounts of ASOs in the outer areas of the brain would suppress mHTT without affecting wtHTT levels or inducing toxicity.

Analogous to other drugs, ASOs have the risk of causing unintended toxicity, which may result from three different mechanisms; the reduction of the target to an extent that leads to adverse outcomes, hybridisation independent events such as nucleic acid-protein interactions, and/or hybridisation-dependent events such as binding to unrelated RNA targets [65]. Currently, there are no algorithms to predict these events and each ASO has

to be fully evaluated independently for safety through in vivo studies in animals and subsequently in carefully controlled human clinical trials [65]. Contingent on pre-clinical validation, the translation into analogous human clinical studies could be rapid, especially considering the latest ASO trials. The first human clinical trial using antisense therapy for a neurodegenerative disease was completed last year for amyotrophic-lateral-sclerosis using intrathecal delivery of ASO. No safety or tolerability concerns were found [48]. Similarly, no safety issues have been reported for an ongoing spinal muscular atrophy trial using intrathecal injection of ASO (ClinicalTrials.gov Identifier: NCT01494701). So far, two ASO drugs have been approved by the FDA, fomivirsen, given intraocularly, and mipomersen, given systemically, and numerous others currently in clincal trials [46,66]. Since the first initial experiments with ASOs targeting HTT more than a decade ago, antisense technologies have come a long way and we are entering a new era of gene silencing. The path from ASO development to the clinic is steadly becoming more feasible with increasing knowledge.

Materials and Methods

Genotyping of patient material

We have previously designed a genotyping panel of 96 SNPs using a Goldengate assay on the Illumina BeadArray platform [33]. Briefly, 96 SNPs were selected for the genotyping assay based on LD patterns from Hapmap, dbSNP and in-house sequencing. DNA samples from the Huntington Disease BioBank at the University of British Columbia from 390 different HD pedigrees were collected. 1151 samples were genotyped using Illumina GenomeStudio v2011 and subsequently phased based on information from family trios using the PHASE 2.0 software.

Ethics statement

Consent and access procedures were in accordance with institutional ethics approval for human research (UBC certificate H05-70532). Publically available human fibroblasts cell lines were obtained from NIGMS Human Genetic Cell Repository at the Coriell Institute for Medical Research (http://ccr.coriell.org). Animal experiments were performed with the approval of the animal care committee at the University of British Columbia.

Fibroblasts

Fibroblast line GM04022, which is heterozygous at SNP rs7685686_A, was used to measure the in vitro potency of the modified ASOs at the mRNA level according to previous protocols [34]. In short, the cells were transfected with 2 μM ASO (or 3 μM for ASOs A15 and A21) by electroporation (Harvard Apparatus ECM830, 115 V, 6 msec) and RNA was extracted 24 h later using the Qiagen RNeasy96 kit according to the manufacturer's specifications. Expression of human HTT mRNA alleles was quantified using a qPCR assay at SNP rs362331 (C_2231945_10, Life Technologies). Quantitative RT-PCR reactions were run on the ABI 7900HT instrument using the Quantitect Probe RT-PCR kit following the manufacturer's instructions. Total RNA content measured by Ribogreen was used for normalization.

Mice and breeding

Mice were housed under a 12 hour light and dark cycle in a clean facility with free access to food and water. Hu18/18 and Hu97/18 [51] timed matings were established, producing offspring of 50% each genotype. Hu97/18 embryos were used to set up primary neuronal cultures. YAC128 (line 53) [67] mice were crossed with FVB mice, and the transgene positive embryos were used for neuronal cultures.

Genotyping of mice

Embryos were collected on day 15.5–16.5 of gestation. Brains were extracted and transferred to Hibernate E (Invitrogen) for 24 hrs, allowing maintenance of neuron viability until genotyping was completed. Tail tissue for genotyping was collected from each embryo, and DNA was extracted using the QuickLyse Miniprep Kit (Qiagen). For Hu97/18 embryos, a PCR across the CAG expansion was used to distinguish between the two human HTT transgenes (forward primer: 5′ - ATTGCCCCGGTGCT-GAGCG -3′ and reverse primer: 5′ - GCGGGCCCAAACT-CACGGTC-3′) yielding product sizes of 351bp and 588bp for the YAC18 and BACHD alleles, respectively. For the YAC128 embryos, two PCRs at each of the YAC arms were used to confirm the presence of the full YAC insert. Actin was used as positive PCR control. Left YAC arm PCR (forward primer: 5′ - CCTGCTCGCTTCGCTACTTGGAGC-3′ and reverse primer: 5′ - GTCTTG CGCCTTAAACCAACTTGG-3′) yielding a product size of 230bp. Right YAC arm PCR (forward primer: 5′ - CTTGAGATCGGGCGTTCGACTCGC-3′ and reverse primer: 5′ - GTCTTGCCGCACCTGTGGCGCCGGT-GATGC-3′) yielding product size of 170bp. Actin PCR (forward primer: 5′ - AGCCTCAGGGCATCGGAACC-3′ and reverse primer: 5′ - GGAGACGGGGTCACCCACAC-3′) yielding product size of 450bp.

Primary neuronal culture and ASO treatment

Embryonic brains were removed from Hibernate E, and the forebrains microdissected in ice-cold Hank's Balanced Salt Solution (HBSS+; Gibco) to remove the hippocampi, isolating the cortex and striatum, which was used to set up neuronal cultures. The tissue was minced and digested with 0.05% Trypsin-EDTA (Invitrogen) at 37°C for 8 minutes, and trypsin was subsequently neutralized with 10% Fetal Calf Serum (FCS; Gibco) in Neuro Basal Medium (NBM; Gibco). Cells were resuspended in complete culture media (NBM+), NBM containing 2% B27 (Gibco), 100 U/ml PS, and 0.5 mM L-Glutamine (Gibco), and treated with DNAse I (153 U/µl) (Invitrogen). Tissue was triturated 5–6 times with a 5 ml serological pipette, and cells were counted and seeded at 1.2×10^6 cells/well on poly-D-lysine coated 6-well plates in 2 ml of NBM+. Primary neuronal cultures were maintained in a humidified incubator at 37°C and 5% CO_2. Neurons were treated with 200 µl ASOs in fresh medium on the second day in vitro (DIV) and fed with 200 µl fresh medium every fifth day post treatment. Images were taken with EVOS XL Core Imaging System from Life Technologies with a 10X objective. Size marker was added to the images using a calibration grid slide (250 uM grids) from MBF Bioscience. As a positive control for spectrin cleavage, we used camptothecin, a topoisomerase inhibitor, to induce apoptosis. At DIV8 increasing concentrations of campthothecin were added to Hu97/18 neurons and spectrin cleavage was evaluated after 24 hours of stress.

Western blotting

Cortical and striatal neurons were collected from the culture dish on DIV 8, 12, or 17 by scraping in ice cold PBS and pelleting by centrifugation at 2400 g for 5 min at 4°C. Dry pellets were then stored at −80°C. Proteins were extracted by lysis with SDP+ buffer and 20–40 µg of total protein was resolved on 10% low-BIS acrylamide gels and transferred to 0.45 µm nitrocellulose membrane as previously described [33]. Membranes were blocked with 5% milk in PBS, and then blotted with the anti-HTT antibody

2166 (Millipore) for detection of HTT. Anti-calnexin (Sigma C4731) immunoblotting was used as a loading control. Membranes were scanned and HTT and Calnexin levels were quantified. Subsequently, the membranes were reprobed with anti-spectrin antibody (Enzo BML-FG6090) and the caspase-3 cleaved 120-kDa fragment of alpha-II-spectrin was quantified. Spectrin cleavage was used as a readout for apoptosis induction to evaluate toxicity of each ASO. Representative images for HTT and spectrin were chosen to best match the data. Proteins were detected with IR dye 800 CW goat anti-mouse (Rockland 610-131-007) and AlexaFluor 680 goat anti-rabbit (Molecular Probes A21076)-labeled secondary antibodies using the LiCor Odyssey Infrared Imaging system. Licor Image Studie Lite was used to quantify the intensity of the individual bands.

Data analysis

Data are expressed as means±SD. Results were analysed using non-linear regression with normalized response and a variable curve. The IC_{50} values were compared using the extra-sum-of-squares F test and the F distribution and degrees of freedom F (DFn, DFd) and the associated p-values have been calculated. Allele specificity was calculated by dividing the IC_{50} for wtHTT by the IC_{50} for mHTT. If the IC_{50} for reducing wtHTT was greater than the highest ASO concentration tested, then allele specificity was calculated by dividing the highest ASO concentration tested by the IC_{50} for mHTT reduction and expressed as >fold. Two way ANOVA with Bonferroni post hoc test have been performed to determine if mHTT expression is different from wtHTT levels at each individual dose of oligo tested. Analyses were performed using GraphPad Prism Ver.5. Differences were considered statistically significant when $p < 0.05$.

Supporting Information

Figure S1 Spectrin cleavage assay. To enable a successful triage and exclusion of toxic ASOs, we measured the level of the 120 kDa spectrin cleavage fragment normalized to calnexin loading control, and then to the untreated sample. Camptothecin induced spectrin cleavage was used as a positive control. Representative Western blots and spectrin quantification from a non-toxic and a toxic ASO are shown. n = 4–6 per data point. Data is presented as mean ± SD. The red dashed line represents the toxicity threshold.

Figure S2 Selection of favourable SNP targets – HTT levels. Hu97/18 neurons were treated with 5e-9-5e ASOs targeted to 10 HD-SNPs and HTT protein level was analyzed. HTT levels were normalized to calnexin and then to the untreated sample for each allele. Representative images are shown. n = 4–6 per data point. Data are presented as mean ± SD. The PS backbone is represented by black; MOE modifications are illustrated by orange. The SNP is illustrated by the underlined nucleotide.

Figure S3 Selection of favourable SNP targets – Spectrin cleavage. Hu97/18 neurons were treated with 5e-9-5e ASOs targeted to 10 HD-SNPs and spectrin cleavage was analyzed. The 120 kDa fragment was normalized to calnexin and then to the untreated sample. HTT membranes were reprobed for spectrin. Representative images are shown. n = 4–6 per data point. Data are presented as mean ± SD. The # denotes two ASOs that induced rearrangement of the neurons. The PS backbone is represented by black; MOE modifications are illustrated by orange. The SNP is illustrated by the underlined nucleotide. The red dashed line represents the toxicity threshold.

Figure S4 Altered neuronal morphology after treatment with some ASOs. Treatment with ASOs E1 and G1 caused marked morphological changes at the highest doses tested (1000 nM) resulting in rearrangement of neuronal cell bodies into an organized network. Representative images are shown of treated and untreated neurons. Black arrows indicate cell bodies grouped together connecting to other cell clusters. Images were taken with EVOS XL Core Imaging System from Life Technologies using the 10X objective. A calibration grid slide with 250 uM grids from MBF Bioscience was used to add a size marker to the images.

Figure S5 Targeting 4 SNPs using two different cEt motifs – HTT levels. Hu97/18 neurons were treated with ASOs with cEt modified wings and HTT protein was analyzed. HTT levels were normalized to calnexin and then to the untreated sample for each allele. Representative images are shown. n = 6–10 per data point. Data are presented as mean ± SD. The PS backbone is represented by black; MOE and cEt modifications are illustrated by orange and blue, respectively. The SNP is illustrated by the underlined nucleotide.

Figure S6 ASO screen at 4 SNPs using two different cEt motifs – Spectrin. Hu97/18 neurons were treated with ASO with cEt modified wings and spectrin cleavage was analyzed. The 120 kDa fragment was normalized to calnexin and then to the untreated sample. HTT membranes were reprobed for spectrin. Representative images are shown. n = 6–8 per data point. Data are presented as mean ± SD. The PS backbone is represented by black; MOE and cEt modifications are illustrated by orange and blue, respectively. The SNP is illustrated by the underlined nucleotide. The red dashed line represents the toxicity threshold.

Figure S7 Wing SAR study. Hu97/18 neurons were treated with ASO with cEt modified wings and HTT protein and spectrin cleavage was analyzed. HTT levels were normalized to calnexin and then to the untreated sample for each allele. The 120 kDa fragment was normalized to calnexin and then to the untreated sample. Membranes were probed for HTT and reprobed for spectrin. Representative images are shown. n = 4–6 per data point. Data are presented as mean ± SD. The PS backbone is represented by black; MOE and cEt modifications are illustrated by orange and blue, respectively. The SNP is illustrated by the

underlined nucleotide. The red dashed line represents the toxicity threshold.

Figure S8 Shortening the gap to 7 nucleotides – HTT levels. Replacing PS-nucleotides with RNase H resistant nucleotides and shortening the gap increases selectivity by preventing cleavage at secondary cleavage sites and restricting cleavage to the main site next to the targeted SNP. Hu97/18 neurons were treated with ASOs and HTT protein was analyzed. HTT levels were normalized to calnexin and then to the untreated sample for each allele. Representative images are shown. n = 6–10 per data point. Data are presented as mean ± SD. The PS backbone is represented by black; MOE and cEt modifications are illustrated by orange and blue, respectively. The SNP is illustrated by the underlined nucleotide.

Figure S9 Shortening the gap to 7 nucleotides – Spectrin cleavage. Hu97/18 neurons were treated with ASOs and spectrin cleavage was analyzed. The 120 kDa fragment is normalized to calnexin and then to the untreated sample. HTT membranes were reprobed for spectrin. Representative images are shown. n = 6–8 per data point. Data are presented as mean ± SD. The PS backbone is represented by black; MOE and cEt modifications are illustrated by orange and blue, respectively. The SNP is illustrated by the underlined nucleotide. The red dashed line represents the toxicity threshold.

Table S1 Summary of ASO RNA screen in human fibroblasts. MOE and cEt modifications are annotated by e and k, respectively. The SNP is underlined.

Acknowledgments

We thank Mahsa Amirabassi and Mark Wang for excellent animal care and Daisy Cao, Lili Liu, and Sheng Yu for assistance with neuronal cultures.

Author Contributions

Conceived and designed the experiments: NHS ALS MEØ JBC SCW SMF GH PPS CFB EES MRH. Performed the experiments: NHS ALS CND EP KV MEO HK ATW. Analyzed the data: NHS ALS CND EP KV MEO HK ATW. Contributed reagents/materials/analysis tools: HK ATW SMF GH PPS CFB EES MRH. Contributed to the writing of the manuscript: NHS MRH. Participated in revisions: NHS ALS MEØ JBC SCW CND EP KV HK ATW SMF GH PPS CFB EES MRH.

References

1. Fisher ER, Hayden MR (2013) Multisource ascertainment of Huntington disease in Canada: Prevalence and population at risk. Mov Disord 29: 105–114. doi:10.1002/mds.25717.
2. Semaka A, Kay C, Doty C, Collins JA, Bijlsma EK, et al. (2013) CAG size-specific risk estimates for intermediate allele repeat instability in Huntington disease. J Med Genet 50: 696–703. doi:10.1136/jmedgenet-2013-101796.
3. Zuccato C, Valenza M, Cattaneo E (2010) Molecular Mechanisms and Potential Therapeutical Targets in Huntington's Disease. Physiological Reviews 90: 905–981. doi:10.1152/physrev.00041.2009.
4. Trottier Y, Biancalana V, Mandel JL (1994) Instability of CAG repeats in Huntington's disease: relation to parental transmission and age of onset. J Med Genet 31: 377–382.
5. Squitieri F, Andrew SE, Goldberg YP, Kremer B, Spence N, et al. (1994) DNA haplotype analysis of Huntington disease reveals clues to the origins and mechanisms of CAG expansion and reasons for geographic variations of prevalence. Hum Mol Genet 3: 2103–2114.
6. Rubinsztein DC, Leggo J, Coles R, Almqvist E, Biancalana V, et al. (1996) Phenotypic characterization of individuals with 30–40 CAG repeats in the Huntington disease (HD) gene reveals HD cases with 36 repeats and apparently normal elderly individuals with 36–39 repeats. The American Journal of Human Genetics 59: 16–22.
7. Gusella JF, Wexler NS, Conneally PM, Naylor SL, Anderson MA, et al. (1983) A polymorphic DNA marker genetically linked to Huntington's disease. Nature 306: 234–238.
8. The Huntington's Disease Collaborative Research Group (1993) A novel gene containing a trinucleotide repeat that is expanded and unstable on Huntington''s disease chromosomes. The Huntington''s Disease Collaborative Research Group. Cell 72: 971–983.
9. Nance MA (2007) Comprehensive care in Huntington''s disease: a physician''s perspective. Brain Research Bulletin 72: 175–178. doi:10.1016/j.brainresbull.2006.10.027.
10. Videnovic A (2013) Treatment of huntington disease. Curr Treat Options Neurol 15: 424–438. doi:10.1007/s11940-013-0219-8.
11. Frank S (2010) Tetrabenazine: the first approved drug for the treatment of chorea in US patients with Huntington disease. Neuropsychiatr Dis Treat 6: 657–665. doi:10.2147/NDT.S6430.

12. Weir DW, Sturrock A, Leavitt BR (2011) Development of biomarkers for Huntington's disease. Lancet Neurol 10: 573–590. doi:10.1016/S1474-4422(11)70070-9.

13. Graham RK, Slow EJ, Deng Y, Bissada N, Lu G, et al. (2006) Levels of mutant huntingtin influence the phenotypic severity of Huntington disease in YAC128 mouse models. Neurobiology of Disease 21: 444–455. doi:10.1016/j.nbd.2005.08.007.

14. Yamamoto A, Lucas JJ, Hen R (2000) Reversal of neuropathology and motor dysfunction in a conditional model of Huntington's disease. Cell 101: 57–66. doi:10.1016/S0092-8674(00)80623-6.

15. Nasir J, Floresco SB, O'Kusky JR, Diewert VM, Richman JM, et al. (1995) Targeted disruption of the Huntington's disease gene results in embryonic lethality and behavioral and morphological changes in heterozygotes. Cell 81: 811–823.

16. Duyao MP, Auerbach AB, Ryan A, Persichetti F, Barnes GT, et al. (1995) Inactivation of the mouse Huntington's disease gene homolog Hdh. Science 269: 407–410.

17. Zeitlin S, Liu JP, Chapman DL, Papaioannou VE, Efstratiadis A (1995) Increased apoptosis and early embryonic lethality in mice nullizygous for the Huntington's disease gene homologue. Nature Genetics 11: 155–163. doi:10.1038/ng1095-155.

18. White JK, Auerbach W, Duyao MP, Vonsattel JP, Gusella JF, et al. (1997) Huntingtin is required for neurogenesis and is not impaired by the Huntington's disease CAG expansion. Nature Genetics 17: 404–410. doi:10.1038/ng1297-404.

19. Dragatsis I, Levine MS, Zeitlin S (2000) Inactivation of Hdh in the brain and testis results in progressive neurodegeneration and sterility in mice. Nature Genetics 26: 300–306. doi:10.1038/81593.

20. Harper SQ, Staber PD, He X, Eliason SL, Martins IH, et al. (2005) RNA interference improves motor and neuropathological abnormalities in a Huntington's disease mouse model. Proc Natl Acad Sci USA 102: 5820–5825. doi:10.1073/pnas.0501507102.

21. McBride JL, Pitzer MR, Boudreau RL, Dufour B, Hobbs T, et al. (2011) Preclinical Safety of RNAi-Mediated HTT Suppression in the Rhesus Macaque as a Potential Therapy for Huntington's Disease. Molecular Therapy 19: 2152–2162. doi:10.1038/mt.2011.219.

22. DiFiglia M, Sena-Esteves M, Chase K, Sapp E, Pfister E, et al. (2007) Therapeutic silencing of mutant huntingtin with siRNA attenuates striatal and cortical neuropathology and behavioral deficits. Proc Natl Acad Sci USA 104: 17204–17209. doi:10.1073/pnas.0708285104.

23. Kordasiewicz HB, Stanek LM, Wancewicz EV, Mazur C, McAlonis MM, et al. (2012) Sustained Therapeutic Reversal of Huntington's Disease by Transient Repression of Huntingtin Synthesis. Neuron 74: 1031–1044. doi:10.1016/j.neuron.2012.05.009.

24. Boudreau RL, McBride JL, Martins I, Shen S, Xing Y, et al. (2009) Nonallele-specific Silencing of Mutant and Wild-type Huntingtin Demonstrates Therapeutic Efficacy in Huntington'ns Disease Mice. Molecular Therapy 17: 1053–1063. doi:10.1038/mt.2009.17.

25. Drouet V, Perrin V, Hassig R, Dufour N, Auregan G, et al. (2009) Sustained effects of nonallele-specific Huntingtin silencing. Ann Neurol 65: 276–285. doi:10.1002/ana.21569.

26. Hu J, Matsui M, Gagnon KT, Schwartz JC, Gabillet S, et al. (2009) Allele-specific silencing of mutant huntingtin and ataxin-3 genes by targeting expanded CAG repeats in mRNAs. Nat Biotechnol 27: 478–484. doi:10.1038/nbt.1539.

27. Gagnon KT, Pendergraff HM, Deleavey GF, Swayze EE, Potier P, et al. (2010) Allele-Selective Inhibition of Mutant Huntingtin Expression with Antisense Oligonucleotides Targeting the Expanded CAG Repeat. Biochemistry 49: 10166–10178. doi:10.1021/bi101208k.

28. Hu J, Liu J, Corey DR (2010) Allele-Selective Inhibition of Huntingtin Expression by Switching to an miRNA-like RNAi Mechanism. Chemistry & Biology 17: 1183–1188. doi:10.1016/j.chembiol.2010.10.013.

29. Zhang Y, Engelman J, Friedlander RM (2009) Allele-specific silencing of mutant Huntington's disease gene. Journal of Neurochemistry 108: 82–90. doi:10.1111/j.1471-4159.2008.05734.x.

30. van Bilsen PHJ, Jaspers L, Lombardi MS, Odekerken JCE, Burright EN, et al. (2008) Identification and Allele-Specific Silencing of the Mutant Huntingtin Allele in Huntington's Disease Patient-Derived Fibroblasts. Human Gene Therapy 19: 710–718. doi:10.1089/hum.2007.116.

31. Lombardi MS, Jaspers L, Spronkmans C, Gellera C, Taroni F, et al. (2009) A majority of Huntington's disease patients may be treatable by individualized allele-specific RNA interference. Experimental Neurology 217: 312–319. doi:10.1016/j.expneurol.2009.03.004.

32. Pfister EL, Kennington L, Straubhaar J, Wagh S, Liu W, et al. (2009) Five siRNAs Targeting Three SNPs May Provide Therapy for Three-Quarters of Huntington•s Disease Patients. Current Biology 19: 774–778. doi:10.1016/j.cub.2009.03.030.

33. Carroll JB, Warby SC, Southwell AL, Doty CN, Greenlee S, et al. (2011) Potent and Selective Antisense Oligonucleotides Targeting Single-Nucleotide Polymorphisms in the Huntington Disease Gene/Allele-Specific Silencing of Mutant Huntingtin. Molecular Therapy 19: 2178–2185. doi:10.1038/mt.2011.201.

34. Ostergaard ME, Southwell AL, Kordasiewicz H, Watt AT, Skotte NH, et al. (2013) Rational design of antisense oligonucleotides targeting single nucleotide polymorphisms for potent and allele selective suppression of mutant Huntington in the CNS. Nucleic Acids Research 41: 9634–9650. doi:10.1093/nar/gkt725.

35. Hu J, Matsui M, Corey DR (2009) Allele-Selective Inhibition of Mutant Huntingtin by Peptide Nucleic Acid-Peptide Conjugates, Locked Nucleic Acid, and Small Interfering RNA. Annals of the New York Academy of Sciences 1175: 24–31. doi:10.1111/j.1749-6632.2009.04975.x.

36. Yu D, Pendergraff H, Liu J, Kordasiewicz HB, Cleveland DW, et al. (2012) Single-stranded RNAs use RNAi to potently and allele-selectively inhibit mutant huntingtin expression. Cell 150: 895–908. doi:10.1016/j.cell.2012.08.002.

37. Liu J, Pendergraff H, Narayanannair KJ, Lackey JG, Kuchimanchi S, et al. (2013) RNA duplexes with abasic substitutions are potent and allele-selective inhibitors of huntingtin and ataxin-3 expression. Nucleic Acids Research 41: 8788–8801. doi:10.1093/nar/gkt594.

38. Hu J, Liu J, Yu D, Aiba Y, Lee S, et al. (2014) Exploring the Effect of Sequence Length and Composition on Allele-Selective Inhibition of Human Huntingtin Expression by Single-Stranded Silencing RNAs. Nucleic Acid Therapeutics 24: 199–209. doi:10.1089/nat.2013.0476.

39. van Dijk JG, van der Velde EA, Roos RA, Bruyn GW (1986) Juvenile Huntington disease. Hum Genet 73: 235–239.

40. Quarrell O, O'Donovan KL, Bandmann O, Strong M (2012) The Prevalence of Juvenile Huntington's Disease: A Review of the Literature and Meta-Analysis. PLoS Curr 4: e4f8606b742ef3. doi:10.1371/4f8606b742ef3.

41. Kay C, Skotte NH, Southwell AL, Hayden MR (2014) Personalized gene silencing therapeutics for Huntington disease. Clin Genet. doi:10.1111/cge.12385.

42. Sun X, Marque LO, Cordner Z, Pruitt JL, Bhat M, et al. (2014) Phosphorodiamidate morpholino oligomers suppress mutant huntingtin expression and attenuate neurotoxicity. Hum Mol Genet. doi:10.1093/hmg/ddu349.

43. Hu J, Matsui M, Gagnon KT, Schwartz JC, Gabillet S, et al. (2009) Allele-specific silencing of mutant huntingtin and ataxin-3 genes by targeting expanded CAG repeats in mRNAs. Nat Biotechnol 27: 478–484. doi:10.1038/nbt.1539.

44. Warby SC, Montpetit A, Hayden AR, Carroll JB, Butland SL, et al. (2009) CAG Expansion in the Huntington Disease Gene Is Associated with a Specific and Targetable Predisposing Haplogroup. The American Journal of Human Genetics 84: 351–366. doi:10.1016/j.ajhg.2009.02.003.

45. Southwell AL, Skotte NH, Bennett CF, Hayden MR (2012) Antisense oligonucleotide therapeutics for inherited neurodegenerative diseases. Trends in Molecular Medicine 18: 634–643. doi:10.1016/j.molmed.2012.09.001.

46. Bennett CF, Swayze EE (2010) RNA Targeting Therapeutics: Molecular Mechanisms of Antisense Oligonucleotides as a Therapeutic Platform. Annu Rev Pharmacol Toxicol 50: 259–293. doi:10.1146/annurev.pharmtox.010909.105654.

47. Passini MA, Bu J, Richards AM, Kinnecom C, Sardi SP, et al. (2011) Antisense oligonucleotides delivered to the mouse CNS ameliorate symptoms of severe spinal muscular atrophy. Science Translational Medicine 3: 72ra18. doi:10.1126/scitranslmed.3001777.

48. Miller TM, Pestronk A, David W, Rothstein J, Simpson E, et al. (2013) An antisense oligonucleotide against SOD1 delivered intrathecally for patients with SOD1 familial amyotrophic lateral sclerosis: a phase 1, randomised, first-in-man study. Lancet Neurol 12: 435–442. doi:10.1016/S1474-4422(13)70061-9.

49. Boado RJ, Kazantsev A, Apostol BL, Thompson LM, Pardridge WM (2000) Antisense-mediated down-regulation of the human huntingtin gene. J Pharmacol Exp Ther 295: 239–243.

50. Nellemann C (2000) Inhibition of Huntingtin Synthesis by Antisense Oligodeoxynucleotides. Molecular and Cellular Neuroscience 16: 313–323. doi:10.1006/mcne.2000.0872.

51. Southwell AL, Warby SC, Carroll JB, Doty CN, Skotte NH, et al. (2013) A fully humanized transgenic mouse model of Huntington disease. Hum Mol Genet 22: 18–34. doi:10.1093/hmg/dds397.

52. Zhang Z, Larner SF, Liu MC, Zheng W, Hayes RL, et al. (2009) Multiple alphaII-spectrin breakdown products distinguish calpain and caspase dominated necrotic and apoptotic cell death pathways. Apoptosis 14: 1289–1298. doi:10.1007/s10495-009-0405-z.

53. Teplova M, Minasov G, Tereshko V, Inamati GB, Cook PD, et al. (1999) Crystal structure and improved antisense properties of 2′-O-(2-methoxyethyl)-RNA. Nat Struct Biol 6: 535–539. doi:10.1038/9304.

54. Smirnova IV, Zhang SX, Citron BA, Arnold PM, Festoff BW (1998) Thrombin is an extracellular signal that activates intracellular death protease pathways inducing apoptosis in model motor neurons. J Neurobiol 36: 64–80.

55. Seth PP, Siwkowski A, Allerson CR, Vasquez G, Lee S, et al. (2009) Short Antisense Oligonucleotides with Novel 2′−4′ Conformationaly Restricted Nucleoside Analogues Show Improved Potency without Increased Toxicity in Animals. J Med Chem 52: 10–13. doi:10.1021/jm801294h.

56. Murray S, Ittig D, Koller E, Berdeja A, Chappell A, et al. (2012) TricycloDNA-modified oligo-2′-deoxyribonucleotides reduce scavenger receptor B1 mRNA in hepatic and extra-hepatic tissues–a comparative study of oligonucleotide length, design and chemistry. Nucleic Acids Research 40: 6135–6143. doi:10.1093/nar/gks273.

57. Nowotny M, Gaidamakov SA, Ghirlando R, Cerritelli SM, Crouch RJ, et al. (2007) Structure of Human RNase H1 Complexed with an RNA/DNA Hybrid: Insight into HIV Reverse Transcription. Molecular Cell 28: 264–276. doi:10.1016/j.molcel.2007.08.015.

58. Monia BP, Lesnik EA, Gonzalez C, Lima WF, McGee D, et al. (1993) Evaluation of 2''-modified oligonucleotides containing 2-''deoxy gaps as antisense inhibitors of gene expression. J Biol Chem 268: 14514–14522.

59. Rigo F, Chun SJ, Norris DA, Hung G, Lee S, et al. (2014) Pharmacology of a Central Nervous System Delivered 2′-O-Methoxyethyl-Modified Survival of Motor Neuron Splicing Oligonucleotide in Mice and Nonhuman Primates. Journal of Pharmacology and Experimental Therapeutics 350: 46–55. doi:10.1124/jpet.113.212407.

60. Liu J, Yu D, Aiba Y, Pendergraff H, Swayze EE, et al. (2013) ss-siRNAs allele selectively inhibit ataxin-3 expression: multiple mechanisms for an alternative gene silencing strategy. Nucleic Acids Research 41: 9570–9583. doi:10.1093/nar/gkt693.

61. Aiba Y, Hu J, Liu J, Xiang Q, Martinez C, et al. (2013) Allele-Selective Inhibition of Expression of Huntingtin and Ataxin-3 by RNA Duplexes Containing Unlocked Nucleic Acid Substitutions. Biochemistry 52: 9329–9338. doi:10.1021/bi4014209.

62. Kauffmann AD, Campagna RJ, Bartels CB, Childs-Disney JL (2009) Improvement of RNA secondary structure prediction using RNase H cleavage

and randomized oligonucleotides. Nucleic Acids Research 37: e121–e121. doi:10.1093/nar/gkp587.

63. Lima WF (1997) The Influence of Antisense Oligonucleotide-induced RNA Structure on Escherichia coli RNase H1 Activity. Journal of Biological Chemistry 272: 18191–18199. doi:10.1074/jbc.272.29.18191.

64. Smith RA (2006) Antisense oligonucleotide therapy for neurodegenerative disease. J Clin Invest 116: 2290–2296. doi:10.1172/JCI25424.

65. Lindow M, Vornlocher H-P, Riley D, Kornbrust DJ, Burchard J, et al. (2012) Assessing unintended hybridization-induced biological effects of oligonucleotides. Nat Biotechnol 30: 920–923. doi:10.1038/nbt.2376.

66. Watts JK, Corey DR (2011) Silencing disease genes in the laboratory and the clinic. J Pathol 226: 365–379. doi:10.1002/path.2993.

67. Hodgson JG, Agopyan N, Gutekunst CA, Leavitt BR, LePiane F, et al. (1999) A YAC mouse model for Huntington's disease with full-length mutant huntingtin, cytoplasmic toxicity, and selective striatal neurodegeneration. Neuron 23: 181–192.

18

Phonatory Dysfunction as a Preclinical Symptom of Huntington Disease

Jan Rusz[1,2*◐], Carsten Saft[3◐], Uwe Schlegel[4], Rainer Hoffman[3], Sabine Skodda[4]

1 Department of Circuit Theory, Faculty of Electrical Engineering, Czech Technical University in Prague, Prague, Czech Republic, 2 Department of Neurology and Centre of Clinical Neuroscience, First Faculty of Medicine, Charles University in Prague, Prague, Czech Republic, 3 Department of Neurology, Huntington-Centre NRW, St. Josef Hospital, Ruhr-University of Bochum, Bochum, Germany, 4 Department of Neurology, Knappschaftskrankenhaus, Ruhr-University of Bochum, Bochum, Germany

Abstract

Purpose: Although dysphonia has been shown to be a common sign of Huntington disease (HD), the extent of phonatory dysfunction in gene positive premanifest HD individuals remains unknown. The aim of the current study was to explore the possible occurrence of phonatory abnormalities in prodromal HD.

Method: Sustained vowel phonations were acquired from 28 premanifest HD individuals and 28 healthy controls of comparable age. Data were analysed acoustically for measures of several phonatory dimensions including airflow insufficiency, aperiodicity, irregular vibration of vocal folds, signal perturbations, increased noise, vocal tremor and articulation deficiency. A predictive model was built to find the best combination of acoustic features and estimate sensitivity/specificity for differentiation between premanifest HD subjects and controls. The extent of voice deficits according to a specific phonatory dimension was determined using statistical decision making theory. The results were correlated to global motor function, cognitive score, disease burden score and estimated years to disease onset.

Results: Measures of aperiodicity and increased noise were able to significantly differentiate between premanifest HD individuals and controls ($p < 0.01$). The combination of these aspects of dysphonia led to a sensitivity of 91.5% and specificity of 79.2% to correctly distinguish speakers with premanifest HD from healthy individuals. Some form of disrupted phonatory function was revealed in 68% of our premanifest HD subjects, where 18% had one affected phonatory dimension and 50% showed impairment of two or more dimensions. A relationship between pitch control and cognitive score was also observed ($r = -0.50$, $p = 0.007$).

Conclusions: Phonatory abnormalities are detectable even the in premotor stages of HD. Speech investigation may have the potential to provide functional biomarkers of HD and could be included in future clinical trials and therapeutic interventions.

Editor: Pedro Gonzalez-Alegre, University of Iowa Carver College of Medicine, United States of America

Funding: This study was supported by the Czech Science Foundation (GACR 102/12/2230) and Charles University in Prague (PRVOUK-P26/LF1/4). The funders had no role in study design, data collection and analysis, decision to publish, or preparation of the manuscript.

Competing Interests: The authors have declared that no competing interests exist.

* Email: rusz.mz@gmail.com

◐ These authors contributed equally to this work.

Introduction

Huntington disease (HD) is an autosomal-dominantly inherited neurodegenerative disorder caused by an expansion in the number of CAG repeats in the IT15 gene [1], leading to widespread neuronal atrophy of both white and grey matter. Clinically, HD is associated with the progressive decline of both motor and cognitive function, as well as psychiatric disturbances. There is a growing body of evidence that progressive functional (e.g., tapping), cognitive and structural changes in the brain precede the clinical onset of HD by many years [2–7]. As predictive testing is available, there is great potential for the development and management of early treatment strategies in HD. Yet, the premanifest period is likely the most suitable period for the

introduction of disease-modifying therapies in order to delay or even prevent symptomatic disease onset [8].

Motor manifestations of HD are generally characterized by involuntary movements termed chorea, which predominate in the initial and middle stages of the disease and are frequently later supplanted by rigidity and dystonia [9]. In addition, abnormalities of voluntary motor function such as problems with planning, initiation, tracing and termination of movements accompany chorea but may already be present in preclinical stages [10].

Speech impairment is a component of the common motor manifestations of HD, occurring in more than 90% of affected patients [11]. Typical signs of dysarthria in HD include voice dysfunction, articulation deficits, irregular loudness variation and abnormalities in speech timing [11–15]. As speech production

Table 1. Clinical characteristics of PreHD subjects.

n = 28 (14 men)	Mean (SD)	Range
Age (years)	37.1 (9.3)	20–55
UHDRS motor score	2.2 (2.4)	0–8
Cognitive score	337 (44)	242–411
Tapping ⸶	189 (23)	142–229
Pegboard ᵠ	4492 (805)	3469–7519
Disease burden score	251 (82)	116–413
Years to onset (years)	16.7 (8.2)	5–36

UHDRS = Unified Huntington's Disease Rating Scale.
⸶Number of taps within a time period of 32 seconds, average value of the dominant and non-dominant hand.
ᵠTime period of peg insertion in 100 ms, average value of the dominant and non-dominant hand.

requires the overall integrity of the central nervous system [16], one may hypothesize that subtle changes in speech may precede the clinical onset of HD. Accordingly, preliminary studies have reported greater incidence of low-frequency segments and decreased oral motor efficiency in subjects at risk for HD [17,18]. While these findings appear promising, only one study sought patterns of subtle preclinical speech abnormalities in genetically proven premanifest HD (PreHD) [13]. This study focused mainly on aspects of speech timing and showed that speech performance tends to decrease with disease progression, however, comparison among groups revealed no significant differences between PreHD individuals and healthy controls [13]. In general, very little is known about different aspects of speech in the preclinical stages of HD and the potential of speech tests as a marker of clinical HD onset.

Considering that complex voice function has never been investigated in gene positive PreHD thus far, the purpose of the present study was to objectively identify phonatory changes that may occur in the premotor stages of HD by assessing a wide range and novel combination of dysphonia measurements. We hypothesized that PreHD patients should manifest subtle voice deficits during sustained vowel phonation, in agreement with previous observations suggesting that certain phonatory deficits are related to the subtle impairment of voluntary movements [14]. Furthermore, we investigated possible relationships between dysphonia features and clinical parameters such as global motor function, cognitive score, disease burden score and estimated years to disease onset to provide deeper insight into the pathophysiology of voice function in PreHD.

Methods

Subjects

A total of twenty-eight German native speakers (14 men, 14 women) with gene positive PreHD volunteered for the present study. Their ages ranged from 20 to 55 years (mean 37.1, standard deviation [SD] 9.3). Classification as PreHD was based on expert rater assessment of motor signs insufficient for a diagnosis of HD (Diagnostic Confidence Level, item 17 of the UHDRS Motor Assessment) [19], suggesting no substantial motor signs. Each PreHD participant underwent extensive neurological and neuropsychological evaluation. In addition to the motor UHDRS score, overall cognitive score (CS) including verbal fluency test, symbol digit modalities test, Stroop colour, Stroop word and Stroop interference subtests were calculated [19]. Subsequently, fine motor performance was assessed by a simple tapping test where

higher motor performance leads to lower scores [20], as well as a more complex pegboard test where higher motor impairment leads to higher scores [21]. In addition, a disease burden score was computed using the formula (age × [CAG repeat - 35.5]) [22]. Years to onset of diagnostic motor manifestations were estimated on the basis of the survival analysis formula introduced by Langbehn et al. [23]. Clinical characteristics of the PreHD group are listed in Table 1.

Twenty-eight healthy German speakers with no history of neurological and/or communication disorders were recruited as a control group (15 men, 13 women), of comparable age ranging from 24 to 55 years (mean 39.7, SD 9.3). No difference in age distribution was found between the PreHD and control groups ($p = 0.31$). The study was in compliance with the Helsinki Declaration and was approved by the Ethics Committee of Ruhr University Bochum. Written informed consent was obtained from each participant.

Speech Data and Acoustic Analyses

Speech samples were digitally recorded in a quiet room using commercial audio software (WaveLab©, Steinberg, Hamburg, Germany) and a head-set microphone (Platronics Audio 550 DSP©, Platronics Inc., California, USA) positioned approximately 5 cm from the subject's lips. The audio data were sampled at 44.1 kHz with 16-bit resolution. During the recording, the participants performed various speaking tasks as a part of a larger protocol. For the current study, only recording of sustained phonation was used for further analyses, where each participant was instructed to take a deep breath and perform sustained phonation of the vowel/a/at a comfortable loudness and pitch, as constant and long as possible. All PreHD individuals performed the sustained vowel phonation twice with a high test-retest reliability ($r = 0.71$–0.94, $p < 0.001$); the first trial of phonation was considered for final analysis.

For evaluation of voice deficits, acoustic analyses were preferred as they offer a non-invasive, valid and reliable method to precisely assess voice abnormalities. Recently, several dysphonia measurements were designed to examine HD-related voice dysfunction [14]. We further extended and elaborated this previous methodology, allowing the assessment of seven specific dimensions of phonatory dysfunction in PreHD individuals. To assess airflow insufficiency, we examined maximum phonation time (MPT) and time to first occurrence of voice break (FOVB) [14]. To investigate aperiodicity, we evaluated number of voice breaks (NVB), degree of pitch breaks (DPB) and degree of vocal arrest (DVA) [24]. With respect to irregular vibration of the vocal folds, we extracted pitch

Table 2. Overview of applied phonatory measurements.

Abbreviation		Description
Airflow insufficiency		
MPT (s)	Maximum phonation time	Aerodynamic efficiency of the vocal tract measured as the maximum duration of the prolonged vowel. This measure includes all voice breaks occurring during the entire vowel phonation.
FOVB (s)	First occurrence of voice break	Maximum duration of the prolonged vowel until the first occurrence of the first voice break, present after at least 250 ms of modal phonation.
Aperiodicity		
NVB (−)	Number of voice breaks	Overall count of voice breaks. A voice break is defined as the distance between consecutive pulses longer than 1.25 divided by the bottom of the pitch range. The segment was defined as a voice break only if it occurred after at least 250 ms of modal phonation and 1 s preceding the termination of phonation. Voice breaks may be associated with both low frequency drop and vocal arrest.
DPB (%)	Degree of pitch breaks	The fraction of pitch frames marked as unvoiced. A frame was considered unvoiced if it had voicing strength below the voicing threshold of 0.45 (autocorrelation function). Silent periods were not considered in analyses.
DVA (%)	Degree of vocal arrests	The fraction of silent periods in the analysed voice signal.
Irregular vibrations of vocal folds		
F0 SD (st)	Standard deviation of fundamental frequency (F0)	Variation in frequency of vocal fold vibration. The F0 sequence was converted to a semitone scale to avoid differences in gender.
RPDE (−)	Recurrence period density entropy	Ability of the vocal folds to sustain simple vibration. RPDE quantifies the deviations from periodicity, representing the uncertainty in the measurement of the pitch period.
Signal perturbations		
Jitter (%)	Frequency perturbation	Extent of variation of the voice range. Jitter is defined as the variability of the fundamental frequency of speech from one cycle to the next.
Shimmer (%)	Amplitude perturbation	Extent of variation of expiratory flow. Shimmer is defined as the sequence of maximum extent of the signal amplitude within each vocal cycle.
Increased noise		
HNR (dB)	Harmonics-to-noise ratio	The amount of noise in the speech signal, mainly due to incomplete vocal fold closure. HNR is defined as the amplitude of noise relative to tonal components in speech.
DFA (−)	Detrended fluctuation analysis	The extent of turbulent noise in the speech signal. DFA measures the stochastic self-similarity of the noise caused by turbulent airflow through the vocal folds.
Vocal tremor		
FTRI (%)	Frequency tremor intensity index	Average ratio of the frequency magnitude of the most intense low-frequency modulating components to the total frequency magnitude of the analysed voice signal.
ATRI (%)	Amplitude tremor intensity index	Average ratio of the amplitude of the most intense low-frequency amplitude modulating components to the total amplitude of the analyzed voice signal.
Articulation deficiency		
MFCC (−)	Mel-frequency cepstral coefficients	Vocal tract transfer function reflecting potential problems with subtle motion of the articulators (jaw, tongue, lips). The MFCC parameter here was defined as the mean of the standard deviations of the 1st-12th MFCCs. It was designed to represent overall stability of individual vocal tract elements, as the individual MFCCs overlap the partitions of the frequency domain.
ΔMFCC (−)	Delta MFCCs	The ΔMFCC parameter represents a similar function as MFCC and was defined as the mean of the standard deviations of the 1st-12th delta MFCCs multiplied by 10.

variability (F0 SD) and recurrence period density entropy (RPDE) [14,25]. To examine signal perturbations, we investigated frequency instability (jitter) and amplitude instability (shimmer) [24]. To capture problems with increased noise, we calculated the harmonics-to-noise ratio (HNR) and detrended fluctuation analysis (DFA) [24,25]. Considering vocal tremor, we applied frequency tremor intensity index (FTRI) and amplitude tremor intensity index (ATRI) [26]. To elucidate articulation deficiency,

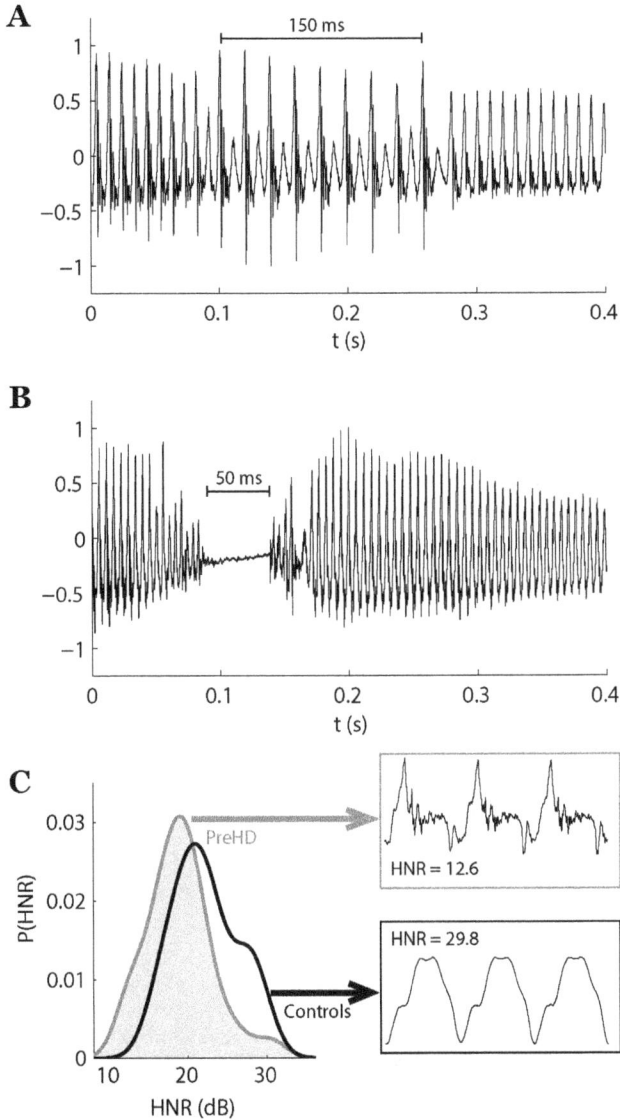

Figure 1. Most salient signs associated with phonatory dysfunction in PreHD individuals: (A) drop in the fundamental frequency to half of its original value over a short period of time; (B) short vocal arrest produced with no vibration of vocal folds; (C) probability density for ratio between harmonics and noise components in voice, with detail of three pitch periods for healthy and disordered voice.

we proposed measures of articulator stability using Mel-frequency cepstral coefficients (MFCC) and delta MFCCs (ΔMFCC) [14]. All acoustic parameters were designed to be gender independent and to provide reliable automated assessment in clinical practice. Table 2 provides a detailed description of the measurements used in the present study.

Statistics

Statistical analyses were performed in Matlab© (Mathworks, Massachusetts, USA). The Kolmogorov-Smirnov test was applied to test for normality and revealed that all acoustic parameters had a normal distribution with the exception of aperiodicity. To evaluate group differences, a two-sample t-test was used for normally distributed data while the nonparametric Mann-Whitney

U-test was performed in other cases. The Pearson and Spearman correlations were applied to test for significant relationships of normally and non-normally distributed data, respectively. Post-hoc Bonferroni adjustment was applied to correct for the number of all tests performed according to specific phonatory dimension; the level of significance after adjustment was set to $p < 0.05$. Effect sizes were determined with Cohens d, with $d > 0.5$ indicating a medium and $d > 0.8$ indicating a large effect.

Wald decision theory was applied to compare the probability distributions between PreHD and healthy subjects and estimate the percentage of affected PreHD individuals according to the specific phonatory dimension [27]. Furthermore, classification experiment based on support vector machine (SVM) with Gaussian radial basis kernel was performed to find the combination of acoustic markers allowing the best discrimination (sensitivity/specificity) between PreHD individuals and controls. To validate reproducibility of SVM classifier, 4-fold cross-validation scheme was used where original data were randomly split into a training subset composed of 75% and testing subset composed of 25% of the data; this cross-validation process was repeated twenty times for each combination. Comprehensive details on classification procedure have been provided elsewhere [28,29].

Results

Table 3 lists the numerical data and comparisons between the PreHD and control groups. From all investigated phonatory dimensions, the voice of PreHD individuals was mainly affected by the presence of aperiodicity and increased noise. In comparison to controls, the PreHD group showed significantly increased NVB ($p = 0.007$), DPB ($p = 0.002$), DFA ($p = 0.0002$) and decreased HNR ($p = 0.007$). Figure 1 provides visual guidance in recognizing the three main features identified (pitch break, vocal arrest and increased noise components) that are associated with early phonatory dysfunction in PreHD.

Figure 2 highlights the percentage of affected subjects according to the specific phonatory dimension (Wald analysis). We observed that 19 PreHD subjects (68%) featured at least one affected phonatory dimension. One disrupted phonatory dimension was also observed in 6 controls (21%). Two or more affected phonatory dimensions were found in 14 PreHD subjects (50%), whereas no control speaker demonstrated more than one disrupted speech dimension. In the majority of individuals with two or more affected phonatory dimensions, at least one dimension was connected with aperiodicity or increased noise. In addition, using SVM classification model, we found that the combination of two aperiodicity measurements (DPB, DVA) and two noise measurements (HNR, DFA) leads to a sensitivity of 91.5±9.9% and specificity of 79.2±11.2% in discriminating PreHD from control participants.

We further observed significant relationships between cognitive score and both measures related to irregular vibration of the vocal folds (F0 SD: $r = -0.43$, $p = 0.02$; RPDE: $r = -0.50$, $p = 0.007$). No relationship was found between phonatory metrics and predicted years to disease onset or disease burden score, although there was a trend where PreHD subjects with some detected phonatory impairment were closer to the predicted age of disease onset (mean 16.1, SD 7.8 years) and showed higher disease burden scores (mean 258, SD 80) than those with a clear voice (years to onset: mean 17.8, SD 9.5 years; disease burden score: mean 238, SD 89). No other significant correlations were detected between phonatory and clinical parameters.

Table 3. Results of voice analyses in PreHD individuals and appropriate controls.

Parameter	Group				Effect size [†]
	PreHD		Controls		PreHD
	Mean (SD)	Range	Mean (SD)	Range	vs. controls
Airflow insufficiency					
MPT (s)	16.9 (7.6)	6.7–43.2	14.1 (4.3)	9.9–25.4	0.44
FOVB (s)	12.4 (6.8)	0.7–30.8	13.9 (4.4)	9.9–25.4	−0.26
Aperiodicity					
NVB (−)	1.11 (2.04)	0–7	0.04 (0.19)	0–1	0.74*
DPB (%)	0.63 (1.14)	0–4.50	0.09 (0.05)	0–0.24	0.77*
DVA (%)	0.09 (0.27)	0–1.14	0 (0)	0–0	0.46
Irregular vibrations of vocal folds					
F0 SD (st)	0.30 (0.16)	0.11–0.79	0.30 (0.13)	0.16–0.67	−0.02
RPDE (−)	0.28 (0.07)	0.14–0.41	0.26 (0.05)	0.18–0.38	0.48
Signal perturbations					
Jitter (%)	0.80 (0.55)	0.16–2.25	0.61 (0.29)	0.28–1.51	0.41
Shimmer (%)	3.69 (1.25)	1.03–8.05	3.18 (1.42)	1.47–8.39	0.38
Increased noise					
HNR (dB)	19.0 (4.1)	12.4–30.5	22.3 (4.0)	15.8–29.8	−0.81*
DFA (−)	0.64 (0.02)	0.59–0.66	0.62 (0.02)	0.58–0.66	1.15**
Vocal tremor					
FTRI (%)	0.37 (0.17)	0.07–0.73	0.42 (0.24)	0.07–1.05	−0.22
ATRI (%)	4.60 (3.39)	1.09–16.59	4.74 (2.27)	0.96–10.13	−0.05
Articulation deficiency					
MFCC (−)	0.43 (0.07)	0.32–0.61	0.41 (0.08)	0.31–0.65	0.26
ΔMFCC (−)	0.45 (0.06)	0.36–0.58	0.44 (0.07)	0.31–0.57	0.12

*$p<0.01$;
**$p<0.001$.
[†]Cohen's d: Effect size 0.8 is considered large, 0.5 is considered medium, and 0.2 is considered small.
MPT = maximum phonation time; FOVB = first occurrence of voice break; NVB = number of voice breaks; DPB = degree of pitch breaks; DVA = degree of vocal arrests; F0 SD = variability of fundamental frequency; RPDE = recurrence period density entropy; HNR = harmonics-to-noise ratio; DFA = detrended fluctuation analysis; FTRI = frequency tremor intensity index; ATRI = amplitude tremor intensity index; MFCC = Mel-frequency cepstral coefficients; ΔMFCC = delta Mel-frequency cepstral coefficients.

Discussion

We detected phonatory dysfunction as a component of the subtle speech motor abnormalities occurring in the prodromal stages of HD. Measures of aperiodicity and increased noise were the most reliable in the prediction of PreHD group membership with 91.5% sensitivity and 79.2% specificity. Some form of disrupted phonatory function was revealed in 68% of our PreHD subjects while 18% had one affected phonatory dimension and 50% showed impairment in two or more dimensions. A relationship between pitch control and cognitive score was also observed. These findings provide new insight into the pathophysiology of speech disorders in premotor HD and may significantly contribute to existing assessment batteries.

Previous studies have shown that patients with manifest HD feature deficits at all phonatory levels, primarily reduced phonation time, aperiodicity, pitch fluctuations, increased noise and problems with articulator coordination [14,30]. Only measures related to aperiodicity and increased noise were significantly aggravated than in controls in our PreHD group; we may thus hypothesize that most phonatory deficits observed in HD arise with the onset of worsening motor function. This hypothesis is further supported by our findings that PreHD speakers are free of markedly increased pitch variations as well as misplacement of articulators, which were previously found to be closely related to the extent of chorea [14]. In addition, respiratory problems associated with markedly reduced phonation time have been found to be pronounced with overall disease severity [30]. Nevertheless, increased addition of noise components in speech already seems to be present in the premotor stages of HD. Elevated noise is likely due to limited control of laryngeal muscles and incomplete vocal fold closure, resulting in inaccuracies in vibratory periods. In particular, similar pathophysiological mechanisms have also been suggested to be responsible for increased signal perturbations and irregular vocal fold vibrations, which were observed in several of our PreHD speakers.

Another manifestation of phonatory dysfunction in the prodromal stages of HD is the occurrence of voice breaks, which are associated with both short pitch drops and vocal arrests. Voice breaks have been hypothesized to be a consequence of hyperadduction of the vocal folds and abnormal muscle tone [14,30]. Conversely, a more reasonable explanation of voice breaks is motor impersistence, which is the inability to sustain certain simple voluntary motor actions such as maintaining a protruded tongue.

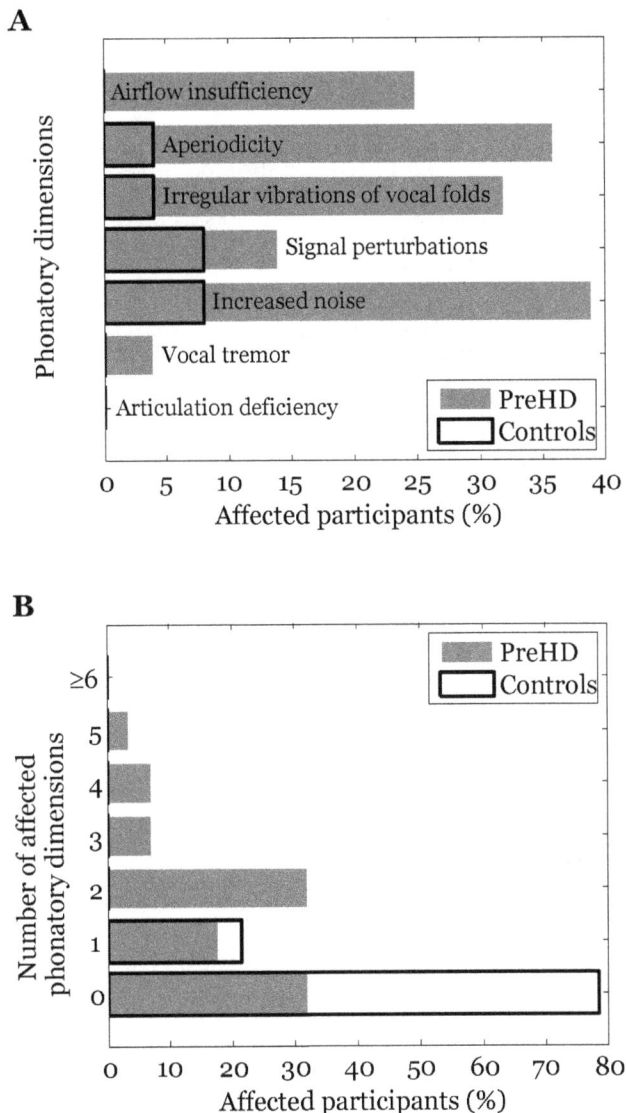

Figure 2. Results of voice analyses: (A) percentage of affected participants according to the specific phonatory dimension; (B) number of affected phonatory dimensions across participants.

enough to detect a motor phenotype early in prodromal HD stages [2], the sensitivity of both methods cannot be compared. On the other hand, when compared to controls, the tongue protrusion method reached a medium effect size [3], while our dysphonia measures showed large effect sizes. Indeed, phonatory tests may provide additional information as sustained phonation requires more sophisticated coordination of the vocal folds, jaw, tongue, palate and facial movements. Furthermore, the advantage of sustained phonation resides in fact that the subject's native language has no or a very small effect on dysphonia parameters, and therefore our findings in German language should be widely applicable to other languages.

However, contrary to previous research [2], we did not detect a relationship between the extent of phonatory dysfunction and disease burden score. One possible explanation is that some PreHD individuals already manifested certain phonatory abnormalities as a part of their habitual vocal behaviour. It is well known that the quality of speech differs among normal speakers and some isolated phonatory deficits were also seen in a few of our healthy controls. In addition, phonatory impairment in 94% of HD patients has recently been reported [14], suggesting that dysphonia do not develop in every individual in the course of premotor HD stages. Therefore, future longitudinal studies are needed to confirm and further elaborate our findings and to show the sensitivity of phonatory measurements as a potential marker of disease onset and progression.

The pathophysiological mechanism responsible for the phonatory deficits in PreHD revealed in the present study still has to be elucidated. Dysphonia with increased noise may be part of various types of motor speech disorders and therefore is likely a rather non-specific marker of neuronal dysfunction [16]. Conversely, recent imaging data have shown involvement of the putamen during the sustained phonation task [32], and putaminal gray matter loss had been detected in PreHD individuals several years before the estimated manifestation of the disease [2]. Notably, we also observed correlations between the cognitive score and measures of irregular vocal fold vibrations, which may be related to dysfunction of the frontostriatal pathways [2].

Although the healthy control group was without previous history of neurological or communication disorders, one potential limitation of the current study is that controls did not undergo rigorous neurological evaluation including UHDRS motor score, cognitive score, tapping, and pegboard. On the other hand, possible subclinical neurological symptoms of any kind that could have been missed in our control group would rather lead to an attenuation of the differences between preHD and controls.

In conclusion, we provide the first objective assessment of a wide range of voice dimensions in prodromal HD, revealing a significant pattern of dysphonia with effect sizes comparable to those found in other studies investigating PreHD subjects. As speech tests are easy to perform, non-invasive and inexpensive, and acoustic analysis of speech can provide objective and quantifiable measures, speech investigations may have the potential to provide functional biomarkers of HD and could be included in future clinical trials and therapeutic interventions.

Author Contributions

Conceived and designed the experiments: JR CS SS. Performed the experiments: CS RH SS. Analyzed the data: JR. Contributed reagents/materials/analysis tools: JR. Wrote the paper: JR. Review and critique: CS US RH SS.

Although short pitch drops may also be present in the vocalizations of the healthy population, their incidence was substantially increased in our PreHD group when compared to controls. Moreover, pitch drops in PreHD individuals frequently appeared in the first seconds of phonation, whereas they typically occur after a long period of phonation in healthy speakers [14]. Conversely, a few PreHD subjects produced short vocal arrests (about 50–300 ms in the present study), which can rarely appear in healthy vocalizations. Accordingly, vocal arrests seem to be a distinctive sign of HD although they have also been reported in certain cases of essential tremor [31].

Our current findings of early phonatory dysfunction are in agreement with data on impaired tongue force performance in a group of PreHD individuals approximately 16 years from expected disease onset [2], which is very similar to the predicted years to diagnosis in our PreHD group (17 years on average). Although deficits in tongue protrusion force coordination were sensitive

References

1. Kremer B, Goldberg P, Andrew SE, Theilmann J, Telenius H, et al. (1994) A worldwide study of the Huntington's disease mutation: The sensitivity and specificity of measuring CAG repeats. New Engl J Med 330: 1401–1406.
2. Tabrizi SJ, Langbehn DR, Leavitt BR, Roos RA, Durr A, et al. (2009) Biological and clinical manifestations of Huntington's disease in the longitudinal TRACK-HD study: cross-sectional analysis of baseline data. Lancet Neurol 8: 791–801.
3. Tabrizi SJ, Scahill RI, Owen G, Durr A, Leavitt BR, et al. (2013) Predictors of phenotypic progression and disease onset in premanifest and early-stage Huntington's disease in the TRACK-HD study: analysis of 36-month observational data. Lancet Neurol 12: 637–649.
4. Feigin A, Tang C, Ma Y, Mattis P, Zgaljardic D, et al. (2007) Thalamic metabolism and symptom onset in preclinical Huntington's disease. Brain 130: 2858–2867.
5. Stout JC, Paulsen JS, Queller S, Solomon AC, Whitlock KB, et al. (2011) Neurocognitive signs in prodromal Huntington disease. Neuropsychology 25: 1–14.
6. Weir DW, Sturrock A, Leavitt BR (2011) Development of biomarkers for Huntington's disease. Lancet Neurol 10: 573–590.
7. Beste C, Stock AK, Ness V, Hoffmann R, Lukas C, Saft C (2013) A novel cognitive-neurophysiological state biomarker in premanifest Huntington's disease validated on longitudinal data. Sci Rep 3: 1997.
8. Tabrizi SJ, Scahill RI, Durr A, Roos RAC, Leavitt BR, et al. (2011) Biological and clinical changes in premanifest and early stage Huntington's disease in the TRACK-HD study: the 12-month longitudinal analysis. Lancet Neurol 10: 31–42.
9. Penney JB Jr, Young AB, Shoulson I, Starosta-Rubenstein S, Snodgrass SR, et al. (1990) Huntington's disease in Venezuela: 7 years of follow-up on symptomatic and asymptomatic individuals. Mov Disord 5: 93–99.
10. Kirkwood SC, Siemers E, Hodes ME, Conneally PM, Christian JC, Foroud T (2000) Subtle changes among presymptomatic carriers of the Huntington's disease gene. J Neurol Neurosurg Psychiatry 69: 773–779.
11. Rusz J, Klempir J, Tykalova T, Baborova E, Cmejla R, et al. (2014) Characteristics and occurrence of speech impairment in Huntington's disease: possible influence of antipsychotic medication. J Neural Transm: in press. DOI 10.1007/s00702-014-1229-8.
12. Hartelius L, Carlstedt A, Ytterberg M, Lillvik M, Laakso K (2003) Speech disorders in mild and moderate Huntington's disease: Results of dysarthria assessment of 19 individuals. J Med Speech-Lang Pa 1: 1–14.
13. Vogel AP, Shirbin C, Andrew J, Churchyard AJ, Stout JC (2012) Speech acoustic markers of early stage and prodromal Huntington disease: A marker of disease onset? Neuropsychologia 50: 3273–3278.
14. Rusz J, Klempir J, Baborova E, Tykalova T, Majerova V, et al. (2013) Objective acoustic quantification of phonatory dysfunction in Huntington's disease. PLoS One 8: e65881.
15. Skodda S, Schlegel U, Hoffman R, Saft C (2014) Impaired motor speech performance in Huntington's disease. J Neural Transm 121: 399–407.
16. Duffy JR (2013) Motor Speech Disorders: Substrates, Differential Diagnosis and Management, 3rd ed., Mosby, St. Louis.
17. Ramig LA (1986) Acoustic analysis of phonation in patients with Huntington's disease. Preliminary report. Ann Otol Rhinol Laryngol 95: 288–293.
18. Coleman R, Anderson D, Lovrien E (1990) Oral motor dysfunction in individuals at risk of Huntington disease. Am J Med Genet 37: 36–39.
19. Huntington Study Group (1996) Unified Huntington's Disease Rating Scale: reliability and consistency. Movement Disord 11: 136–142.
20. Saft C, Andrich J, Meisel NM, Przuntek H, Muller T (2006) Assessment of simple movements reflects impairments in Huntington's disease. Mov Disord 21: 1208–1212.
21. Saft C, Andrich J, Meisel NM, Przuntek H, Muller T (2003) Assessment of complex movements reflects dysfunction in Huntington's disease. J Neurol 250: 1469–1474.
22. Penney JB Jr, Vonsattel JP, MacDonald ME, Gusella JF, Myers RH (1997) CAG repeat number governs the development rate of pathology in Huntington's disease. Ann Neurol 41: 689–692.
23. Langbehn DR, Brinkman RR, Falush D, Paulsen JS, Hayden MR, et al. (2004) A new model for prediction of the age of onset and penetrance for Huntington's disease based on CAG length. Clin Genet 65: 267–277.
24. Boersma P, Weenink D (2001) PRAAT, a system for doing phonetics by computer. Glot International 5: 341–345.
25. Little MA, McSharry PE, Roberts SJ, Costello DA, Moroz IM (2007) Exploiting Nonlinear recurrence and Fractal scaling properties for voice disorder detection. Biomedical Engineering Online 6: 23.
26. Kay Elemetrics Corp (2003) Multi-Dimensional Voice Program (MDVP): Software Introduction Manual. Lincon Park, Kay Elemetrics.
27. Rusz J, Megrelishvili M, Bonnet C, Okujava M, Brozova H, et al. (2014) A distinct variant of mixed dysarthria reflects parkinsonism and dystonia due to ephedrone abuse. J Neural Transm 121: 655–664.
28. Tsanas A, Little MA, McSharry PE, Spielman J, Ramig LO (2012) Novel speech signal processing algorithm for high-accuracy classification of Parkinson's disease. IEEE T Bio-Med Eng 59: 1264–1271.
29. Novotny M, Rusz J, Cmejla R, Ruzicka E (2014) Automatic evaluation of articulatory disorders in Parkinson's disease. IEEE/ACM T Audio Speech Lang Process 22: 1366–1378.
30. Velasco Garcia MJ, Cobeta I, Martin G, Alonso-Navarro H, Jimenez-Jimenez FJ (2011) Acoustic analysis of voice in Huntington's disease. J Voice 25: 208–217.
31. Gamboa J, Jimenez-Jimenez FJ, Nieto A, Cobeta I, Vegas A, et al (1998) Acoustic voice analysis in patients with essential tremor. J Voice 12: 444–452.
32. Peck KK, Galgano JF, Branski RC, Bogomolny D, Ho M, et al. (2009) Event-related functional MRI investigation of vocal pitch variation. NeuroImage 44: 175–181.

19

Direct Reprogramming of Huntington's Disease Patient Fibroblasts into Neuron-Like Cells Leads to Abnormal Neurite Outgrowth, Increased Cell Death, and Aggregate Formation

Yanying Liu[1], Yuanchao Xue[2], Samantha Ridley[1], Dong Zhang[1], Khosrow Rezvani[1], Xiang-Dong Fu[2], Hongmin Wang[1]*

1 Division of Basic Biomedical Sciences, University of South Dakota Sanford School of Medicine, Vermillion, South Dakota, United States of America, 2 Department of Cellular and Molecular Medicine, University of California San Diego, The Palade Laboratories Room 231, La Jolla, California, United States of America

Abstract

Recent advances in trans-differentiation of one type cell to another have made it possible to directly convert Huntington's disease (HD) patient fibroblasts into neurons by modulation of cell-lineage-specific transcription factors or RNA processing. However, this possibility has not been examined. Here, we demonstrate that HD patient-derived fibroblasts can be directly trans-differentiated into neuron-like cells by knockdown of the expression of a single gene encoding the polypyrimidine-tract-binding protein. The directly converted HD neuron-like cells were positive in expression of Tuj1, NeuN, DARPP-32, and γ-aminobutyric acid and exhibited neuritic breakdown, abnormal neuritic branching, increased cell death, and aggregation of mutant huntingtin. These observations indicate that the neuron-like cells directly converted from HD patient fibroblasts recapitulate the major aspects of neuropathological characteristics of HD and thus provide an additional model for understanding the disorder and validation of therapeutic reagents.

Editor: Wanli Smith, University of Maryland School of Pharmacy, United States of America

Funding: This work was supported by Start-up Funds from the University of South Dakota. HW was supported in part by the NIH grant 1R15NS071459-01A1. The funders had no role in study design, data collection and analysis, decision to publish, or preparation of the manuscript.

Competing Interests: The authors have declared that no competing interests exist.

* Email: Hongmin.Wang@usd.edu

Introduction

Huntington's disease (HD) is a progressive neurodegenerative disorder caused by expansion of polyglutamine (polyQ) repeats in the N-terminus of the huntingtin (Htt) protein [1,2]. The disease is neuropathologically characterized by neuronal loss in the striatum and cortex and formation of protein aggregates (inclusions), resulting in motor and behavioral dysfunction [3]. To understand the pathogenesis of HD, a number of HD cell models have been created and applied in many studies over the last two decades [4,5]. Although these HD cells exhibit at least some of the pathological features of HD, most of them do not express full-length human mutant Htt and neuronal markers and thus are not ideal for modeling HD. Induced pluripotent stem cells from HD patient or animal fibroblasts provide a new model for studying HD [6–9]. However, the neuronal induction process is usually time-consuming and tedious. Recently, trans-differentiation of one type cell to another has been made it possible to directly convert HD patient fibroblasts into neuron-like cells by modulation of cell-lineage-specific transcription factors or RNA processing [10–12]. However, it remains unknown whether HD patient-derived fibroblasts can be directly reprogrammed into the neuron-like cells that reproduce the major aspect of HD pathological features.

The polypyrimidine-tract-binding (PTB) is an RNA-binding protein that regulates RNA splicing, stability, and localization [13]. During neuronal differentiation, the expression of PTB is switched to its neuronal homolog, nPTB [14]. Forced expression of PTB blocks neuronal differentiation [15], whereas knockdown of PTB expression by PTB-RNA interactions dramatically promotes conversion of diverse cell types into neurons [12,16]. Here, we demonstrate that following PTB knockdown, HD patient-derived fibroblasts can be directly reprogrammed to neuron-like cells that exhibit the major HD pathological characteristics.

Materials and Methods

Ethics statement

The following cell lines were obtained from the NIGMS Human Genetic Cell Repository at the Coriell Institute for Medical Research: AG07095, GM04281, and GM05539. The Coriell Institute and ATCC maintain the written consent forms and privacy of the donors of the fibroblast samples, and the authors had no contact or interaction with the donors. All human fibroblast cells and protocols in the present study were carried out in accordance with the guidelines approved by the University of South Dakota Institutional Review Board.

Cell culture, preparation and infection of PTB1 small-hairpin (sh) RNA lentiviral particles

Human fibroblasts were maintained in DMEM supplemented with 10% defined FBS, non-essential amino acids, Glutamax, β-mercaptoethanol and 100 ng/mL bFGF at 37°C, 5% CO_2. The CAG repeat number information in the htt gene was obtained from Coriell and confirmed by PCR using a PCR kit (Genelink).

Preparation of lentiviral particles of the shRNAs against human PTB1 and infection of fibroblasts were performed as previously described [12]. Sixteen hours after the shRNA treatment, the cells were selected either with 2 μg/ml puromycin or 100 ng/μl of hygromycin B for 48 h. Selected cells were switched into N3 medium (DMEM/F12, 25 μg/ml insulin, 50 μg/ml human transferrin, 30 nM sodium selenite, 20 nM progesterone, and 100 nM putrescine) supplemented with FGF2 (10 ng/ml) for 3 days and then switched to N3 medium for 10 days. Finally, cells were maintained in N3 medium supplemented with BDNF, GDNF, NT3 and CNTF as previously described [12] until being used for different analyses.

Immunocytochemistry and fluorescence and confocal microscopy

Immunocytochemical staining was performed according to our previously described method [17]. Primary antibodies used include anti-Tuj1 (1:100, Millipore), anti-NeuN (1:100, Millipore), anti-gamma amminobutyric acid (GABA) (1:1000, Millipore), anti-DARPP-32 (1:50, Santa Cruz Biotechnology), and Htt EM48 (1:100, Millipore). Nuclei were stained with Hoechst 33342 (Life Technologies) as previously described [18,19]. Images were acquired with a Carl Zeiss fluorescence microscope equipped with the Axiocam HRM ZEISS camera and AxioVision software. For cells stained with Htt EM48 antibody, images were captured with an Olympus confocal laser scanning microscope equipped with an argon laser and two HeNe lasers and FluoView 1000 software.

Cell counting

If a Tuj1-positive cell had lost all neurites or showed neurite breakdown, the cell would be treated as a cell with neuritic degeneration. Tuj1-positive cells with less than 20 μm in length of neurites or showing apparent thin neurites were regarded as cells with abnormal neuritic branching. GABA-positive cells with neurite breakdown and/or shrunken nuclei/cell bodies were counted as degenerated cells. If a cell had a nucleus containing one or more Htt aggregates, the cell would be counted as the positive for nuclear inclusion. If a cell contains aggregate(s) in the non-nuclear soma region or inside a neurite, the cell would be counted as the positive for non-nuclear (soma/neuropil) aggregate. At least 50 cells were counted in each experiment group and three independent experiments were performed.

Detection of apoptotic cells

Apoptotic cell death was examined as previously described [20] by utilizing a TUNEL (terminal deoxynucleotidyl transferase dUTP nick end labeling, TUNEL) based apoptosis detection kit (Millipore). Stained cells were observed with a fluorescence microscope. Apoptotic cell rate was calculated as follows: apoptotic (or TUNEL positively stained cell) rate (%) = number of TUNELpositively stained cells/number of total cells (assessed by Hoechst 33342 staining) × 100%.

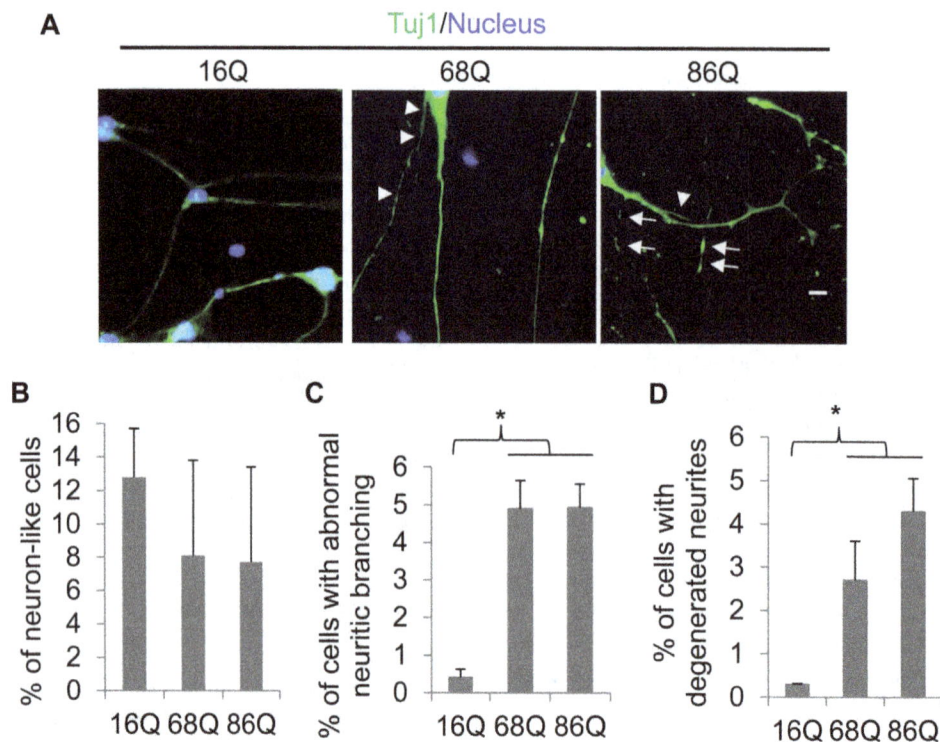

Figure 1. Direct conversion of HD patient fibroblasts into neuron-like cells. Human fibroblasts derived from a normal individual (16Q) or HD patients (68Q and 86Q) were infected with lentiviral shRNAs against human PTB. Nineteen days following the treatment, cells were used for analyses. (A) Immunostaining of the trans-differentiated cells with a neuron-specific marker, Tuj1, antibody. Arrow heads indicate thin or short neurites and arrows show broken neurites. Scale bar, 10 μm. Cell counting results showing the percentage of cells with neuron-like morphology positive in Tuj1 staining (B), with abnormal neurites (C), or with degenerated (breakdown) neurites (D). Data are shown as mean ± SD; n = 3. *p<0.05.

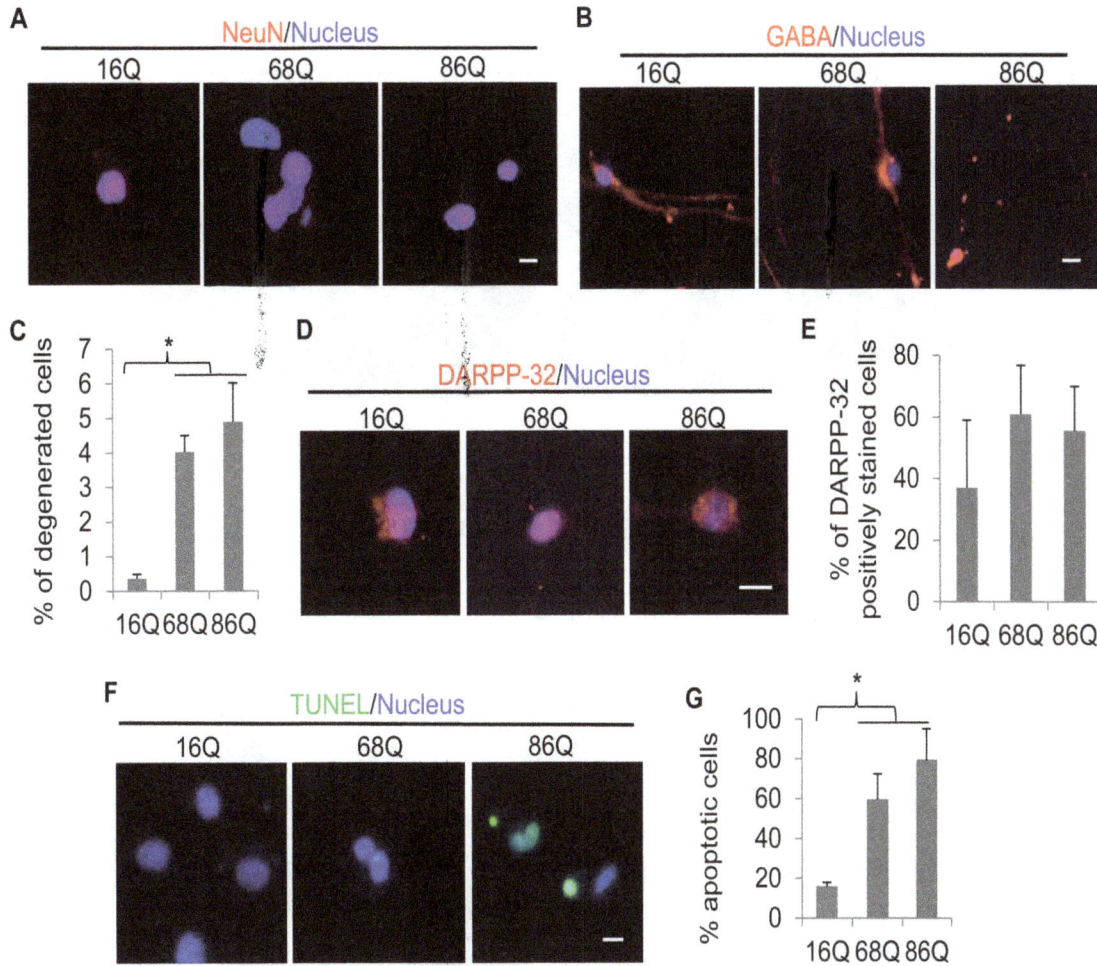

Figure 2. The directly converted HD neuron-like cells are positive in NeuN, GABA, and DARPP-32 expressions and show progressive cell death. Immunostaining of the trans-differentiated cells with a NeuN (*A*) or GABA (*B*) antibody at nineteen days following PTB knockdown. Scale bar, 10 μm. (*C*) Quantification results showing the percentage of degenerated GABA-positive cells derived from the three types of fibroblasts at nineteen days. (*D*) Immunostaining of the trans-differentiated cells with a DARPP-32 antibody at thirty days. Scale bar, 10 μm. (*E*) Graph showing the percentage of DARPP-32 positive cells at thirty days following PTB knockdown. (*F*) TUNEL staining of the converted cells at thirty days following the reprogramming. Scale bar, 10 μm. (*G*) Graph showing the percentage of apoptotic cells assessed by TUNEL staining shown in (*F*). All quantitative data are shown as mean ± SD; n=3 for each group of cells. *p<0.001.

Statistical analysis

Statistical comparisons between two groups were evaluated using two-tailed student's t test. P<0.05 was regarded as statistically significant.

Results and Discussion

To reprogram the fibroblasts derived from HD patients into neuron-like cells, we employed a recently described method to knock down PTB protein [12] by infecting HD patient fibroblasts expressing Htt containing either 16Q, 68Q, or 86Q with lentiviral shRNAs against human PTB. Nineteen days following PTB knockdown, the cells exhibited a typical neuron-like morphology and showed positive immunoreactivity with Tuj1, a neuron-specific cytoskeleton protein present in newly generated immature postmitotic neurons and differentiated neurons [20,21] (Fig. 1A). Cell counting showed that the HD patient-derived fibroblasts did not significantly differ from the normal fibroblasts in the capability of conversion to Tuj1-positive neuron-like cells (Fig. 1B). Those undifferentiated cells did not show Tuj1 staining and only showed the nuclear staining (Fig. 1A). The Tuj1-positive cells converted from HD patients (referred to as 68Q and 86Q, respectively) showed different neuritic morphology from the cells derived from a normal individual (16Q). The normal fibroblast-converted cells extended from one to several relatively thick neurites directly from the cell body (Fig. 1A, left panel). In addition to the thick neurites, however, the HD fibroblasts-derived cells frequently grew out thin neurites either directly from their cell bodies or from thick neurites (Figs. 1A, middle and right panels, pointed by arrow heads). Interestingly, some of the neurites derived from HD neuron-like cells were broken down and degenerated into small fragments positive in Tuj1 staining (Fig. 1A, pointed by arrows). Additionally, cell counting results indicated that more HD neuron-like cells (68Q and 86Q) exhibited abnormal neuritic branching (Fig. 1C) and neuritic breakdown (Fig. 1D) than the wild-type of neuron-like cells (16Q). These results indicate that the trans-differentiation of HD patient's fibroblasts into neuron-like cells leads to abnormal neuritic branching and degeneration.

As the neuronal nuclear antigen (NeuN) is a nuclear protein widely expressed in the mature postmitotic neurons, it has been

A

B

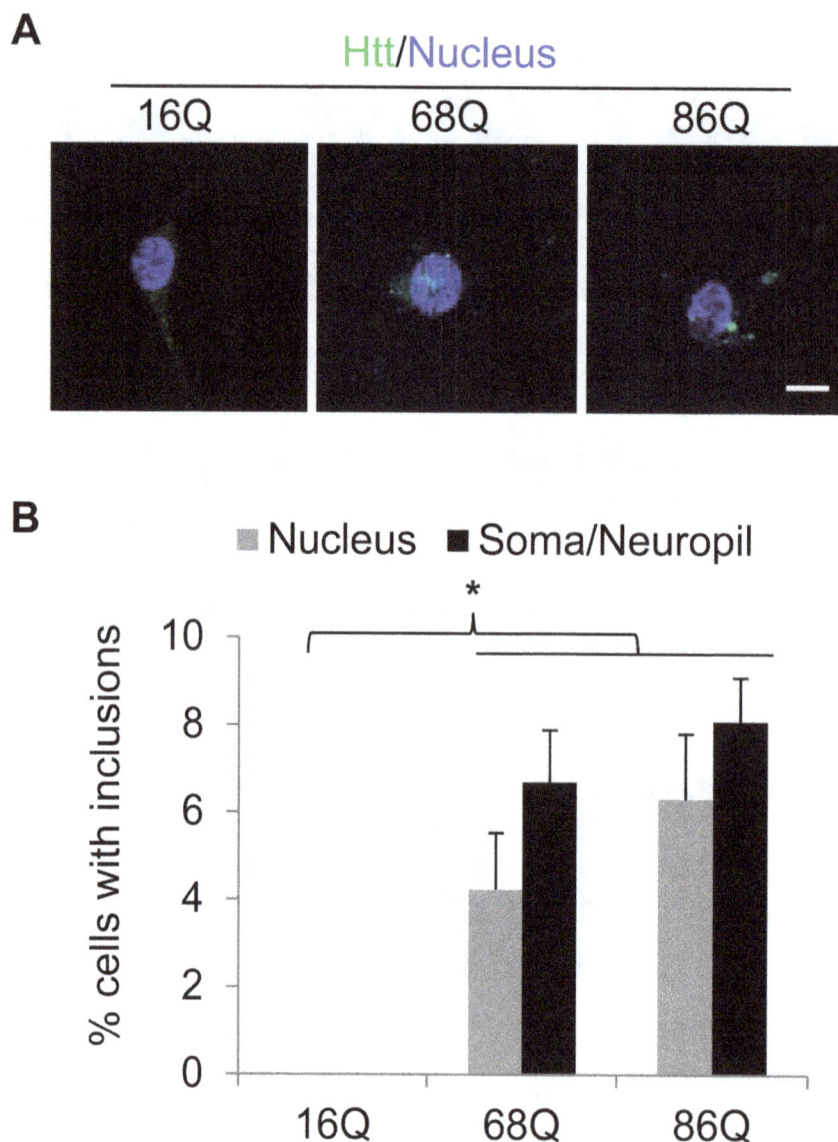

Figure 3. The directly converted HD neuron-like cells show Htt inclusions at nineteen days following PTB knockdown. *(A)* Immunostaining of the trans-differentiated cells with the EM48 antibody indicates the presence of Htt inclusions in the HD cells. Scale bar, 10 μm. *(B)* Cell counting results showing the percentage of cells with aggregates in the nucleus or non-nuclear regions (soma and/or neuropil). Data are shown as mean ± SD; *p<0.001. n = 3.

commonly used as a neuron-specific marker for mature neurons [22]. We thus stained the cells with a NeuN specific antibody and found that at least 10% cells were positive in NeuN expression in each of the three converted cell types after nineteen days of the reprogramming (Fig. 2A). Since one major pathological feature of HD is selective loss of GABAergic neurons in the striatum [23], we next examined whether the trans-differentiated neuron-like cells express γ-aminobutyric acid (GABA), an inhibitory neurotransmitter. As shown in Fig. 2B, GABA was strongly expressed in both the normal and HD neuron-like cells nineteen days after shRNA knockdown of PTB. Compared to the normal fibroblast-derived GABA-positive cells, some HD GABA-positive cells showed degenerating neurites and shrunken cell bodies (Fig. 2B, right panel). Cell counting indicates that neurodegeneration was significantly more in the HD neuron-like cells than in the normal cells (Fig. 2C). Additionally, as degenerated neurons in HD striatum are DARPP-32 positive cells [23], we examined whether

the trans-differentiated neuron-like cells are also positively stained with the protein. As shown in Figs. 2D and 2E, thirty days following the reprogramming, many cells expressed DARPP-32. At this time point, however, degenerated cells were dramatically increased to 59% and 79% in the 68Q and 86Q HD cells, respectively (Figs. 2F, 2G). Taken together, these data suggest that the HD patient fibroblasts can be trans-differentiated to GABA and DARPP-32-positive neuron-like cells and the reprogramming triggers increased cell death in the HD fibroblast-derived cells.

We next examined whether trans-differentiation of HD patient fibroblasts to neuron-like cells leads to mutant Htt aggregation. We therefore immunostained the three types of converted neuron-like cells with the well-documented EM48 Htt antibody, which selectively binds to the toxic N-terminal fragment of the mutant Htt protein [24], and then assessed the cells positive with inclusions in the nucleus, soma, and neuropil by confocal microscopy. There was no EM48-positive nuclear inclusion in the neuron-like cells trans-converted from the normal fibroblasts, whereas most of the neuron-like cells converted from the two types of HD fibroblasts contained Htt inclusions in their nuclei and non-nuclear regions (soma and neuropils) (Figs. 3A, 3B). These results indicate that the mutant Htt proteins preferentially form aggregates in both the nucleus and non-nuclear regions upon conversion to neuron-like cells.

One interesting observation from this research is that direct conversion of HD patient fibroblasts to neuron-like cells leads to abnormal neurite outgrowth and branching, characterized by frequently short or thin neurite outgrowth. This is in accordance with a previous *in vivo* study, in which abnormal dendritic arbors and increased dendritic branching in spiny striatal neurons were identified in post-mortem HD patients' brain sections [25]. Although it remains unclear why the HD neuron-like cells selectively exhibit this dysmorphic alteration, mutant Htt-caused intracellular trafficking dysfunction may be, at least partially, responsible for abnormal neurite outgrowth and branching [26]. Additionally, mutant Htt also impairs mitochondrial integrity [27] and disrupts production and trafficking of neurotrophic factors [28], which may also affect neurite outgrowth and branching. As a

further direction, it is interesting to explore the biological significance underlying this dysmorphic alteration. In addition to showing increased cell death, the directly trans-converted HD cells also form aggregates not only in the nucleus but also in non-nuclear regions such as neuropils, which is in accordance with previous *in vivo* studies using HD patient brain tissues [29]. Thus, the directly converted neuron-like cells from HD fibroblasts provide a reliable model for studying pathogenic mechanisms of HD and may be a useful tool for validation of therapeutic target or drugs in the future.

Acknowledgments

We would like to thank Dr. Fran Day at the Imaging Core Facility of the University of South Dakota for assistance in confocal microscopy.

Author Contributions

Conceived and designed the experiments: YL HW. Performed the experiments: YL YX SR HW. Analyzed the data: YL HW. Contributed reagents/materials/analysis tools: XDF KR DZ. Wrote the paper: YL HW.

References

1. The-Huntington-disease-collaborative-research-group (1993) A novel gene containing a trinucleotide repeat that is expanded and unstable on Huntington's disease chromosomes. The Huntington's Disease Collaborative Research Group. Cell 72: 971–983.
2. Li SH, Li XJ (2004) Huntingtin and its role in neuronal degeneration. Neuroscientist 10: 467–475.
3. Reiner A, Albin RL, Anderson KD, D'Amato CJ, Penney JB, et al. (1988) Differential loss of striatal projection neurons in Huntington disease. Proc Natl Acad Sci U S A 85: 5733–5737.
4. Wyttenbach A, Swartz J, Kita H, Thykjaer T, Carmichael J, et al. (2001) Polyglutamine expansions cause decreased CRE-mediated transcription and early gene expression changes prior to cell death in an inducible cell model of Huntington's disease. Hum Mol Genet 10: 1829–1845.
5. Sipione S, Cattaneo E (2001) Modeling Huntington's disease in cells, flies, and mice. Mol Neurobiol 23: 21–51.
6. Park IH, Arora N, Huo H, Maherali N, Ahfeldt T, et al. (2008) Disease-specific induced pluripotent stem cells. Cell 134: 877–886.
7. Chan AW, Cheng PH, Neumann A, Yang JJ (2010) Reprogramming Huntington monkey skin cells into pluripotent stem cells. Cell Reprogram 12: 509–517.
8. The-HD-iPSC-Consortium (2012) Induced pluripotent stem cells from patients with Huntington's disease show CAG-repeat-expansion-associated phenotypes. Cell Stem Cell 11: 264–278.
9. Kaye JA, Finkbeiner S (2013) Modeling Huntington's disease with induced pluripotent stem cells. Mol Cell Neurosci 56: 50–64.
10. Ambasudhan R, Talantova M, Coleman R, Yuan X, Zhu S, et al. (2011) Direct reprogramming of adult human fibroblasts to functional neurons under defined conditions. Cell Stem Cell 9: 113–118.
11. Vierbuchen T, Ostermeier A, Pang ZP, Kokubu Y, Sudhof TC, et al. (2010) Direct conversion of fibroblasts to functional neurons by defined factors. Nature 463: 1035–1041.
12. Xue Y, Ouyang K, Huang J, Zhou Y, Ouyang H, et al. (2013) Direct conversion of fibroblasts to neurons by reprogramming PTB-regulated microRNA circuits. Cell 152: 82–96.
13. Valcarcel J, Gebauer F (1997) Post-transcriptional regulation: the dawn of PTB. Curr Biol 7: R705–708.
14. Boutz PL, Stoilov P, Li Q, Lin CH, Chawla G, et al. (2007) A post-transcriptional regulatory switch in polypyrimidine tract-binding proteins reprograms alternative splicing in developing neurons. Genes Dev 21: 1636–1652.
15. Makeyev EV, Zhang J, Carrasco MA, Maniatis T (2007) The MicroRNA miR-124 promotes neuronal differentiation by triggering brain-specific alternative pre-mRNA splicing. Mol Cell 27: 435–448.
16. Xue Y, Zhou Y, Wu T, Zhu T, Ji X, et al. (2009) Genome-wide analysis of PTB-RNA interactions reveals a strategy used by the general splicing repressor to modulate exon inclusion or skipping. Mol Cell 36: 996–1006.
17. Dong G, Ferguson JM, Duling AJ, Nicholas RG, Zhang D, et al. (2011) Modeling pathogenesis of Huntington's disease with inducible neuroprogenitor cells. Cell Mol Neurobiol 31: 737–747.
18. Dong G, Gross K, Qiao F, Ferguson J, Callegari EA, et al. (2012) Calretinin interacts with huntingtin and reduces mutant huntingtin-caused cytotoxicity. J Neurochem 123: 437–446.
19. Dong G, Callegari EA, Gloeckner CJ, Ueffing M, Wang H (2012) Prothymosin-alpha interacts with mutant huntingtin and suppresses its cytotoxicity in cell culture. J Biol Chem 287: 1279–1289.
20. Menezes JR, Luskin MB (1994) Expression of neuron-specific tubulin defines a novel population in the proliferative layers of the developing telencephalon. J Neurosci 14: 5399–5416.
21. von Bohlen Und Halbach O (2007) Immunohistological markers for staging neurogenesis in adult hippocampus. Cell Tissue Res 329: 409–420.
22. Lavezzi AM, Corna MF, Matturri L (2013) Neuronal nuclear antigen (NeuN): a useful marker of neuronal immaturity in sudden unexplained perinatal death. J Neurol Sci 329: 45–50.
23. Vonsattel JP, DiFiglia M (1998) Huntington disease. J Neuropathol Exp Neurol 57: 369–384.
24. Zhou H, Cao F, Wang Z, Yu ZX, Nguyen HP, et al. (2003) Huntingtin forms toxic NH2-terminal fragment complexes that are promoted by the age-dependent decrease in proteasome activity. J Cell Biol 163: 109–118.
25. Ferrante RJ, Kowall NW, Richardson EP Jr. (1991) Proliferative and degenerative changes in striatal spiny neurons in Huntington's disease: a combined study using the section-Golgi method and calbindin D28k immunocytochemistry. J Neurosci 11: 3877–3887.
26. Rong J, McGuire JR, Fang ZH, Sheng G, Shin JY, et al. (2006) Regulation of intracellular trafficking of huntingtin-associated protein-1 is critical for TrkA protein levels and neurite outgrowth. J Neurosci 26: 6019–6030.
27. Wang H, Lim PJ, Karbowski M, Monteiro MJ (2009) Effects of overexpression of huntingtin proteins on mitochondrial integrity. Hum Mol Genet 18: 737–752.
28. Ferrer I, Goutan E, Marin C, Rey MJ, Ribalta T (2000) Brain-derived neurotrophic factor in Huntington disease. Brain Res 866: 257–261.
29. Gutekunst CA, Li SH, Yi H, Mulroy JS, Kuemmerle S, et al. (1999) Nuclear and neuropil aggregates in Huntington's disease: relationship to neuropathology. J Neurosci 19: 2522–2534.

20

Deep White Matter in Huntington's Disease

Owen Phillips[1], Ferdinando Squitieri[2]*, Cristina Sanchez-Castaneda[3], Francesca Elifani[2], Carlo Caltagirone[1,4], Umberto Sabatini[3], Margherita Di Paola[1]*

1 Clinical and Behavioural Neurology Dept, IRCCS Santa Lucia Foundation, Rome, Italy, **2** IRCSS Neuromed, Pozzilli, Italy, **3** Radiology Dept, IRCCS Santa Lucia Foundation, Rome, Italy, **4** Neuroscience Dept, University of Rome "Tor Vergata", Rome, Italy

Abstract

White matter (WM) abnormalities have already been shown in presymptomatic (Pre-HD) and symptomatic HD subjects using Magnetic Resonance Imaging (MRI). In the present study, we examined the microstructure of the long-range large deep WM tracts by applying two different MRI approaches: Diffusion Tensor Imaging (DTI) -based tractography, and T2*weighted (iron sensitive) imaging. We collected Pre-HD subjects (n = 25), HD patients (n = 25) and healthy control subjects (n = 50). Results revealed increased axial (AD) and radial diffusivity (RD) and iron levels in Pre-HD subjects compared to controls. Fractional anisotropy decreased between the Pre-HD and HD phase and AD/RD increased and although impairment was pervasive in HD, degeneration occurred in a pattern in Pre-HD. Furthermore, iron levels dropped for HD patients. As increased iron levels are associated with remyelination, the data suggests that Pre-HD subjects attempt to repair damaged deep WM years before symptoms occur but this process fails with disease progression.

Editor: David Blum, Inserm U837, France

Funding: This work was supported by the Italian Ministry of Health grant 204/GR-2009-1606835. Also, support was provided by the European Commission: Marie Curie Fellowship for career development to CS (FP7-PEOPLE-2011-IEF). The authors are grateful for the support they received from the Italian Ministry of Health (Ricerca Corrente), European Huntington's Disease Network for the Registry Study, by the "Italian League for Huntington and related diseases onlus (www.lirh.it)" to FS. The funders had no role in study design, data collection and analysis, decision to publish, or preparation of the manuscript. The authors are grateful to all patients for contributing to the work.

Competing Interests: The authors have declared that no competing interests exist.

* Email: m.dipaola@hsantalucia.it (MDP); ferdinando.squitieri@lirh.it (FS)

Introduction

Huntington's disease (HD) is a neurodegenerative autosomal dominate disorder caused by increased CAG repeats, this leads to increased accumulation of mutant huntingtin, and formation of intranuclear inclusions and eventually to brain damage. Damage has long been thought to start in the striatum (for review see: [1]), however, most areas of the brain show abnormalities. Of the abnormalities found in the HD brain, the changes to white matter in particular have been become a major focus of research.

A model for the white matter changes in HD has been formulated [2], which suggests that the pathogenesis of HD begins with a deleterious effect of the mutant huntingtin on myelin. Indeed mutant huntingtin is not found in higher levels in the neurons that degenerate first, rather the mutated protein is expressed throughout the nervous system and periphery [3]. This implies that its primary impact may not be on neurons. The myelin breakdown is, in turn, associated with increased density of oligodendrocytes in the brain, which are involved in repairing myelin damage. As the oligodendrocytes have the highest iron content, when they increase in number, iron content increases [2].

Abnormalities in white matter cause downstream effects through a complex physiological process that is still being uncovered (see [4] for a summary). In short, oligodendrocytes and myelin abnormalities can slow or stop fast axon transport, which can result in synaptic loss and eventually axonal degeneration in a retrograde, ("Dying back") fashion [5].

In the last decades in-vivo Magnetic Resonance Imaging (MRI) investigations have revealed the extent of changes to white matter in HD. MRI research has reported extensive white matter volume loss in the whole brain [6], in the frontal lobe [7] and across the total cerebrum [8], as well as changes to white matter microstructure; the motor cortico-striatal circuit [9–12], sensorimotor cortex, [10], corpus callosum [11,13], and across extensive distributed white matter fibers (corpus callosum, superior and inferior longitudinal fasciculi and external capsule) [12]) years before symptoms occur.

The increasing evidence that white matter is negatively impacted in HD even before disease onset (Pre-HD) has led us to investigate the changes in the large white matter tracts in Pre-HD and HD and how these changes were related to the iron content. We first investigated the corpus callosum and found that early callosal white matter demyelination damage characterizes HD in the pre-symptomatic stage [11]. At that clinical stage, the myelin breakdown starts at the level of the early and heavily myelinated callosal fibres [14]. Changes in iron content (reduction) manifest in the early stages of HD, likely indicating a failure of the remyelination processes at that time. Then we focused on the cortical spinal tract, which is the brain's main motor fiber [15]. We found that a likely active repair mechanism (as indicated by increased iron) helps keep the cortical spinal tract at a normal functional level in the presymptomatic stage. However, this repair seems to fail with disease progression and cortical spinal white matter tract damage becomes extensive in HD patients. The damage to the cortical spinal white matter tract appears to occur in a retrograde ("Dying back") fashion, similar to what happens in striatal and cortical projection neurons [5,16].

In the present study we were interested in making a step forward, by investigating the whole deep white matter in HD, definable as the large easily identifiable association white matter tracts, i.e. the arcuate fasciculus (AF), the superior longitudinal fasciculus (SLF), the cingulate (Cing), the inferior longitidinal fasciculus (ILF), the inferior occipital fasciculus (IFO), the anterior thalamic radiation (ATR) and the uncinate fasciculus (UF). We studied the deep white matter tracts both as a combined whole (called from now on "total deep white matter") in order to investigate the disease effect on deep white matter in general and as single tracts (AF, SLF, Cing, ILF, IFO, ATR, and UF; we will refer to them as "individual deep white matte tracts") in order to identify possible regional variations in the disease process.

With the white matter model in mind, we adopted two different MRI approaches to investigate the deep white matter in HD: Diffusion Tensor Imaging (DTI)-based tractography and T2*weighted imaging.

DTI is the MRI technique most frequently used to study white matter fiber changes. It is a non-invasive technique that uses local water diffusion in the brain tissue. Although the biological determinants of diffusion parameters (fractional anisotropy-FA, axial diffusivity-AD and radial diffusivity-RD) are not yet fully understood (for a discussion on diffusion imaging see [17], it is agreed that this approach is sensitive to microstructural tissue properties. Indeed, it has been used in numerous studies to investigate everything from the effects of age on white matter in healthy subjects [18] to disease effects in Alzheimer's disease [19] and schizophrenia [20].

T2* weighted volumes, which are sensitive to iron/ferritin [21,22] are useful to investigate the iron content that is associated with the remyelination process [2]. The few studies present in literature show a non-univocal picture of the regional white matter iron content changes in HD, with no iron level differences in the callosal splenium, but decreased iron levels in the frontal lobe white matter [2], the callosal isthmus [14] and the cortical spinal white matter tract [15]. However, no studies to date in HD have combined the sensitivity of DTI tractography to identify the deep white matter in-vivo with T2* weighted volume images. By combining these imaging methods in a large cohort of subjects (25 HD patients, 25 Pre-HD and 50 healthy subjects), we can assess the effect HD has on the deep white matter tissue microstructure (total and individual tracts).

The main aims of our study were the following: 1) to examine total deep white matter microstructure in Pre-HD subjects and HD patients; 2) to investigate whether variations in connectivity parameters (FA, AD, RD) and in iron level within the deep white matter provide evidence for the white matter demyelination and remyelination model in HD; 3) to explore whether white matter microstructural properties vary by individual deep white matter tract in a particular manner.

Methods

Subjects

Subject demographics and clinical assessments are outlined in Table 1. HD patients (n = 25) and Pre-HD subjects (n = 25), underwent a genetic test (abnormal CAG repeats ≥36) and were examined clinically by the same neurologist (FS) with expertise in HD. All individuals were assessed using the Unified Huntington's Disease Rating Scale (UHDRS), which includes motor, cognitive, behavioral, and functional subscales [23]. Each section consists of a multistep subscale. The motor section measures eye movements, limb coordination, tongue impersistence and movement disorders (such as rigidity, bradykinesia, dystonia, chorea, and gait disturbances). A higher score means more motor impairment. The cognitive scale mainly evaluates executive function. A higher score means better cognitive performance. The behavioral section investigates the presence of depression, aggressiveness, obsessions/compulsions, delusions/hallucinations and apathy. A higher score means more impairment. The functional assessments include the HD functional capacity scale (HDFCS), the independence scale and a checklist of common daily tasks. All three scales mainly investigate independence in daily life activities. The HDFCS is reported as the total functional capacity (TFC) score (range 0–13) and is the only functional subscale with established psychometric properties (including inter-rater reliability and validity), which are based on radiographic measures of disease progression. Thus, the TFC score is used worldwide to determine patients' HD stage. On the independence scale, the investigator indicates whether the patient can perform the task that evaluates independence level (range 10–100). The checklist (functional assessment) is summed by giving a score of 1 to all "yes" answers (range 0–25). Pre-HD are defined as those subjects whom the suspected clinical diagnosis is confirmed by DNA analysis, which revealed (CAG)(n) expansion into the range characteristic of Huntington disease (>36 or repeats), but who do not have manifested Huntington's disease symptoms yet defined by a total motor score of <5 in the UHDRS and cognitive and behavioral assessment within the normality. The Disease Burden index, a measure of disease severity, was used according to the already described formula (age×[CAG-35.5]), where CAG is the number of CAG repeats [24]. A higher score reflects increased disease severity. The Mini Mental State Examination (MMSE) [25], which measures global cognitive functioning, was administered to Pre-HD subjects and HD patients. A lower score reflects greater impairment.

Fifty individually healthy subjects were recruited from the community. Patients in the advanced stages of disease (Stages III and IV) and/or with traumatic brain injury or focal lesions were excluded.

Ethics Statement

Presymptomatic test, genetic diagnosis and clinical exams were performed at Neurological Research Institute IRCCS Neuromed. All participants had the cognitive capacity to understand the research protocol and gave their oral and written consent. Cognitive capacity to consent was determined the MMSE. No subjects had cognitive impairment (see score on Table 1). In no case was there a surrogate consent procedure consented on the behalf of participants. Consent was obtained according to the Declaration of Helsinki and the Santa Lucia Foundation Research Ethics Committee approved the study.

MRI Data Acquisition

All MRI data was acquired on a 3T Allegra MRI system (Siemens, Germany) using a birdcage head coil. Scans were collected in a single session, with the following pulse sequences: 1) proton density and T2-weighted double turbo spin echo (SE) acquired in transverse planes (time repetition [TR]: 4500 ms, time echo [TE]: 12 ms, time to inversion [TI]: 112 ms, field of view [FOV]: 230×172 mm, matrix: 320×240, slice thickness: 5 mm, number of slices: 24); 2) fluid-attenuated inversion recovery in the same planes as the SE sequence (TR/TE/TI: 8500/109/

Table 1. Sociodemographic and clinical characteristics of patients and control subjects.

Characteristics	Pre-HD (n = 25)	HD (n = 25)	Controls (n = 25)	Fisher's Exact Test; F or T Test	df	p
Gender male/female	16/9	14/11	30/20	0.367	2	0.833
Age (years ± SD)	37.44±7.01	47.40±14.53	42.88±12.48	4.349	2	0.012[a††]
CAG repetition length	43.28±2.17	46.68±6.80	NA	−2.380	48	0.021[a††]
MMSE	27.82±1.24	24.97±3.23	NA	3.682	38	0.001[b††]
UHDRS Motor	8.00±9.28	37.22±13.18	NA	−8.695	44	0.001[a††]
UHDRS Cognitive	257.80±42.34	142.65±50.35	NA	8.046	41	0.001[b††]
UHDRS Behavioural	7.67±7.84	18.39±9.13	NA	−4.160	42	0.001[a††]
UHDRS Functional	25±0	17.91±5.68	NA	5.984	44	0.001[b††]
TFC	13±0	8.39±2.37	NA	9.329	44	0.001[b††]
Independence scale	99.8±1.04	78.04±12.49	NA	8.312	44	0.001[b††]
Disease burden	292.3±87.52	458.6±104.75	NA	−6.091	48	0.001[a††]

Legend. HD = Huntington's disease; Pre-HD = gene-positive, without motor symptoms; SD = standard deviation; df = degrees of freedom; CAG, trinucleotide repeat number; MMSE = Mini Mental State Examination; UHDRS = Unified Huntington's Disease Rating Scale; TFC = Total Functional Capacity; NA = Not Available; [††]T-student, Bonferroni correction.
[a]Pre-HD<HD (when referred to a cognitive scale comparison or CAG repetition, higher punctuations mean greater impairment).
[b]Pre-HD>HD (when referred to a cognitive scale comparison, higher punctuations mean lesser impairment).
*MMSE: Missing data for 5 Pre-HD & 5 HD subjects.
*UHDRS Motor: Missing data for 2 Pre-HD & 2 HD subjects.
*UHDRS Cognitive: Missing data for 5 Pre-HD & 2 HD subjects.
*UHDRS Behavioral: Missing data for 4 Pre-HD & 2 HD subjects.
*UHDRS Functional: Missing data for 2 Pre-HD & 2 HD subjects.
*TFC: Missing data for 2 Pre-HD & 2 HD subjects.

2000 ms; FOV: 230×168 mm, matrix: 256×256, slice thickness: 5 mm, number of slices: 24); 3) T1-weighted 3D images, with partitions acquired in the sagittal plane, using a modified driven equilibrium Fourier transform [26] sequence (TE/TR/TI: 2.4/7.92/910 ms, flip angle: 15°, 1 mm3 isotropic voxels); and 4) diffusion-weighted volumes were also acquired using SE echo-planar imaging (TE/TR: 89/8500 ms, bandwidth: 2126 Hz/voxel, matrix: 128×128, 80 axial slices, voxel size: 1.8×1.8×1.8 mm) with 30 isotropically distributed orientations for the diffusion sensitizing gradients at a b value of 1000 s/mm2 and 6 b = 0 images. Scanning was repeated 3 times to increase the signal-to-noise ratio.

Six consecutive T2*-weighted gradient echo-planar whole-brain volumes were acquired at different time of echo (TE) (TEs: 6, 12, 20, 30, 45 and 60 ms; TR = 5000; bandwidth = 1116 Hz/vx; matrix size 128×128×80; flip angle 90°; voxel size of 1.5×1.5×2 mm3).

Images were visually inspected for gross anatomical abnormalities by 2 experienced observers (a neuropsychologist expert in neuroimaging and a neuroradiologist) blind to participant identities.

Images were also visually inspected for movement artifacts, which are a common source of concern while studying HD. Since movement can compromise tracking, we excluded subjects who had excessive movement in their scans.

DTI Processing

Diffusion-weighted images were processed with FMRIB's Software Library (FSL 4.1 www.fmrib.ox.ac.uk/fsl/). Images were corrected for eddy current distortion. The non-diffusion-weighted images were skull stripped using FSL's Brain Extraction Tool (BET) (http://www.fmrib.ox.ac.uk/fsl/bet2/index.html), and used to mask all diffusion-weighted images. A diffusion tensor model was fitted at each voxel using Diffusion Toolkit, generating FA, AD, and RD maps. RD was defined as the average of the second and third eigenvalues of the diffusion tensor, while AD corresponded to the first eigenvalue.

T2*weighted images processing

T2*weighted volumes were post processed accordingly to previously published methods [21,27]. Briefly the six T2*weighted volumes were averaged in order to generate a mean T2*-weighted volume. A full affine 3D alignment was calculated between each of the six T2*-weighted volumes and the mean T2*-weighted volume. For each subject we performed a voxel-by-voxel nonlinear least-squares fitting of the data acquired at the six TEs to obtain a mono-exponential signal decay curve. In order to facilitate analysis of relaxation results, we considered the inverse of relaxation times, i.e. relaxation rates $R2* = 1/T2* \times 1000$.

Iron images (R2*) were registered into subject DTI space using FSL Flirt 12 degree of freedom transformation with the DTI B0 image used as the reference image. Registrations were visually inspected for accuracy.

Tractography

Tractography methods are outlined in more detail in [28], however, the tractography and ROI drawing was modified to use TrackVis, an interactive environment for fiber tracking reconstruction, display and analysis developed at the Harvard Medical School Martinos Center for Biomedical Imaging at Massachusetts General Hospital (www.trackvis.org). The FACT approach was used to reconstruct fiber paths. A track angle threshold of 35° was used as well as an image mask based on the B0 image to restrict tracking to biologically plausible results.

Tractography of the total deep white matter was performed by manually drawing regions of interest on each individuals FA color map by a single expert (O.P.) who was blinded to subject age, gender, and diagnosis. To determine intra-rater reliability, fiber tracts were identified in 10 randomly chosen brain volumes. Reliability was assessed using the intraclass correlation coefficient (2-way mixed for intra-rater). The advantage of DTI-based tractography is that the tracts can be precisely mapped within subjects without the reliance on registration prodedures to align imaging data across subjects [28].

Region of interest placement for the AF, SLF, Cing, ILF, IFO, ATR, and UF was based on Wakana, et al [28]. The total deep white matter was for the present study considered to be the combined white matter of the individual tracts (AF, SLF, Cing, ILF, IFO, ATR, and UF). FA, AD, RD, and iron were calculated for each subject by averaging all voxels over the total deep white matter and separately for each individual tract, counting each voxel only once. Excellent intra-reliability was achieved for ROI placement, as determined by computing the intra-class correlation coefficients for tract volume and mean FA, AD, RD and Iron (Table S1). It is important to note, that the specific anatomical delineations for the deep white matter tracts are still emerging. For example, the ILF in [28], may include the middle longitudinal fasciculus (see [29] and the specific delineations of the SLF and AF (temporal component of the SLF) has been a source on contention, [30].

Statistical Analysis

Demographic differences were assessed using chi-square, independent sample t-tests or Anova as appropriate. All statistical analyses were performed using SPSS 14.0.

To test for total deep white matter differences among groups, a Multivariate Analysis of Variance (Manova) was applied to all three groups (healthy controls, HD patients and Pre-HD subjects). Sex and age were included as covariates in the model. After that, contrasts were run to individuate the significant difference between groups.

In order to localize differences in individual deep white matter tracts between groups, a Multivariate Analysis of Variance (Manova) was applied to all three groups (healthy controls, HD patients and Pre-HD subjects). Sex and age were included as covariates in the model. After that, contrasts were run to individuate the significant difference between groups.

All results were corrected using a False Discovery Rate (FDR) correction, where order ranked p-values less than the resulting q-value were considered significant. Practically, results with a p-value less than 0.03 were considered significant.

Results

Subject demographics are reported in Table 1. Pre-HD subjects and HD patients differed in age and CAG repetition length, but not in gender. Additionally, as expected, HD patients had significantly poorer performances with respect to all measures assessed by the UHDRS, and also a significantly higher score of Disease Burden.

Total Deep White Matter Findings

Results are shown in Figure 1.

Statistical details are outlined in Table 2.

FA: Pre-HD subjects did not have significantly reduced FA. HD patients had reduced FA compared to Pre-HD subjects and controls.

AD: Pre-HD subjects had increased AD compared to controls. HD patients had increased AD compared to Pre-HD and control subjects.

RD: Pre-HD subjects showed increased RD compared to controls. HD patients also had increased RD compared to Pre-HD subjects and controls.

R2*: R2* values were elevated in Pre-HD subjects both compared to controls and HD patients. HD patients did not have different values of R2* compared to controls.

We explored the individual covariates' effect on white matter parameters, we found that age has an impact on diffusivity differences (AD and RD) between Controls and Pre-HD subjects, that results in the loss of statistical significance. All other results remain significant in the same direction. We did not find any effect of gender on the white matter parameters.

Hemisphere Deep White Matter

Results are shown in Figure 2.

Hemisphere deep white matter is the combined total of the deep white matter tracts for the left and, separately, for the right hemisphere. Statistical details are outlined in Table 2.

FA: Pre-HD subjects had reduced FA in the right hemisphere deep white matter and HD patients had reduced FA in both the left and right hemisphere deep white matter compared to both Pre-HD and control subjects.

AD: Pre-HD subjects had increased right hemisphere AD compared to controls. HD patients had increased AD compared to Pre-HD and control subjects in both hemispheres.

RD: Pre-HD subjects showed bilateral increases in RD compared to controls and HD patients had elevated bilateral RD compared to Pre-HD subjects and controls.

R2*: R2* values were elevated in both hemispheres within Pre-HD subjects compared to both controls and HD patients. HD patients did not have different values of R2* compared to controls.

Individual Deep White Matter tract Findings

Results are shown in Figure 2 and Figure 3.

Statistical details of tractography analysis of the individual deep white matter tracts are in Table 3 and Table S2.

FA: Pre-HD subjects revealed, compared to controls, lower FA in the right SLF, IFO and UF for Pre-HD subjects. In comparisons to controls, HD patients had lower FA bilaterally in the AF, SLF, Cing, IFO, ILF, and UF. Finally, FA analyses between Pre-HD subjects and HD patients revealed reductions in HD patients bilaterally in the AF, SLF, Cing, IFO as well as the right ILF.

AD: Pre-HD subjects exhibited, compared to controls, increased AD bilaterally in the SLF and ATR. AD analysis between HD patients and controls revealed increased AD bilaterally in the AF, SLF, IFO, and ATR as well as the left ILF and right UF. Furthermore, when comparing Pre-HD subjects with HD patients, HD patients had increased AD bilaterally in AF, SLF, IFO, and ATR as well as the left ILF.

RD: Pre-HD subjects, compared to healthy controls, showed significant increased RD in the SLF, and ATR bilaterally, as well as the right IFO. HD patients also showed increased RD compared to healthy controls bilaterally in the AF, SLF, Cing, ILF, IFO, ATR, and UF. Finally, Pre-HD subjects had lower RD compared to HD patients bilaterally in the AF, SLF, Cing, ILF, IFO, ATR and right UF.

R2*: The analysis between Pre-HD subjects and controls revealed increased R2* values in Pre-HD subjects in the left AF and right Cing and IFO. There were no differences in R2* values between HD patients and controls. However, when comparing

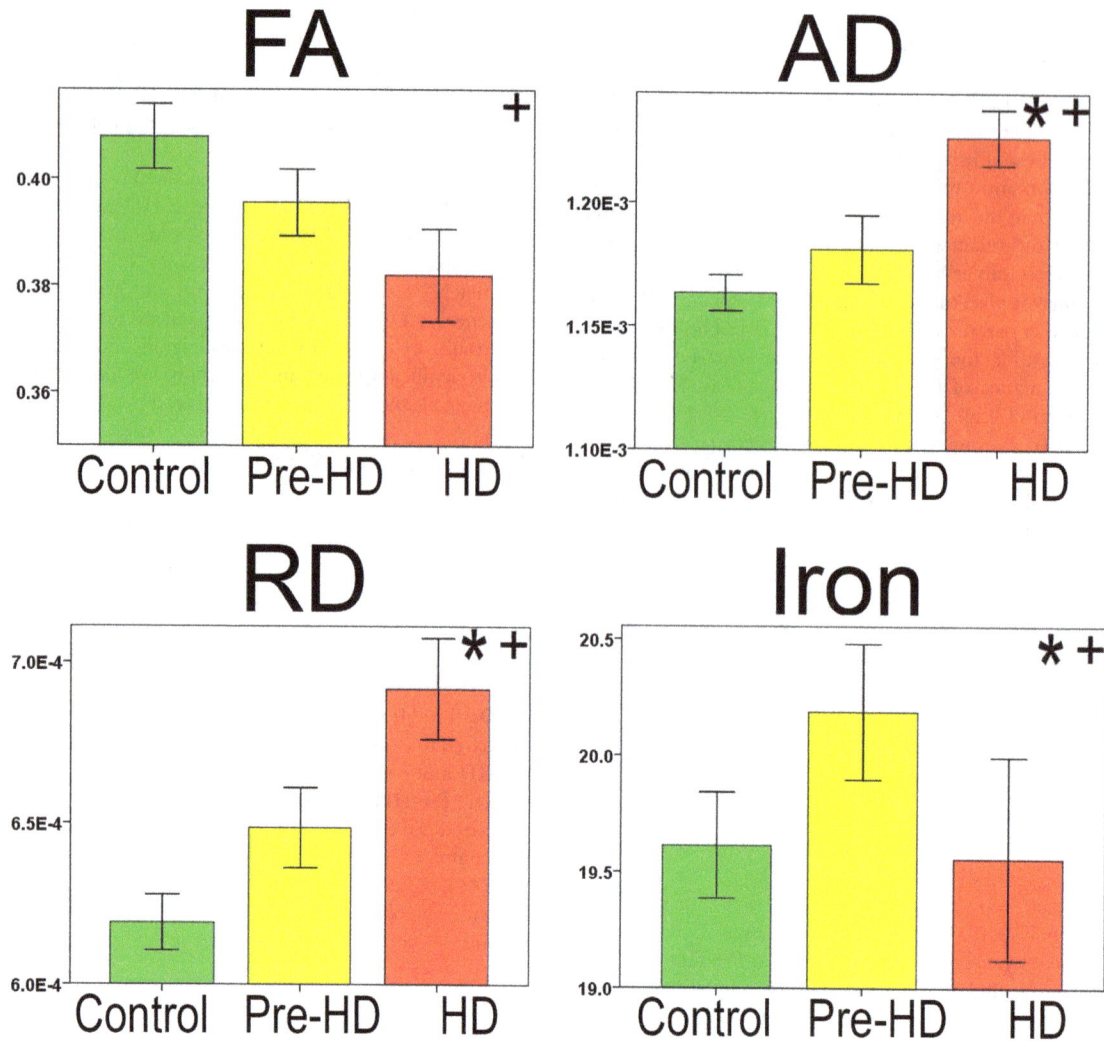

Figure 1. Total Deep White Matter Tractography and Group Comparison. Bar graphs show differences between Total Deep White Matter FA, AD, RD, and Iron. The error bars represent the Standard Error Mean (SEM). Legend. FA = Fractional Anisotropy; AD = Axial Diffusivity; RD = Radial Diffusivity. (AD/RD Mean units: 10^{-3} mm^2/s, R2* (10^{-3} mm^1/s). * Significant difference between Pre-HD and Controls+ Significant difference between Pre-HD and HD.

Pre-HD subjects and HD patients, Pre-HD subjects had increased R2* values bilaterally in the IFO as well as in the left AF, SLF and right Cing, ILF and ATR.

Discussion

This study sought to identify variations in the deep white matter (total and individual tracts) of Pre-HD subjects and HD patients compared to each other and to healthy controls. A number of major findings emerged from the results: (1) increases in AD and RD in total deep white matter are present in Pre-HD subjects before disease onset; (2) Pre-HD subjects show increased total deep white matter iron content (R2* values) compared to both controls and HD patients; (3) changes in individual white matter tracts in Pre-HD are pervasive and become worse as the disease progresses.

Postmortem studies have repeatedly demonstrated the striking myelin breakdown and white matter atrophy in HD [31]. Furthermore, a HD mouse model [32], found thinner myelin sheaths and increased myelin periodicity (that is less compacted the white matter). Also, an increasing number of white matter DTI

studies on human subjects have found extensive distributed changes to white matter microstructure both in Pre-HD and HD subjects [9–13,33–36]

Our current findings on total deep white matter are in line with these previous works. We found an increase in AD and RD in Pre-HD subjects compared to healthy controls and abnormalities become significantly worse in HD. The precise biological meaning of the DTI parameters is still unclear [17] and caution should be used in interpreting the results. However, AD a measure of how fast diffusion occurs in the preferred direction, has been shown to be sensitive to the number of axons, as well as their coherence [37]. Increased AD is related to white matter axonal atrophy likely associated with Wallerian degeneration [38]. RD is a measure of how fast diffusion occurs in the perpendicular direction. Increased RD is thought to reflect reductions in myelination [39].

These white matter changes can be interpreted as a manifestation of the pathology's evolution. Indeed, our data suggests that the deep white matter incurs early axonal atrophy (increased AD) and myelin damage (increased RD) even before measurable symptoms appear (Pre-HD stage), and this insult to deep white

Table 2. Total Deep White Matter Tractography Group Comparisons.

Region		Pre-HD	HD	Control	MANOVA			Control vs Pre-HD	Control vs HD	Pre-HD vs HD
					F	df	p	p	p	p
Total Deep White Matter (mean value ± SD)	FA	0.399±0.017	0.378±0.022	0.408±0.023	14.81	2,95	0.001	0.048	**0.001**	**0.005**
	AD	1.118E-03±3.00E-05	1.234E-03±3.00E-05	1.116E-03±3.00E-05	41.52	2,95	0.001	**0.013**	**0.001**	**0.001**
	RD	6.38E-04±4.00E-0	7.01E-04±4.00E-05	6.19E-04±3.00E-05	42.132	2,95	0.001	**0.002**	**0.001**	**0.001**
	R2*	20.19±0.75	19.54±1.08	19.62±0.71	4.383	2,85	0.011	**0.010**	0.676	**0.010**

Legend. FA = Fractional Anisotropy; AD = Axial Diffusivity; RD = Radial Diffusivity. (AD/RD Mean units: 10^{-3} mm^2/s, R2* (10^{-3} mm^1/s).
*Significant FDR corrected results are in **BOLD**.

matter increases progressively as the disease progresses (stage I and II). However, it is important to keep in mind the hypothesis that abnormal brain development may contribute to the pathogenesis of HD, as a precursor to the more global neurodegeneration process [40]. Future longitudinal studies are needed to examine if deep white matter changes are already in place in young Pre-HD subjects.

In order to explore the underlying mechanism of deep white matter abnormalities in HD, we examined the iron content. We found a significant increase in iron content within Pre-HD subjects compared to both healthy controls and HD patients. This suggests that a repair mechanism is active in Pre-HD subjects, and it may lead to an increase in oligodendrocytes before disease onset. The data is in line with previous reports on iron levels in Pre-HD subjects. In fact, extremely elevated numbers of oligodendrocytes have been reported years before symptom appearance [41–43]. The ability to repair appears to keep the brain working with minimal symptoms early in the disease and may be why white matter damage has not been identified to be a central part of HD. The repair mechanism may mask the downstream effects the damage causes.

Furthermore, because HD patients have substantially impaired total deep white matter compared to Pre-HD subjects, it may indicate that the repair process is failing. There are two likely reasons for this. One, the oligodendrocytes themselves may be abnormal and thus they do not function correctly and/or the accumulation of oligodendrocytes could be helpful at first, but may be harmful once the levels become too high by causing neuronal excitotoxicity and promoting free radical toxicity [2]. Either of these possibilities fit with the idea that the HD brain is continually trying to remyelinate in a losing attempt to compensate for the disease-related myelin loss [2]. In HD, these remyelination processes may successfully compensate during younger years, which usually correspond to the beginning of the pathology or to the years before onset (Pre-HD stage), but eventually begin failing in older years as brain myelin volume continues to grow and the maintenance of this expanding volume becomes increasingly difficult. This is similar to what happens in healthy older individuals [44] and likely explains the decrease in iron content that we found between Pre-HD and HD subjects.

Interestingly, myelin may play a role in producing adenosine triphosphate (ATP) [46], if this is the case, damage to the total deep white matter could have a substantial impact on the brain's available energy, however, future studies will be needed to verify this.

The R2* measurement has some limitations. Indeed it is sensitive to increases in tissue iron, which increases the R2* value [45] but it is not a specific measure of iron. In fact, many other tissue changes, including myelination, calcifications, blood flow, and increased tissue water, can influence the R2* measure.

Although R2* is not an exclusive measure of iron, combined with diffusivity parameters it helps us reach a conclusion regarding the data. This is because as our DTI findings in Pre-HD subjects indicate tissue damage with more water and myelin damage (see changes in diffusivity Figure 1 and 2), both factors should lower the R2* values in our data. However, we still found higher R2* values in Pre-HD group (Figure 2). This suggests that higher R2* values reflect greater iron in our Pre-HD group.

Furthermore, shimming effects were controled for using the protocol outlined in Peran et al. [27].

However, in the future, higher Tesla strengths, such as 7T or above, and phase images (more related to the iron content) or quantitative susceptibility mapping should be investigated to confirm this data.

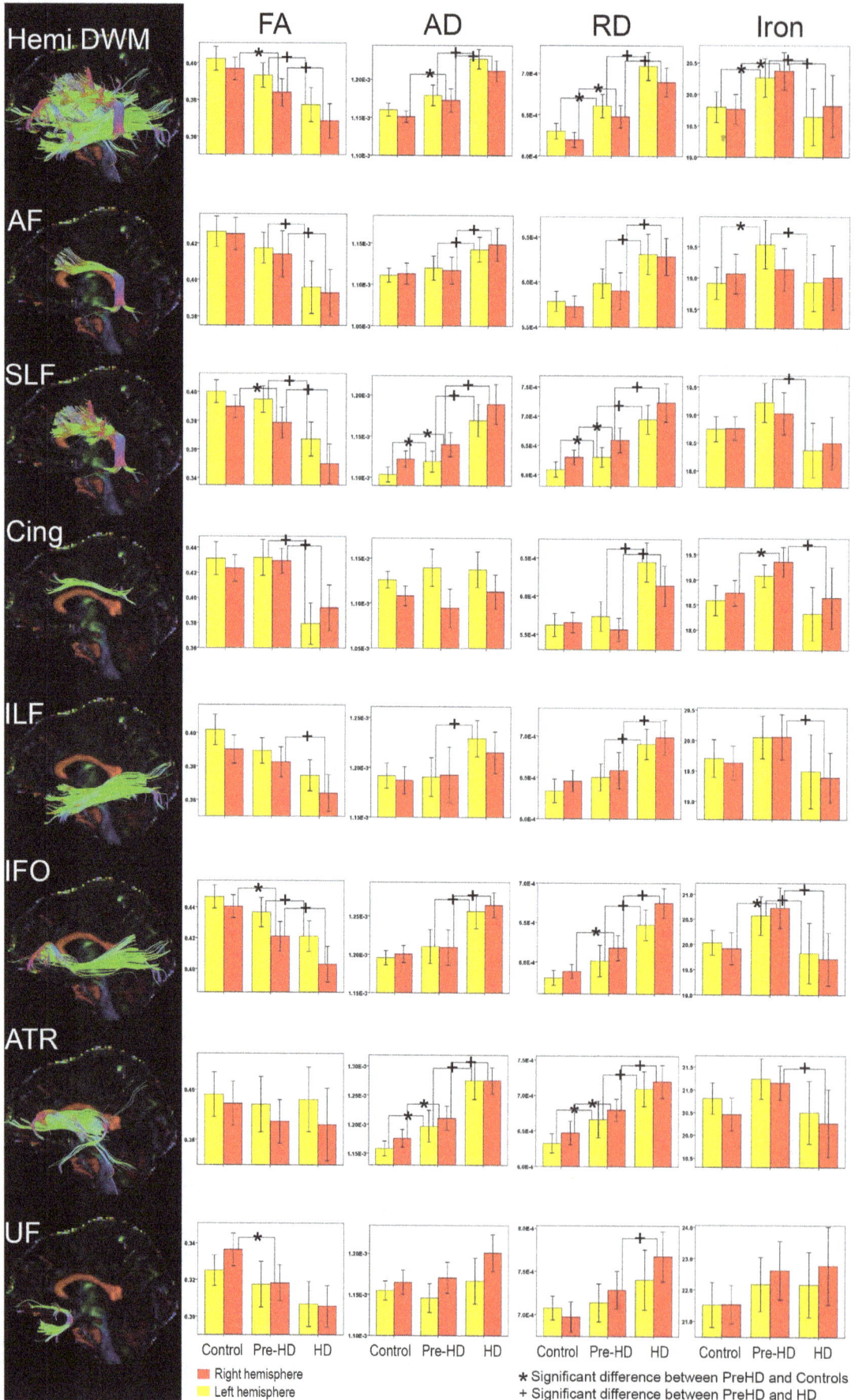

Right hemisphere
Left hemisphere

* Significant difference between PreHD and Controls
+ Significant difference between PreHD and HD

Figure 2. Individual Deep White Matter Tractography and Group Comparison. Bar graphs show differences between Deep White Matter Tracts FA, AD, RD, and Iron. The error bars represent the Standard Error Mean (SEM). Legend. FA = Fractional Anisotropy; AD = Axial Diffusivity; RD = Radial Diffusivity. (AD/RD Mean units: 10^{-3} mm^2/s, R2* (10^{-3} mm^1/s) Tracts are from a representative single subject. Legend. Hemi DWM = total Deep White Matter for each hemisphere, it is the result of the individual white matter tracts combined, AF = Arcuate Fasciculus, SLF = Superior Longitudinal Fasciculus, Cing = Cingulate, ILF = Inferior Longitudinal Fasciculus, IFO = Inferior Frontal Occipital fasciculus, ATR = Anterior Thalamic Radiation, UF = Uncinate Fasciculus.

In order to identify whether the changes in the deep white matter were localized to individual tracts or presented in a pattern, we examined each tract's microstructure. When comparing controls and Pre-HD subjects, we found the ILF tract was spared in Pre-HD subjects (no difference in FA, AD, RD and iron level). We also found that the AF and Cing did not show any microstructure changes (no difference in FA, AD, RD) but they present a higher level of iron unilaterally (left side for the AF, right side for the Cing) which indicates that the repair mechanism is working in these fibers, hiding the microstructural damage. We further found the IFO and UF were damaged unilaterally (decreased right FA, and increased RD for the IFO, decreased right FA for the UF) and increased iron level in the right IFO which indicates that the repair mechanism is at a breaking point, with both high level of iron and microstructural damage detectable. Finally, we found that the SLF and the ATR were the most damaged tracts at the microstructural level (increased of AD and RD bilaterally) and no difference in iron, which indicates

that the repair mechanism already failed in those fibers, and the damage progressed to impair both sides of the tracts.

Thus, it seems that individual white matter tracts are impaired in a specific manner in Pre-HD subjects, and it is possible to describe a pattern in the tract damage, going from spared (ILF), to more damaged (SLF and ATR), passing through those only partially damaged (IFO and UF) to those damaged and under repair (AF and Cing).

When we compare Pre-HD subjects with HD patients, the fibers already damaged in the Pre-HD phase, proceed in a peculiar way. The ILF, initially spared in Pre-HD, becomes impaired in HD (increased AD on the left side; increased RD bilaterally; increased iron on the right side); the AF and Cing, initially with a spared microstructure in Pre-HD, show bilateral microstructural changes in HD; the IFO, damaged unilaterally in Pre-HD, becomes impaired bilaterally in HD; the UF remains stable and relatively spared in both Pre-HD and HD; the SLF and the ATR, already damaged in the Pre-HD phase, become increasingly impaired. We found a high level of iron in Pre-HD compared to HD at the level of the SLF and the ATR, which was not present when Pre-HD subjects were compared with controls, which suggests a repair mechanism was active but is no longer working in HD patients.

Thus it seems that in our sample group: the SLF and ATR are fibers involved in the early phase of the pathology (Pre-HD) while the IFO is relatively spared early but worsens quickly unlike the UF which is more spared throughout the course of the pathology.

The difference in the individual white matter tracts damage (i.e. unilateral or bilateral involvement, early or late involvement in the course of the pathology) may be due to their different function and/or structure. As for the function, it seems there is a link between the fibers we have found damaged or spared (as the UF) and some aspects of the disease. For example, the ATR is involved in executive function and planning complex behaviours and working memory and encoding of new stimuli [47]. The SLF, with its three subcomponents SLFI SLFII and SFLII, is involved in regulation of higher aspects of motor behavior, in spatial attention and in gesture [48,49]. The IFO is involved in the awareness and use of visual information for the purpose of guiding movements and in the preparation and release of reaching-grasping arm movement [50] as well as the execution of language processing [49]. The UF, which is the spared one, is linked with the regulation of auditory stimuli and recognition memory [50] and likely plays a role in the language network [49]. However, despite our growing understanding of the deep white matter tracts, there is still much we do not yet know about their function thus, cautious consideration is warranted before drawing conclusions between the HD symptomology and specific tracts.

As for the structure, there is some evidence that HD might preferentially damage large early myelinating fibers such as those in the isthmus/splenium of the corpus callosum, which connect to the occipital lobe [13,14,33]. Large fibers can be advantageous because they encode more information but even a simple doubling in firing rate appears to more than quadruple an axon's energy use [51]. Large early myelinating high caliber fibers might thus be particularly susceptible. However, all the tracts had significantly worse microstructure as the disease progressed, with changes in

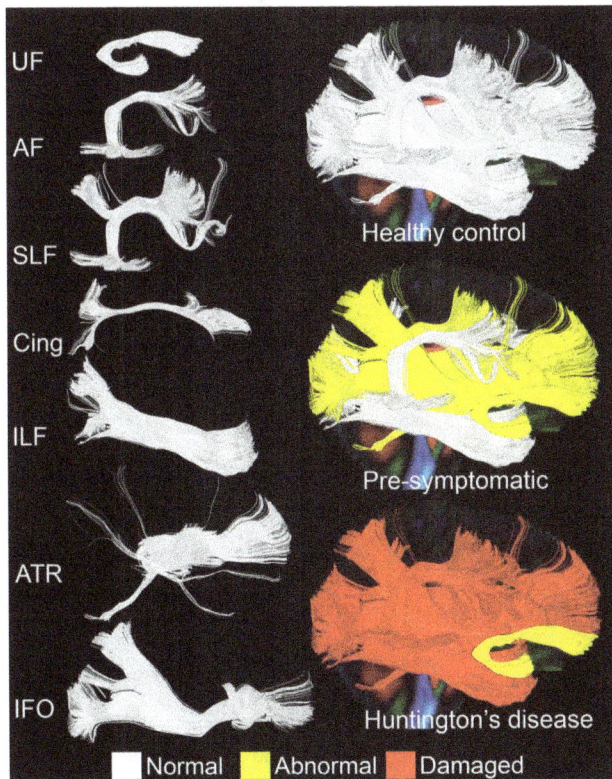

Figure 3. Deep White Matter Microstructure for Each Group. Tracts shown use colour to represent the overall microstructure for each tract within each group. White = Normal, Yellow = Abnormal, Red = Damaged. Tracts Legend. AF = Arcuate Fasciculus, SLF = Superior Longitudinal Fasciculus, Cing = Cingulate, ILF = Inferior Longitudinal Fasciculus, IFO = Inferior Frontal Occipital fasciculus, ATR = Anterior Thalamic Radiation, UF = Uncinate Fasciculus.

Table 3. Individual Deep White Matter Tractography Group Comparisons.

Region	Parameters	MANOVA			Control vs Pre-HD	Control vs HD	Pre-HD vs HD
		F	df	P	P	P	P
	FA	11.72	2,95	0	0.128	**0.001**	**0.007**
Hemi DWM L	AD	41.226	2,95	0	0.033	**0.001**	**0.001**
	RD	42.081	2,95	0	**0.002**	**0.001**	**0.001**
	R2*	3.956	2,85	0.023	**0.027**	0.392	**0.009**
	FA	15.459	2,95	0	**0.025**	**0.001**	**0.008**
Hemi DWM R	AD	32.857	2,95	0	**0.013**	**0.001**	**0.001**
	RD	33.854	2,95	0	**0.004**	**0.001**	**0.001**
	R2*	4.217	2,85	0.018	**0.007**	0.945	**0.023**
	FA	9.489	2,95	0.000	0.284	**0.001**	**0.008**
AF L	AD	7.662	2,95	0.001	0.358	**0.001**	**0.014**
	RD	12.412	2,95	0.001	0.097	**0.001**	**0.007**
	R2*	4.184	2,85	0.018	**0.009**	0.921	**0.018**
	FA	9.259	2,95	0.001	0.204	**0.001**	**0.013**
AF R	AD	5.869	2,95	0.004	0.832	**0.001**	**0.011**
	RD	12.739	2,95	0.001	0.183	**0.001**	**0.003**
	R2*	0.106	2,85	0.899	0.773	0.809	0.647
	FA	10.908	2,95	0	0.132	**0.001**	**0.010**
SLF L	AD	25.772	2,95	0	**0.007**	**0.001**	**0.001**
	RD	26.074	2,95	0	**0.003**	**0.001**	**0.001**
	R2*	5.118	2,85	0.008	0.035	0.133	**0.002**
	FA	14.621	2,95	0	**0.023**	**0.001**	**0.013**
SLF R	AD	18.941	2,95	0	**0.020**	**0.001**	**0.002**
	RD	22.77	2,95	0	**0.002**	**0.001**	**0.004**
	R2*	2.184	2,85	0.119	0.194	0.276	0.040
	FA	11.218	2,95	0	0.453	**0.001**	**0.001**
Cing L	AD	1.282	2,95	0.282	0.131	0.366	0.603
	RD	18.397	2,95	0	0.052	**0.001**	**0.001**
	R2*	2.331	2,85	0.103	0.092	0.499	0.042
	FA	5.607	2,95	0.005	0.852	**0.002**	**0.006**
Cing R	AD	0.573	2,95	0.566	0.343	0.850	0.339
	RD	7.015	2,95	0.001	0.904	**0.001**	**0.003**
	R2*	3.669	2,85	0.03	**0.018**	0.721	**0.019**
	FA	8.587	2,95	0	0.089	**0.001**	0.050
ILF L	AD	7.036	2,95	0.001	0.768	**0.001**	**0.002**
	RD	12.574	2,95	0	0.218	**0.001**	**0.002**
	R2*	1.804	2,85	0.171	0.193	0.395	0.064
	FA	7.896	2,95	0.001	0.337	**0.001**	**0.014**
ILF R	AD	2.333	2,95	0.102	0.764	0.035	0.129
	RD	10.176	2,95	0	0.381	**0.001**	**0.003**
	R2*	3.79	2,85	0.027	0.056	0.235	**0.008**
	FA	8.716	2,95	0	0.146	**0.001**	**0.027**
IFO L	AD	15.865	2,95	0	0.277	**0.001**	**0**
	RD	23.041	2,95	0	0.064	**0.001**	**0**
	R2*	3.781	2,85	0.027	0.050	0.262	**0.008**
	FA	17.85	2,95	0	**0.006**	**0.001**	**0.014**
IFO R	AD	19.794	2,95	0	0.595	**0.001**	**0**
	RD	47.271	2,95	0	**0.005**	**0.001**	**0**
	R2*	7.113	2,85	0.001	**0.003**	0.327	**0.001**

Table 3. Cont.

Region	Parameters	MANOVA			Control vs Pre-HD	Control vs HD	Pre-HD vs HD
		F	df	P	P	P	P
	FA	0.148	2,95	0.862	0.593	0.803	0.810
ATR L	AD	32.937	2,95	0	**0.022**	**0.001**	**0.001**
	RD	16.961	2,95	0	**0.022**	**0.001**	**0.005**
	R2*	2.368	2,85	0.100	0.160	0.283	0.033
	FA	0.848	2,95	0.431	0.344	0.263	0.887
ATR R	AD	30.096	2,95	0	**0.019**	**0.001**	**0.001**
	RD	15.608	2,95	0	**0.025**	**0.001**	**0.008**
	R2*	3.577	2,85	0.032	0.032	0.463	**0.014**
	FA	3.174	2,95	0.046	0.352	**0.014**	0.193
UF L	AD	1.214	2,95	0.302	0.413	0.306	0.124
	RD	2.577	2,95	0.081	0.757	**0.027**	0.110
	R2*	0.893	2,85	0.413	0.274	0.282	0.997
	FA	10.228	2,95	0	**0.017**	**0.001**	0.114
UF R	AD	4.421	2,95	0.015	0.753	**0.004**	0.032
	RD	10.889	2,95	0	0.064	**0.001**	**0.024**
	R2*	2.673	2,85	0.075	0.087	0.046	0.785

Legend. AF = Arcuate Fasciculus, SLF = Superior Longitudinal Fasciculus, Cing = Cingulate, ILF = Inferior Longitudinal Fasciculus, IFO = Inferior Frontal Occipital fasciculus, ATR = Anterior Thalamic Radiation, UF = Uncinate Fasciculus; Hemi DWM = total left and right Deep White Matter, it is the result of the individual white matter tracts combined for each hemisphere; FA = Fractional Anisotropy; AD = Axial Diffusivity; RD = Radial Diffusivity; R = Right; L = Left.
*Significant FDR corrected results are in **BOLD**.

FA, AD and RD involving the tracts bilaterally. In particular though, across the DTI parameters (FA, AD, RD), the parameter that was most sensitive to disease effects was RD, indeed each individual tract (AF, SLF; Cing, ILF, IFO and UF) presented an increase in RD for HD patients.

Again our data is in line with the accumulating number of DTI studies of Pre-HD and HD subjects that have looked at white matter. For example, a very recent paper showed extensive alterations to white matter in HD that effects many different anatomical regions [12] and others are rapidly uncovering similar findings [9–11]. Because these abnormalities in white matter are being reliably found despite different populations and different methodological approaches, it strongly suggests that there may be a common mechanism damaging white matter across the whole brain in HD. This is important because damage to white matter is extremely detrimental to the brain. There are extensive reasons for this and they are covered in detail by Bartzokis [16]). In short, 1) synapses depends on axonal transport for survival and this is disrupted when white matter is damaged; 2) repair is extremely energetically expensive; 3) repaired myelin is not as good (thinner sheaths, increased number of internodes) as the original undamaged one.

Conclusions

White matter is critical to the human brain's complexity [16] and we have shown that it is damaged in Pre-HD years before symptoms occur in a specific pattern. Furthermore, Pre-HD subjects attempt to repair this damage but fail as the disease progresses. Finally, the data presented supports the conclusion that changes to deep white matter are a central component of HD.

Supporting Information

Table S1   Intra-rater Reliability Coefficient.

Table S2   Tract Measures.

Author Contributions

Analyzed the data: OP. Wrote the paper: OP. Interpreted the data: OP MDP. Revised the manuscript: MDP US FS CC. Performed the experiment: CSC FE. Collected the data: CSC FE.

References

1. Esmaeilzadeh M, Ciarmiello A, Squitieri F (2011) Seeking brain biomarkers for preventive therapy in Huntington disease. CNS Neurosci Ther 17: 368–386.
2. Bartzokis G, Lu PH, Tishler TA, Fong SM, Oluwadara B, et al. (2007) Myelin breakdown and iron changes in Huntington's disease: pathogenesis and treatment implications. Neurochem Res 32: 1655–1664.
3. Ehrlich ME (2012) Huntington's disease and the striatal medium spiny neuron: cell-autonomous and non-cell-autonomous mechanisms of disease. Neurotherapeutics 9: 270–284.
4. Bartzokis G (2012) Neuroglialpharmacology: myelination as a shared mechanism of action of psychotropic treatments. Neuropharmacology 62: 2137–2153.
5. Han I, You Y, Kordower JH, Brady ST, Morfini GA (2010) Differential vulnerability of neurons in Huntington's disease: the role of cell type-specific features. J Neurochem 113: 1073–1091.
6. Squitieri F, Cannella M, Simonelli M, Sassone J, Martino T, et al. (2009) Distinct brain volume changes correlating with clinical stage, disease progression rate, mutation size, and age at onset prediction as early biomarkers of brain atrophy in Huntington's disease. CNS Neurosci Ther 15: 1–11.
7. Aylward EH, Anderson NB, Bylsma FW, Wagster MV, Barta PE, et al. (1998) Frontal lobe volume in patients with Huntington's disease. Neurology 50: 252–258.

8. Paulsen JS, Magnotta VA, Mikos AE, Paulson HL, Penziner E, et al. (2006) Brain structure in preclinical Huntington's disease. Biol Psychiatry 59: 57–63.

9. Kloppel S, Draganski B, Golding CV, Chu C, Nagy Z, et al. (2008) White matter connections reflect changes in voluntary-guided saccades in pre-symptomatic Huntington's disease. Brain 131: 196–204.

10. Dumas EM, van den Bogaard SJ, Ruber ME, Reilman RR, Stout JC, et al. (2012) Early changes in white matter pathways of the sensorimotor cortex in premanifest Huntington's disease. Hum Brain Mapp 33: 203–212.

11. Di Paola M, Luders E, Cherubini A, Sanchez-Castaneda C, Thompson PM, et al. (2012) Multimodal MRI analysis of the corpus callosum reveals white matter differences in presymptomatic and early Huntington's disease. Cereb Cortex 22: 2858–2866.

12. Novak MJ, Seunarine KK, Gibbard CR, Hobbs NZ, Scahill RI, et al. (2013) White matter integrity in premanifest and early Huntington's disease is related to caudate loss and disease progression. Cortex.

13. Phillips O, Sanchez-Castaneda C, Elifani F, Maglione V, Di Pardo A, et al. (2013) Tractography of the Corpus Callosum in Huntington's Disease. PLoS One 8: e73280.

14. Di Paola M, Phillips OR, Sanchez-Castaneda C, Di Pardo A, Maglione V, et al. (2014) MRI measures of corpus callosum iron and myelin in early Huntington's disease. Hum Brain Mapp 35: 3143–3151.

15. Phillips O, Squitieri F, Sanchez-Castaneda C, Elifani F, Griguoli A, et al. (2014) The Corticospinal Tract in Huntington's Disease. Cereb Cortex.

16. Bartzokis G (2011) Alzheimer's disease as homeostatic responses to age-related myelin breakdown. Neurobiol Aging 32: 1341–1371.

17. Jones DK, Knosche TR, Turner R (2012) White matter integrity, fiber count, and other fallacies: The do's and don'ts of diffusion MRI. Neuroimage.

18. Phillips OR, Clark KA, Luders E, Azhir R, Joshi SH, et al. (2013) Superficial white matter: effects of age, sex, and hemisphere. Brain Connect 3: 146–159.

19. Di Paola M, Luders E, Di Iulio F, Cherubini A, Passafiume D, et al. (2010) Callosal atrophy in mild cognitive impairment and Alzheimer's disease: different effects in different stages. Neuroimage 49: 141–149.

20. Phillips OR, Nuechterlein KH, Asarnow RF, Clark KA, Cabeen R, et al. (2011) Mapping corticocortical structural integrity in schizophrenia and effects of genetic liability. Biol Psychiatry 70: 680–689.

21. Cherubini A, Peran P, Caltagirone C, Sabatini U, Spalletta G (2009) Aging of subcortical nuclei: microstructural, mineralization and atrophy modifications measured in vivo using MRI. NeuroImage 48: 29–36.

22. Cherubini A, Peran P, Hagberg GE, Varsi AE, Luccichenti G, et al. (2009) Characterization of white matter fiber bundles with T2* relaxometry and diffusion tensor imaging. Magn Reson Med 61: 1066–1072.

23. Kieburtz K, Penney JB, Como P, Ranen N, Shoulson I, et al. (1996) Unified Huntington's disease rating scale: Reliability and consistency. Movement Disorders 11: 136–142.

24. Penney JB Jr, Vonsattel JP, MacDonald ME, Gusella JF, Myers RH (1997) CAG repeat number governs the development rate of pathology in Huntington's disease. Ann Neurol 41: 689–692.

25. Folstein MF, Folstein SE, McHugh PR (1975) "Mini-mental state". A practical method for grading the cognitive state of patients for the clinician. J Psychiatr Res 12: 189–198.

26. Deichmann R, Schwarzbauer C, Turner R (2004) Optimisation of the 3D MDEFT sequence for anatomical brain imaging: technical implications at 1.5 and 3 T. Neuroimage 21: 757–767.

27. Peran P, Hagberg G, Luccichenti G, Cherubini A, Brainovich V, et al. (2007) Voxel-based analysis of R2* maps in the healthy human brain. J Magn Reson Imaging 26: 1413–1420.

28. Wakana S, Caprihan A, Panzenboeck MM, Fallon JH, Perry M, et al. (2007) Reproducibility of quantitative tractography methods applied to cerebral white matter. Neuroimage 36: 630–644.

29. Makris N, Preti MG, Asami T, Pelavin P, Campbell B, et al. (2013) Human middle longitudinal fascicle: variations in patterns of anatomical connections. Brain Struct Funct 218: 951–968.

30. Dick AS, Bernal B, Tremblay P (2013) The Language Connectome: New Pathways, New Concepts. Neuroscientist.

31. de la Monte SM, Vonsattel JP, Richardson EP Jr (1988) Morphometric demonstration of atrophic changes in the cerebral cortex, white matter, and neostriatum in Huntington's disease. J Neuropathol Exp Neurol 47: 516–525.

32. Xiang Z, Valenza M, Cui L, Leoni V, Jeong HK, et al. (2011) Peroxisome-proliferator-activated receptor gamma coactivator 1 alpha contributes to dysmyelination in experimental models of Huntington's disease. J Neurosci 31: 9544–9553.

33. Rosas HD, Lee SY, Bender AC, Zaleta AK, Vangel M, et al. (2010) Altered white matter microstructure in the corpus callosum in Huntington's disease: implications for cortical "disconnection". Neuroimage 49: 2995–3004.

34. Bohanna I, Georgiou-Karistianis N, Sritharan A, Asadi H, Johnston L, et al. (2011) Diffusion tensor imaging in Huntington's disease reveals distinct patterns of white matter degeneration associated with motor and cognitive deficits. Brain Imaging Behav 5: 171–180.

35. Marrakchi-Kacem L, Delmaire C, Guevara P, Poupon F, Lecomte S, et al. (2013) Mapping cortico-striatal connectivity onto the cortical surface: a new tractography-based approach to study Huntington disease. PLoS One 8: e53135.

36. Matsui JT, Vaidya JG, Johnson HJ, Magnotta VA, Long JD, et al. (2013) Diffusion weighted imaging of prefrontal cortex in prodromal huntington's disease. Hum Brain Mapp.

37. Takahashi M, Ono J, Harada K, Maeda M, Hackney DB (2000) Diffusional anisotropy in cranial nerves with maturation: quantitative evaluation with diffusion MR imaging in rats. Radiology 216: 881–885.

38. Hasan KM, Sankar A, Halphen C, Kramer LA, Brandt ME, et al. (2007) Development and organization of the human brain tissue compartments across the lifespan using diffusion tensor imaging. Neuroreport 18: 1735–1739.

39. Schmierer K, Wheeler-Kingshott CA, Tozer DJ, Boulby PA, Parkes HG, et al. (2008) Quantitative magnetic resonance of postmortem multiple sclerosis brain before and after fixation. Magn Reson Med 59: 268–277.

40. Nopoulos PC, Aylward EH, Ross CA, Johnson HJ, Magnotta VA, et al. (2010) Cerebral cortex structure in prodromal Huntington disease. Neurobiol Dis 40: 544–554.

41. Gomez-Tortosa E, MacDonald ME, Friend JC, Taylor SA, Weiler LJ, et al. (2001) Quantitative neuropathological changes in presymptomatic Huntington's disease. Ann Neurol 49: 29–34.

42. Myers RH, Vonsattel JP, Paskevich PA, Kiely DK, Stevens TJ, et al. (1991) Decreased neuronal and increased oligodendroglial densities in Huntington's disease caudate nucleus. J Neuropathol Exp Neurol 50: 729–742.

43. Sotrel A, Paskevich PA, Kiely DK, Bird ED, Williams RS, et al. (1991) Morphometric analysis of the prefrontal cortex in Huntington's disease. Neurology 41: 1117–1123.

44. Bartzokis G, Lu PH, Heydari P, Couvrette A, Lee GJ, et al. (2012) Multimodal magnetic resonance imaging assessment of white matter aging trajectories over the lifespan of healthy individuals. Biol Psychiatry 72: 1026–1034.

45. Browne SE (2008) Mitochondria and Huntington's disease pathogenesis: insight from genetic and chemical models. Ann N Y Acad Sci 1147: 358–382.

46. Ravera S, Panfoli I, Calzia D, Aluigi MG, Bianchini P, et al. (2009) Evidence for aerobic ATP synthesis in isolated myelin vesicles. Int J Biochem Cell Biol 41: 1581–1591.

47. Zoppelt D, Koch B, Schwarz M, Daum I (2003) Involvement of the mediodorsal thalamic nucleus in mediating recollection and familiarity. Neuropsychologia 41: 1160–1170.

48. Makris N, Kennedy DN, McInerney S, Sorensen AG, Wang R, et al. (2005) Segmentation of subcomponents within the superior longitudinal fascicle in humans: a quantitative, in vivo, DT-MRI study. Cereb Cortex 15: 854–869.

49. Muthusami P, James J, Thomas B, Kapilamoorthy TR, Kesavadas C (2013) Diffusion tensor imaging and tractography of the human language pathways: Moving into the clinical realm. J Magn Reson Imaging.

50. Schmahmann JD, Pandya DN (2006) Fiber pathways of the brain. Oxford; New York: Oxford University Press. xviii, 654 p. p.

51. Perge JA, Niven JE, Mugnaini E, Balasubramanian V, Sterling P (2012) Why do axons differ in caliber? J Neurosci 32: 626–638.

21

Differential Effect of HDAC3 on Cytoplasmic and Nuclear Huntingtin Aggregates

Tatsuo Mano[1], Takayoshi Suzuki[2,3], Shoji Tsuji[1], Atsushi Iwata[1,3]*

1 Department of Neurology, Graduate School of Medicine, The University of Tokyo, Tokyo, Japan, **2** Department of Graduate School of Medical Science, Kyoto Prefectural University of Medicine, Kyoto, Japan, **3** Japan Science and Technology Agency, Precursory Research for Embryonic Science and Technology (PRESTO), Saitama, Japan

Abstract

Histone deacetylases (HDACs) are potential therapeutic targets of polyglutamine (pQ) diseases including Huntington's disease (HD) that may function to correct aberrant transcriptional deactivation caused by mutant pQ proteins. HDAC3 is a unique class 1 HDAC found in both the cytoplasm and in the nucleus. However, the precise functions of HDAC3 in the two cellular compartments are only vaguely known. HDAC3 directly binds to huntingtin (Htt) with short pQ and this interaction is important for suppressing neurotoxicity induced by HDAC3. With long pQ Htt, the interaction with HDAC3 is inhibited, and this supposedly promotes neuronal death, indicating that HDAC3 would be a good therapeutic target for HD. However, the knockout of one HDAC3 allele did not show any efficacy in reducing neurodegenerative symptoms in a mouse model of HD. Therefore, the role of HDAC3 in the pathogenesis of HD has yet to be fully elucidated. We attempted to resolve this issue by focusing on the different roles of HDAC3 on cytoplasmic and nuclear Htt aggregates. In addition to supporting the previous findings, we found that HDAC3 preferentially binds to nuclear Htt over cytoplasmic ones. Specific HDAC3 inhibitors increased the total amount of Htt aggregates by increasing the amount of nuclear aggregates. Both cytoplasmic and nuclear Htt aggregates were able to suppress endogenous HDAC3 activity, which led to decreased nuclear proteasome activity. Therefore, we concluded that Htt aggregates impair nuclear proteasome activity through the inhibition of HDAC3. Our findings provide new insights regarding cross-compartment proteasome regulation.

Editor: Yoshitaka Nagai, National Center of Neurology and Psychiatry, Japan

Funding: This study was supported by Kakenhi (KB: 24390220, JSPS, Tokyo, Japan), JST PRESTO (Kawaguchi, Saitama), the Cell Science Research Foundation (Osaka, Japan), the Ichiro Kanehara Foundation for the Promotion of Medical Sciences and Medical Care (Tokyo, Japan), the Takeda Science Foundation (Osaka, Japan), Janssen Pharmaceutical K.K. (Tokyo, Japan), and Eisai Co. (Tokyo, Japan). The funders had no role in study design, data collection and analysis, decision to publish, or preparation of the manuscript.

Competing Interests: The authors have declared that no competing interests exist.

* Email: Iwata-tky@umin.ac.jp

Introduction

In polyglutamine (pQ) diseases, the gene transcription machinery required for proper neuronal function is impaired, and this may result from the sequestration of essential proteins for transcription [1–4] and/or the abnormal hypo-acetylation of the genome [5]. The up-regulation of transcription by histone deacetylase (HDAC) inhibitors was shown to be an effective treatment in a fly model of pQ disease [6]. Since then, multiple studies have shown that HDAC inhibitors ameliorate symptoms and pathology in various models of Huntington's disease (HD), one of the major pQ diseases [7–11]. However, broad-spectrum HDAC inhibitors used in these studies have multiple targets and should therefore be avoided for therapeutic purposes. Indeed, considering that the inhibition of HDAC6 has a negative effect on pQ degradation [12], caution is needed when interpreting data from these broad-spectrum inhibitor studies. Moreover, these broad-spectrum inhibitors are not suitable for use as actual medicines to be administered to human subjects because of the potential for unwanted side effects.

There are four classes of HDACs and among them, class I or IIa HDACs have been previously suggested as therapeutic targets for

pQ diseases [13]. Classes I and IIa each contain four HDACs, and in order to narrow down the therapeutic target, various studies using specific inhibitors or genetic ablation strategies have been performed. The results seem to consistently show that inhibition of HDAC1, 2, or 4 leads to some improvement [11,14–16] and inhibition of HDAC6 or 7 has no effect, at least at doses that can be administered without any negative effects in animal models [17,18]. The results for HDAC3 inhibition are mixed. While one study using a specific HDAC3 inhibitor showed phenotypic improvement in a fly model [16], another study showed no effect in the offspring of crossbred HDAC3 knockout and HD model mice [19]. One possibility for this discrepancy is that the HDAC3 inhibitor used in the first study was not specific enough and that the observed improvement was a result of the inhibition of other HDACs. In addition, it is possible that the genetic ablation in the second study did not achieve enough inhibition since the study was performed using hemi-zygote HDAC3 knockout mice because the full knockout resulted in embryonic lethality.

Another possible cause of this discrepancy is that unlike HDAC1 or 2, which only functions at the nucleus, HDAC3 can shuttle between the cytoplasm and the nucleus where it can have different roles. Therefore, the effect of HDAC3 inhibition on HD models can depend on the balance of nuclear vs. cytoplasmic aggregates. In the case of pQ diseases, nuclear aggregates exhibit a far higher toxicity than cytoplasmic aggregates [20,21] and there are cellular machineries that can only facilitate aggregate degradation in either the cytoplasm or in the nucleus [22,23]. Inhibitors against proteins that shuttle between the cytoplasm and the nucleus might have a differential effect on aggregate degradation in different cellular compartments.

To overcome these issues, we utilized highly specific HDAC3 inhibitors made by a click chemistry-based combinatorial fragment assembly technique (Table S1) [24]. These HDAC3 inhibitors have an IC50 for HDAC3 that is at least 100-fold higher than that for other HDACs. By utilizing these reagents, we used cell lines that stably express pQ aggregates in different cellular compartments [23] to precisely analyze the role of HDAC3. Here, we show that these specific HDAC3 inhibitors affect cytoplasmic and nuclear huntingtin (Htt) aggregates differently. Moreover, the presence of intracellular aggregates also affected HDAC3 activity, indicating that HDAC3 could be an indirect regulator of proteasome function.

Materials and Methods

Cell culture and transfection of mammalian cells

HeLa and 293T cells were grown in 95% air and 5% CO_2 at 37°C. Cells were transfected with plasmids using Lipofectamine 2000 (Life Technologies, Carlsbad, CA, USA) following the manufacturer's protocol. The transfection efficiency was 60–75% for HeLa cells and >90% for 293T cells.

Cell viability assay

Cells were incubated with CellTiter 96 Aqueous solution for an hour and absorbance at 490 nm was measured by the Spectra Max 384 Plus colorimetric plate reader (Molecular Devices, Sunnyvale, CA, USA).

Filter trap assay

The filter trap assay was performed as previously described [12].

HDAC3 constructs

HDAC3 cDNA was cloned from a cDNA library with oligonucleotide primers 5′ -CATGGCCAAGACCGTG- 3′ and 5′ -AAAGAAATTCCTTGGGACACA-3′. The HDAC3 knock-down construct was made with oligonucleotide primers, 5′-GATCCCCGATGCTGAACCATGCACCTTTCAAGA-GAAGGTGCATGGTTCAGCATCTTTTTA-3′ and 5′-AGCTTAAAAAGATGCTGAACCATGCACCTTCTCTT-GAAAGGTGCATGGTTCAGCATCGGG-3′ and was inserted into the pSuper vector (Oligoengine, Seattle, WA, USA). HDAC3 inactive mutants were PCR generated with oligonucleotide primers 5′ -TCGGGTGCTCTACATTGCCATTGCCATC-CACCATGGTGA-3′ and 5′ -TCACCATGGTGGATGG-CAATGGCAATGTAGAGCACCCGA-3′.

HDAC3 inhibitors

Details about HDAC3 inhibitors T130, T247, and T326 were previously published [24]. Trichostatin A and suberoylanilide hydroxamic acid (SAHA) were purchased from Sigma Aldrich (St. Louis, MO, USA).

HDAC activity assay

Pan-HDAC activity was assayed using the Flour-de-lys HDAC assay kit (Enzo Life Sciences, Farmingdale, NY, USA). The fluorometric assay was performed using the Spectramax Gemini XS (Molecular Devices) with an excitation wavelength of 360 nm and emission at 460 nm. HDAC3 activity was assayed using the HDAC3 activity assay kit (Sigma Aldrich) with excitation at 380 nm and emission at 500 nm.

Image quantitation

Western blot images were obtained using a LAS 3000 Mini (Fujifilm, Tokyo, Japan). Digital images were analyzed by Multi Gauge software (Fujifilm).

Immunoprecipitation and GST pull down analysis

To prepare lysates for immunoprecipitation, cells were sonicated in 50 mM Tris, pH 7.5, 150 mM NaCl, 1% NP40, 1 mM ethylenediaminetetraacetic acid (EDTA), and Complete protease inhibitor cocktail (Roche, Basel, Switzerland) and centrifuged at 20,000×g for 15 min. Lysates were incubated with 1 µg of anti-FLAG M2 antibody immobilized agarose beads (Sigma) for 4 h at 4°C and washed for four times with lysis buffer and subjected to SDS-PAGE and Western blot analysis. For the glutathione S-transferase (GST) pull-down assay, cells were lysed in 20 mM HEPES, pH 7.5, 100 mM NaCl, 0.1% Triton X-100, 10% glycerol, and Complete protease inhibitor cocktail (Roche). GST or GST-HDAC3 (500 ng) was mixed with glutathione sepharose beads (Amersham Biosciences, Uppsala, Sweden) and incubated with the lysates for 2 h at 4°C. Beads were washed four times with the lysis buffer and subjected to SDS-PAGE and Western blot analysis.

Microscopic imaging

Cells were fixed with 4% paraformaldehyde and a standard immunocytochemistry procedure was performed. Visualization of the primary anti-HDAC3 antibody (Imgenex, San Diego, CA, USA). was done with the Alexa 546 secondary antibodies (Life Technologies). Nucleus was visualized by Hoechst 33258 (Sigma Aldrich). Images were obtained using an Axioplan 2 fluorescent microscope and Axiocam HRc CCD camera system (Zeiss, Göttingen, Germany).

Proteasome activity assay

Proteasome activity was measured using a 20S Proteasome Activity Assay Kit (Merck, Darmstadt, Germany) following the manufacturer's protocol. The fluorometric assay was performed using a Spectramax Gemini XS (Molecular Devices) with an excitation wavelength of 380 nm and emission at 460 nm.

Proteasome purification

Proteasomes were purified using the Proteasome purification kit (Enzo Life Sciences) following the manufacturer's instructions.

Quantitative PCR

Total RNA was extracted with TRIzol (Life Technologies) and cDNA was generated by ReverTra Ace qPCR RT Kit (Toyobo, Osaka, Japan). Quantitative PCR (qPCR) was performed with the HT-7900 system (Applied Biosystems, Foster City, CA, USA). For qPCR, the probe set Mr04097229_mr was used to measure EGFP mRNA, and HuGAPDH and HuACTB (Applied Biosystems) were used as internal controls.

SDS-PAGE and western blot

Samples were incubated at 60°C in 4×LDS buffer (Life Technologies) for 15 min and subjected to SDS-PAGE with Mini-PROTEAN TGX gels (Bio-RAD, Hercules, CA, USA) and

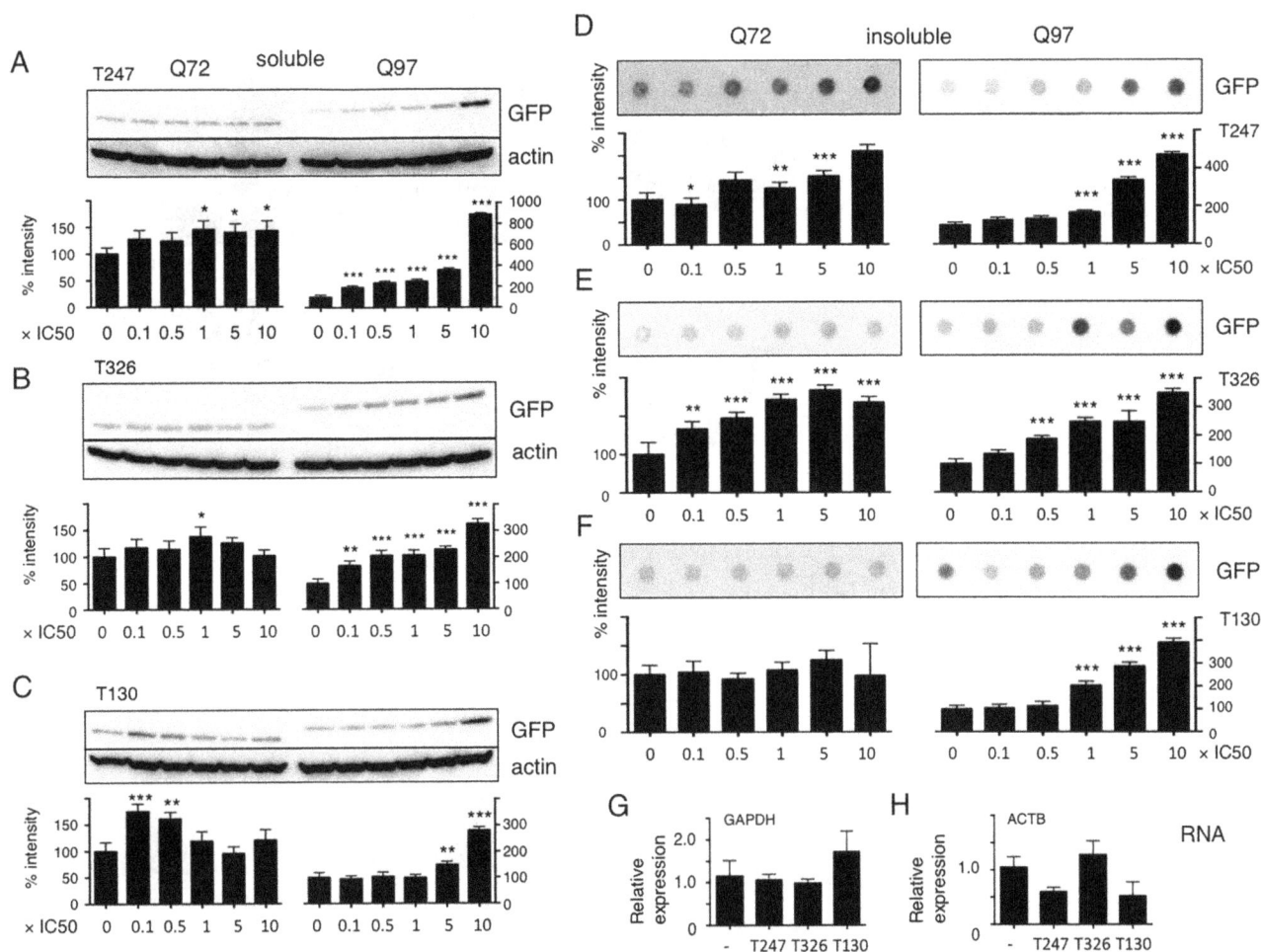

Figure 1. HDAC3 inhibitors increase both soluble and insoluble Htt-ex1s but prefer long Qs. A–F: Indicated amounts of HDAC3 inhibitors T247, T326, and T130 were added to C3 or C4 HeLa stable cell lines. The cells were harvested after 48 h of incubation and the fraction soluble in 1% Triton X-100 was subjected to western blot analysis (A–C). The insoluble fraction was subjected to a filter trap assay (D–E). Signals were detected by anti-GFP antibodies and chemiluminescence. Signal intensities were normalized to no inhibitors (DMSO only) = 100. The band from an anti-actin blot is shown as a loading control. Panels A, D: T247, B, E: T326, C, F: T130. *P≤0.05, **P≤0.01, ***P≤0.001 vs. 0×IC50 by ANOVA with multiple comparisons. N = 3. **G, H:** HDAC3 inhibitors do not increase Htt-ex1 mRNA levels. Effect of HDAC3 inhibitors on Htt-ex1 expression levels were assayed by qPCR. G: internal control = GAPDH, H: internal control = ACTB. Expression level was normalized to no inhibitor = 1.0. There was no statistical significance by ANOVA with multiple comparisons. N = 3.

transferred to PVDF membrane with the Trans-Blot Turbo Blotting System and Trans-Blot Turbo Transfer Pack (Bio-RAD). For the primary antibodies, Anti-GFP (Roche), anti-20S protea- some antibody (Abcam, Cambridge, UK), anti-actin antibody (Millipore, Billerica, MA, USA), anti-FLAG antibody (Sigma Aldrich), anti-HDAC3 antibody (Abcam and Imgenex, San Diego, CA, USA), anti-GST antibody (Millipore), anti-HSP90 antibody (Millipore), anti-SP1 antibody (Millipore), anti-acetylated lysine antibody (Cell Signaling, Boston, MA, USA), anti-HSP70 antibody (StressMarq, Victoria, BC, Canada) were used.

Stable cell lines

Stable HeLa cell lines expressing green fluorescent protein (GFP) fused to huntingtin exon-1 (Htt-ex1) with a nuclear export signal (NES), or nuclear localization signal (NLS) was previously published [23]. Cells with NES and CAG repeat lengths of 25, 47, and 72 were named E1, E2, E3, respectively, and cells with NLS were designated N1, N2, and N3, respectively. Cells without any localizing signals were named C1, C2, C3, and C4 with their CAG

repeat lengths in ascending order (Table S2). The expressed protein sequence of Htt exon-1 (Htt-ex1) was "MATLEKLMKA-FES-LKSF(Q)$_n$PPPPPPPPPPPQLPQPPPQAQPLLPQPQPPPPPPPP-PPGPAVAEEPLHRP" which was followed by an EGFP sequence.

Statistical analysis

Statistical analysis was performed using the GraphPad Prism 6 software (GraphPad, San Diego, CA, USA). The significance was tested with t-tests or ANOVA with Dunnett's multiple compar- isons.

Subcellular fractionation

Cytoplasmic and nuclear fractions were extracted using NE-PER Nuclear and Cytoplasmic Extraction Kit (Thermo Scientific, Rockford, IL, USA).

Inclusion body count

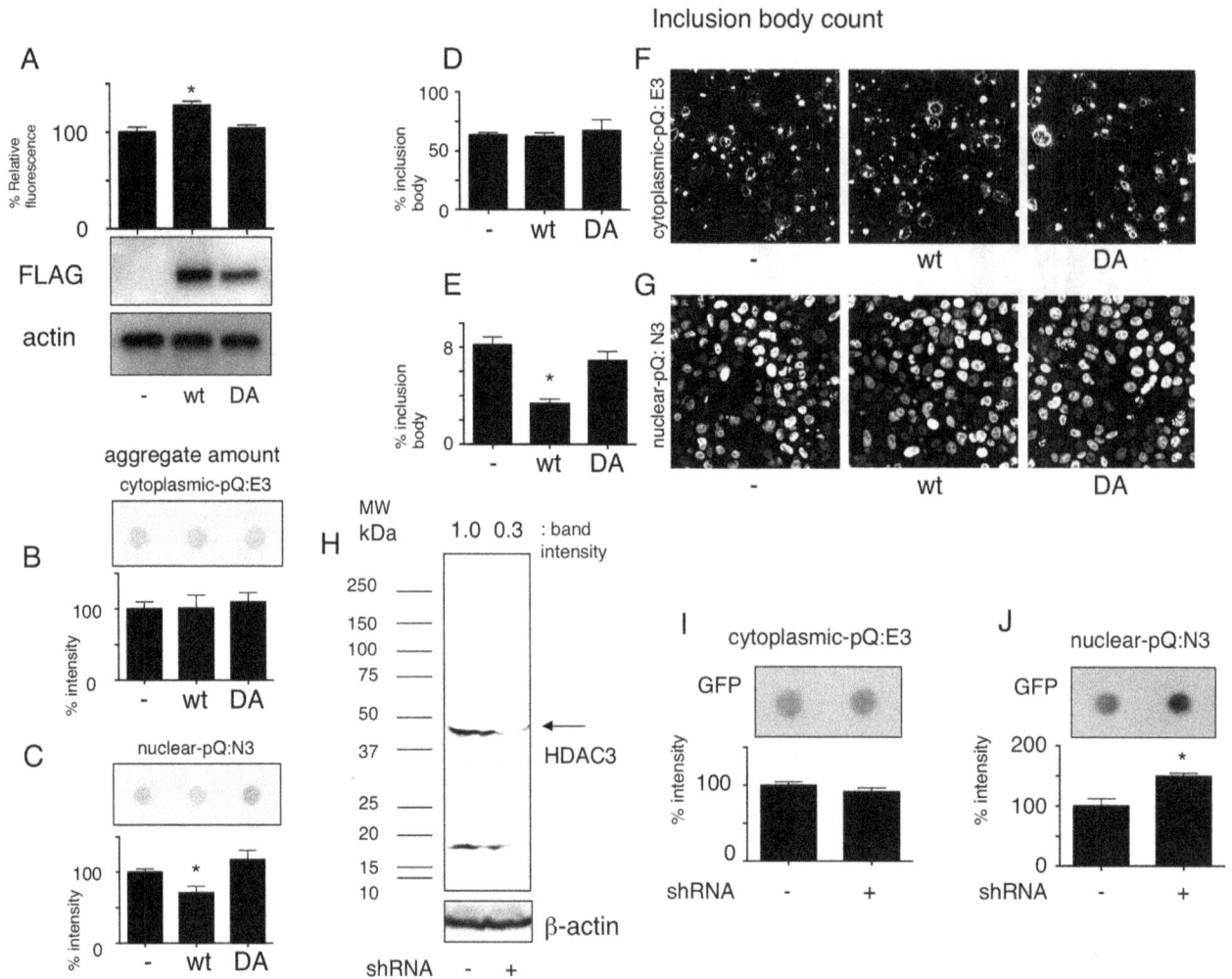

Figure 2. Effect of HDAC3 on cytoplasmic and nuclear Htt aggregates. A: Aspartate at the 166th and 168th amino acid of HDAC3 is crucial for its activity. An empty plasmid (–), FLAG tagged wild-type (wt), or D166A + D168A mutant (DA) of HDAC3 were overexpressed in 293T cells. After immunoprecipitation using anti-FLAG antibodies, pan-histone deacetylase activity was measured by fluorometric analysis. *P≤0.05 vs. empty plasmid by ANOVA and multiple comparisons. N = 3. Anti-FLAG and anti-actin western blots from cell lysates are shown below. **B–C:** HDAC3 overexpression reduces nuclear Htt-ex1 aggregates. Empty vector (–), FLAG-tagged wild-type or DA mutant HDAC3 were transfected to E3 and N3 cells. Amount of aggregate measured by filter trap assay are shown in B and C. *significant against – and DA by ANOVA and multiple comparisons. N = 3. **D–G:** Empty vector (–), FLAG-tagged wild-type or DA mutant HDAC3 were transfected to E3 and N3 cells. Cells harboring inclusion bodies are counted and their fraction in total cells was plotted in 2D and E. Representative GFP images of low powered magnification fields are shown in 2F and 2G. *significant against – and DA by ANOVA and multiple comparisons. **H:** HDAC3 shRNA reduces HDAC3 amount by 70%. Molecular weight markers are shown at the left side. **I–J:** HDAC3 knockdown increases nuclear aggregates. HDAC3 shRNA was transfected into E3 or N3 cells and the 1% TritonX-100 insoluble fraction was subjected to filter trap assay. *P = 0.0003 by *t*-test. N = 3.

Results

HDAC3-specific inhibitors affect the degradation of aggregation-prone Htt-ex1

Generation of aggregated over soluble species is essential for Htt toxicity. To understand the effect of HDAC3 inhibition on the amount of Htt aggregates, we used stable HeLa cell lines that express Htt exon-1 (Htt-ex1) with various pQ lengths (Table S2) [23]. Three HDAC3 inhibitors had no effect on Htt-ex1 Q25 (C1 cells) and Htt-ex1 Q46 (C2 cells) (Figure S1), increased soluble Htt-ex1 Q72 to some extent, and significantly increased insoluble Htt-ex1 Q72 (C3 cells), and also significantly increased both soluble and insoluble Htt-ex1 Q97 (C4 cells) (Fig. 1A–F). None of the HDAC3 inhibitors showed a significant effect on Htt-ex1 mRNA levels (Fig. 1G, H); therefore, we concluded that HDAC3

inhibition affected the intracellular Htt-ex1 aggregate degradation pathway.

HDAC3 activity reduces the amount of nuclear Htt-ex1 aggregates

To confirm that HDAC3 activity was important for the results of the previous experiments, and to see the effect of HDAC3 inhibition independently in the cytoplasm and the nucleus, we first generated plasmid constructs with either wild-type HDAC3 or a deacetylase activity-defective HDAC3 mutant. The key amino acids for HDAC3 activity were predicted to be the 166th and 168th aspartates; therefore, we mutated these amino acids to alanine, which successfully resulted in the loss of deacetylase activity (Fig. 2A). We then transfected these constructs into cell lines that stably express Htt-ex1 Q72 in the cytoplasm (E3 cells) or in the

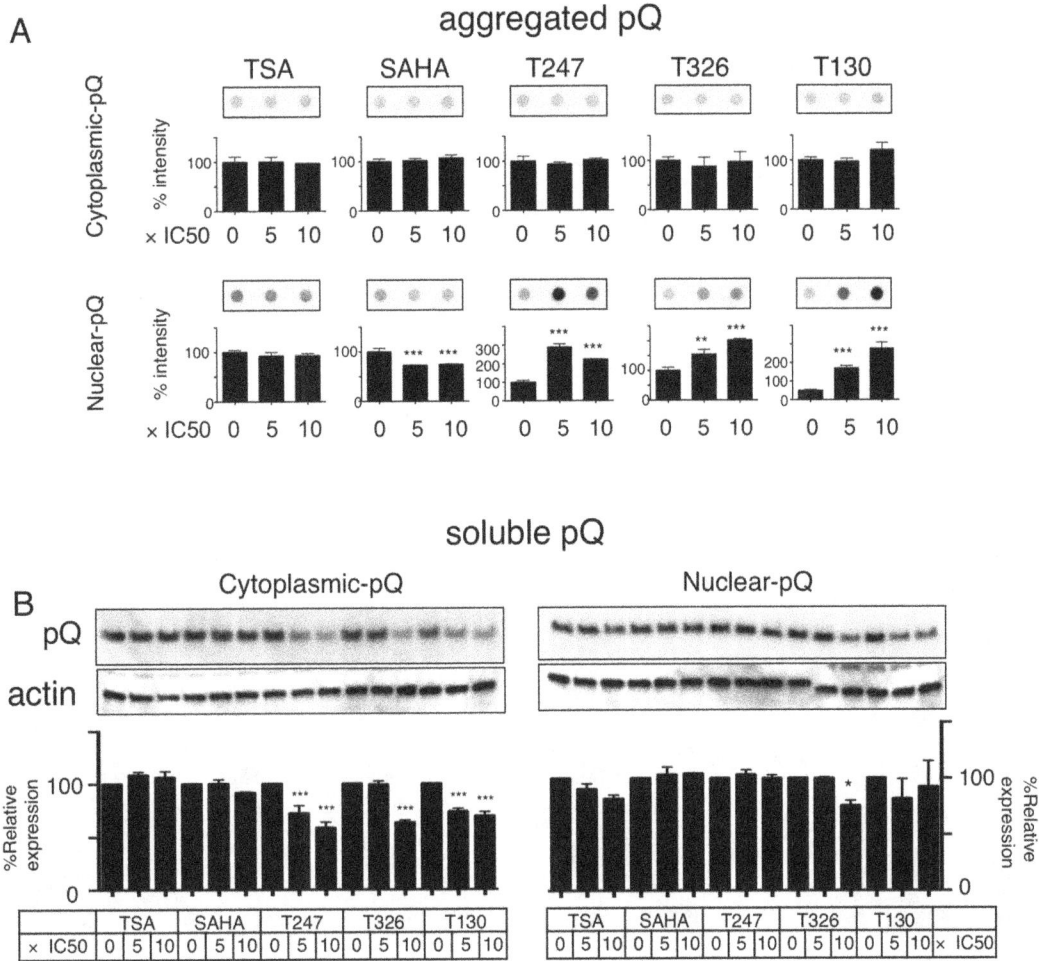

Figure 3. HDAC3 inhibitors have differential effects on cytoplasmic and nuclear Htt-ex1 aggregates. A: HDAC3 inhibitors increase aggregated nuclear Htt-ex1. For filter trap analysis, three independently made insoluble fractions were analyzed on one single membrane; thus, there are error bars shown for 0×IC50s. *P≤0.05, ***P≤0.001 vs. each 0×IC50 by ANOVA and multiple comparisons. N = 3. **B:** HDAC3 inhibitors reduce cytoplasmic soluble Htt-ex1s. The effect of various HDAC inhibitors on 1% TritonX-100 soluble cytoplasmic Htt-ex1s. Indicated amount of HDAC inhibitors were added to E3 (cytoplasmic) or N3 (nuclear) cells for 48 h. Quantitated band intensity was normalized to each band without HDAC inhibitors (0×IC50); thus, there are no error bars. **P≤0.01, ***P≤0.001 vs. each 0×IC50 by ANOVA with multiple comparisons. N = 3. Anti-actin blots are shown for loading control.

nucleus (N3 cells) and observed a significant decrease of biochemically (Fig. 2B, C) or microscopically (Fig. 2D–G) aggregated nuclear Htt-ex1 in accordance with HDAC3 activity. We also generated an HDAC3 knockdown construct that was able to reduce the amount of HDAC3 by 70% (Fig. 2H). We transfected these constructs into E3 and N3 cells and observed a significant increase of aggregated Htt-ex1 only in the N3 cells upon HDAC3 knockdown (Fig. 2I, J). These results show that HDAC3 activity negatively affected the amount of nuclear Htt-ex1 aggregates.

We then used HDAC3 specific inhibitors on the E3 and N3 cells. The results clearly showed that the HDAC3 inhibitors specifically increased the amount of nuclear Htt-ex1 aggregates and had no effect on cytoplasmic Htt-ex1 aggregates. Non-specific HDAC inhibitors TSA and SAHA had very little to no effect on the amount of either cytoplasmic or nuclear Htt-ex1 aggregates (Fig. 3A). HDAC3 inhibitors decreased soluble cytoplasmic Htt-ex1 (Fig. 3B).

HDAC3 preferably binds to nuclear pQs

HDAC3 was previously reported to associate with pQ-containing proteins [25,26]. We tested whether this association was a direct one using a GST pull-down assay. From sonicated lysates of E1, E2, E3, N1, N2, and N3 cells, GST-HDAC3 successfully pulled down both NES- and NLS-attached Htt-ex1s (Fig. 4A). We then performed immunoprecipitation using E1, E3, N1, and N3 cell lysates transfected with FLAG-tagged HDAC3. Interestingly, FLAG-tagged HDAC3 preferably co-immunoprecipitated with nuclear Htt-ex1s (Fig. 4B) and HDAC3 exhibited increased binding to 25Qs over 72Qs. This was confirmed with immunocytochemistry. Nuclear inclusion bodies in N3 cells displayed positive signals for endogenous HDAC3; however, cytoplasmic inclusion bodies from E3 cells were negative for HDAC3 (Fig. 4C). Thus, we concluded that HDAC3 binds to Htt-ex1s preferably inside the nucleus.

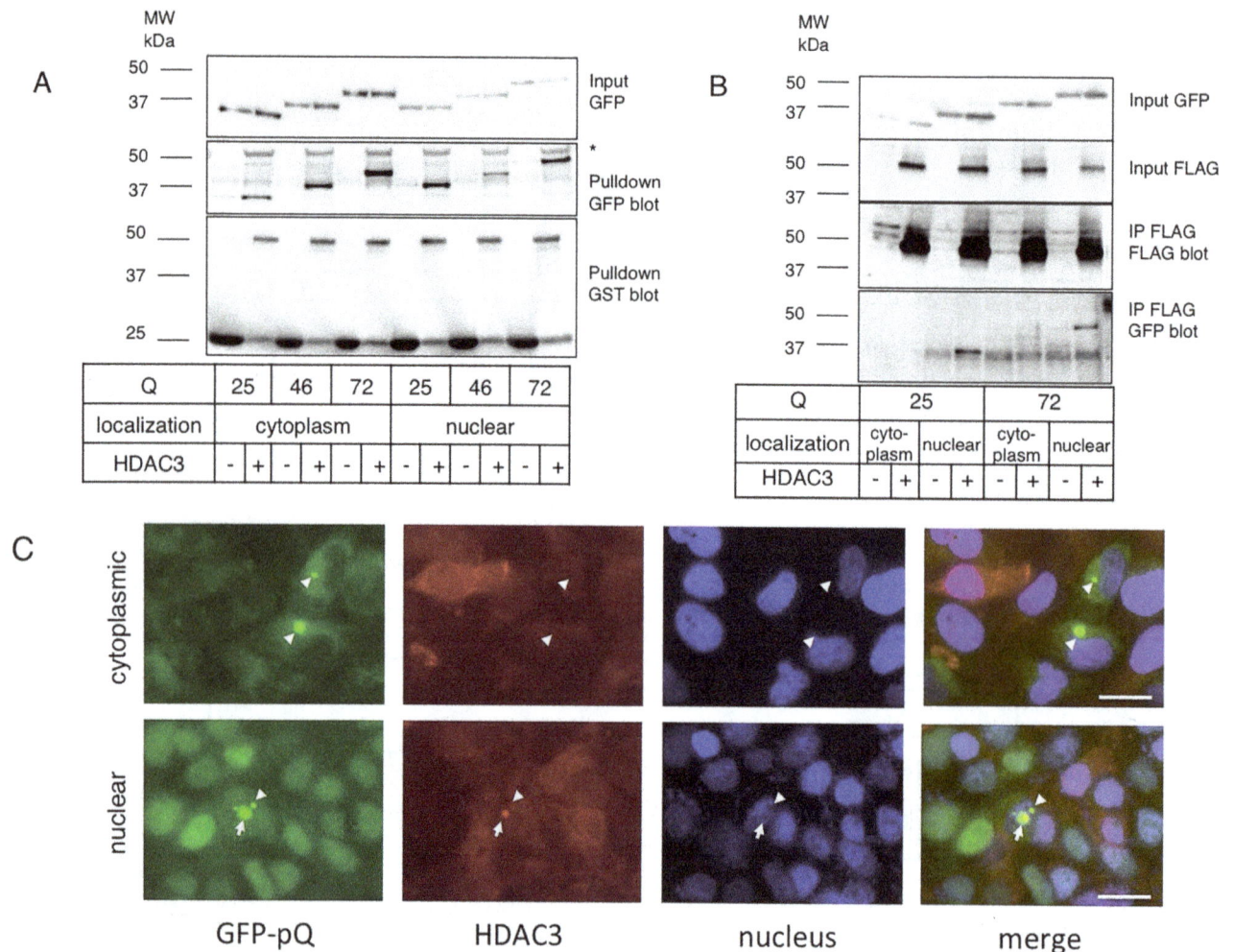

Figure 4. HDAC3 preferably binds to nuclear Htt with long Qs. A: GST-HDAC3 binds directly to either cytoplasmic or nuclear Htt-ex1. GST pull-down assay of E1, E2, E3 (cytoplasm), and N1, N2, N3 (nuclear) HeLa cell lysates is shown. Pulled-down fraction was analyzed by anti-GFP or GST antibodies. *Non-specific band. **B:** HDAC3 immunoprecipitates almost exclusively with nuclear Htt-ex1s. E1, E3 (cytoplasm), N1, and N3 (nuclear) HeLa cells were transfected with FLAG-tagged HDAC3 and those lysates were immunoprecipitated with anti-FLAG antibodies immobilized to protein G agarose beads. The pre-IP fraction and the IPed fraction were analyzed using anti-FLAG or anti-GFP antibodies. Molecular weight markers are shown on the left. **C:** HDAC3 associates exclusively with nuclear inclusion bodies. E3 or N3 cells were fixed and stained with anti-HDAC3 antibodies and visualized by Alexa 546 conjugated secondary antibodies. Arrowheads: inclusion bodies with no HDAC3 signals associated. Arrows: HDAC3 signal-associated inclusion bodies. Bar = 20 μm.

HDAC3 inhibition caused by Htt-ex1 aggregates affects nuclear proteasome activity

As shown in Figure 1, specific HDAC3 inhibitors increased Htt-ex1. It was either possible that HDAC3 inhibited its degradation or promoted its stability. Therefore we tested if HDAC3 inhibitors had any direct effect on the function of proteasomes, the major degradation machinery in the cell. We added HDAC3 inhibitors to HeLa cells and measured proteasome activity using a fluorometric assay. HDAC3 inhibitors impaired proteasome activity by 10–30%, even at a very low dose, with no further effect at higher doses (Fig. 5A–C). We then determined if these inhibitors had different effects on cytoplasmic and nuclear proteasome activity. As expected, HDAC3 inhibitors impaired nuclear proteasome activity but had no effect on cytoplasmic proteasomes (Fig. 5D, E). HDAC3 inhibitors did not directly inhibit proteasome activity (Fig. 5F). HDAC3 inhibitors did not affect the localization of the proteasome (Fig. S2), the acetylation level of Htt-ex1s or the proteasome (Fig. S3A, B, S4A). HDAC3

inhibitors did not affect the expression levels of HSP70, a chaperone that facilitates Htt-ex1 degradation by the proteasome (Fig. S4B). HDAC3 also does not bind to the proteasome and act as a scaffold between Htt-ex1 aggregates and the proteasome (Fig. S5). Thus, we speculated that proteasome function was impaired through an indirect pathway and hypothesized that the Htt-ex1 aggregates themselves affected HDAC3 activity. Therefore, we measured HDAC3 activity in the presence or absence of cellular aggregates. We showed that HDAC3 activity was suppressed by the overexpression of aggregate-prone Htt-ex1, regardless of its cellular localization (Fig. 6A). This effect was relatively specific to HDAC3 since pan-HDAC activity was not significantly affected by the same Htt-ex1 overexpression (Fig. 6B).

Discussion

Role of HDAC3 in pQ disease pathogenesis

The effect of HDAC3 inhibition in studies using pQ model animals has been controversial. While injection of an HDAC3

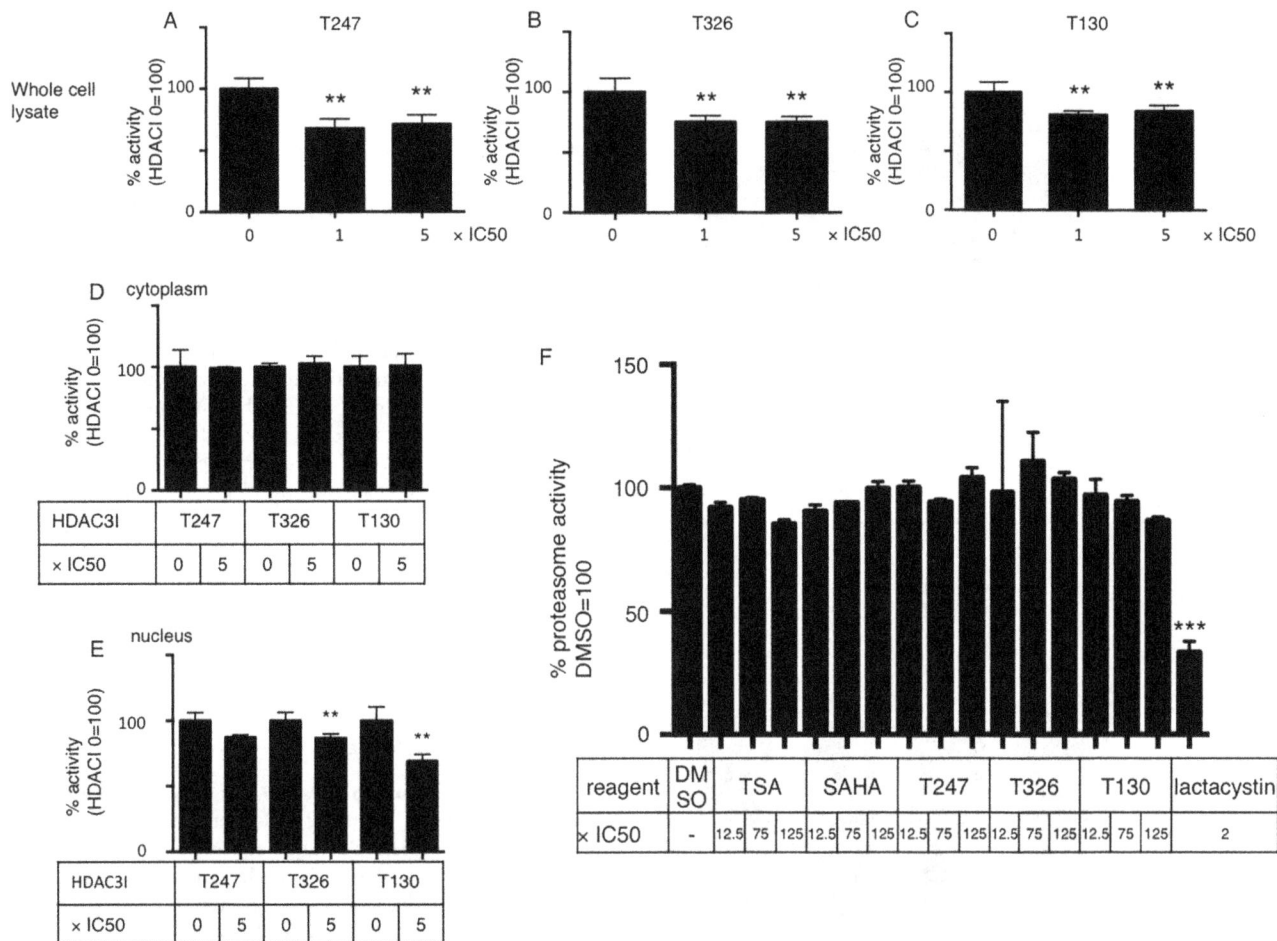

Figure 5. HDAC3 inhibitors affect proteasome activity. A–C: HDAC3 inhibitors inhibit proteasome activity. Three different HDAC3 inhibitors were added to HeLa cell cultures at the indicated concentrations. After 48 h of incubation, the proteasome activity of 5 μg total protein in a PBS lysate was measured using a fluorometric assay. A: T247, B: T326, C: T130. *P≤0.05 vs. each 0×IC50 by ANOVA with multiple comparisons. N = 3. **D, E:** HDAC3 inhibitors show a differential effect on cytoplasmic and nuclear proteasome activity. After incubating with the indicated amount of HDAC3 inhibitors for 48 h, cells were fractionated and the proteasome activity of 5 μg total protein from each fraction was independently measured. *P< 0.05, **P<0.001 0×IC50 vs. 5×IC50 by t-tests N = 3. **F:** HDAC inhibitors have little or no direct proteasome inhibitory effect. Total protein (5 μg) from a HeLa cell PBS extract was subjected to the proteasome activity assay. During the incubation period for activity measurement, the indicated amount of HDAC inhibitors, or lactacystin as positive control, were added. Relative activity was shown with DMSO = 100%. ***P≤0.001 vs. DMSO by ANOVA with multiple comparisons. N = 3.

inhibitor into R62 mice seems to be effective in restoring the expression of genes that have been compromised by HD [16], the genetic knockdown of HDAC3 did not alter the phenotypic and pathological appearance of the same mice [19]. The latter study used HDAC3 hemizygote knockdowns that only achieved 10–20% reduction in the amount of HDAC3 at a protein level possibly being an insufficient inhibition. This discrepancy could also be due to specificity of the HDAC3 inhibitor used in the earlier study. Another possibility is that HDAC3 could have a particular function in HD pathogenesis, such that its inhibition might have multiple effects on the pathway and make the results difficult to interpret.

Then how is HDAC3 involved in HD pathogenesis? Previous studies have emphasized that HDAC3 itself is a neurotoxic protein that was neutralized by normal Htt when they are bound to each other. Since it prefers Htt with short Q as a binding partner (Figure 4B), unbound HDAC3 in the presence of long Q Htt exhibits its neurotoxicity [25] [27]. HDAC3 interacts with ataxin-7, another nuclear pQ protein, and stabilizes its post-translational

modification [26]. HDAC3 is a class I HDAC that is abundantly expressed in the brain [28]. It is known to associate with and to be activated by a nuclear receptor co-repressor in order to control circadian metabolic physiology [29]. HDAC3 is also thought to have cytoplasmic function upon axonal injury [30], but its precise role is still unclear. The molecule has both a nuclear localization signal and a nuclear export signal [31], suggesting that it has different roles in the cytoplasm and the nucleus.

Our results indicate that HDAC3 inhibition could be beneficial in accelerating cytoplasmic Htt-ex1 pQ aggregation, but it inhibits the degradation of nuclear Htt-ex1 aggregates. In our study, we could not find an ideal dosage of HDAC3 inhibitors that would accelerate cytoplasmic aggregate degradation and not affect nuclear aggregate degradation, indicating that the therapeutic window for using HDAC3 inhibitors to treat HD could be very narrow, if it exists.

A previous report showed that HDAC inhibitors targeting HDAC1/3 prevent the formation of Htt aggregates in the brains of N171-82Q HD transgenic mice [32]. It is possible that this

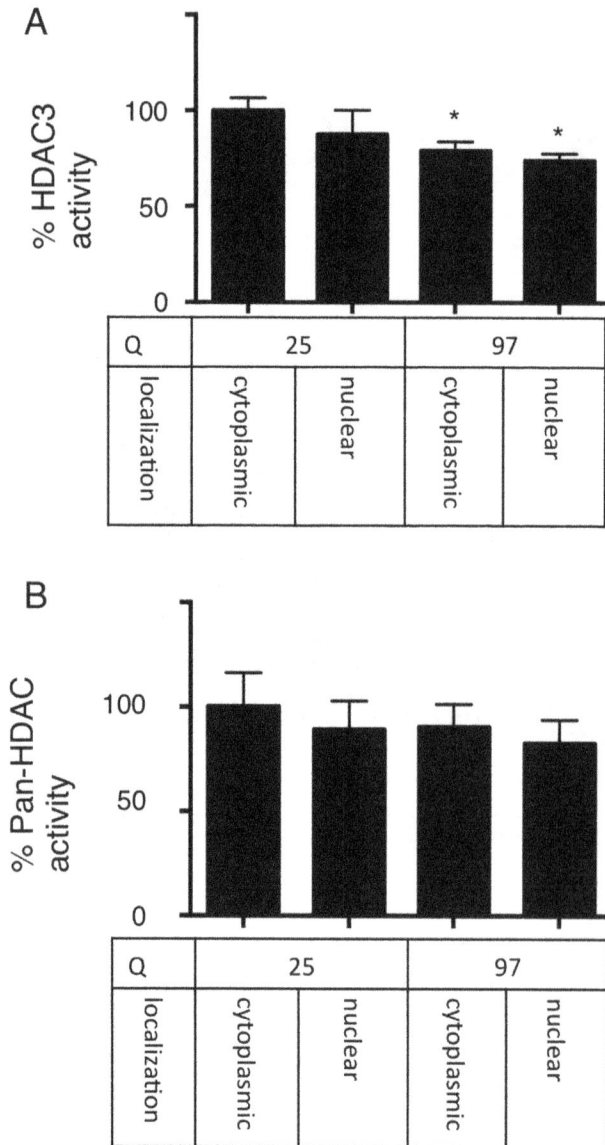

Figure 6. Htt aggregates inhibit HDAC3 activity. A: HDAC3 activity is suppressed upon either cytoplasmic or nuclear Htt-ex1 expression. After two days of transfection in 293T cells, the HDAC3 activity of cellular lysates was measured using a fluorescence-based assay. **B:** Htt-ex1 overexpression does not alter pan-HDAC activity. After two days of transfection in 293T cells, the pan-HDAC activity was measured using a fluorescence-based assay.

effect could be mediated by HDAC1 since acetylation of Htt can promote its autophagic clearance [33]. Thus the effect of HDAC3 could differ between cytoplasmic and nuclear aggregates.

Indirect proteasome inhibition by Htt-ex1 aggregates could be linked to HDAC3

Our results clearly indicated that HDAC3 inhibitors impaired nuclear proteasome activity. Since direct incubation of the proteasome activity assay with HDAC3 inhibitors did not show any decrease in activity, this inhibition was determined to be an indirect effect of the inhibitors. Although there could be some non-specific background protease activity that was detected by our method, our results (Fig. 5F) show that this background activity

could be negligible. We sought the mechanism of the inhibitory pathway and showed that it did not result from changes in the acetylation of the substrate Htt-ex1s or the proteasome itself. The localization of the proteasome was not affected by the inhibitors. In addition, we showed that HSP70, a chaperone that accelerates Htt degradation, was not affected by HDAC3 inhibitors. Thus, proteasome impairment was not a direct effect of HDAC3 inhibitors, but there was an indirect signaling pathway through HDAC3 to be discovered. We measured HDAC3 activity upon Htt-ex1 transfection and showed that both cytoplasmic and nuclear Htt-ex1 aggregates reduced endogenous HDAC3 activity.

In cellular models of HD, it has been reported that proteasome function has been impaired [34]. This inhibition is not a direct effect of the aggregates but rather an indirect effect where the full players are still unknown [35]. This inhibitory effect bi-directionally crosses the nuclear envelope [36], that is, nuclear aggregates inhibit cytoplasmic proteasome activity and vice versa. The mechanism of this phenomenon is unknown but our results suggest that at least nuclear proteasome function is impaired through the inhibition of HDAC3 by Htt-ex1s.

Our findings clearly demonstrate that HDAC3 inhibition is not a reasonable therapeutic target for HD. However, our results can lead to a better understanding of the regulation of proteasome function in different cellular compartments and provide new insight into proteasome inhibition by aggregated proteins.

Supporting Information

Figure S1 HDAC3 inhibitors do not have any effect on soluble Htt-ex1s. C1 and C2 cells were incubated with the indicated amount of HDAC3 inhibitors for 48 h. The fractions soluble in 1% Triton X-100 from the filter trap assay were subjected to western blot analysis. There were no detectable filter trapped aggregates in these cells. Molecular weight markers are shown at the left side.

Figure S2 The amount of 20S proteasome in each cellular compartment was not affected by HDAC3 inhibition HeLa cells were incubated with indicated amount of HDAC3 inhibitors for 48 h, and nuclear and cytoplasmic fractions were extracted. HSP90 and Sp1 blots are shown for the purity of the fractions. There was a slight increase of cytoplasmic HDAC3 and a slight decrease of nuclear HDAC3 upon addition of inhibitors. Molecular weight markers are shown at the left side.

Figure S3 A, B: HDAC3 inhibitor does not alter the acetylation level of Htt-ex1s. E3 (NES) or N3 (NLS) cells were incubated with indicated amount of T326 for 48 h. Cells were lysed and immunoprecipitated by anti-GFP antibodies immobilized to protein G agarose beads. After a rigorous wash, they were run on SDS-PAGE and western blotted by anti-GFP (upper panel) or anti-acetylated lysine antibodies (lower panel). *are non-specific bands.

Figure S4 A: HDAC3 inhibitor does not affect the acetylation of the proteasome. The 293T and HeLa cells were incubated with indicated HDAC inhibitors at 10×IC50, and the proteasome was extracted from sonicated cell lysates. Purified proteasomes were analyzed by western blotting using anti-20S proteasome antibody (upper panel) or anti-acetylated lysine antibodies (lower panel). The "beads" lane indicates the negative control without any cell lysates. *are non-specific bands. **B:** HDAC3 inhibitors do not affect the amount of HSP70 chaperone. Indicated amounts of HDAC3 inhibitors were added to HeLa cells and the cell lysates were analyzed by western blotting by anti-HSP70 antibody. Anti-actin blot is shown for loading control. Molecular weight markers are shown at the left side.

Figure S5 HDAC3 does not bind to the proteasome. Proteasome was purified from extracts of HeLa cells sonicated in PBS and analyzed with anti-HDAC3 or 20S proteasome antibody. Molecular weight markers are shown at the left side.

Table S1 IC50 of HDAC3 inhibitors used in this study and previously reported studies.

Table S2 Name of HeLa cell lines used in this study.

Acknowledgments

We are grateful for the technical support provided by Yuki Inukai.

Author Contributions

Conceived and designed the experiments: TM AI ST. Performed the experiments: TM AI. Analyzed the data: TM AI. Contributed reagents/materials/analysis tools: TS. Contributed to the writing of the manuscript: TM AI ST.

References

1. Boutell JM, Thomas P, Neal JW, Weston VJ, Duce J, et al. (1999) Aberrant interactions of transcriptional repressor proteins with the Huntington's disease gene product, huntingtin. Hum Mol Genet 8: 1647–1655.
2. Steffan JS, Kazantsev A, Spasic-Boskovic O, Greenwald M, Zhu YZ, et al. (2000) The Huntington's disease protein interacts with p53 and CREB-binding protein and represses transcription. Proc Natl Acad Sci U S A 97: 6763–6768.
3. Shimohata T, Nakajima T, Yamada M, Uchida C, Onodera O, et al. (2000) Expanded polyglutamine stretches interact with TAFII130, interfering with CREB-dependent transcription. Nat Genet 26: 29–36.
4. Nucifora FC Jr., Sasaki M, Peters MF, Huang H, Cooper JK, et al. (2001) Interference by huntingtin and atrophin-1 with cbp-mediated transcription leading to cellular toxicity. Science 291: 2423–2428.
5. Sadri-Vakili G, Cha JH (2006) Mechanisms of disease: Histone modifications in Huntington's disease. Nat Clin Pract Neurol 2: 330–338.
6. Steffan JS, Bodai L, Pallos J, Poelman M, McCampbell A, et al. (2001) Histone deacetylase inhibitors arrest polyglutamine-dependent neurodegeneration in Drosophila. Nature 413: 739–743.
7. Ferrante RJ, Kubilus JK, Lee J, Ryu H, Beesen A, et al. (2003) Histone deacetylase inhibition by sodium butyrate chemotherapy ameliorates the neurodegenerative phenotype in Huntington's disease mice. J Neurosci 23: 9418–9427.
8. Hockly E, Richon VM, Woodman B, Smith DL, Zhou X, et al. (2003) Suberoylanilide hydroxamic acid, a histone deacetylase inhibitor, ameliorates motor deficits in a mouse model of Huntington's disease. Proc Natl Acad Sci U S A 100: 2041–2046.
9. Gardian G, Browne SE, Choi DK, Klivenyi P, Gregorio J, et al. (2005) Neuroprotective effects of phenylbutyrate in the N171-82Q transgenic mouse model of Huntington's disease. J Biol Chem 280: 556–563.
10. Pallos J, Bodai L, Lukacsovich T, Purcell JM, Steffan JS, et al. (2008) Inhibition of specific HDACs and sirtuins suppresses pathogenesis in a Drosophila model of Huntington's disease. Hum Mol Genet 17: 3767–3775.
11. Mielcarek M, Landles C, Weiss A, Bradaia A, Seredenina T, et al. (2013) HDAC4 reduction: a novel therapeutic strategy to target cytoplasmic huntingtin and ameliorate neurodegeneration. PLoS Biol 11: e1001717.
12. Iwata A, Riley BE, Johnston JA, Kopito RR (2005) HDAC6 and microtubules are required for autophagic degradation of aggregated huntingtin. J Biol Chem 280: 40282–40292.
13. Kazantsev AG, Thompson LM (2008) Therapeutic application of histone deacetylase inhibitors for central nervous system disorders. Nat Rev Drug Discov 7: 854–868.
14. Thomas EA, Coppola G, Desplats PA, Tang B, Soragni E, et al. (2008) The HDAC inhibitor 4b ameliorates the disease phenotype and transcriptional abnormalities in Huntington's disease transgenic mice. Proc Natl Acad Sci U S A 105: 15564–15569.
15. Hathorn T, Snyder-Keller A, Messer A (2011) Nicotinamide improves motor deficits and upregulates PGC-1alpha and BDNF gene expression in a mouse model of Huntington's disease. Neurobiol Dis 41: 43–50.
16. Jia H, Pallos J, Jacques V, Lau A, Tang B, et al. (2012) Histone deacetylase (HDAC) inhibitors targeting HDAC3 and HDAC1 ameliorate polyglutamine-elicited phenotypes in model systems of Huntington's disease. Neurobiol Dis 46: 351–361.
17. Benn CL, Butler R, Mariner L, Nixon J, Moffitt H, et al. (2009) Genetic knock-down of HDAC7 does not ameliorate disease pathogenesis in the R6/2 mouse model of Huntington's disease. PLoS One 4: e5747.
18. Bobrowska A, Paganetti P, Matthias P, Bates GP (2011) Hdac6 knock-out increases tubulin acetylation but does not modify disease progression in the R6/2 mouse model of Huntington's disease. PLoS One 6: e20696.
19. Moumne L, Campbell K, Howland D, Ouyang Y, Bates GP (2012) Genetic knock-down of HDAC3 does not modify disease-related phenotypes in a mouse model of Huntington's disease. PLoS One 7: e31080.
20. Katsuno M, Adachi H, Kume A, Li M, Nakagomi Y, et al. (2002) Testosterone reduction prevents phenotypic expression in a transgenic mouse model of spinal and bulbar muscular atrophy. Neuron 35: 843–854.
21. Klement IA, Skinner PJ, Kaytor MD, Yi H, Hersch SM, et al. (1998) Ataxin-1 nuclear localization and aggregation: role in polyglutamine-induced disease in SCA1 transgenic mice. Cell 95: 41–53.
22. Iwata A, Christianson JC, Bucci M, Ellerby LM, Nukina N, et al. (2005) Increased susceptibility of cytoplasmic over nuclear polyglutamine aggregates to autophagic degradation. Proc Natl Acad Sci U S A 102: 13135–13140.
23. Iwata A, Nagashima Y, Matsumoto L, Suzuki T, Yamanaka T, et al. (2009) Intranuclear degradation of polyglutamine aggregates by the ubiquitin-proteasome system. J Biol Chem 284: 9796–9803.
24. Suzuki T, Kasuya Y, Itoh Y, Ota Y, Zhan P, et al. (2013) Identification of highly selective and potent histone deacetylase 3 inhibitors using click chemistry-based combinatorial fragment assembly. PLoS One 8: e68669.
25. Bardai FH, Verma P, Smith C, Rawat V, Wang L, et al. (2013) Disassociation of histone deacetylase-3 from normal huntingtin underlies mutant huntingtin neurotoxicity. J Neurosci 33: 11833–11838.
26. Duncan CE, An MC, Papanikolaou T, Rugani C, Vitelli C, et al. (2013) Histone deacetylase-3 interacts with ataxin-7 and is altered in a spinocerebellar ataxia type 7 mouse model. Mol Neurodegener 8: 42.
27. Bardai FH, D'Mello SR (2011) Selective toxicity by HDAC3 in neurons: regulation by Akt and GSK3beta. J Neurosci 31: 1746–1751.
28. Broide RS, Redwine JM, Aftahi N, Young W, Bloom FE, et al. (2007) Distribution of histone deacetylases 1–11 in the rat brain. J Mol Neurosci 31: 47–58.
29. Alenghat T, Meyers K, Mullican SE, Leitner K, Adeniji-Adele A, et al. (2008) Nuclear receptor corepressor and histone deacetylase 3 govern circadian metabolic physiology. Nature 456: 997–1000.
30. Cho Y, Sloutsky R, Naegle KM, Cavalli V (2013) Injury-induced HDAC5 nuclear export is essential for axon regeneration. Cell 155: 894–908.
31. Yang WM, Tsai SC, Wen YD, Fejer G, Seto E (2002) Functional domains of histone deacetylase-3. J Biol Chem 277: 9447–9454.
32. Jia H, Kast RJ, Steffan JS, Thomas EA (2012) Selective histone deacetylase (HDAC) inhibition imparts beneficial effects in Huntington's disease mice: implications for the ubiquitin-proteasomal and autophagy systems. Hum Mol Genet 21: 5280–5293.
33. Jeong H, Then F, Melia TJ Jr., Mazzulli JR, Cui L, et al. (2009) Acetylation targets mutant huntingtin to autophagosomes for degradation. Cell 137: 60–72.
34. Bence NF, Sampat RM, Kopito RR (2001) Impairment of the ubiquitin-proteasome system by protein aggregation. Science 292: 1552–1555.
35. Hipp MS, Patel CN, Bersuker K, Riley BE, Kaiser SE, et al. (2012) Indirect inhibition of 26S proteasome activity in a cellular model of Huntington's disease. J Cell Biol 196: 573–587.
36. Bennett EJ, Bence NF, Jayakumar R, Kopito RR (2005) Global impairment of the ubiquitin-proteasome system by nuclear or cytoplasmic protein aggregates precedes inclusion body formation. Mol Cell 17: 351–365.

Permissions

List of Contributors

Valérie Drouet, Marta Ruiz, Gwennaëlle Auregan, Karine Cambon, Johann Carpentier, Raymonde Hassig, Noëlle Dufour, Philippe Hantraye and Nicole Déglon
Institute of Biomedical Imaging (I2BM) and Molecular Imaging Research Center (MIRCen), Atomic Energy Commission (CEA), Fontenay-aux-Roses, France
URA2210, Centre National de Recherché Scientifique (CNRS), Fontenay-aux-Roses, France

Diana Zala and Frédéric Saudou
Institut Curie, Orsay, France
UMR3306, Centre National de Recherché Scientifique (CNRS), Orsay, France
U1005, Institut National de la Santé et de la Recherche Médicale (INSERM), Orsay France

Maxime Feyeux, Fany Bourgois-Rocha and Anselme L. Perrier
U861, Institut National de la Santé et de la Recherche Médicale (INSERM), AFM, Evry, France
UEVE U861, I-STEM, AFM, Evry, France

Sophie Aubert
CECS, I-STEM, AFM, Evry, France

Laetitia Troquier, Nicolas Merienne, Maria Rey and Nicole Déglon
Department of Clinical Neurosciences (DNC), Lausanne University Hospital (CHUV), Lausanne, Switzerland

Yun-Beom Choi and Eric R. Kandel
Department of Neuroscience, College of Physicians and Surgeons of Columbia University, New York, New York, United States of America
Department of Psychiatry, College of Physicians and Surgeons of Columbia University, New York, New York, United States of America

Eric R. Kandel
Howard Hughes Medical Institute, College of Physicians and Surgeons of Columbia University, New York, New York, United States of America
Kavli Institute for Brain Science, College of Physicians and Surgeons of Columbia University, New York, New York, United States of America

Beena M. Kadakkuzha, Xin-An Liu, Komolitdin Akhmedov and Sathyanarayanan V. Puthanveettil
Department of Neuroscience, The Scripps Research Institute, Scripps Florida, Jupiter, Florida, United States of America

Shaun S. Sanders, Katherine K. N. Mui, Liza M. Sutton and Michael R. Hayden
Department of Medical Genetics and Centre for Molecular Medicine and Therapeutics, Child and Family Research Institute, University of British Columbia, Vancouver, British Columbia, Canada

Ekaterina I. Galkina, Aram Shin, Ihn Sik Seong, Vanessa C. Wheeler, James F. Gusella, Marcy E. MacDonald and Jong-Min Lee
Center for Human Genetic Research, Massachusetts General Hospital, Boston, Massachusetts, United States of America

Kathryn R. Coser and Toshi Shioda
Massachusetts General Hospital Cancer Center, Charlestown, Massachusetts, United States of America

Isaac S. Kohane
Children's Hospital Informatics program, Children's Hospital, Boston, Massachusetts, United States of America
Center for Biomedical Informatics, Harvard Medical School, Boston, Massachusetts, United States of America
i2b2 National center for Biomedical Computing, Boston, Massachusetts, United States of America

Shuhua Mu, Wenda Peng, Junle Qu and Jian Zhang
College of Optoelectronics Engineering, Shenzhen University, Shenzhen, China

Shuhua Mu, Jiachuan Wang, Guangqian Zhou, Zhendan He, Zhenfu Zhao, CuiPing Mo and Jian Zhang
School of Medicine, Shenzhen University, Shenzhen, China

Gaëlle Désaméricq and Guillaume Dolbeau
Equipe 01, U955, Inserm, Créteil, France
Faculté de médecine, Université Paris Est, Créteil, France

Gaëlle Désaméricq
Service de Pharmacologie Clinique, Hôpital H. Mondor – A.Chenevier, AP-HP, Créteil, France
Déspartement d'Etudes Cognitives, Ecole Normale Supérieure, Paris, France

Guillaume Dolbeau
Unité de recherche clinique, Hôpital H. Mondor – A. Chenevier, AP-HP, Créteil, France

Christophe Verny
Centre de référence des maladies neurogénétiques, service de neurologie, CHU d'Angers, Angers, France
UMR CNRS 6214 – INSERM U1083, Angers, France

Katrin S. Lindenberg, Patrick Weydt, Hans-Peter Müller, Albert C. Ludolph, G. Bernhard Landwehrmeyer and Jan Kassubek
Department of Neurology, Ulm University, Ulm, Germany

Axel Bornstedt, Wolfgang Rottbauer and Volker Rasche
Department of Internal Medicine II, Ulm University, Ulm, Germany

Volker Rasche
Core Facility Small Animal Imaging, Ulm University, Ulm, Germany

Douglas Macdonald and Ignacio Munoz-Sanjuan
CHDI Management/CHDI Foundation, Los Angeles, California, United States of America

Michela A. Tessari and Kristiina Pulli
Galapagos B.V., Leiden, The Netherlands

Melanie Smith, Marieke B. A. C. Lamers and George McAllister
BioFocus, a Charles River company, Saffron Walden, United Kingdom

Ivette Boogaard, Agnieszka Szynol, Faywell Albertus, Sipke Dijkstra and David F. Fischer
BioFocus, a Charles River company, Leiden, The Netherlands

Daniel Kordt, Wolfgang Reindl and Frank Herrmann
Evotec AG, Hamburg, Germany

Silvia Corrochano, Sarah Carter, Michelle Stewart, Joel May, Steve D. M. Brown and Abraham Acevedo-Arozena
MRC Mammalian Genetics Unit, Harwell, Oxfordshire, United Kingdom

Maurizio Renna and David C. Rubinsztein
Department of Medical Genetics, Cambridge Institute for Medical Research, University of Cambridge, Wellcome/MRC Building, Addenbrooke's Hospital, Cambridge, United Kingdom

Georgina Osborne and Gillian P. Bates
Department of Medical and Molecular Genetics, King's College London, London, United Kingdom

Qiqi Feng, Yuxin Ma, Shuhua Mu, Jiajia Wu, Si Chen, Lisi OuYang and Wanlong Lei
Department of Anatomy, Zhongshan School of Medicine, Sun Yat-sen University, Guangzhou, China

Qiqi Feng
Department of Nephrology, The Third Affiliated Hospital of Sun Yat-sen University, Guangzhou, China

Yuxin Ma
Department of Anatomy, School of Basic Medicine, Guangdong Pharmaceutical University, Guangzhou, China

Liliana B. Menalled, Andrea E. Kudwa, Steve Oakeshott, Andrew Farrar, Neil Paterson, Igor Filippov, Sam Miller, Mei Kwan, Michael Olsen, Jose Beltran, Justin Torello, Jon Fitzpatrick, Richard Mushlin, Kimberly Cox, Kristi McConnell, Matthew Mazzella, Dansha He, Dani Brunner, Afshin Ghavami and Sylvie Ramboz
PsychoGenics Inc., Tarrytown, New York, United States of America

Georgina F. Osborne, Rand Al-Nackkash and Gill P. Bates
Department of Medical and Molecular Genetics, King's College London, London, United Kingdom

Pasi Tuunanen and Kimmo Lehtimaki
Charles River Discovery Research Services, Kuopio, Finland

Larry Park, Douglas Macdonald, Ignacio Munoz-Sanjuan and David Howland
CHDI Management/CHDI Foundation, Princeton, New Jersey, United States of America

Erik Karl Håkan Jansson, Laura Emily Clemens, Olaf Riess and Huu Phuc Nguyen
Institute of Medical Genetics and Applied Genomics, University of Tuebingen, Tuebingen, Germany; and Centre for Rare Diseases, University of Tuebingen, Tuebingen, Germany

Karolina Kolodziejczyk, Matthew P. Parsons and Lynn A. Raymond
Department of Psychiatry, Brain Research Centre, University of British Columbia, Vancouver, British Columbia, Canada

Amber L. Southwell and Michael R. Hayden
Centre for Molecular Medicine and Therapeutics, Child and Family Research Institute, University of British Columbia, Vancouver, British Columbia, Canada

Albino Carrizzo, Alba Di Pardo, Vittorio Maglione, Antonio Damato, Enrico Amico, Carmine Vecchione and Ferdinando Squitieris
IRCCS Neuromed, Pozzilli (IS), Italy

Luigi Formisano
Department of Science and Technology, University of Sannio, Benevento, Italy

Carmine Vecchione
Department of Medicine and Surgery, University of Salerno, Salerno, Italy

Jane S. Sutcliffe, James M. Watson, Chang Sing Chew and Daniel M. Hutcheson
Dept. of Neuroscience and CNS Safety Pharmacology, Maccine Pte Ltd, Singapore, Singapore

Vahri Beaumont, Maria Beconi, Celia Dominguez and Ignacio Munoz-Sanjuan
CHDI Foundation/CHDI Management Inc., Los Angeles, California, United States of America

Maria Angeles Fernandez-Estevez, Maria Jose Casarejos, Ana Gomez, Juan Perucho and Maria Angeles Mena
Department of Neurobiology, Ramóny Cajal Hospital, Madrid, Spain

Jose López Sendon, Juan Garcia Caldentey, Carolina Ruiz and Justo García de Yebenes
Department of Neurology, Ramóny Cajal Hospital, Madrid, Spain

Maria Angeles Fernandez-Estevez, Maria Jose Casarejos, Jose López Sendon, Carolina Ruiz, Ana Gomez, Juan Perucho, Justo García de Yebenes and Maria Angeles Mena
CIBERNED, Instituto de Salud Carlos III, Madrid, Spain

Niels H. Skotte, Amber L. Southwell, Crystal N. Doty, Eugenia Petoukhov, Kuljeet Vaid and Michael R. Hayden
Centre for Molecular Medicine and Therapeutics, Child and Family Research Institute, University of British Columbia, Vancouver, British Columbia, Canada

Michael E. Østergaard, Holly Kordasiewicz, Andrew T. Watt, Susan M. Freier, Gene Hung, Punit P. Seth, C. Frank Bennett and Eric E. Swayze
ISIS Pharmaceuticals, Carlsbad, California, United States of America

Jeffrey B. Carroll
Behavioral Neuroscience Program, Department of Psychology, Western Washington University, Bellingham, Washington, United States of America

Simon C. Warby
Center for Advanced Research in Sleep Medicine, Department of Psychiatry, University of Montréal, Montréal, Quebec, Canada

Jan Rusz
Department of Circuit Theory, Faculty of Electrical Engineering, Czech Technical University in Prague, Prague, Czech Republic
Department of Neurology and Centre of Clinical Neuroscience, First Faculty of Medicine, Charles University in Prague, Prague, Czech Republic

Carsten Saft and Rainer Hoffman
Department of Neurology, Huntington-Centre NRW, St. Josef Hospital, Ruhr-University of Bochum, Bochum, Germany

Uwe Schlegel and Sabine Skodda
Department of Neurology, Knappschaftskrankenhaus, Ruhr-University of Bochum, Bochum, Germany

Yanying Liu, Samantha Ridley, Dong Zhang, Khosrow Rezvani and Hongmin Wang
Division of Basic Biomedical Sciences, University of South Dakota Sanford School of Medicine, Vermillion, South Dakota, United States of America

Yuanchao Xue and Xiang-Dong Fu
Department of Cellular and Molecular Medicine, University of California San Diego, The Palade Laboratories Room 231, La Jolla, California, United States of America

Owen Phillips, Carlo Caltagirone and Margherita Di Paola
Clinical and Behavioural Neurology Dept, IRCCS Santa Lucia Foundation, Rome, Italy

Ferdinando Squitieri and Francesca Elifani
IRCSS Neuromed, Pozzilli, Italy

Cristina Sanchez-Castaneda and Umberto Sabatini
Radiology Dept, IRCCS Santa Lucia Foundation, Rome, Italy

Carlo Caltagirone
Neuroscience Dept, University of Rome "Tor Vergata", Rome, Italy

Tatsuo Mano, Shoji Tsuji and Atsushi Iwata
Department of Neurology, Graduate School of Medicine, The University of Tokyo, Tokyo, Japan,

Takayoshi Suzuki
Department of Graduate School of Medical Science, Kyoto Prefectural University of Medicine, Kyoto, Japan

Takayoshi Suzuki and Takayoshi Suzuki
Japan Science and Technology Agency, Precursory Research for Embryonic Science and Technology (PRESTO), Saitama, Japan

Index

Index